A Textbook of Pharmaceutical Analysis

About the Book—

Written for junior or senior-level undergraduate courses in pharmaceutical analysis, this unique book adequately describes modern pharmaceutical analysis so that students understand most analytical methods in principle, and many of them in detail. Each of the text's systematically selected topics is first treated theoretically, then practically—so that both principles and practice are described.

Some of the many changes in this new edition include:

- expanded sections on rate constants and their application
- new material on treatments of ion-selective membrane electrodes, nuclear magnetic resonance, mass spectrometry, circular dichroism and optical rotatory dispersion, high pressure liquid chromatography, and analytical toxicology
- changes in potentiometry, acid-base titrations, chromatography, voltammetry, and spectrophotometry

The text also discusses volumetric laboratory techniques and methods of calculation, as well as analytical literature and how to use it. It makes modern methods of drug analysis clear to students and provides many experimental procedures geared to student use for experiments or in practical analysis.

With this text, both student and teacher find a comprehensive, essentially complete course in modern pharmaceutical analysis.

A Textbook of Pharmaceutical Analysis

Second Edition

Kenneth A. Connors
Professor of Pharmacy
The University of Wisconsin

A Wiley-Interscience Publication

John Wiley & Sons New York London Sydney Toronto

Library of Congress Cataloging in Publication Data:
Connors, Kenneth Antonio, 1932–
A textbook of pharmaceutical analysis.

"A Wiley-Interscience publication."
Includes bibliographical references and index.
1. Drugs—Adulteration and analysis. I. Title
[DNLM: QV744 C753t]
RS189.C63 1975 615'.1901 74-34134
ISBN 0-471-16853-X

Printed in the United States of America

10 9 8 7 6 5 4

About the Author—

KENNETH A. CONNORS is a Professor of Pharmacy at the University of Wisconsin. He was also Assistant Dean of its School of Pharmacy from 1968-1972. The author of *Reaction Mechanisms in Organic Analytical Chemistry* (Wiley-Interscience, 1973), Dr. Conners received his Ph.D. in pharmacy from the University of Wisconsin in 1959.

Element	Symbol	Atomic Number	Atomic Weight
Magnesium	Mg	12	24.305
Manganese	Mn	25	54.9380
Mendelevium	Md	101	255.0906
Mercury	Hg	80	200.59
Molybdenum	Mo	42	95.94
Neodymium	Nd	60	144.24
Neon	Ne	10	20.179
Neptunium	Np	93	237.0482
Nickel	Ni	28	58.71
Niobium	Nb	41	92.9064
Nitrogen	N	7	14.0067
Nobelium	No	102	255
Osmium	Os	76	190.2
Oxygen	O	8	15.9994
Palladium	Pd	46	106.4
Phosphorus	P	15	30.9738
Platinum	Pt	78	195.09
Plutonium	Pu	94	242.0587
Polonium	Po	84	208.9825
Potassium	K	19	39.102
Praseodymium	Pr	59	140.9077
Promethium	Pm	61	145
Protactinium	Pa	91	231.0359
Radium	Ra	88	226.0254
Radon	Rn	86	222.0175
Rhenium	Re	75	186.2
Rhodium	Rh	45	102.9055
Rubidium	Rb	37	85.4678
Ruthenium	Ru	44	101.07
Samarium	Sm	62	150.4
Scandium	Sc	21	44.9559
Selenium	Se	34	78.96
Silicon	Si	14	28.086
Silver	Ag	47	107.868
Sodium	Na	11	22.9898
Strontium	Sr	38	87.62
Sulfur	S	16	32.06
Tantalum	Ta	73	180.9479
Technetium	Tc	43	98.9062
Tellurium	Te	52	127.60
Terbium	Tb	65	158.9254
Thallium	Tl	81	204.37
Thorium	Th	90	232.0381
Thulium	Tm	69	168.9342
Tin	Sn	50	118.69
Titanium	Ti	22	47.90
Tungsten	W	74	183.85
Uranium	U	92	238.029
Vanadium	V	23	50.9414
Xenon	Xe	54	131.30
Ytterbium	Yb	70	173.04
Yttrium	Y	39	88.9059
Zinc	Zn	30	65.37
Zirconium	Zr	40	91.22

To Some of My Students

Preface

The course in pharmaceutical analysis ("drug assay") retains a place in the undergraduate curriculum, despite its apparent inutility to the practicing pharmacist, for two reasons. The pharmacist is primarily an expert on drugs, and an important aspect of the development, production, distribution, and use of drugs is their analysis. His education should reveal to him this component of his professional field, even though few practicing pharmacists will ever need to analyze a drug sample. The second reason is that much of the subject matter of pharmaceutical analysis is fundamental to techniques and results of other fields in the curriculum, such as biochemistry, medicinal chemistry, and pharmaceutics. This is a preparatory or service function of the course.

Because pharmaceutical analysis deals with bulk materials, dosage forms, and more recently, biological samples in support of biopharmaceutical and pharmacokinetic studies, I regard it as a branch of pharmaceutics rather than of pharmaceutical chemistry (its traditional assignment). This is important only in that students and teachers should keep in mind the close relationship between the analytical support and drug delivery, and pharmaceutics is the study of drug delivery systems.

In this book I try to give a sufficiently systematic and detailed account of modern pharmaceutical analysis to permit the pharmacy student and the pharmacist to understand most analyses in principle and many of them in detail. In some sections I have gone beyond this level, and I think that this further treatment will be helpful to graduate students and research analysts without lessening the value of the book in the undergraduate course. The material in this book will enable the student to approach with understanding the official compendia, reference works in analysis, specialized monographs, and advanced textbooks in analytical chemistry. On the other hand, this is not a catalog of assay methods for specific drugs, nor is it a commentary on the official volumes. It is a textbook.

Since the appearance of the first edition in 1967, I have had to recognize that in most schools of pharmacy changing curricula have left a single required analytical course; it is no longer possible to assume that students come to the drug assay course with a background in classical quantitative analysis. I have therefore provided much of the basic information in an appendix on volumetric techniques, but space limitations prevent a full treatment, and instructors may wish to supplement this discussion. Instructors will also find opportunities for contributing to the design of the laboratory experiments, particularly in the nature of unknown samples, which I often have not specified very closely. The capabilities for preparing and using these samples will vary with the school, depending upon the availability of a manufacturing facility, the number of students, and the time available.

This edition differs from the first primarily in its presentation of new sections or chapters on ion-selective electrodes, optical rotatory dispersion and circular dichroism, nuclear magnetic resonance and electron spin resonance, mass spectrometry, high-pressure liquid chromatography, and analytical toxicology. A fuller treatment of chromatographic theory is given. More chemical structures have been used to develop facility in thinking structurally because, although a pharmacist's first question upon hearing of a new drug may be "What is its pharmacological action?," his second should be "What is its chemical structure?" This is what he needs to know to make reasonable estimates of behavior bearing on important pharmaceutical decisions relating to solubility, stability, and bioavailability (and, of course, analysis). Answers have been included for most of the problems as a result of experience with the first edition. In adding new material it has been necessary, in order to keep the book reasonable in length, to discard some of the earlier material, and I hope I have done this wisely.

I am indebted to many of my students and colleagues for suggesting changes and corrections in the first edition. For providing new data and experimental work I especially want to thank Kenneth S. Albert, Elizabeth Chang, Jordan L. Cohen, Harriet P. Corrick, Jay Knutowski, Judith M. Ludy, Richard Minkley, Joseph A. Mollica, and Albert Wong.

Kenneth A. Connors

Madison, Wisconsin
October, 1974

Contents

A Textbook of Pharmaceutical Analysis

Part One: Titrimetric Analysis

The basic experimental operation in titrimetric analysis is called a *titration*. In a titration, a solution of one reactant of accurately known concentration (the *titrant*, or *standard solution*) is added to a second reactant, the solution of sample whose amount or concentration is to be determined. Titrant is added to the sample until the reaction is just complete, that is, until the amount of titrant added is equivalent chemically to the amount of sample. The stage at which this equivalence occurs is called the equivalence point of the titration, and its experimental estimate is called the titration *end point*. From the amount of titrant used to reach the end point, from its concentration, and from the known stoichiometry of the titration reaction, the amount of sample substance can be calculated. Usually the volume of titrant is measured, and then titrimetric analysis is also called volumetric analysis.

This part of the book describes many of the chemical reactions that form the basis of successful titrations, and methods for end point detection. Titrimetry is a classical method of analysis, but even in modern analytical practice it is very important, as can be seen by browsing through the latest revisions of *The United States Pharmacopeia* and *The National Formulary*. Later chapters describe newer methods of end point detection and applications of titrimetry to more complicated analytical problems.

A brief description of the experimental technique and calculational basis of volumetric analysis is given in Appendix A. Chapter 27 includes a discussion of the statistical treatment of experimental data; this material is useful in interpreting the results of titrimetric analysis, and it probably should be reviewed several times during one's progress through this book, since it applies to all kinds of quantitative experimentation.

1 AQUEOUS ACID-BASE TITRATIONS

1.1 Acid-Base Equilibria

Definitions of Acids and Bases. The first successful acid-base theory is due to Arrhenius, who defined an acid as a substance that when dissolved in water gives rise to hydrogen ions, and a base as a substance that in water yields hydroxide ions.

$$\underset{\text{Acid}}{HA} \rightleftharpoons H^+ + A^-$$

$$\underset{\text{Base}}{BOH} \rightleftharpoons B^+ + OH^-$$

This theory was broadened to include those substances that increase the hydroxide ion concentration of a solution but that do not themselves contain the hydroxyl group; amines, for example, are such substances. The concept of hydrolysis, or reaction with water, was adopted to account for this behavior, and these substances were referred to as pseudo bases.

$$B + H_2O \rightleftharpoons BH^+ + OH^-$$

The Arrhenius theory, which was introduced just before the turn of the century, leads to an adequate quantitative description of acid-base behavior in aqueous solution and is still widely taught and used. It lacks generality, however; in particular, it does not account for manifestations of acid-base reactions in nonaqueous solvents. In 1923 Bronsted (and, independently, Lowry) proposed new definitions of great generality, as follows: an acid is a species that can yield a proton, and a base is a species that can accept a proton.

$$\underset{\text{Acid}}{HA} \rightleftharpoons H^+ + A^-$$

$$\underset{\text{Base}}{B} + H^+ \rightleftharpoons BH^+$$

This definition of acid is slightly different from that in the Arrhenius theory.

In the older theory, the acid yields a hydrogen ion in aqueous solution (that is, the definition requires water as the solvent), whereas a Bronsted acid yields a proton, and this definition is independent of the solvent. A major difference between the theories is in their concepts of the base. Notice that in the system $HA \rightleftharpoons H^+ + A^-$ the anion A^- is acting as a base, since it accepts a proton. Also, in the reaction $B + H^+ \rightleftharpoons BH^+$, the cation BH^+ acts as a Bronsted acid. In general, we may write

$$\text{Acid} \rightleftharpoons \text{Base} + H^+ \tag{1.1}$$

and an acid-base pair related by this equation is known as a *conjugate acid-base pair*.

One result of this definition is that an acid or a base can have any charge, the only limitation being that the charge of an acid is greater than that of its conjugate base by one positive unit. For example, each of the following equilibria fits the general Eq. 1.1; acids and bases that are neutral, positive, and negative are shown:

Acid		Base
CH_3COOH	$\rightleftharpoons$	$CH_3COO^- + H^+$
$CH_3NH_3{}^+$	$\rightleftharpoons$	$CH_3NH_2 + H^+$
$H_2PO_4{}^-$	$\rightleftharpoons$	$HPO_4{}^{2-} + H^+$
${}^+H_3NCH_2CH_2NH_3{}^+$	$\rightleftharpoons$	$H_2NCH_2CH_2NH_3{}^+ + H^+$

Notice that the solvent has not yet been invoked in these descriptions. In fact, Eq. 1.1 will not be observable in the absence of a substance to accept the proton because of the great reactivity of the proton. This second proton-accepting substance is a base by definition. Thus two conjugate acid-base systems are necessary in order to observe a reaction, and an acid-base reaction is a proton transfer from one system to the other.

1st system:

$$\underset{\text{Acid 1}}{HA} \rightleftharpoons \underset{\text{Base 1}}{A^-} + H^+$$

2nd system:

$$H^+ + \underset{\text{Base 2}}{B^-} \rightleftharpoons \underset{\text{Acid 2}}{BH}$$

Overall reaction:

$$HA + B^- \rightleftharpoons A^- + BH$$

Often the solvent assumes the role of the second acid-base pair if it has acid-base properties. Water is such a solvent.

$$\underset{\text{Acid}}{H_2O} \rightleftharpoons \underset{\text{Base}}{OH^-} + H^+$$

But water can act as both an acid and a base (it is *amphoteric*).

$$H^+ + \underset{\text{Base}}{H_2O} \rightleftharpoons \underset{\text{Acid}}{H_3O^+}$$

This duel behavior means that water can be the second conjugate acid-base system for solutes that are acids and for solutes that are bases.

$$\underset{\text{Acid 1}}{HA} + \underset{\text{Base 2}}{H_2O} \rightleftharpoons \underset{\text{Base 1}}{A^-} + \underset{\text{Acid 2}}{H_3O^+}$$

and

$$\underset{\text{Base I}}{B} + \underset{\text{Acid II}}{H_2O} \rightleftharpoons \underset{\text{Acid I}}{BH^+} + \underset{\text{Base II}}{OH^-}$$

The Bronsted acid-base theory is very useful in describing reactions in many solvents besides water. Throughout this book acid-base phenomena will be considered in terms of this theory.

A third theory of acid-base behavior was suggested by G. N. Lewis in 1923. An acid is defined as an electron-pair acceptor and a base as an electron-pair donor. This involves no change in the concept of a base, since every proton acceptor is also an electron-pair donor. The concept of the acid is altered markedly, however, to include some substances that do not contain hydrogen. In the Lewis sense the reaction

$$\underset{\text{Base}}{:NH_3} + \underset{\text{Acid}}{BF_3} \rightleftharpoons H_3N:BF_3$$

is an acid-base reaction. It has become common to refer to such nonprotonic acids as "Lewis acids." The Lewis theory has helped to describe many phenomena (such as indicator color changes) that can take place in non-protonic systems but that exhibit all the characteristics of acid-base reactions.

Table 1.1 gives a comparison of these three important theories, with equivalent definitions enclosed by dashed lines (actually, the Arrhenius and Bronsted definitions of acid are not precisely equivalent, as was pointed out previously).

Acid-Base Dissociation Constants. For a reversible chemical reaction

$$aA + bB \rightleftharpoons cC + dD$$

TABLE 1.1
Comparison of Acid-Base Theories

Theory	Acid	Base
Arrhenius	Proton donor	Hydroxide donor
Bronsted	Proton donor	Proton acceptor
Lewis	Electron-pair acceptor	Electron-pair donor

the quantity K, defined by Eq. 1.2, is a constant at constant temperature and pressure.*

$$K = \frac{[C]^c[D]^d}{[A]^a[B]^b} \tag{1.2}$$

In this equation $[A]$ represents the equilibrium molar concentration of A, etc. It is customary to write the expression for K with the products (that is, the species on the right-hand side of the equation) in the numerator.

The concept of the equilibrium constant can be applied profitably to the quantitative description of all types of chemical equilibria, and much of this book is devoted to such applications. In the present case acid-base equilibria in aqueous solution are treated. Consider the dissociation of the weak acid HA,

$$HA \rightleftharpoons H^+ + A^-$$

where the symbol H^+ represents the hydrated proton. By analogy with Eq. 1.2 we define the *acid dissociation constant*† K_a.

$$K_a = \frac{[H^+][A^-]}{[HA]} \tag{1.3}$$

This symbolism implies that the second conjugate acid-base pair is the solvent, water, which is usually not explicitly written. The K_a is always written with the hydrogen ion concentration in the numerator.

In a similar manner, an equilibrium constant K_b, called the *base dissociation constant*, can be defined for all weak bases.‡

$$B + H_2O \rightleftharpoons BH^+ + OH^-$$

$$K_b = \frac{[BH^+][OH^-]}{[B]} \tag{1.4}$$

* This statement is not strictly true. For K to be a constant, each concentration c must be replaced by the corresponding activity a, where $a = fc$. The proportionality constant f is called the activity coefficient; its deviation from unity is a measure of the deviation of the solution from ideal behavior. A more detailed discussion of this effect is given in Chapter 6. In this chapter we assume that all activity coefficients equal unity.

† *Ionization* is the formation of ions, whereas *dissociation* is the separation of species. These terms are usually used as synonyms in discussions of aqueous solutions, since in dilute aqueous solution every ionized species dissociates. (See p. 50 for a discussion of nonaqueous electrolyte behavior.) Sometimes ionization is restricted to those reactions in which charged species are formed; that is, separation of a neutral molecule into a cation and an anion is called ionization, whereas separation of a cation into another cation and a neutral molecule is called dissociation. We shall usually use the term dissociation.

‡ In the Arrhenius theory, K_b was labelled K_h and called the hydrolysis constant, since it represented reaction with water. In the Bronsted theory, the concept of hydrolysis (in this sense) is unnecessary.

Here $[H_2O]$, which may be taken as a constant quantity in dilute aqueous solution, is absorbed into K_b.

Water, too, is capable of dissociation.

$$H_2O \rightleftharpoons H^+ + OH^-$$

This equilibrium is characterized by the constant $K = [H^+][OH^-]/[H_2O]$. It is conventional to absorb the constant quantity $[H_2O]$ into the constant, thus giving the important relation

$$K_w = [H^+][OH^-] \tag{1.5}$$

K_w is the *ion product*, or auto-protolysis constant, of water. This is a very valuable quantity because it relates the K_a of a weak acid and the K_b of its conjugate base. Consider the acid HA and its conjugate base A^-:

$$K_a = \frac{[H^+][A^-]}{[HA]}$$

$$K_b = \frac{[HA][OH^-]}{[A^-]}$$

Multiplying these two constants gives

$$K_w = K_a K_b \tag{1.6}$$

which holds for any conjugate acid-base pair. Since K_w is accurately known over a wide range of temperature, this means that it is necessary only to know *either* K_a *or* K_b for a conjugate pair; the unknown constant may then be calculated with the aid of Eq. 1.6. It is, of course, essential that all quantities in this equation refer to the same temperature.

The numerical values of most dissociation constants are very small numbers; hence it is convenient to employ logarithms when manipulating them. The symbolism

$$\text{pK} = -\log K$$

is widely used. Thus Eq. 1.6 may be written

$$\text{pK}_w = \text{pK}_a + \text{pK}_b$$

for any conjugate acid-base pair. Table 1.2 lists values of pK_w at numerous temperatures; the effect of temperature upon pK_w is very marked.

For weak acids it is usual to express the acid dissociation constant as either K_a or pK_a. It is *not* common, however, to find the K_b or pK_b of weak bases tabulated. Rather, we usually encounter the K_a or pK_a of the conjugate acid of the weak base. (This is often referred to, erroneously, as the "pK_a of the base.")

TABLE 1.2
Ion Product of Water as a Function of Temperature[a]

t (°C)	pK_w
0	14.94
10	14.54
20	14.17
25	14.00
30	13.83
40	13.54
50	13.26
60	13.02

[a] From Harned, H. S. and B. B. Owen, *The Physical Chemistry of Electrolytic Solutions*, 3rd ed., Reinhold Publishing, New York, 1958, p. 638.

The formulation of acid dissociation constants for some specific substances is shown below.* All these equations have the form of Eq. 1.3.

Benzoic acid $C_6H_5COOH \rightleftharpoons C_6H_5COO^- + H^+$

$$K_a = \frac{[H^+][C_6H_5COO^-]}{[C_6H_5COOH]}$$

Phenol $C_6H_5OH \rightleftharpoons C_6H_5O^- + H^+$

$$K_a = \frac{[H^+][C_6H_5O^-]}{[C_6H_5OH]}$$

* An acid with a single dissociable proton is called a monoprotic acid or a monobasic acid, the latter designation indicating that one molecule of the acid can transfer one proton to a base; similarly a base that can accept a single proton is a monoacidic base. Polybasic acids (and polyacidic bases) can donate (or accept) more than one proton per molecule.

Anilinium ion $C_6H_5NH_3^+ \rightleftharpoons C_6H_5NH_2 + H^+$

$$K_a = \frac{[H^+][C_6H_5NH_2]}{[C_6H_5NH_3^+]}$$

If an acid or base possesses more than one ionizable group, a separate dissociation constant can be defined for each. These dissociation constant expressions will be simultaneously satisfied in any solution of the substance. If the groups are chemically equivalent, as in ethylenediamine (below), it is irrelevant which dissociation constant is assigned to which group, but K_1 will always be larger than K_2 for reasons to be considered later.

$$^+H_3NCH_2CH_2NH_3^+ \rightleftharpoons H^+ + H_2NCH_2CH_2NH_3^+$$

$$K_1 = \frac{[H^+][H_2NCH_2CH_2NH_3^+]}{[^+H_3NCH_2CH_2NH_3^+]}$$

$$H_2NCH_2CH_2NH_3^+ \rightleftharpoons H^+ + H_2NCH_2CH_2NH_2$$

$$K_2 = \frac{[H^+][H_2NCH_2CH_2NH_2]}{[H_2NCH_2CH_2NH_3^+]}$$

If the two groups are not equivalent, independent evidence must be used to assign the measured K_a values to the dissociation of the appropriate group. In salicyclic acid, for example, it is known that K_1 describes the dissociation of the carboxylic acid group and K_2 corresponds to the phenolic dissociation.

Salicyclic acid $C_6H_4(OH)COOH \overset{K_1}{\rightleftharpoons} C_6H_4(OH)COO^- + H^+$

$C_6H_4(OH)COO^- \overset{K_2}{\rightleftharpoons} C_6H_4(O^-)COO^- + H^+$

Table 1.3 gives values of K_a and the corresponding pK_a for the equilibria listed above. Note that of two K_a values, the larger one implies a stronger acid, and so a smaller pK_a also means a stronger acid. Because of the relationship pK_w = pK_a + pK_b, this means that a larger pK_a value for the conjugate acid of a base corresponds to a stronger base. Thus ethylenediamine is a stronger base than is aniline, and benzoic acid is a much stronger acid than is

TABLE 1.3
Some Acid Dissociation Constants at 25°C

Substance[a]	K_a	pK_a
Benzoic acid	6.25×10^{-5}	4.20
Phenol	1.00×10^{-10}	10.00
Aniline	2.51×10^{-5}	4.60
Ethylenediamine	1.41×10^{-7}	6.85
	1.18×10^{-10}	9.93
Salicylic acid	1.05×10^{-3}	2.98
	4×10^{-14}	13.40

[a] That is, the conjugate acid in each case. See text for definitions of the K_a.

phenol. The assignment of the 2.98 value (pK_1) of salicyclic acid to the carboxylic acid dissociation and the 13.40 to the phenol group is based in part on comparisons like that between benzoic acid and phenol.

pH. In the preceding discussion we introduced the operator p, which operates on a quantity to give its negative logarithm; for example, $pK_a = -\log K_a$. Since the hydrogen ion concentration in most aqueous solutions is much smaller than one equivalent per liter, it is convenient to deal with the logarithmic quantity pH.

$$pH = -\log [H^+] = \log \frac{1}{[H^+]} \tag{1.7}$$

The larger the value of pH, the smaller is the hydrogen ion concentration. Of two solutions, the one with the lower pH is more acidic, and the one with the higher pH is more alkaline.

From Eq. 1.5 we note that if the hydrogen ion concentration is known, the hydroxide ion concentration of the solution can be calculated. Frequently this can be done most easily by means of the equivalent relation:

$$pK_w = pH + pOH \tag{1.8}$$

A solution in which pH = pOH is said to be neutral. Evidently, the pH of a neutral solution is equal to $pK_w/2$; thus at 25°C (but *only* at 25°) neutrality corresponds to pH 7.00.

It is possible to calculate successfully the pH of solutions of acids or bases. Such calculations can be made at several levels of accuracy, depending upon the assumptions made to simplify the computations. Although the calculation of pH is frequently necessary, very seldom is the highest accuracy required. In part this is because the calculations need not be more accurate than the experimental accuracy, which is about ± 0.01 pH unit. Moreover, some of the mathematical simplifications used to achieve an easier calculation are chemically very reasonable. Examples will be given as the equations are developed. Methods will be shown at this point for the calculation of pH in aqueous solutions of strong and weak acids and bases.

Strong acid or base: a strong acid is one that is essentially completely dissociated into its component ions in dilute aqueous solution. The concept of the dissociation constant is therefore not applicable. The common strong acids are hydrochloric, perchloric, sulfuric, and nitric acids. Sodium hydroxide and potassium hydroxide are the most common strong bases. (Note that we are here using the traditional Arrhenius nomenclature, in which NaOH is a base; in the Bronsted definitions it is OH^- that is the base.)

Let c be the total analytical (formal) concentration of a strong acid HX, where c is expressed in molarity (M) or normality (N). Since the solution as a whole is electrically neutral, it must contain as many positive charges as negative charges. Because of this *electroneutrality rule*, we can write

$$[H^+] = [OH^-] + [X^-] \tag{1.9}$$

In Eq. 1.9, the source of the hydroxide ion is the dissociation of water. If the total acid concentration c is greater than about 10^{-6} M, then $[OH^-]$ will be very much less than $[X^-]$, and it is a good approximation to write

$$[H^+] = [X^-] \tag{1.10}$$

But $[X^-] = c$, so we have $[H^+] = c$. That is, the hydrogen ion concentration (more properly, the hydronium ion concentration) is equal to the total strong acid concentration.

Similarly for a strong base MOH the electroneutrality equation is

$$[H^+] + [M^+] = [OH^-] \tag{1.11}$$

which simplifies to $c = [OH^-]$, where c is the analytical concentration of the strong base.

EXAMPLE 1.1. (*a*) What is the pH of a solution 0.0154 N in HCl?

By Eq. 1.10, $[H^+] = 0.0154$ N, so pH = 1.81. (*b*) What is the pH of 0.01 N KOH?

We have $[OH^-] = 0.01$ N, so pOH = 2.00 and pH = 12.00 (at 25°C).

Since these calculations ignore activity coefficient effects, they are not highly accurate. For example, the calculated pH of 0.10 N HCl is 1.00, whereas the measured pH is 1.10. It is therefore not feasible to analyze such solutions by measuring their pH and calculating the concentration. Activity coefficient effects can be taken into account if desired, as described in Chapter 6.

Weak acid: A weak acid is one that is not completely dissociated; that is, the undissociated species can be detected in solution. The extent of dissociation is characterized by K_a. Consider weak acid HA in solution at total solute concentration c. The dissociation reaction is

$$HA \rightleftharpoons H^+ + A^-$$

The acid dissociation constant is defined

$$K_a = \frac{[H^+][A^-]}{[HA]} \tag{1.12}$$

An exact calculation would start with the electroneutrality condition, $[H^+] = [OH^-] + [A^-]$, and the material balance condition, $c = [HA] + [A^-]$. Usually it will be possible to neglect the dissociation of water, giving $[H^+] = [A^-]$. This result is also obtained by noting that each molecule of HA dissociates to yield one H^+ and one A^-; hence $[H^+] = [A^-]$. Combining this with the material balance gives, for the equilibrium concentration, $[HA] = c - [H^+]$. Substituting into 1.12,

$$K_a = \frac{[H^+]^2}{c - [H^+]} \tag{1.13}$$

Equation 1.13 is a quadratic equation in $[H^+]$; it can be rearranged to

$$[H^+]^2 + K_a[H^+] - K_a c = 0$$

and $[H^+]$ can be found by applying the quadratic formula.

$$[H^+] = \frac{-K_a \pm \sqrt{K_a^{\,2} + 4K_a c}}{2} \tag{1.14}$$

Although Eq. 1.14 is accurate enough for most work, it is not exact because it does not take into account the dissociation of water.

If $[H^+]$ is negligible relative to c, Eq. 1.13 becomes $K_a = [H^+]^2/c$, or

$$[H^+] = \sqrt{K_a c} \tag{1.15}$$

This very simple expression is widely applicable. If $[H^+]$ is less than about 5% of c, Eq. 1.15 probably will yield an answer sufficiently accurate for most purposes. In nearly every case Eq. 1.15 will be used for a preliminary estimate of $[H^+]$ to determine if the approximation $c - [H^+] \approx c$ is valid. Obviously the larger c is, the better is this approximation [1].

Recall that the charge type of an acid is irrelevant to these considerations, so Eqs. 1.14 and 1.15 apply to neutral acids (for example, acetic acid), positively charged acids (for example, ammonium ion), and negatively charged acids (for example, biphthalate ion).

Weak base: the reaction may be written

$$B + H_2O \rightleftharpoons BH^+ + OH^-$$

and the base dissociation constant is

$$K_b = \frac{[BH^+][OH^-]}{[B]}$$

By the same type of reasoning used above, the hydroxide ion concentration is given by

$$K_b = \frac{[OH^-]^2}{c - [OH^-]} \tag{1.16}$$

where c is the formal concentration of the base. When $[OH^-]$ is very much smaller than c, this reduces to

$$[OH^-] = \sqrt{K_b c} \tag{1.17}$$

These equations apply to neutral bases (for example, amines), positively charged bases (for example, ethylenediamine monohydrochloride), and negatively charged bases (for example, benzoate ion). The hydrogen ion concentration (and from this the pH) of these solutions can be obtained from the hydroxide ion concentration by utilizing the fundamental relationship $K_w = [H^+][OH^-]$.

EXAMPLE 1.2. What is the pH of 0.01 *M* acetic acid? ($pK_a = 4.76$.)
First applying the approximate Eq. 1.15 with $c = 0.01$ and $K_a = 1.75 \times 10^{-5}$ gives $[H^+] = 4.18 \times 10^{-4}$ *N*, or pH = 3.38. A more accurate solution is found with Eq. 1.14, which yields $[H^+] = 4.10 \times 10^{-4}$ *N*, pH = 3.39. For most purposes the simpler calculation would, in this instance, be adequate.

The Bronsted concept of the conjugate acid-base pair is helpful in treating the problem of solutions of salts. The salt of a weak acid and a strong base is nothing more than the conjugate base of the weak acid, and Eqs. 1.16 and 1.17 are applicable. Sodium acetate is an example. The dissociation reaction is

$$CH_3COO^- + H_2O \rightleftharpoons CH_3COOH + OH^-$$

and the analytical concentration c of acetate ion is identical with the analytical concentration of sodium acetate, since the *salt* (but not CH_3COO^-) is completely dissociated.

Analogously the salt of a weak base and a strong acid is equivalent to the conjugate acid of the base, as with ammonium chloride. In this case Eqs. 1.14 and 1.15 apply.

EXAMPLE 1.3. Calculate the pH of 0.025 *M* potassium benzoate at 25°C.

The salt is completely dissociated into potassium and benzoate ions, and the pH is determined by the subsequent acid-base equilibrium

$$C_6H_5COO^- + H_2O \rightleftharpoons C_6H_5COOH + OH^-$$

The total concentration c of benzoate species is 0.025 *M*, and $pK_a = 4.20$ for benzoic acid (Table 1.3). It follows that $pK_b = 9.80$ and $K_b = 1.60 \times 10^{-10}$. Using Eq. 1.17 we get $[OH^-] = 2.00 \times 10^{-6}$ *N* or pOH = 5.70. Therefore pH = 8.30.

It is helpful to check that the calculated pH is on the correct side of neutrality. Thus in Example 1.3 the pH must be greater than 7 because potassium benzoate is a base.

Distribution of Acid-Base Species with pH. A better insight into the composition of a solution containing acids and bases can be obtained by studying the dependence of each species on the pH of the medium. Consider the weak monobasic acid HA with acid dissociation constant K_a. We define the fractions of total solute in the conjugate acid and base forms by

$$F_{HA} = \frac{[HA]}{c} \tag{1.18}$$

$$F_A = \frac{[A^-]}{c} \tag{1.19}$$

where c represents, as usual, the formal concentration of the solute; that is,

$$c = [HA] + [A^-] \tag{1.20}$$

Equations 1.18, 1.19, and 1.20 are combined with the dissociation constant expression to give the following equations:

$$F_{HA} = \frac{[H^+]}{[H^+] + K_a} \tag{1.21}$$

$$F_A = \frac{K_a}{[H^+] + K_a} \tag{1.22}$$

which relate the fractions of solute in the conjugate acid and base forms to the acid dissociation constant and the hydrogen ion concentration of the medium. Figure 1.1 shows F_{HA} and F_A plotted against pH for a weak acid of $pK_a = 4.0$. Such a function is called an S-shaped or sigmoid curve.

These curves have some interesting properties. At any given hydrogen ion concentration, $F_{HA} + F_A = 1$. At the point where the two curves cross, evidently $F_{HA} = F_H = 0.5$, and from Eqs. 1.21 and 1.22 it can be seen that at

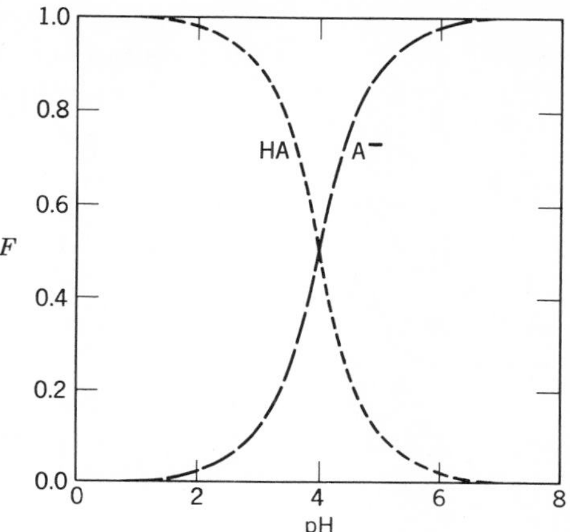

Fig. 1.1. Variation with pH of the fraction F_{HA} (conjugate acid) and F_A (conjugate base) for an acid with $pK_a = 4.0$.

this point $[H^+] = K_a$, or $pH = pK_a$. In the limit as $[H^+]$ becomes much greater than K_a, F_{HA} approaches unity and F_A approaches zero (though theoretically they never attain these limiting values). Similarly, as $[H^+]$ becomes less than K_a, F_{HA} approaches zero and F_A, unity. These same curves apply to any monofunctional conjugate acid-base pair merely by sliding the curves along the horizontal axis until the pH of intersection is equal to the pK_a.

From such a curve it is a simple matter to calculate the concentrations of each species at any pH. Rearranging 1.18 and 1.19 gives $[HA] = cF_{HA}$ and $[A^-] = cF_A$. Thus if the analytical concentration c of solute is known, the concentration of each species is found by multiplying c by the fraction corresponding to the given pH; the fraction is calculated with Eq. 1.21 or 1.22. As in all such calculations, the charge type of the acid is irrelevant.

The situation is more complicated with a dibasic acid (for example, H_2A). Now three species may exist. We define fractions as before.

$$F_{H_2A} = \frac{[H_2A]}{c}$$

$$F_{HA} = \frac{[HA^-]}{c}$$

$$F_A = \frac{[A^{2-}]}{c}$$

where $c = [H_2A] + [HA^-] + [A^{2-}]$. Combining these relations with the

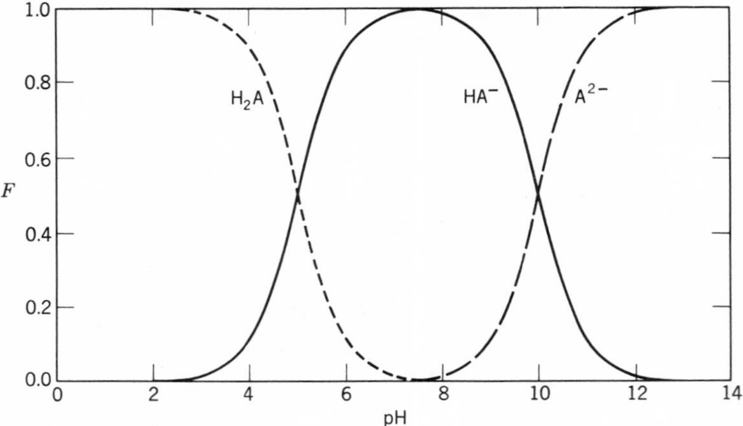

Fig. 1.2. Species distribution diagram for a dibasic acid H_2A with $pK_1 = 5.0$ and $pK_2 = 10.0$.

two dissociation constants gives

$$F_{H_2A} = \frac{[H^+]^2}{[H^+]^2 + K_1[H^+] + K_1K_2} \tag{1.23}$$

$$F_{HA} = \frac{K_1[H^+]}{[H^+]^2 + K_1[H^+] + K_1K_2} \tag{1.24}$$

$$F_{A} = \frac{K_1K_2}{[H^+]^2 + K_1[H^+] + K_1K_2} \tag{1.25}$$

and $F_{H_2A} + F_{HA} + F_A = 1$. Three terms that appear in each fraction vary in relative importance as the pH changes. At high values of hydrogen ion concentration the term $[H^+]^2$ becomes important to the exclusion of the others. As $[H^+]$ becomes smaller the middle term, $K_1[H^+]$, assumes primary importance. At very small values of $[H^+]$, the term K_1K_2 controls the magnitude of these functions. Figure 1.2 is a plot of F_{H_2A}, F_{HA}, and F_A calculated for a dibasic acid with $pK_1 = 5.0$ and $pK_2 = 10.0$. Because the pK's are widely separated, the successive dissociations are practically independent, and the solution contains only two species at any given pH.* This is evident from the figure. The pH at which the maximum concentration of the monoanion occurs can be found by differentiating Eq. 1.24 with respect to $[H^+]$ and setting the derivative equal to zero; this gives

$$pH = \frac{(pK_1 + pK_2)}{2} \tag{1.26}$$

* Actually, of course, all three species are present, but one of them is always at vanishingly low concentration.

as the maximum in F_{HA}. Another general relationship is found by setting $F_{H_2A} = F_{HA}$; at this point, corresponding to the intersection of the two curves, solution of the equality shows that pH = pK_1. Also, at the point where the F_{HA} and F_A curves cross, pH = pK_2.

A more complicated picture develops if pK_1 and pK_2 are not very widely separated, for now it is possible that all three species may coexist in significant fractions at a given pH. In Fig. 1.3 F_{H_2A}, F_{HA}, and F_A are plotted for a dibasic acid with pK_1 = 7.0 and pK_2 = 8.0. The general relationships already developed apply in this system, but a significant difference is apparent between Figs. 1.2 and 1.3. At no pH, in the system depicted in Fig. 1.3, does the fraction of solute in the monoanion form approach unity. As the pH is raised through pK_1 the acid form H_2A is converted to monoanion, but continued pH increase soon converts HA^- into the dianion because of the proximity of the two pK values.

These principles can be extended to acids and bases with any number of acid-base groups. The form of the expressions for the fractions are seen to take on a predictable pattern, and it is possible to write these expressions down without derivation. For the tribasic acid H_3A they become

$$F_{H_3A} = \frac{[H^+]^3}{[H^+]^3 + K_1[H^+]^2 + K_1K_2[H^+] + K_1K_2K_3}$$

$$F_{H_2A} = \frac{K_1[H^+]^2}{[H^+]^3 + K_1[H^+]^2 + K_1K_2[H^+] + K_1K_2K_3}$$

and so on.

It will be clear from these considerations that, for a given acid or base, the fractional composition of the solution is governed only by the solution pH.

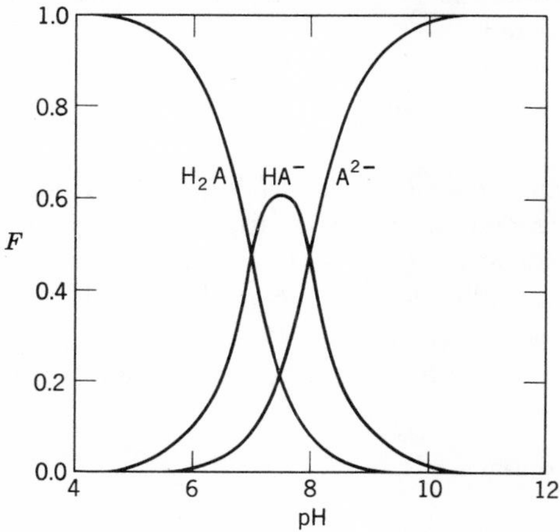

Fig. 1.3. Species distribution diagram for a dibasic acid H_2A with pK_1 = 7.0 and pK_2 = 8.0.

If the pH, the total concentration of solute, and the dissociation constant(s) are known, the concentrations of individual conjugate acid-base species can be calculated.

Buffer Solutions. Consider an aqueous solution prepared to contain a moles/liter of a weak acid HA and b moles/liter of its conjugate base A^-. The actual equilibrium concentrations of these species will be slightly different from the formal concentrations a and b because of the dissociation equilibrium $HA \rightleftharpoons H^+ + A^-$. That is, the equilibrium concentration [HA] will be slightly smaller than a because of this dissociation. Since each HA molecule dissociates to give one H^+ and one A^-, the concentrations are given by*

$$[HA] = a - [H^+] \tag{1.27}$$

$$[A^-] = b + [H^+] \tag{1.28}$$

The dissociation constant expression,

$$K_a = \frac{[H^+][A^-]}{[HA]} \tag{1.29}$$

can be placed in the convenient logarithmic form

$$pK_a = pH - \log \frac{[A^-]}{[HA]} \tag{1.30}$$

Combining Eqs. 1.27, 1.28, and 1.30,

$$pK_a = pH - \log \frac{b + [H^+]}{a - [H^+]} \tag{1.31}$$

In most practical situations $[H^+]$ is much smaller than a or b, and the simple Eq. 1.32 can be written.

$$pK_a = pH - \log \frac{b}{a} \tag{1.32}$$

Equation 1.32 is the *Henderson-Hasselbalch equation*, which relates the pH of a solution containing comparable and appreciable concentrations of a conjugate acid-base pair to the ratio of these concentrations.

Such a solution is called a *buffer solution* because it resists a change in pH upon the addition of a small amount of acid or base. This phenomenon can be demonstrated with an example. Suppose a solution is prepared to be 0.1 M

* Actually Eqs. 1.27 and 1.28 are still approximations because they neglect the dissociation of water; the rigorous equations are

$$[HA] = a - [H^+] + [OH^-] \quad \text{and} \quad [A^-] = b + [H^+] - [OH^-]$$

These can be derived via the electroneutrality and material balance conditions.

in acetic acid and 0.1 *M* in sodium acetate. Then $b/a = 1.00$ and, according to Eq. 1.32, pH = pK_a, or pH = 4.76. Now let 1.0 ml of 0.1 *N* NaOH be added to 100 ml of this solution; what will be the new value of pH? It may be assumed that the sodium hydroxide converts an equivalent amount of acetic acid to sodium acetate. The solution therefore contains, after addition of the sodium hydroxide, $(100)(0.1) - (1)(0.1) = 9.9$ meq (milliequivalents) of acetic acid, and $(100)(0.1) + (1)(0.1) = 10.1$ meq of acetate, all in 101 ml of solution. The ratio b/a is now 1.02, its logarithm is 0.01, and Eq. 1.32 shows that the new pH is 4.77. Addition of the alkali has resulted in a pH change of only 0.01 unit. If the same volume of the sodium hydroxide solution has been added to 100 ml of pH 4.76 strong acid, the pH would have changed to about 11.

The user of Eq. 1.32 or 1.30 should always derive it as needed from the appropriate acid dissociation constant expression, such as Eq. 1.29; this will prevent the otherwise inevitable confusion of signs, ratios, and transposed terms that will result from memorizing Eq. 1.30. The student will encounter the Henderson-Hasselbalch equation in many places, for it has application in describing (besides the solution behavior considered in this chapter) solubilities of acids and bases, stability of organic compounds, measurement of dissociation constants, transport across biological membranes, and other situations. Some of the forms in which the equation will be encountered may at first appear different from Eq. 1.32, because some authors consider that a weak acid, upon treatment with a strong base, is converted to its salt; thus the equation could be written pH = pK_a + log (salt/acid); when a weak base is treated with a strong acid to form its salt, the equivalent form is pH = pK_a + log (base/salt). Because of the possible confusion resulting from this terminology, we will adhere to the Bronsted concept, thus speaking of conjugate acid and base species. All the above equations then have the same form, namely, Eq. 1.33, in which the charge types of the species are irrelevant.

$$\mathrm{pH} = \mathrm{p}K_a + \log \frac{[\text{conjugate base}]}{[\text{conjugate acid}]} \qquad (1.33)$$

The Henderson-Hasselbalch equation relates three quantities: pH, pK_a, and the ratio b/a. In practical situations two of these are often known and the third may then be calculated.

EXAMPLE 1.4. Calculate the pH of a buffer solution prepared by dissolving 242.2 mg of tris(hydroxymethyl)aminomethane in 10.0 ml of 0.170 *N* HCl and diluting to 100 ml with water. The molecular weight of the solute is 121.1. It is a primary amine of structure $(HOCH_2)_3CNH_2$, with $pK_a = 8.08$ for the conjugate acid.

A total of 2.0 meq of solute was weighed out, and 1.7 meq of HCl was added. Since the HCl reacts with the amine to convert an equivalent amount to its conjugate acid (protonated) form, this means that $a = 1.7/100\ M$ and $b = (2.0 - 1.7)/100\ M$. Using these figures in the Henderson-Hasselbalch equation,

$$\text{pH} = \text{pK}_a + \log \frac{0.003}{0.017} = 8.08 - \log \frac{0.017}{0.003}$$

$$\text{pH} = 8.08 - \log 5.67 = 7.25$$

In this calculation the ratio was inverted merely to give a value greater than unity, for ease in taking the logarithm.

EXAMPLE 1.5. Calculate the pH of a buffer prepared to contain 0.09 *M* NaH_2PO_4 and 0.01 *M* K_2HPO_4. $\text{pK}_1 = 2.23$, $\text{pK}_2 = 7.21$, $\text{pK}_3 = 12.32$ for phosphoric acid.

In general a buffer of a polyprotic acid may be a very complex mixture, and a species distribution diagram is helpful in clarifying the problem. Figure 1.4 shows this diagram for phosphoric acid. The pK values of this acid are widely spaced, and phosphoric acid behaves essentially as if it were an equimolar mixture of three monobasic acids of the given pK values. From the experimental values $a = 0.09\ M$ and $b = 0.01\ M$, Fig. 1.4 clearly shows that the pH will be approximately 6.3 and that the solution contains practically no H_3PO_4 or PO_4^{3-} at this pH. We have now simplified the problem to that of a monobasic acid ($H_2PO_4^-$) and its conjugate base (HPO_4^{2-}), with the dissociation constant $\text{pK}_2 = 7.21$. Applying the Henderson-Hasselbalch equation gives pH = 7.21 − log 9 = 6.26.

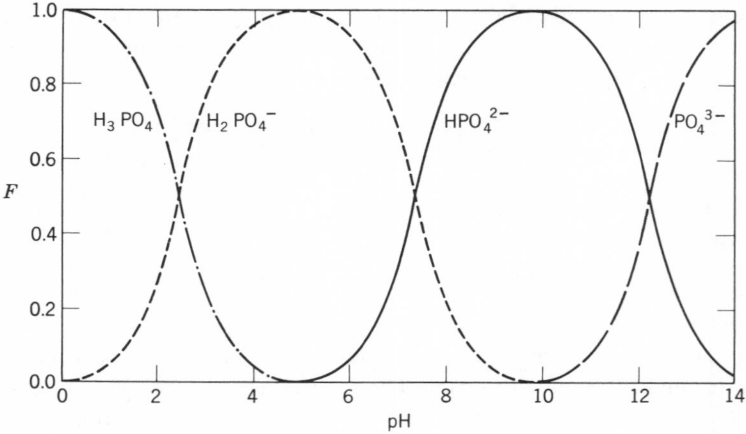

Fig. 1.4. Species distribution diagram for phosphoric acid: $\text{pK}_1 = 2.23$, $\text{pK}_2 = 7.21$, $\text{pK}_3 = 12.32$.

Since the function of a buffer is to minimize changes in pH, it is of practical importance to determine how this buffer capacity depends upon the buffer solution properties. The *buffer index* β is the measure of buffering capacity. If b is the concentration of strong base added to a solution containing total concentration c of a weak acid, the buffer index is defined by

$$\beta = \frac{db}{d\text{pH}} \tag{1.34}$$

β is evidently the concentration of strong base required to change the pH by a given amount. A simple graphical interpretation of β is given in Section 1.2 of this chapter. The higher the value of β, the greater is the buffer capacity of the solution. Since the strong base converts the weak acid to its conjugate base, b has the same meaning given to it earlier, and we can write, from Eq. 1.22, $F_A = b/c = K_a/([H^+] + K_a)$. It can then be shown [2] that $\beta = 2.3cF_{HA}F_A$. The maximum value of β occurs when pH = pK_a of the buffering acid, and acceptable capacity is achieved when the solution pH is within the range p$K_a \pm 1$. The capacity is also directly proportional to the buffer concentration c.

The choice of buffer substance for a particular application will therefore depend upon the pH desired for the solution. In the very low or very high pH regions strong acids and bases, respectively, are good buffers. Some of the common buffers in the intermediate range* are acetate, phosphate, borate, phthalate, carbonate, citrate, and tris(hydroxymethyl)aminomethane (TRIS). Directions for their preparation will be found in many reference works and other sources [3, 4], and of course the user can design buffers with the aid of the treatment given in this section.

Acid-Base Strength and Chemical Structure. The dissociation constant K_a is a quantitative measure of acid strength. Since K_a is an equilibrium constant for a proton transfer between two conjugate acid-base pairs, some ambiguity is associated with its interpretation. This is resolved, as shown earlier, by choosing one of the conjugate pairs to be the solvent system, water. This factor therefore remains constant, and aqueous K_a (or pK_a) values can be interpreted as measures of acid strength of the conjugate acid. We will briefly examine the relationship of pK_a to chemical structure [5].

The equilibrium described by K_a is

$$\text{Conjugate acid} + H_2O \rightleftharpoons \text{Conjugate base} + H_3O^+$$

* It is common to refer to a buffer as, for example, an acetate buffer, whereas of course it really is an acetic acid-acetate mixture. A typical description might, for instance, specify a 0.1 M pH 7.5 phosphate buffer; the concentration given is the total concentration of the buffer species.

Structural effects that are acid-strengthening (increase K_a, decrease pK_a) might be interpreted as rendering either the conjugate acid less stable, or the conjugate base more stable, or both; in any case, the equilibrium has been shifted to the right. Among the most clear-cut of these effects (at least in a qualitative sense) are those caused by electronic charges. In the dissociation reaction a proton, H^+, is leaving the acid molecule. A simple electrostatic argument therefore predicts that if the conjugate acid is already positively charged, loss of the proton will be easier (require less energy) than from a neutral molecule, because of charge repulsion. Further, if the acid is negatively charged, dissociation of the proton will be more difficult because of charge attraction. These predictions are consistent with the following data:

$$H_3\overset{+}{N}—CH_2COOH \rightleftharpoons H_3\overset{+}{N}—CH_2COO^- + H^+ \qquad pK_a = 2.31$$

$$H_3C—CH_2COOH \rightleftharpoons H_3C—CH_2COO^- + H^+ \qquad pK_a = 4.88$$

$$^-O_2C—CH_2COOH \rightleftharpoons {}^-O_2C—CH_2COO^- + H^+ \qquad pK_a = 5.69$$

This is why pK_2 of a diprotic acid is always larger than pK_1. The difference between them becomes smaller as the distance between the two acidic groups increases, because the electrostatic effect depends on distance.*

It is not necessary to introduce a discrete charge into a molecule to observe acid-strengthening or acid-weakening effects. Substitution of a functional group capable of electron donation or electron withdrawal by the inductive (polar) or resonance effects can also lead to significant changes in acid strength. Some of the best illustrations are seen in the *m*- and *p*-substituted benzoic acids. In fact, much of our knowledge of the electronic effects of substituent groups is derived from such pK_a values. Table 1.4 gives pK_a values for some monosubstituted benzoic acids [5]. It is immediately apparent that the nitro group is acid-strengthening, and therefore it must be electron-withdrawing, and that the amino group is acid-weakening and electron-donating. Some of these effects can be attributed to inductive effects, as in *m*- and *p*-methylbenzoic acids; the methyl group is slightly acid-weakening relative to hydrogen. Other substituents are capable of both inductive and resonance effects, and these can act in the same or opposite directions. These phenomena can be seen especially well in substituted phenols, since in these compounds the phenolic group can enter into direct conjugation with the ring. Table 1.5 shows some pK_a data for substituted phenols. Note that the nitro group is acid-strengthening in both benzoic acid and phenol, but the effect is much more pronounced in phenol, and it is greater in the *para* than

* The reader may have noticed that multiple K values appear as products or quotients, so pK values always appear as sums or differences. There is a more fundamental meaning to this observation, which is made clear in Chapter 6.

TABLE 1.4
pK_a *Values for Monosubstituted Benzoic Acids in Water*

	Position		
Substituent	*ortho*	*meta*	*para*
—H	4.20	4.20	4.20
—NO_2	2.17	3.45	3.44
—Cl	2.94	3.83	3.99
—OCH_3	4.09	4.09	4.47
—CH_3	3.91	4.24	4.34
—$C(CH_3)_3$	3.46	4.28	4.40
—COOH	2.95	3.54	3.51
—COO^-	5.41	4.60	4.82
—OH	2.98	4.08	4.58
—NH_2	4.98	4.79	4.92

in the *meta* position. This can be rationalized in terms of the resonance hybrid **1**, which stabilizes the conjugate base (relative to $C_6H_5O^-$ itself).

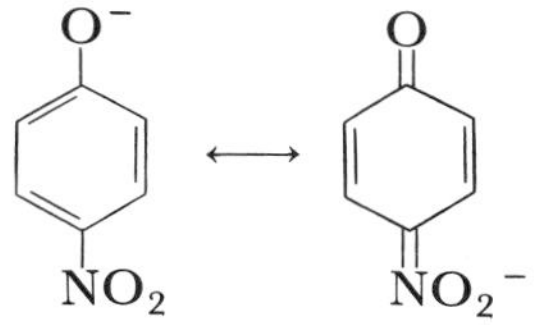

O^- $\longleftrightarrow$ O

NO_2 NO_2^-

1

In *p*-nitrophenol the electron-withdrawing properties of the nitro group by the inductive and resonance effects cooperate to cause a large increase in acid

TABLE 1.5
pK_a *Values for Monosubstituted Phenols in Water*

	Position		
Substituent	*ortho*	*meta*	*para*
—H	10.00	10.00	10.00
—NO_2	7.23	8.35	7.14
—Cl	8.48	9.02	9.35
—OCH_3	9.93	9.65	10.20
—CH_3	10.28	10.08	10.19
—NH_2	9.71	9.87	10.30

strength. In *m*-nitrophenol the resonance effect cannot be brought into play, and the pK_a is accordingly intermediate to that of phenol and *p*-nitrophenol.

In the methoxyphenols the inductive and resonance effects are in opposition. The methoxy group is electron-withdrawing by the inductive effect but electron-donating by the resonance effect. In *m*-methoxyphenol, where the resonance effect cannot operate, this group is therefore acid-strengthening (relative to phenol), but in *p*-methoxyphenol the resonance effect apparently overcomes the inductive effect (see **2**), and *p*-methoxyphenol is a weaker acid than is phenol.

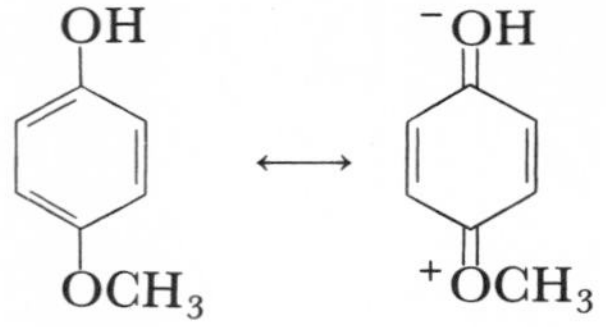

OH ⟷ $^{-}$OH

OCH_3 $^{+}OCH_3$

2

ortho-Substituted aromatic compounds are more complicated because they include the possibility of steric effects by direct interaction between the two groups. For example, the methyl group is slightly acid-weakening in *m*- and *p*-methyl benzoic acids, because of its inductive electron release. In the *ortho* position it is acid-strengthening, presumably by a steric effect. Moreover, *o*-*tert*-butylbenzoic acid exhibits this behavior to even a greater degree. These appear to be examples of the steric inhibition of resonance [5]. The benzoic acid (conjugate acid) may be stabilized by the resonance shown in **3**. The

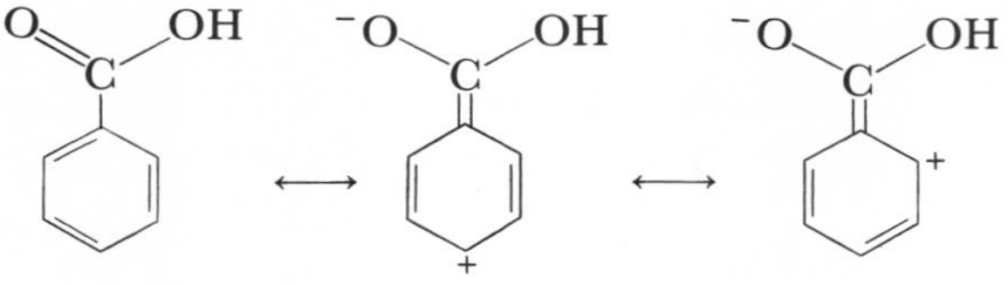

O=C–OH ⟷ $^{-}$O–C–OH ⟷ $^{-}$O–C–OH

3

resonance structures require the carboxyl group and the aromatic ring to be coplanar. Substitution of a bulky group in the *ortho* position will force the carboxyl out of coplanarity with the ring, thus decreasing resonance stabilization of the conjugate acid and increasing acid strength.*

Another kind of *ortho* effect is seen in salicylic acid (*o*-hydroxybenzoic acid), whose pK_1 value, for ionization of the carboxyl group, is much lower than in the electronically comparable *p*-hydroxybenzoic acid. This is thought to be a

* The same argument could be applied to the conjugate base, but the comparable resonance contributions should be less in the anion because they would place charges on both oxygens, so the net effect is acid-strengthening.

consequence of stabilization of the conjugate base by intramolecular hydrogen bonding, as in **4**.

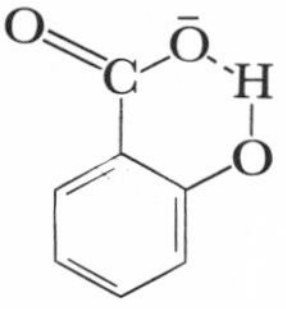

4

Table 1.6 lists pK_a values of some bases, or rather of their conjugate acids. A larger pK_a means a stronger base. Thus methylamine, CH_3NH_2, is a stronger base than ammonia, as expected with the introduction of the electron-donating methyl group. A comparison of aniline, **5**, with its saturated analogue cyclohexylamine, **6**, shows how the electron-withdrawing property of the phenyl ring decreases base strength by more than five orders of magnitude ($pK_{\text{cyclohexylamine}} - pK_{\text{aniline}} = 5.47$).

5 **6**

A similar effect is seen for pyridine, **7**, and piperidine, **8**.

7 **8**

TABLE 1.6
pK_a *Values for Amines in Water*

Amine	pK_a
Ammonia	9.25
Methylamine	10.66
Dimethylamine	10.73
Trimethylamine	9.75
Cyclohexylamine	10.68
Piperidine	11.12
Pyridine	5.21
Aniline	4.60

The series ammonia, methylamine, dimethylamine, and trimethylamine presents an anomalous order of basicity. Increasing substitution (replacement of hydrogen by methyl) should result in increasing basicity. This is observed for the series NH_3, CH_3NH_2, and $(CH_3)_2NH$. Trimethylamine, however, reverses this trend. This reversal indicates that some other (opposing) factor is also involved, and several proposals have been made to explain this basicity series. It now appears that the reversal is a consequence of small changes in solvation properties within the series [6].

Amides, R′CONHR, are very much weaker bases than are the corresponding amines, RNH_2, because of the strongly electron-withdrawing property of the acyl group.

1.2 Acid-Base Titrations

Titration Curves. An acid-base titration curve is a graph of pH against volume of titrant added during a titration. These curves can be calculated and they can be determined experimentally. The calculation of titration curves uses the equations and methods already described, since at any point in a titration the sample solution can be described as a solution of an acid, a base, or a mixture of the two.

Strong acid-strong base titration: when a strong acid and a strong base are mixed together, as in the titration of one by the other, the reaction that occurs is $H^+ + OH^- \rightleftharpoons H_2O$. Since this is the reverse of the ionization of water, its equilibrium constant is very large. This is a requirement for a reaction to form the basis of a good titration. The calculation of a titration curve is illustrated with Example 1.6.

EXAMPLE 1.6. Calculate the titration curve for the titration of 50 ml of 0.1 *N* HCl with 0.5 *N* NaOH.

The pH before the titration begins is the pH of 0.1 *N* HCl; therefore $[H^+] = 0.1\ N$, or pH = 1.00.

After the addition of 1.0 ml of titrant, the volume is 51 ml. Initially the solution contained 5.0 meq of acid ($V \times N =$ meq), and 0.5 meq of base has been added. Therefore the solution now contains $5.0 - 0.5 = 4.5$ meq of acid in 51 ml, or 4.5/51 eq/liter; $[H^+] = 0.0833\ N$, and pH = 1.08. In this manner the calculation is made for several points throughout the titration. A few results are: at 2 ml, pH = 1.11; at 4 ml, 1.26; at 6 ml, 1.45; at 8 ml, 1.76; and at 9 ml, 2.07.

When 10 ml of NaOH has been added, all of the HCl has been neutralized. The total volume is 60 ml and the only solute is sodium chloride. In the absence of carbon dioxide the pH $= \frac{1}{2}pK_w$, or 7.00 in water at 25°C.

When 11 ml of NaOH has been added, the total volume is 61 ml and the solution contains 1.0 ml of excess NaOH, or 0.5 meq. The hydroxide ion concentration is 0.5/61 N, or 8.20×10^{-3} N. The pOH is 2.09 and pH = 11.91.

Titration of weak acid with strong base: it is possible to derive an exact equation that describes the entire course of the titration, but the calculation is just as convenient with the approximate equations introduced earlier. Then the titration is considered in four stages.

1. Before titration begins. At this point the sample solution contains only the weak acid, and the pH is calculated with Eq. 1.14 or 1.15.
2. During titration. After some strong base has been added, its reaction with the weak acid will produce an equivalent amount of the conjugate weak base. The solution now is a mixture of the weak acid and its conjugate base—in fact it is a buffer solution—and the Henderson-Hasselbalch equation, Eq. 1.32, applies.
3. At the end point. Now an amount of strong base has been added that is exactly equivalent to the amount of weak acid initially present. The solution now contains only the conjugate base of the weak acid, and its pH can be calculated via Eq. 1.16 or 1.17.
4. After the end point. An excess of titrant has now been added, and the pH is determined essentially by this excess, the appropriate dilution within the solution being taken into account. It is true that the conjugate weak base produced by the titration also contributes to the solution pOH, but its contribution is small relative to the effect of the excess titrant; moreover, the hydroxide added as excess titrant will repress the dissociation of the weak base.

The titration of a weak base by a strong acid is completely analogous, as shown in Example 1.7.

EXAMPLE 1.7. Calculate the titration curve for the titration of 24 ml of 0.2 M n-butylamine ($pK_a = 10.60$) with 0.3 N HCl.

The calculation will be divided into the four stages suggested above.

1. The controlling equilibrium is

$$RNH_2 + H_2O \rightleftharpoons RNH_3^+ + OH^-$$

Eq. 1.17 can be used, with $c = 0.2$ M and $K_b = 4.0 \times 10^{-4}$, giving pOH = 2.05 and pH = 11.95.

2. Suppose 2.0 ml of titrant has been added. Then

$$\begin{aligned}
\text{meq of base initially present} &= (24)(0.2) = 4.8\\
\text{meq of HCl added} &= (2)(0.3) = 0.6\\
\text{meq of base left} &= 4.2
\end{aligned}$$

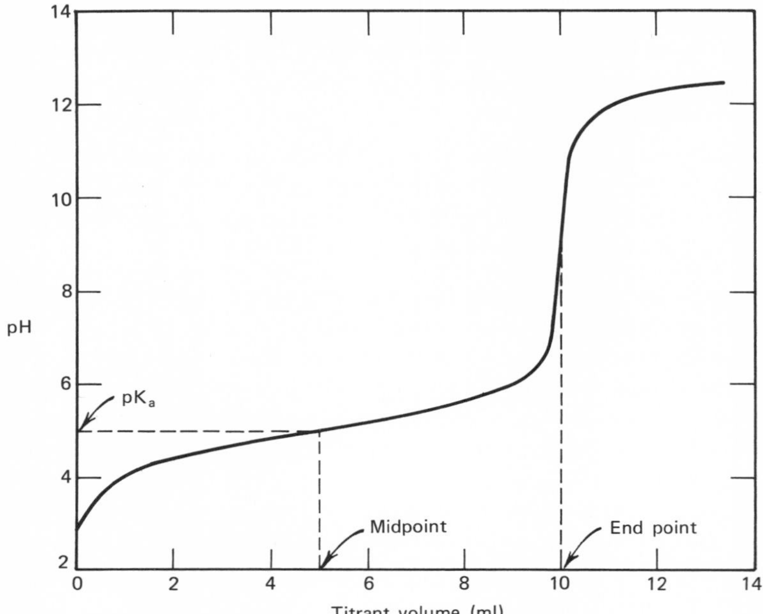

Fig. 1.5. Calculated curve for the titration of 10.0 ml of 0.2 *N* weak acid (pK_a = 5.00) with 0.2 *N* strong base.

The Henderson-Hasselbalch equation is

$$pH = pK_a + \log \frac{4.2}{0.6} = 11.45$$

The calculation can be carried out similarly for more points during the titration, with these results: at 5 ml, pH = 10.94; at 8 ml, 10.60; at 12 ml, 10.12.

3. The end point titrant volume is readily calculated to be 16.0 ml. The solution now contains the conjugate acid of *n*-butylamine, and Eq. 1.15 is appropriate. The total solution volume is now 40 ml, so the value of c has decreased, solely because of this dilution, from 0.2 to 0.12 *M*. The calculated pH is 5.76.

4. Suppose 18 ml of titrant has been added, so a 2 ml excess of titrant is present. This means that (2)(0.3) = 0.6 meq of strong acid is present in 42 ml, so $[H^+] = 1.43 \times 10^{-2}$ *M* and pH = 1.84.

Figure 1.5 is a calculated titration curve for the titration of 10 ml of 0.2 *N* weak acid (pK_a 5.00) with 0.2 *N* strong base. Several features are of interest.*

* The reader may encounter the term "neutralization" used as a synonym for "titration." It is evident, from these calculations, that the pH at the end point is not usually at neutrality, so this usage is not accurate, but it is widespread.

The end point volume is 10 ml, and it can be seen that this occurs at an inflection point and at the point of the curve with the steepest slope. Also, since at the end point all the weak acid has been converted to its conjugate base, then at the midpoint of the titration (when one-half of the end point volume has been added), evidently one-half of the weak acid has been converted to its conjugate base, so their concentrations are equal. According to Eq. 1.33, pH = pK_a at this point. This relationship is indicated in Fig. 1.5.

The slope of the titration curve at any point is a measure of the rate of change of pH upon the addition of a given volume of titrant. It is evident from Fig. 1.5 that this slope is a maximum at the end point and it is a minimum at the midpoint. In fact, it can be seen that the slope of the titration curve is the reciprocal of the buffer index β (Eq. 1.34). Figure 1.5 shows that buffer capacity is maximal when pH = pK_a (that is, when the concentrations of conjugate acid and base are equal) and remains substantial in the pH range $pK_a \pm 1$, for within this range the titration curve is very flat.

Titration of polyfunctional acids and bases: thus far we have considered solutions of monofunctional acids and bases. Polyfunctional solutes yield more complicated titration curves with, in general, each acidic or basic group leading to a "break" in the curve. Usually successive pK values differ by at least 3 units, so the successive dissociations can be treated independently. This simple circumstance does not always hold.

We shall consider the titration of the dibasic acid H_2A with a strong base. Before any titrant has been added the pH of the solution can be calculated as if the solute were a monobasic acid, according to the dissociation

$$H_2A \overset{K_1}{\rightleftharpoons} H^+ + HA^-$$

with Eq. 1.15 being used. This calculation assumes that the secondary dissociation,

$$HA^- \overset{K_2}{\rightleftharpoons} H^+ + A^{2-}$$

does not occur to a significant extent. This assumption is valid for two reasons: (1) the hydrogen ion produced in the primary dissociation represses the secondary dissociation; and (2) K_2 is usually several orders of magnitude smaller than K_1.

During the first phase of the titration, when the titration reaction may be written

$$H_2A + OH^- \rightleftharpoons HA^- + H_2O$$

the Henderson-Hasselbalch equation may be used and the secondary dissociation may be ignored in most cases. As the first end point is approached, however, it may be necessary to take account of the second titration reaction

$$HA^- + OH^- \rightleftharpoons A^{2-} + H_2O$$

which can occur simultaneously with the titration of H_2A if K_2 is not very much smaller than K_1.

From the analytical point of view it is most important to be able to calculate the pH at the first end point. This calculation requires recognition of both acidic functions on the molecule, for as the titration passes through the first end point the pH will be controlled by both acid-base equilibria. At the first end point the principal species present is HA^-, which dissociates as follows:

$$HA^- \rightleftharpoons H^+ + A^{2-}$$

For each A^{2-} formed one H^+ is formed. However, some of the H^+ is consumed by the reaction

$$H^+ + HA^- \rightleftharpoons H_2A$$

Each H^+ thus consumed yields one H_2A. Therefore we can write, at the first end point,

$$[A^{2-}] = [H^+] + [H_2A] \qquad (1.35)$$

Substituting the dissociation constant expressions for K_1 and K_2 into Eq. 1.35 leads to

$$[H^+]^2 = \frac{K_1K_2[HA^-]}{K_1 + [HA^-]}$$

It will be reasonably accurate to set the equilibrium concentration $[HA^-]$ equal to its formal concentration c,

$$[H^+]^2 = \frac{K_1K_2c}{K_1 + c} \qquad (1.36)$$

If, as is often the case, c is much larger than K_1, Eq. 1.36 becomes

$$[H^+]^2 = K_1K_2$$

or

$$\text{pH} = \frac{\text{p}K_1 + \text{p}K_2}{2} \qquad (1.37)$$

at the first end point.

The pH at the second end point may be calculated by ignoring the primary dissociation. In the titration of H_2A to the second end point, the pH is controlled, at this point, by the reaction

$$A^{2-} + H_2O \rightleftharpoons HA^- + OH^-$$

and the hydroxide ion concentration is calculated with Eq. 1.17; the pertinent basic dissociation constant is of course given by K_w/K_2.

EXAMPLE 1.8. Calculate the pH at both end points in the titration of 20 ml of 0.1 *M* phthalic acid with 0.1 *N* NaOH. $\text{p}K_1 = 2.95$, $\text{p}K_2 = 5.41$.

At the first end point $c = 0.05\ M$, so c is about 50 times as large as K_1. Equation 1.37 may therefore be used, giving pH = 4.18 at the first end point.

At the second end point the total volume of the solution is 60 ml. The concentration of phthalate ion is 0.0333 M and the appropriate basic dissociation constant is the one describing the reaction

$$P^{2-} + H_2O \rightleftharpoons HP^- + OH^-$$

This is K_w/K_2, or 2.57×10^{-9}. Using Eq. 1.17 gives $[OH^-] = 9.25 \times 10^{-6}$ or pOH = 5.03, so pH = 8.97 at the second end point.

Acid-Base Indicators. An acid-base indicator is a compound whose conjugate acid and base forms exhibit different colors. There is no limitation on the charge type of the indicator. Indicators are used to detect the end point in a titration, the selection of an indicator being based on the simple principles to be discussed here.

Consider the indicator acid HI. This acid will undergo dissociation in aqueous solution.

$$HI \rightleftharpoons H^+ + I^-$$

The acid dissociation constant has the form of Eq. 1.3, but it is often symbolized K_I.

$$K_I = \frac{[H^+][I^-]}{[HI]} \tag{1.38}$$

The acid form HI is responsible for the acid color of the indicator solution, and I^- shows the base color. The color that our eyes see is related to the relative concentrations of these two forms of the indicator. Rearranging Eq. 1.38 gives

$$\frac{[I^-]}{[HI]} = \frac{K_I}{[H^+]} \tag{1.39}$$

Two important conclusions follow from Eq. 1.39. The color is controlled by the hydrogen ion concentration of the solution; and the color change during a titration is not abrupt but occurs in a continuous manner, since the hydrogen ion concentration changes continuously.

It is characteristic of the typical human eye that in order to detect the first deviation from the pure acid color in a solution of the indicator, the ratio $[I^-]/[HI]$ must be at least $\frac{1}{10}$; that is, about 10% of the indicator must be in the base form. Similarly, about 10% of the indicator must be in the acid form to detect any acid color. (These statements apply to two-color indicators.) In between these limits the eye recognizes that a mixture of colors is present, and that the indicator color change is taking place if a titration is being carried out. It must be realized that these limits for $[I^-]/[HI]$ of 0.1 to 10 have no theoretical significance but are related to the sensitivity of the observer's eyes and to the particular indicator used; some colors are more readily detected than others.

The pH values at which these limits of observable color change occur are easily calculated. From Eq. 1.38,

$$pH = pK_I + \log \frac{[I^-]}{[HI]}$$

For the limit on the acid side, $[I^-]/[HI] = 0.1$, or $pH = pK_I - 1$. For the limit on the base side, $[I^-]/[HI] = 10$, or $pH = pK_I + 1$. The pH range within which the indicator can be observed to be changing color is thus given approximately by $pH = pK_I \pm 1$. This is called the *transition interval* of the indicator, and it clearly depends upon the pK_I of the indicator. This is why indicators of different structure change color at different pH's.

Table 1.7 gives the colors and transition intervals of some useful acid-base indicators. Many of the intervals are less than 2 pH units, suggesting that the limits $pK_I \pm 1$ are rather conservative. One-color indicators, in which only one of the conjugate forms possesses a visible color, will not behave visually in accordance with the above treatment, though of course their equilibria will be described by the same equations. The pK_I of an indicator, and therefore its transition interval, can be affected by the salt concentration of the solution and by organic solvents incorporated into the aqueous medium.

In order to achieve an accurate visual detection of the end point in an acid-base titration, evidently the pH of the solution must change by about 2 units in the immediate vicinity (say, $\pm 0.2\%$) of the end point. Whether this condition is satisfied in any given circumstance can be determined by calculating the titration curve. Figure 1.5 shows the results of such a calculation, indicating that this would be a feasible titration with visual end point detection because of the sharp break in the region of the theoretical equivalence point. Calculations show that this break is greater, the more concentrated the solution and the stronger the acid (for titrations with base).

An indicator should now be chosen such that the pH at the titration equivalence point falls within the transition interval of the indicator. In the titration of a weak acid with a strong base, at the end point the solution contains the conjugate base of the acid, so its pH is in the alkaline range, as shown in Fig. 1.5. Weak acids therefore are usually titrated using thymol blue, phenolphthalein, or thymolphthalein as indicators. In titrations of weak bases with strong acids the end point pH will be in the acidic range (see Example 1.7), and methyl red, methyl orange, and bromcresol green are commonly used indicators.

An empirical, but very useful, method of indicator selection is by conducting a potentiometric titration (see Chapter 6) and incorporating an indicator in

TABLE 1.7
Properties of Acid-Base Indicators[a]

Indicator	Transition Interval	Acid Color	Base Color
m-Cresol purple	0.5–2.5	Red	Yellow
Thymol blue	1.2–2.8	Red	Yellow
Tropaeolin 00	1.4–2.6	Red	Yellow
2,4-Dinitrophenol	2.6–4.0	Colorless	Yellow
Bromphenol blue	3.0–4.6	Yellow	Blue
Methyl orange	3.1–4.4	Red	Yellow
Sodium alizarin sulfonate	3.7–5.2	Yellow	Violet
Bromcresol green	3.8–5.4	Yellow	Blue
Methyl red	4.2–6.2	Red	Yellow
Bromcresol purple	5.2–6.8	Yellow	Purple
Alizarin	5.5–6.8	Yellow	Red
p-Nitrophenol	5.6–7.6	Colorless	Yellow
Bromthymol blue	6.0–7.6	Yellow	Blue
Phenol red	6.8–8.4	Yellow	Red
Cresol red	7.2–8.8	Yellow	Red
m-Cresol purple	7.4–9.0	Yellow	Pink
Tropaeolin 000 no. 1	7.6–8.9	Yellow	Red
Thymol blue	8.0–9.6	Yellow	Blue
Phenolphthalein	8.2–10	Colorless	Red
Thymolphthalein	9.3–10.5	Colorless	Blue
Alizarin yellow R	10.2–12	Yellow	Red
Tropaeolin 0	11–13	Yellow	Orange

[a] From *The Merck Index*, 8th ed., Merck & Co., Rahway, N.J., 1968.

the sample solution. If the visual and potentiometric end points coincide, then the indicator is suitable for the titration.

Some analysts prefer to use *mixed indicators*, which when properly constituted can exhibit a very sharp color change over a small pH interval. The two indicators to be mixed usually have similar transition intervals, and they are selected, when possible, such that their acid colors combine to give a hue that is the complement (see Table 8.2) of the hue resulting from the combination of their base colors. Then a very sharp color change, sometimes passing through a gray or colorless phase, is observed. For example, bromcresol green and methyl red together give a red color in the acid form and green in the base form, the transition being very sharp at pH 5.1. Other mixed indicators are bromthymol blue-phenol red, cresol red-thymol blue, and thymol blue-phenolphthalein [7].

If several indicators are mixed so that their transition intervals overlap, it is possible to observe color changes over a wide range of pH. Then a rough estimate of solution pH can be obtained by observing the indicator color. When such a *universal indicator* is applied to filter paper, the resulting "pH paper" provides a simple means of measuring pH to within about 1 unit by dipping it into the solution and comparing the color with a series of standards.

We now consider the chemical basis for indicator color changes. Without the results of Chapter 8 it is not possible to give an entirely satisfactory discussion, but a simplified approach will still be useful. The essential fact about acid-base indicators is that the acid and base forms have different colors. All acid-base indicators in common use are organic compounds. Apparently the reason for the different colors must be sought in the different structures of the acid and base forms of the indicator. It is possible to account for the fact of color differences on this basis: if two forms of the indicator differ markedly in their electronic distribution, and particularly in their extents of resonance delocalization, two colors will be observed. Color is associated with the capability of the compound to absorb visible light, and this capability can be related to the electronic structure. In the resonance hybrid several factors may contribute, but we can simplify and say that a change in the length of conjugation path or in extent of electronic delocalization will result in absorption of a different color component of white light, with a resultant color change.

Consider tropaeolin 000 no. 1, also called Orange I and α-naphthol orange. The acid (yellow) form is believed to have structure **9**. Conversion of **9** to its

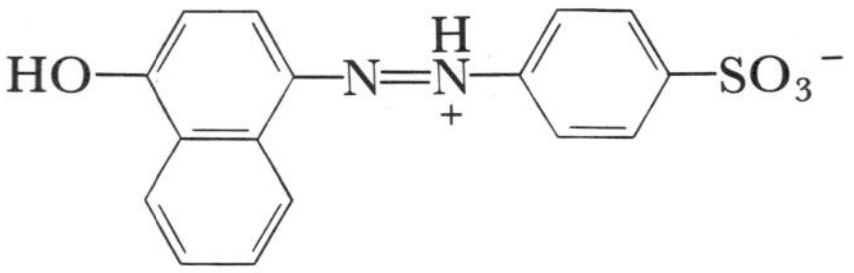

9

conjugate base form by dissociation of the phenolic group leads to the delocalized structure **10,** which is red. The quinoid structure in **10** is often responsible for color changes in indicators possessing a phenolic group. The

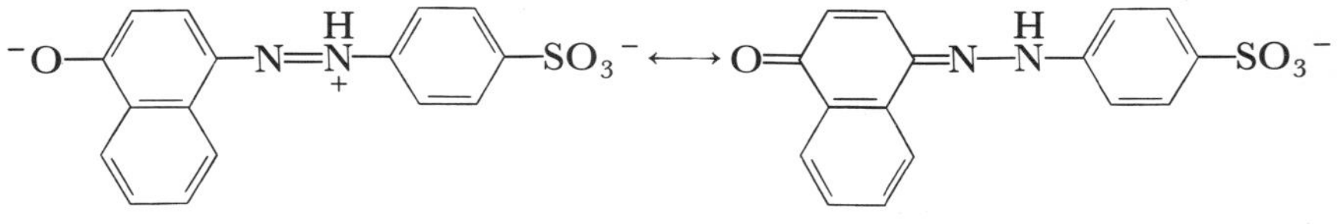

10

phthalein indicators all have such a group. A similar electronic distribution occurs in aminoazo indicators like methyl orange, **11**.

$$(CH_3)_2N-C_6H_4-N{=}N-C_6H_4-SO_3^- \xrightleftharpoons{H^+}$$

Base (yellow)

11

$$(CH_3)_2N-C_6H_4-N{=}\overset{H}{\underset{+}{N}}-C_6H_4-SO_3^-$$

$$\updownarrow$$

$$(CH_3)_2\overset{+}{N}{=}C_6H_4{=}N-\overset{H}{N}-C_6H_4-SO_3^-$$

Acid (red)

1.3 Experimental Titrimetry

Techniques. In its simplest form, an acid-base titration is carried out by adding the standard solution of titrant acid or base, from a buret, to the solution of sample base or acid containing a suitable indicator. The volume of titrant required to reach the end point is read from the calibrated scale of the buret. Many modifications, refinements, and procedures have been developed to improve the method and to extend its utility. The procedure described above is a *direct titration*. Sometimes a *back-titration* (residual titration) is useful, for example, if the sample should be a volatile base. Then a known volume of standard acid, in excess of that required for the stoichiometric reaction, is added to the sample. The excess of acid is back-titrated with standard alkali.

The accuracy of the titrimetric analysis depends upon several factors: (1) the accuracy with which the concentration of the titrant solution is known; (2) the end point detection accuracy; (3) the measurement of titrant volume at the end point; and (4) factors relating to sample preparation. The titrant solution is always a strong acid or a strong base. These substances are not commercially available in forms of accurately known concentration, so titrant solutions are prepared to be approximately the desired concentration, and they are then *standardized*, that is, they are analyzed accurately by titration of a substance (the *primary standard*) whose purity *is* accurately known.

Strong acid solutions commonly are standardized against sodium carbonate, Na_2CO_3; borax, $Na_2B_4O_7 \cdot 10H_2O$; or tris(hydroxymethyl)aminomethane

(TRIS), $(HOCH_2)_3C—NH_2$ [8–10]. Strong bases usually are standardized against potassium biphthalate, $(HOOC)C_6H_4(COOK)$.

If the end point break is great enough, little error will be introduced through titrant consumption by the indicator, if the latter is chosen with an appropriate transition interval. This can be checked by carrying out an indicator blank titration, that is, by titrating a solution containing the indicator and solvent but not the sample substance, in order to ascertain the volume of titrant required to change the indicator. If significant, this volume can be subtracted from the titrant volume. If the end point break is too gradual for a sharp color change, good results may still be obtained by using a comparison solution, which is a solution with the same pH as that expected at the titration end point, the indicator being incorporated to the same concentration in the comparison as in the titration solution. The sample is titrated until its color matches that of the comparison. For example, 1 *N* sodium acetate can be titrated with 1 *N* HCl by using a comparison solution prepared to be 0.5 *N* in acetic acid and 0.5 *N* in sodium chloride.

Many acids and bases are strong enough to be titrated, but are not sufficiently soluble in water. A hydroalcoholic medium will usually increase the solubility. It is important to realize that pK_a and pK_I values (and, indeed, the pH scale itself) are altered by incorporating an organic solvent into the aqueous medium, so indicator selection according to Table 1.7 may not be appropriate. Another way to overcome insolubility of the sample is with a back-titration. Many alkaloids can be titrated in this way. Sometimes the product of the titration is insoluble and precipitates as the titration progresses. This may obscure the visual end point. A "diphasic" titration may be carried out with an immiscible organic solvent, such as chloroform or ether, being added to the titration flask. With vigorous shaking the water-insoluble product of the titration reaction passes into the organic layer.

A pervasive problem in the preparation, storage, and use of standard solutions of alkali is the presence of carbon dioxide (the anhydride of carbonic acid) in the atmosphere. All water used in such solutions or in dissolving sample acids should be freshly boiled and preferably cooled in the absence of air. Solutions of bases must be protected from CO_2 during storage. During titration CO_2 may be absorbed; it is easy to see the effect of this at the end point of a titration using phenolphthalein as indicator. The pink color denoting the end point soon fades to colorless as a consequence of the consumption of alkali by absorbed CO_2, with a consequent drop in pH. Solutions can be titrated at the boiling point to prevent over-titration caused by CO_2 absorption, or a stream of nitrogen can be played over the surface of the solution being titrated.

Acid-base titrations are routinely made on the macro level (sample sizes of the order 100 mg) and semimicro level ($\sim$10 mg) using burets of 50 ml,

25 ml, 10 ml, and 5 ml capacities, the volume readings usually being estimated to within 0.01 ml. With ordinary care, accuracy and precision in the parts per thousand range (that is, tenths of 1%) are attainable. Procedures have been devised extending these methods to the micro ($\sim$1 mg) and submicro ($\sim$1 μg) levels. Fifty microgram samples of carboxylic acids can be titrated using a syringe buret of 0.5 ml capacity graduated in 0.0002 ml intervals [11]. Microtitrations have been performed by a serial dilution technique, using a transfer loop and a spot plate rather than a buret and a titration flask [12]. Very accurate titrations can be made by weighing the titrant rather than measuring its volume [13].

Applications. The straightforward determination of purity by acid-base titration is an obvious application. Sometimes an acid or base of unknown identity is obtained in pure form and, as an aid in its identification, its equivalent weight (also called its neutralization equivalent) is determined by titration. Thus if the identity (and therefore equivalent weight) of the sample compound is known, its purity may be determined, whereas if its purity is known its equivalent weight can be established. The necessary calculations are outlined in Appendix A. Many functional group methods use an acid-base titration as the final step.

Strong acids and bases are analyzed easily by titration. Sulfonic acids, which have pK_a values in the range 1–3, are also titrated readily. Carboxylic acids usually have pK_a's in the range 3–6, and these also can be titrated accurately with strong bases. It will be appreciated, from the earlier considerations in this chapter, that the success of these titrations is dependent also upon the concentrations of the sample solutions. If the pK_a is not greater than about 6, solutions 0.01 N can be accurately titrated with direct visual detection of the end point. More dilute solutions, or samples of weaker acids, often can be accurately titrated using the comparison solution technique.

These same considerations apply also to titration of weak bases with strong acids, except that pK_b (which equals $pK_w - pK_a$) should be 6 or smaller for accurate visual titrations of 0.01 N solutions. At higher concentrations weaker bases can be titrated. Most aliphatic amines, but few aromatic amines, can therefore be titrated in water. Amides cannot be titrated.

Many salts can be titrated by these methods. As shown earlier, a salt is either a conjugate base (for example, sodium acetate) of a weak acid or a conjugate acid (e.g., ammonium chloride) of a weak base, and the above considerations apply.* These titrations are sometimes called displacement titrations, because the titration reaction may be viewed as the displacement of a weaker acid by a stronger one, or as the displacement of a weaker base by

* The salt of a strong acid and a strong base (e.g., sodium chloride) is neutral. The salt of a weak acid and a weak base (e.g., ammonium acetate) may be titratable as either an acid or a base.

a stronger one. Thus when ammonium chloride, NH_4Cl, is titrated with sodium hydroxide, our earlier view was that the weak acid NH_4^+ is being titrated with a strong base OH^-; the same reaction may be described, however, as the displacement of the weak base NH_3 from HCl by the strong base OH^-.

Experiment 1.1. Visual Indicator Titration of Acids

The following directions specify the use of "freshly boiled" water. Ordinary distilled water is supersaturated with respect to carbon dioxide, which acts as an acid:

$$H_2O + CO_2 \rightleftharpoons H_2CO_3$$

$$H_2CO_3 + 2OH^- \rightleftharpoons CO_3^{2-} + 2H_2O$$

If distilled water is boiled for a few minutes to expel most of the CO_2 and is then cooled to room temperature, its carbon dioxide content will be negligible for purposes of acid-base titration.

Appendix A should be consulted before beginning this experiment. Aqueous acid-base titrations with potentiometric detection of the end point are described in Experiment 6.1.

REAGENTS

0.1 N Sodium Hydroxide. Dilute 6 ml of saturated sodium hydroxide solution to 1 liter with freshly boiled water. (This method yields a carbonate-free solution, since sodium carbonate is insoluble in saturated NaOH.) Standardize the solution as follows: accurately weigh about 0.4 g (2 meq) of primary standard potassium biphthalate (previously dried at 105°C for 2 hr) into a 250 ml Erlenmeyer flask. Add about 50 ml of freshly boiled water to dissolve the sample. Add 3 drops of phenolphthalein indicator solution, and titrate with the sodium hydroxide solution from a 25 ml buret. The end point is marked by the first permanent pink color. Carry out an indicator blank titration and subtract the blank titrant volume from the sample titrant volume. Perform 3 or 4 such titrations of biphthalate. Calculate the normality of the sodium hydroxide solution from each titration (this result should be expressed to the fourth decimal place), the mean normality, and the standard deviation. In this titration the equivalent weight of potassium biphthalate is equal to its molecular weight. The relative standard deviation should not be greater than 0.3% (3 parts per thousand).

Phenolphthalein Indicator Solution. Dissolve 1 g of phenolphthalein in 100 ml of alcohol.

Methyl Red Indicator Solution. Dissolve 100 mg of methyl red in 100 ml of alcohol.

PROCEDURES

Determination of an Equivalent Weight. Tartaric acid, HOOC—CH(OH)-CH(OH)—COOH, is a dicarboxylic acid, and this experiment will establish whether one or both acid groups are titrated at the phenolphthalein end point. Accurately weigh samples of tartaric acid in the range 0.1–0.2 g. Dissolve in about 50 ml of freshly boiled water, add 3 drops of phenolphthalein solution, and titrate with standard 0.1 *N* NaOH to the first permanent pink color. Assuming the tartaric acid is pure, calculate its equivalent weight (EW). This will allow you to conclude whether EW = MW or EW = MW/2.

Analysis of a Tartaric Acid Sample. Obtain from your instructor a sample of tartaric acid of unknown purity.* Accurately weigh samples equivalent to about 2 meq of tartaric acid, and analyze them as described in the preceding paragraph. Your estimate of sample size will require the EW of tartaric acid, obtained in the above experiment, and the approximate composition of your sample, which can be obtained by making a rapid rough analysis before performing a careful series of weighings and titrations.

Calculate the percent purity of the sample of tartaric acid. In this calculation use the theoretical equivalent weight, that is, exactly MW or MW/2, as determined in the preceding experiment, rather than your experimental value.

Determination of Total Acidity of Vinegar. Vinegar is an aqueous solution of acetic acid and other substances produced by fermentation of various fruits or vegetables. To be called vinegar the solution must contain at least 4% acetic acid.

Give your instructor a dry, labeled, stoppered flask, into which will be delivered a sample of vinegar. Pipet a 25.0 ml portion of the vinegar into a 250 ml volumetric flask, dilute to the mark with water, and mix well. Withdraw 25.0 ml aliquots of this diluted solution by pipet, transfer to Erlenmeyer flasks, add 3 drops of phenolphthalein solution, and titrate with standard 0.1 *N* NaOH. Calculate the total acid content of the original vinegar sample as w/v percent of acetic acid (that is, the number of grams of acetic acid per 100 ml of vinegar).

Titration of a Strong Acid. Obtain a sample of hydrochloric acid solution from your instructor. Using a suitable volumetric pipet, transfer an accurately known volume to an Erlenmeyer flask. Add 3 drops of methyl red solution and titrate to the yellow color with standard 0.1 *N* NaOH. Perform several titrations and calculate the normality of the hydrochloric acid.

* Such samples can be prepared by mixing tartaric acid with sodium chloride, triturating the mixture well in a mortar, and mixing thoroughly.

Experiment 1.2. Visual Indicator Titration of Bases

REAGENTS

0.1 N Hydrochloric Acid. Dilute about 8 ml of concentrated hydrochloric acid to 1 liter with water. This solution will be standardized against tris(hydroxymethyl)aminomethane (TRIS) [9, 10]. Dry a sample of primary standard TRIS at 100°C for 2 hr, or over P_2O_5 in a desiccator for several days. Accurately weigh about 250 mg into an Erlenmeyer flask, dissolve it in about 25 ml of freshly boiled water, add 3 drops of one of the indicators (A, B, C, or D) listed below, and titrate with the 0.1 *N* HCl. Perform at least three such titrations and an indicator blank titration, and calculate the normality of the HCl solution. The equivalent weight of TRIS is 121.14.

Indicator A. Dissolve 100 mg of ethyl orange in 100 ml of water. The color change is orange to pink.

Indicator B. Triturate 100 ml of 4-(4-dimethylamino-1-naphthylazo)-3-methoxybenzenesulfonic acid with 2.6 ml of 0.10 *N* NaOH in a glass mortar, and dilute to 100 ml with water. The color change is yellow to pink.

Indicator C. Triturate 100 mg of bromcresol green with 1.5 ml of 0.10 *N* NaOH in a glass mortar, and dilute to 100 ml with water. Separately dissolve 100 mg of sodium alizarin sulfonate (alizarin red S) in 100 ml of water. Mix the two solutions. The color change is blue to yellow.

Indicator D. Dissolve 75 mg of bromcresol green and 50 mg of methyl red in 100 ml of alcohol. The color change is green to grey to pink; for the TRIS titration the end point should be taken as the first appearance of pink in the gray background.

Methyl Orange Indicator Solution. Dissolve 100 mg of methyl orange in 100 ml of water.

PROCEDURES

Analysis of Potassium Bicarbonate. First obtain experience with this titration by analyzing some pure $KHCO_3$. Accurately weigh 0.2–0.25 g of $KHCO_3$ into an Erlenmeyer flask, dissolve in about 30 ml of water, add 3 drops of methyl orange solution, and titrate with standard 0.1 *N* HCl until within 0.5–1.0 ml of the end point, as revealed by the transient color change. Boil the solution for 1–3 min, cool to room temperature by setting it in cold water, and then complete the titration, the end point being marked by the orange color. Carry out an indicator titration, including the boiling step. Calculate the purity of the sample of $KHCO_3$.

Obtain a sample of impure $KHCO_3$* from the instructor, weigh out samples corresponding to about 2 meq of $KHCO_3$, and titrate them as above. Calculate the w/w percentage of $KHCO_3$ in the sample.

* Prepared by dilution with NaCl and grinding to a fine powder in a mortar.

Analysis of Triethanolamine Solution. Give a dry stoppered flask to your instructor, who will provide you with an aqueous solution containing triethanolamine, $N(CH_2CH_2OH)_3$, in the approximate concentration range 2–6%. With a volumetric pipet, transfer about 2 meq of triethanolamine to an Erlenmeyer flask. (Try 5.0 or 10.0 ml portions initially.) Add water if needed to produce sufficient volume for good mixing, add 3 drops of methyl red solution (see Experiment 1.1), and titrate to the pink color with 0.1 *N* HCl. Calculate the solution concentration as w/v percent of triethanolamine.

Back-Titration of Ephedrine. Accurately weigh about 0.5 g of ephedrine, dissolve it in 10 ml of alcohol, add 40.00 ml of standard 0.1 *N* HCl and 3 drops of methyl red solution, and back-titrate the excess hydrochloric acid with standard 0.1 *N* NaOH. Calculate the percent purity of the sample as anhydrous ephedrine, MW 165.24.

A blank titration should be carried out and an appropriate correction applied if necessary. This calculation is described in Appendix A.

References

1. House, J. E., Jr., and R. C. Reiter, *J. Chem. Educ.*, **45,** 679 (1968).
2. Freiser, H., *J. Chem. Educ.*, **47,** 809 (1970).
3. Bates, R. G., and V. E. Bower, *Anal. Chem.*, **28,** 1322 (1956).
4. Good, N. E., G. D. Winget, W. Winter, T. N. Connolly, S. Izawa, and R. M. M. Singh, *Biochemistry*, **5,** 467 (1966).
5. Brown, H. C., D. H. McDaniel, and O. Häfliger, Chap. 14 in *Determination of Organic Structures by Physical Methods*, E. A. Braude and F. C. Nachod (eds.), Academic Press, New York, 1955.
6. Arnett, E. M., F. M. Jones, M. Taagepera, W. G. Henderson, J. L. Beauchamp, D. Holtz, and R. W. Taft, *J. Am. Chem. Soc.*, **94,** 4724 (1972).
7. Kolthoff, I. M., *Acid-Base Indicators*, Macmillan, New York, 1937.
8. Kolthoff, I. M., and V. A. Stenger, *Volumetric Analysis*, Vol. II, 2nd ed., Interscience, New York, 1947.
9. Fossum, J. H., P. C. Markunas, and J. A. Riddick, *Anal. Chem.*, **23,** 491 (1951).
10. Whitehead, T. H., *J. Chem. Educ.*, **36,** 297 (1959).
11. Belcher, R., *Submicro Methods of Organic Analysis*, Elsevier, Amsterdam, 1966.
12. Robinson, J. R., H. Stelmach, and S. P. Eriksen, *Anal. Chem.*, **42,** 495 (1970).
13. Butler, E. A., and E. H. Swift, *J. Chem. Educ.*, **49,** 425 (1972).

FOR FURTHER READING

Ricci, J. E., *Hydrogen Ion Concentration*, Princeton University Press, Princeton, N.J., 1952.

Bruckenstein, S., and I. M. Kolthoff, Chap. 12 in *Treatise on Analytical Chemistry*, Part I, Vol. I, I. M. Kolthoff and P. J. Elving (eds.), Interscience, New York, 1959.

Freiser, H., and Q. Fernando, *Ionic Equilibria in Analytical Chemistry*, John Wiley, New York, 1963.

Butler, J. N., *Ionic Equilibrium: A Mathematical Approach*, Addison-Wesley, Reading, Mass., 1964.

Parascandola, J., "L. J. Henderson and the Theory of Buffer Action," *Med. Histor. J.*, **6,** 297 (1971).

Bell, R. P., *The Proton in Chemistry*, Cornell University Press, Ithaca, New York, 1959.

Problems

1. Convert these values of hydrogen ion concentration to pH.
(*a*) $[H^+] = 4.5 \times 10^{-5}$ *N*
(*b*) $[H^+] = 1.00$ *N*
(*c*) $[H^+] = 3.6 \times 10^{-10}$ *N*
(*d*) $[H^+] = 0.88 \times 10^{-7}$ *N*
(*e*) $[H^+] = 0.00143$ *N*

2. Calculate the hydrogen ion concentration of solutions with these pH values.
(*a*) pH = 3.95
(*b*) pH = 6.85
(*c*) pH = 12.52
(*d*) pH = 8.00
(*e*) pH = 8.30

3. (*a*) The pK_a of codeine is 8.21. What is its K_b value?
(*b*) List the compounds in Table 1.6 in order of increasing strength.

4. Calculate the pH of each of these aqueous solutions at 25°C.
(*a*) 2.00×10^{-3} *M* HCl
(*b*) 1.00×10^{-3} *M* H_2SO_4
(*c*) 0.05 *M* ammonia
(*d*) 0.05 *M* ammonium chloride
(*e*) 5.0×10^{-2} *N* NaOH

5. A buffer solution was prepared by adding 50 ml of 0.10 *N* sodium hydroxide to 100 ml of 0.15 *M* acetic acid (pK_a 4.76). What was its pH?

6. A buffer solution was prepared by making 100 ml of a solution 0.05 *M* with respect to acetic acid and 0.10 *M* with respect to potassium acetate. 10.0 ml of 0.5 *N* HCl was then added. What was the change in pH upon the addition of the hydrochloric acid?

7. What is the molar concentration of pure water?

8. What is the pH of 10^{-8} *M* hydrochloric acid (protected from contamination by the air)?

9. The following data were obtained in the standardization of a sodium hydroxide solution. (MW = 204.2 for the primary standard.)

Sample	Weight of potassium biphthalate (g)	Volume of NaOH (ml)
1	1.2771	41.25
2	1.2005	38.84

Calculate the mean normality of the sodium hydroxide solution.

10. 0.7050 g of an acid was dissolved in water and titrated to the phenolphthalein end point with 30.05 ml of the sodium hydroxide solution from Problem 9. Calculate the equivalent weight of the acid.

11. A solution was prepared by dissolving 1.450 g of TRIS (pK_a 8.08, MW 121.1) in 50.0 ml of 0.060 *N* HCl and diluting to 100 ml with water. Calculate the pH.

12. A 1.3540 g sample of potassium biphthalate (MW 204.2) was titrated with 0.1063 *N* NaOH, a total of 48.50 ml being added. The end point was overrun with this volume, however, so the excess was back-titrated with 3.25 ml of 0.0965 *N* HCl.

(*a*) How many grams of potassium biphthalate did the sample contain?

(*b*) What was the percent purity of the sample?

13. Given these pK values: acetic acid, $pK_a = 4.76$; *n*-butylamine, $pK_b = 3.40$; water, $pK_w = 14.00$. Calculate numerical values for the equilibrium constants of these reactions.

(*a*) $CH_3COOH + OH^- \rightleftharpoons CH_3COO^- + H_2O$

(*b*) $CH_3COOH + C_4H_9NH_2 \rightleftharpoons C_4H_9NH_3{}^+ + CH_3COO^-$

14. (*a*) Calculate the pH of 0.100 *N* NaOH at 50°C.

(*b*) K_a is 1.65×10^{-4} for formic acid at 50°C. What is pK_b for formate ion at this temperature?

15. Calculate the pH of a solution prepared by dissolving 10.00 g of dihydrogen potassium phosphate (KH_2PO_4, MW 136.1) in 50.0 ml of 0.50 *N* NaOH and diluting to 500.0 ml.

16. Aspirin (acetylsalicylic acid, pK_a 3.50) is absorbed from the stomach in the conjugate acid form. A patient takes an antacid that brings the pH of his stomach contents to 3.00, and then takes two 5 grain aspirin tablets (0.65 g of aspirin). Calculate the amount of aspirin available for immediate absorption from the stomach.

17. Sorensen buffer solutions are prepared by mixing suitable volumes of the following stock solutions: Stock solution A: 9.21 g of $NaH_2PO_4 \cdot H_2O$ (MW 138.0) is dissolved in water to make 1 liter. Stock solution B: 9.47 g of Na_2HPO_4 (MW 142.0) is dissolved in water to make 1 liter.

(*a*) Calculate the molar concentrations of stock solutions A and B.

(*b*) Calculate the pH of a Sorensen's buffer prepared by mixing 30 ml of A and 70 ml of B. (The effective pK_2 of phosphoric acid may be taken as 6.80 in this solution.)

18. 25.00 ml of sulfuric acid solution reacted quantitatively with excess barium ion to yield a precipitate of $BaSO_4$ weighing 0.4650 g. Calculate the normality of the sulfuric acid solution.

19. Calculate the pH of a solution prepared by mixing equal volumes of 0.20 *M* HCl, 0.16 *M* NaOH, 0.20 *M* Na_2HPO_4, and 0.20 *M* NaH_2PO_4. Use $pK_2 = 6.80$ for phosphoric acid.

20. Calculate and plot the acid-base species distribution curves for these substances.

(*a*) *p*-Nitrophenol ($pK_a = 7.14$)

(*b*) Pyridine ($pK_a = 5.21$)

(*c*) Succinic acid ($pK_1 = 4.21$, $pK_2 = 5.64$)

(*d*) Citric acid ($pK_1 = 3.06$, $pK_2 = 4.74$, $pK_3 = 5.40$)

21. What is the concentration of oxalate dianion in a solution 0.10 *M* in total oxalic acid at pH 4.00? ($pK_1 = 1.19$, $pK_2 = 4.21$.)

22. Write the electroneutrality condition for each of these solutions.

(*a*) Salt of a weak base, BHX

(*b*) Dibasic acid, H_2A

(*c*) Solution of acetic acid partially titrated with potassium hydroxide

23. Consider the titration of a weak acid HA with strong base MOH. Let $b = [M^+]$ and $c = [HA] + [A^-]$. Then derive an *exact* equation relating $[H^+]$, K_a, K_w, b, and

c throughout the entire titration. Suggestion: start by writing the electroneutrality condition.

24. Let K_a° be the acid dissociation constant for benzoic acid, and K_a the constant for a substituted benzoic acid. Then the *Hammett substituent constant* σ is defined

$$\sigma = \log \frac{K_a}{K_a^\circ}$$

and σ is interpreted as a measure of the electron-donating or electron-attracting capacity of the substituent.

(*a*) Derive an equation for σ in terms of pK values.

(*b*) Calculate σ for these substituents: H; *p*-NO_2; *m*-NH_2 (data in Table 1.4).

(*c*) Is an electron-withdrawing substituent characterized by a plus or minus sigma value?

25. What is the approximate concentration of saturated sodium hydroxide solution? (See Experiment 1.1.)

2 NONAQUEOUS ACID-BASE TITRATIONS

2.1 Nonaqueous Acid-Base Chemistry

For many decades it has been known that phenomena analogous to acid-base reactions in water, such as indicator color changes and stoichiometric reactions of compounds clearly regarded as acids and bases, can be observed in nonaqueous solutions. For example, in 1912, Folin and Flanders [1] titrated acids in benzene, chloroform, and chloroform-ethanol mixtures. Perhaps because of the great theoretical and practical successes of the theory of aqueous acid-base chemistry, very little progress was made in the study of the nonaqueous systems. In 1927, Conant and Hall [2, 3] reported their important investigations of the behavior of bases in glacial acetic acid. Although these workers carried out many accurate titrations in this solvent, it was not until the 1940s and 1950s that extensive practical and theoretical studies on acid-base behavior in nonaqueous media were initiated.

Water, of course, recommends itself as a solvent for study because of its widespread occurrence in biological, geological, and man-made systems. Water is a most convenient solvent, for it can act as the second acid-base pair both for acids (in which case it functions as a base) and for bases (when it functions as an acid). The major limitation of water as a titration medium, however, is also due to this amphoteric behavior; recall that the acid-base equilibrium is a competition between two bases for a proton. In aqueous solution one of these bases is water. If the other base is relatively weak, it will not compete effectively with the solvent for the proton. In practical terms, it will not be titratable. In an aqueous solution of a weak acid the titration situation can be described as a competition of the solute acid and the solvent acid for the titrant base. Thus neither weakly acidic nor weakly basic substances can be titrated easily in aqueous solution because of the overwhelming effect of the solvent acting as a competing weak acid or base.

The simplest solution to this problem is to replace the solvent. If the solute is a weakly basic compound, successful titration is blocked by the basic character of the solvent water. If water is replaced by a relatively nonbasic solvent, this undesirable competition is effectively eliminated or at least reduced, and the solute base can now be titrated. A similar situation holds for weakly acidic solutes; in this case, the acidic nature of water renders it an undesirable solvent, and it should be supplanted by a solvent displaying essentially no acid properties.

Dissociating and Nondissociating Solvents. The physical and chemical properties of solvents are a reasonable subject for beginning a discussion of nonaqueous acid-base chemistry. Practical reasons often determine the usefulness of a solvent; thus the solvent should be a liquid at room temperature, and it should not be highly toxic if it is to be widely used in analysis. Of all the properties of a solvent that can affect its utility, three deserve special attention. These are its capability of self-dissociation, its acid-base character, and its dielectric constant.

Solvents may be classified as dissociating or nondissociating; in Chapter 1, for example, we noted that water dissociates according to the reaction

$$H_2O \rightleftharpoons H^+ + OH^-$$

Other pure solvents may dissociate similarly. Ethanol reacts to give the ethoxide ion,

$$EtOH \rightleftharpoons H^+ + OEt^-$$

and glacial acetic acid yields acetate (symbolized OAc^-).

$$HOAc \rightleftharpoons H^+ + OAc^-$$

In each of these equations the symbol H^+ represents the solvated proton; it is therefore a different species in each solvent.

Some solvents dissociate without the production of the solvated proton. Acetic anhydride is such a substance.

$$Ac_2O \rightleftharpoons Ac^+ + OAc^-$$

Ac^+, which is an abbreviation for CH_3CO^+, is called the acetylium ion.

Examples of nondissociating solvents are ethers and hydrocarbons. Actually even these substances may dissociate to a minute extent, but such dissociation is not usually detectable.

As we saw in the case of water, it is possible to define an ion product for a dissociating solvent. If we let the solvent be represented by AB, and the dissociation process by $AB \rightleftharpoons A^+ + B^-$, then the ion product K_s is given by

$$K_s = [A^+][B^-] \tag{2.1}$$

Table 2.1 gives pK_s values for a few important solvents.

The analytical significance of K_s may be developed by comparing water

TABLE 2.1
Ion Products of Some Solvents[a]

Solvent	pK_s
Water	14.00
Methanol	16.7
Ethanol	19.1
Acetic acid	14.45
Acetic anhydride	14.5
Acetonitrile	26.5

[a] At room temperature.

and ethanol. In water, in order to pass from an acidic solution in which pA (that is, pH) = 1 to a basic solution in which pB (pOH) = 1, an acidity range of 12 orders of magnitude must be traversed (since pA + pB = 14). In ethanol, however, to pass from pA = 1 to pB = 1 requires a traverse of 17.1 orders of magnitude. Thus in ethanol a greater range is available in which to titrate substances of varying strengths. The approximate but useful generalization may be given that the smaller is K_s of a solvent, the greater is the potential range available for titration.

Acid-Base Character. Acidity and basicity are relative qualities, requiring for their definition a standard of reference. The Bronsted acid-base theory provides a basis for making such comparisons for many substances. Some terms that are used in describing solvents will often be encountered in discussions of nonaqueous chemistry. *Protogenic* solvents yield a solvated proton upon dissociation. Examples are acetic acid and sulfuric acid. *Protophilic* solvents are those capable of accepting a proton; they may be either dissociating or nondissociating solvents. Acetic anhydride, ether, and pyridine are protophilic solvents. *Amphiprotic* solvents can either accept or donate a proton; water and the alcohols are examples. *Aprotic* solvents have essentially no tendency either to yield or to accept a proton. Chloroform and the hydrocarbons are examples.

Protogenic solvents are essentially acidic solvents having little basic character, whereas the opposite is true of protophilic substances. Amphiprotic solvents are both acidic and basic to significant extents; in the presence of strong acids such solvents would behave as bases, whereas strongly basic solutes would bring out their acidic character. Aprotic solvents have essentially no acid-base properties.

Dissociating solvents, and especially nonprotonic dissociating solvents, may be considered in terms of the solvent theory. A solvent AB dissociates to give the cation A^+ (called the lyonium ion) and the anion B^- (the lyate ion).

The lyonium ion is considered the species responsible for the acidic character of the solvent, and the lyate ion exhibits basic properties. The dissociation of these five solvents, with the proton solvation indicated explicitly, illustrates this point of view.

	Lyonium ion	Lyate ion
$2H_2O$	$\rightleftharpoons H_3O^+$	$+ OH^-$
$2MeOH$	$\rightleftharpoons MeOH_2^+$	$+ OMe^-$
$2HOAc$	$\rightleftharpoons H_2OAc^+$	$+ OAc^-$
$2NH_3$ (liq)	$\rightleftharpoons NH_4^+$	$+ NH_2^-$
Ac_2O	$\rightleftharpoons Ac^+$	$+ OAc^-$

Note that acetate ion in acetic acid performs the same role as hydroxide ion in water; that is, acetate ion is the strongest base capable of existence in acetic acid, just as hydroxide is the strongest base in water. A further conclusion to be drawn from this concept is that an acid is any substance that increases the concentration of lyonium ions when dissolved in a dissociating solvent, whereas a substance that increases the lyate ion concentration is a base. Ammonium chloride should therefore be a strong acid in liquid ammonia. Alkali acetates are strong bases in acetic acid, and so are amines, which increase the acetate concentration by reaction with the solvent.

$$RNH_2 + HOAc \rightleftharpoons RNH_3^+ + OAc^-$$

The Dielectric Constant. If we assume that a solvent is a homogeneous medium and that ions are point charges, the force of attraction between two univalent ions of unlike charge is given by Coulomb's law

$$F = \frac{-e^2}{Dr^2}$$

where e is the electronic charge, D is the dielectric constant of the medium,* and r is the distance between the ions. The work of separating the ions is found by integrating the force over the distance, giving $W = e^2/Dr$. Although this is a very simplified picture of the dissociation process, it leads to the approximately valid generalization that the ease of dissociation of two oppositely charged ions will be greater with an increase in size of the dielectric constant of the solvent. This observation will be pursued later.

Table 2.2 lists the dielectric constants of some common solvents.

The Leveling and Differentiating Effects. The acidic or basic character of a solvent is of critical importance when the solvent is to provide an environment

* The dielectric constant of a solvent is the ratio of the (electrical) capacity of a condenser filled with the solvent to the capacity of the empty condenser. D is therefore a dimensionless number greater than unity.

TABLE 2.2
Dielectric Constants of Some Solvents[a]

Solvent	*D*	Solvent	*D*
Cyclohexane	2.02	Acetone	20.7
Dioxane	2.21	Ethanol	24.3
Benzene	2.27	Methanol	32.6
Ethyl ether	4.34	Acetonitrile	37.5
Chloroform	4.81	Dimethyl sulfoxide	46.7
Acetic acid	6.15	Water	78.5
t-Butyl alcohol	11.5	Sulfuric acid	100

[a] At room temperature.

for a solute that is acidic or basic. The solute will react with the solvent to a degree determined by the relative strengths of the two. There are two possibilities.

1. Essentially the solute reacts completely with the solvent. Suppose the strongly acidic solute HX is dissolved in the basic solvent S. If the reaction

$$HX + S \rightleftharpoons SH^+ + X^-$$

goes to completion—that is, essentially all HX is transformed into SH^+—the solvent is said to be a *leveling solvent* for HX. Evidently it is impossible to compare the strengths of two acids HX and HY in a leveling solvent for these acids, for they will appear to be identical in strength. In fact, these acids will be leveled to the strength of the lyonium ions, which is equivalent to saying that the lyonium ion is the strongest acid that can exist in the solvent. A similar statement can be made about the lyate ion as the strongest possible base. It is in this manner that the mineral acids appear to be of identical strength in water; although they are actually of quite different strengths, they are all strong enough to convert water quantitatively to the hydronium ion. Glacial acetic acid, being fairly acidic, should be a leveling solvent for many bases, and it is observed that all bases that are (in water) stronger than aniline are leveled by acetic acid; they are thus transformed into the strongest possible base in this solvent, which is acetate ion.

2. The other possibility is that the solute does not react completely with the solvent. If the acid HA is dissolved in solvent S, this reaction occurs:

$$HA + S \rightleftharpoons SH^+ + A^-$$

If the reaction does not go completely to the right, the solvent S is called a *differentiating solvent* for HA. The value of such a system will be appreciated by considering a second acid HB for which S is also a differentiating solvent.

The extents of reaction between HA and the solvent and between HB and the solvent are characterized by the constants K_{HA} and K_{HB}. Since the solvent is the same in the two cases, these constants may be taken as indications of the strengths of the acids HA and HB relative to the reference base S. This is precisely the procedure adopted in measuring acid strengths in water, where $S \equiv H_2O$, and the constants are the conventional acid dissociation constants.

Ionization and Dissociation. Ionization is the process of ion production, and dissociation is the separation of species. The general equation representing these processes in the present context is

$$AB \xrightleftharpoons{\text{Ionization}} A^+B^- \xrightleftharpoons{\text{Dissociation}} A^+ + B^- \tag{2.2}$$

The species A^+B^- is called an *ion pair*.

The extent of ionic dissociation is controlled largely by the dielectric properties of the medium. This is why it is not necessary to distinguish between ionization and dissociation of the ions with water, which has an unusually high dielectric constant. As soon as an ion pair is formed in such a solvent, the ions separate. In solvents of low or intermediate dielectric constant, however, the extent of dissociation may be very small and ion pairs may be detectable. The magnitude of this ionic association effect is remarkable; salts that are strong electrolytes (that is, completely dissociated) in water have been shown to have dissociation constants in the range 10^{-7} to 10^{-4} in solvents whose dielectric constants are 6–11.

Because of its importance in titrimetry, glacial acetic acid has been studied carefully as a solvent for acids, bases, and salts [4, 5]. The behavior of solutes in acetic acid may be treated as follows. An acid reacts according to

$$HX + HOAc \rightleftharpoons H_2OAc^+X^- \rightleftharpoons H_2OAc^+ + X^-$$

This is conventionally written without the solvent indicated.

$$HX \rightleftharpoons H^+X^- \rightleftharpoons H^+ + X^- \tag{2.3}$$

These equations should be compared with Eq. 2.2. Ionization constant K_i^{HX} and dissociation constant K_d^{HX} are defined.

$$K_i^{\mathrm{HX}} = \frac{[H^+X^-]}{[HX]} \tag{2.4}$$

$$K_d^{\mathrm{HX}} = \frac{[H^+][X^-]}{[H^+X^-]} \tag{2.5}$$

An overall dissociation constant K_{HX} is given by

$$K_{\mathrm{HX}} = \frac{[H^+][X^-]}{c_{\mathrm{HX}}} \tag{2.6}$$

where $c_{\mathrm{HX}} = [\mathrm{HX}] + [\mathrm{H^+X^-}]$. Combining these gives

$$K_{\mathrm{HX}} = \frac{K_i^{\mathrm{HX}} K_d^{\mathrm{HX}}}{1 + K_i^{\mathrm{HX}}} \tag{2.7}$$

A quantitative theory of acid-base equilibria in acetic acid, based upon these definitions, leads to several important conclusions. For example, it is found that the common practice of estimating pK values from the point of half-neutralization on a titration curve is unsound in acetic acid. Another marked difference between acid-base chemistry in acetic acid and in water is found in the study of indicator behavior. In water, indicator color change is governed by pH, or $-\log [\mathrm{H^+}]$; in acetic acid, however, the free acid concentration c_{HX} is the controlling factor. It is also observed [6] that the sharpness of indicator color changes is not markedly reduced by dilution, so dilute solutions of acids and bases can be titrated.

Similar findings may be expected in other solvents of low dielectric constant. These significant differences between aqueous and nonaqueous solution chemistry are in large part ascribable to the great difference in dielectric constants and therefore in dissociating power.

Measurement of Acid-Base Strength. The quantitative evaluation of acid-base strength of a substance usually involves the determination of the equilibrium constant of its reaction with a reference acid or base. The reference substance may be the solvent, or another substance may be added to the solution to act as the reference acid or base. The nature of the solvent and the kind of information sought will determine which of these approaches is used.

If the solvent is sufficiently acidic or basic to provide a suitable reference reactant for the substances being investigated, and moreover is characterized by a moderate to high dielectric constant, the first method often is employed. The equilibrium constant of the reaction between the solvent and the solute is then taken as a measure of acid-base strength. The determination of acid-base strength in water is an example.

Studies on a low dielectric constant solvent that is itself the reference substance yield data that are more difficult to interpret. Acetic acid is the classic example of this type. As pointed out earlier, the extent of reaction with the solvent may be measured in terms of the ionization constant K_i, the dissociation constant K_d, or the overall dissociation constant. K_d is influenced primarily by the dielectric character of the medium, and is least directly indicative of acid-base strength. K_i gives probably the best estimate, of these three quantities, of acid-base strength. However, the most accessible constant is the overall dissociation constant, and so this constant is often taken as a measure of strength in acetic acid. Table 2.3 gives overall dissociation constants for some acids and bases in acetic acid [7]. Notice that even perchloric acid, the strongest of the common mineral acids, is dissociated to only

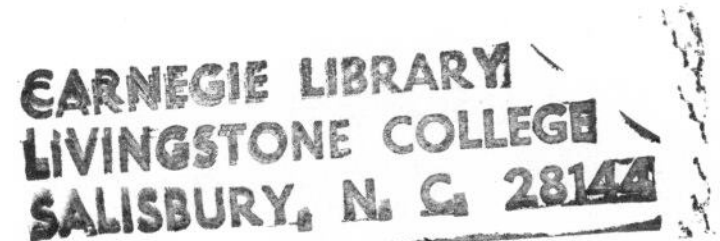

TABLE 2.3
Overall Dissociation Constants for Some Acids and Bases in Acetic Acid [7]

Acid	pK_{HX}	Base	pK_B
Perchloric acid	4.87	Tribenzylamine	5.36
Sulfuric acid	7.24	Diethylaniline	5.78
p-Toluenesulfonic acid	8.46	Potassium acetate	6.10
		Sodium acetate	6.58
		Lithium acetate	6.79
		2,5-Dichloroaniline	9.48
		Urea	10.24

a minute extent in glacial acetic acid. The alkali acetates, which behave titrimetrically as strong bases in this solvent, are nevertheless only slightly dissociated.

By adding a reference acid or base to the system, a wider range of acid-base strengths may be studied than is normally accessible when the solvent functions as the reference. When inert solvents are employed as media for acid-base studies, the addition of a reference substance is necessary because the solvent cannot perform the role of reference. An indicator is a very convenient reference acid or base. If it is desired to study the relative strengths of a series of weak bases, one procedure would be to react each of the bases with the same indicator acid HI, and to determine the extent of reaction.

$$HI + B \rightleftharpoons BHI$$

The equilibrium constant is called the salt formation constant, or association constant.

Perhaps the most general method for measuring acid-base strength involves a reference acid or base selected not for its indicator properties but for its other advantages, in particular its strength. Thus perchloric acid is the best reference acid for the study of weakly basic compounds in acetic acid.

$$B + HClO_4 \rightleftharpoons BH^+ClO_4^-$$

$$K_f^{BHClO_4} = \frac{[BH^+ClO_4^-]}{[B][HClO_4]} \tag{2.8}$$

The perchlorate formation constant then serves as a measure of relative basicity as determined against the reference acid $HClO_4$. Table 2.4 gives values of $K_f^{BHClO_4}$ for some weak bases and indicator bases in acetic acid [8].

The relative acid-base strengths of a series of compounds may depend

TABLE 2.4
Perchlorate Formation Constants for Some Weak Bases in Acetic Acid at 25°C

Base	$\log K_f^{BHClO_4}$
Salicylamide	2.68
Benzamide	2.86
Acetanilid	2.96
Acetophenetidin	3.51
Acetamide	4.04
Urea	4.93
Thiourea	5.18
Caffeine	5.38
Indicators	
Sudan III	2.96
Nile Blue A	4.59
p-Naphtholbenzein	5.04
Malachite green	5.26

upon the particular measure of acidity or basicity and upon the solvent. This means that interpretations of acid-base strength (including aqueous pK_a values) in terms of molecular structure may be ambiguous.

2.2 Determination of Bases

Solvents, Titrants, and Indicators. All the solvents used as media for the titration of weak bases are neutral or acidic, for the reasons presented in Section 2.1. Although almost any such solvent could be used, in practice only a few find wide application.

Glacial acetic acid is the most used solvent for the titration of bases. It is commercially available in reagent grade, which is suitable for use without purification in most applications. Acetic anhydride is used in the analysis of very weak bases, such as amides, that are not easily acylated; the reagent grade product may be used directly. Dioxane is often used as a solvent, sometimes in mixture with acetic acid. Solutions of perchloric acid in technical grade dioxane discolor quickly, so dioxane is often purified before use by treatment with asbestos [9] or an ion-exchange resin [10, 11]. Acetonitrile can be similarly purified [10].

Benzene, chloroform, and similar solvents are available in grades sufficiently pure to use directly. This is also true of alcohols and glycols, which are employed in mixtures called G-H (glycol-hydrocarbon) solvents [12]. Such solvent mixtures may consist of 1 : 1 solutions of propylene glycol and chloroform, ethylene glycol and *n*-butanol, etc. These solvents are used for the titration of difficultly soluble substances, the hydroxy component usually being a good solvent. Incorporation of an aprotic solvent appears to sharpen the indicator end point. A phenol-chloroform-acetonitrile solvent has been recommended [13].

In aqueous titrimetry the selection of one of the mineral acids as a titrant acid is usually a matter of indifference, since they are leveled by water to the same acid strength. Acetic acid, however, is a differentiating solvent for these acids. Therefore, it is desirable to select the strongest of the acids as the titrant, and of the common mineral acids perchloric is found to be the strongest. This acid, dissolved in acetic acid, is the most frequently used titrant for the determination of weak bases. Since perchloric acid is commercially available as a concentrated aqueous solution, and the removal of the weak base water is desirable to increase the sensitivity of titration, a calculated amount of acetic anhydride is customarily added for this purpose. (An excess of anhydride must be avoided because acylable samples such as amines might be converted in its presence to much less basic compounds.)*

Other useful acid titrants are *p*-toluenesulfonic acid and fluorosulfonic acid, HSO_3F [14].

The standardization of acid titrants may be carried out against any substance that is a strong base and is available in a known state of purity. Potassium biphthalate is most commonly used, its titration reaction with perchloric acid being

$$C_6H_4(COOK)(COOH) + HClO_4 \rightleftharpoons C_6H_4(COOH)(COOH) + KClO_4$$

During the titration a crystalline precipitate of $KClO_4$ appears, but this does not interfere with location of the end point. The sulfonic acid titrants do not form such precipitates. Among the other primary standards that have been used for acid titrants are tris(hydroxymethyl)aminomethane, sodium carbonate, and diphenylguanidine.

One disadvantage associated with volumetric analysis employing nonaqueous solutions follows from the large coefficient of cubical expansion of most organic liquids. This means that the normality of a nonaqueous titrant solution will vary more widely with changes in temperature than will the concentration of an aqueous solution. The coefficient of cubical expansion for acetic acid is 1.07×10^{-3} deg^{-1} at 20°C (that for water is 0.21×10^{-3}

* The acetous $HClO_4$ solution should be used as the titrant even when acetic anhydride is the titration solvent; a perchloric acid–acetic anhydride titrant is not stable, probably because of a reaction between acetyl perchlorate and acetic anhydride.

deg^{-1}). Therefore the normality of a standard solution of perchloric acid in glacial acetic acid may be considered to change by 0.1%/deg (Celsius) change in temperature. This is a significant alteration. The solution temperature should be recorded at the time of standardization, and whenever the standard solution is employed thereafter, the appropriate correction (that is, +0.0001 *N* for a 1 deg fall in temperature and −0.0001 *N* for a 1 deg rise, these corrections calculated for a 0.1 *N* solution) should be applied.

Detection of the end point usually is accomplished with indicators or potentiometrically. The basis for the latter method is discussed in Chapter 6. Indicators useful for the titration of bases are themselves very weak bases. It is possible to arrange a series of indicators in order of their basicity as measured by their perchlorate formation constants, as in Table 2.4.

Indicator selection is usually empirical. Stock and Purdy have summarized much of this experience [15]. The most popular indicator for the titration of bases is *crystal violet* (gentian violet). The closely related *methyl violet* behaves similarly. The color change is complex, ranging through violet (base color), blue, blue-green, green, yellow-green, and yellow (acid color). The color change corresponding to the end point will depend upon the particular base and solvent, and should be determined by simultaneous potentiometric and indicator titration. For many bases the violet to blue color change marks the end point.

p-Naphtholbenzein (also called α-naphtholbenzein) is one of the most satisfactory indicators for titrations in glacial acetic acid. The color change is from yellow in the base form to green in the acid form; the color change is sharp for bases leveled by acetic acid. Another good indicator is *quinaldine red*, a much stronger indicator base than *p*-naphtholbenzein; the color change is from pink (base form) to colorless in acid solution. *Malachite green* is a slightly stronger base than is *p*-naphtholbenzein and is similarly useful; the color change is from green to yellow.

Applications. Many hundreds of papers have been published describing applications of nonaqueous acid-base titrations. This literature has been surveyed in books [16–18], and in biennial reviews published in *Analytical Chemistry*. The technique finds wide use in pharmaceutical analysis; many such titrations appear in the USP and NF.

The practical effect of a change in solvent on titration behavior is shown in Fig. 2.1 for the potentiometric titration of the weak base antipyrine in water (which provides no end point break) and in acetic acid. (The pK_a of antipyrine in water is about 1.5.) Figure 2.2 shows titration curves for caffeine, a very weak base, in acetic acid and in acetic anhydride; the inflection point is hardly detectable in acetic acid, but is pronounced in acetic anhydride.

Bases whose pK_a values in water are larger than 4 are leveled by glacial acetic acid, and can be titrated with visual detection of the end point. Bases

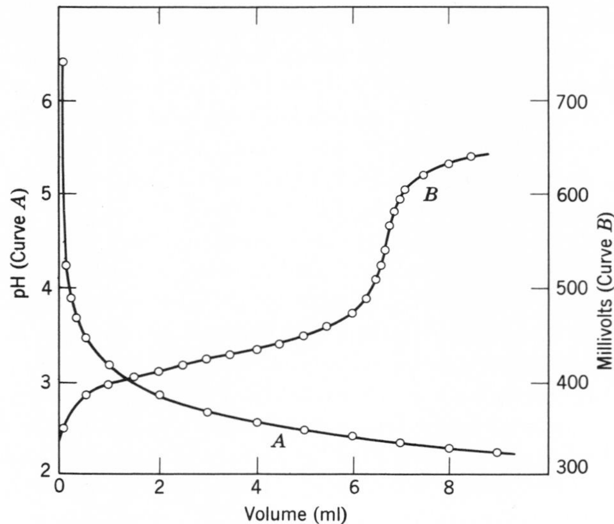

Fig. 2.1. Potentiometric titration of identical samples of antipyrine. Curve *A*, titration in water with 0.1 *N* hydrochloric acid; curve *B*, titration in glacial acetic acid with 0.1 *N* acetous perchloric acid.

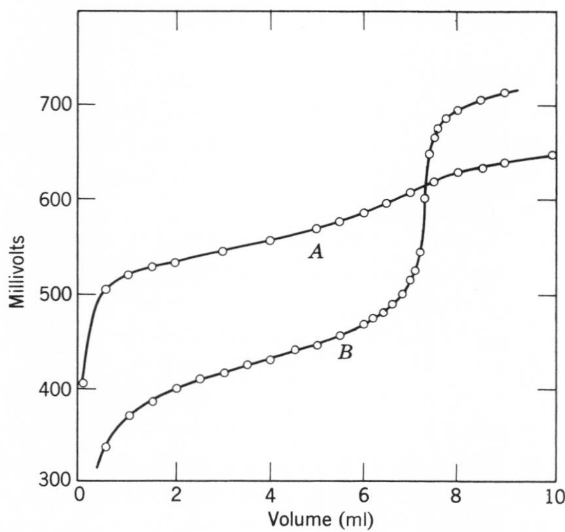

Fig. 2.2. Potentiometric titration of identical samples of caffeine with 0.1 *N* acetous perchloric acid. Curve *A*, titration in glacial acetic acid; curve *B*, titration in acetic anhydride.

whose aqueous pK_a values fall in the approximate range 1–4 cannot be titrated accurately with visual detection of the end point, but may be analyzed by potentiometric titration (see Fig. 2.1). Even weaker bases, such as amides, give good end point breaks in acetic anhydride (Fig. 2.2). Most amines are titratable in acetic acid, and many alkaloids can be determined in this way. Salts of weak acids can be titrated in acetic acid. This is a valuable method for the alkali salts of weak acids; in fact, the standardization of perchloric acid by titration against potassium biphthalate is such a reaction.

Mixtures of bases of different strengths sometimes can be analyzed by selecting a differentiating solvent for the bases. For this purpose the less acidic solvents, such as acetonitrile, are most valuable. Potentiometric titration is the usual form of end point detection.

One of the interesting applications of these methods is in the determination of substances that are not themselves particularly basic, usually by conversion to a basic derivative. The most useful of such procedures, introduced by Pifer and Wollish [19], permits the titration of hydrohalide salts of amines. The amine salt, dissolved in acetic acid, is treated with an excess of mercuric acetate. The amine is freed and can be titrated as a base with perchloric acid.

$$2RNH_3 + Hg(OAc)_2 \rightarrow HgCl_2 + 2RNH_2 + 2HOAc$$

The mercuric chloride and excess mercuric acetate are nonbasic. Quaternary ammonium halides can also be determined with this procedure.

2.3 Determination of Acids

Solvents, Titrants, and Indicators. All the solvents used for the titration of acids are themselves essentially nonacidic. The very basic solvents enhance the acidic character of very weak acids, and neutral solvents are suitable for the differentiating titration of mixtures.

Ethylenediamine, *n*-butylamine, and pyridine are useful basic solvents. Since they readily absorb atmospheric CO_2, they are apt to give high blank titration values. *N,N*-dimethylformamide (DMF) is used extensively. Traces of water in DMF may cause hydrolysis to formic acid, which would be titrated. Commercial DMF is used directly. Other solvents finding wide use are benzene, methanol, ethanol, acetone, methyl ethyl ketone, methyl isobutyl ketone, and *t*-butyl alcohol.

The methoxides of potassium, sodium, or lithium, in methanol-benzene solution, are suitable titrants for the determination of weak acids. They are prepared by dissolving the metal in methanol. Sodium and potassium methoxides lead to the formation of gelatinous precipitates during the course of many titrations, and such gels can obscure visual end points. Lithium methoxide does not form these gels.

Gel formation has also been overcome with the introduction of tetralkylammonium hydroxide titrants [20, 21]. Tetrabutylammonium hydroxide is most frequently used; it can be prepared by reacting tetrabutylammonium iodide with silver oxide. Solutions of tetraalkylammonium hydroxides are commercially available. All basic titrants should be stored in Pyrex or polyethylene containers, and exposure to atmospheric CO_2 should be minimized.

Benzoic acid is the usual primary standard substance. Titrations can be carried out under a nitrogen stream to minimize absorption of CO_2. Blank titrations are essential to correct for titratable impurities in the solvent.

The most important visual indicator for acid determinations is *thymol blue* (thymolsulfonphthalein). The color change is from yellow in the acid form to blue in the base form. It is useful in titrations of carboxylic acids, imides, sulfonamides, etc. *Azo violet* (*p*-nitrobenzeneazoresorcinol) is a weaker indicator acid, so it is effective for the titration of fairly weak acids such as phenols substituted with electron-withdrawing substituents. The color change is from red to blue. For yet weaker acids *o-nitroaniline* can be used, though potentiometric titration is preferable. *Phenolphthalein* and *thymolphthalein* are excellent indicators for titrations in alcohols and in pyridine.

Applications. Acids whose pK_a values in water are not greater than about 7 can be titrated with visual end point detection, using thymol blue, in DMF. Acids in the aqueous pK_a range 7–11 require potentiometric end point detection or, somewhat less precisely, visual detection with azo violet or *o*-nitroaniline. Very generally, carboxylic acids fall into the stronger category and phenols in the weaker class.

It was pointed out in Chapter 1 that acylation of an amine reduces its basicity markedly by electron withdrawal, so that amides are very weak bases. If a second acyl group is introduced, giving an *imide*, the electron density is reduced to a level such that a proton bonded to the nitrogen becomes detectably acidic. Equations 2.9–2.11 show the structural relationships of these compounds and approximate pK_a values. The slashes through reaction arrows indicate equilibria that do not take place to a significant extent in these titrimetric systems.

$$\text{Amine}\quad RNH_3^+ \underset{}{\overset{pK_a\ 8-11}{\rightleftharpoons}} RNH_2 \not\rightleftharpoons RNH^- \tag{2.9}$$

$$\text{Amide}\quad R\overset{O}{\overset{\|}{C}}NH_3^+ \overset{pK_a\ -1\text{ to }1}{\rightleftharpoons} R\overset{O}{\overset{\|}{C}}NH_2 \not\rightleftharpoons R\overset{O}{\overset{\|}{C}}NH^- \tag{2.10}$$

$$\text{Imide}\quad R\overset{O}{\overset{\|}{C}}\underset{+}{N}H_2\overset{O}{\overset{\|}{C}}R \not\rightleftharpoons R\overset{O}{\overset{\|}{C}}NH\overset{O}{\overset{\|}{C}}R \overset{pK_a\ 6-9}{\rightleftharpoons} R\overset{O}{\overset{\|}{C}}-\overset{-}{N}-\overset{O}{\overset{\|}{C}}R \tag{2.11}$$

That is, amines are moderately strong bases (in the sense of this chapter), amides are very weak bases, but imides are moderately strong acids. This is of interest because the imide structure appears in some important drug molecules. Among these are the hydantoins (**1**) and the 5,5-disubstituted barbituric

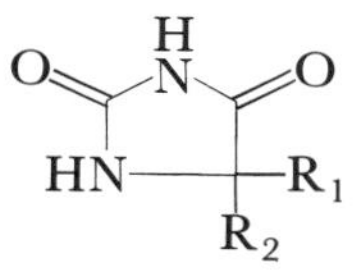

1

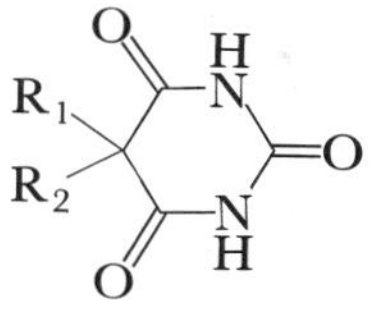

2

acid derivatives, **2**. The barbiturates are cyclic diimides, with aqueous pK_1 values about 8 and pK_2 about 12. Sulfonamides, which have the general structure **3**, are acidic because of the electron-withdrawing ability of the $—SO_2—$ function. Imides and sulfonamides can be titrated in nonaqueous media.

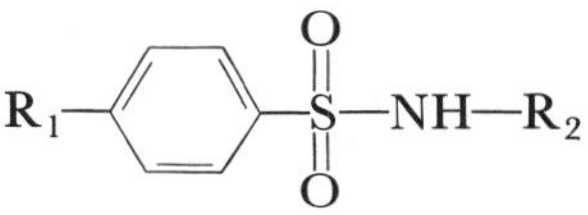

3

Often drugs can be titrated in their dosage forms, without interference from pharmaceutical adjuncts like diluents, binders, and lubricants [22]. Sometimes such components interfere; for example, stearic acid in a tablet formulation will consume base in a direct titration, and this substance must be removed before an acidic active ingredient is titrated.

Experiment 2.1. Nonaqueous Titration of Bases

APPARATUS AND REAGENTS

0.1 N Perchloric Acid. Pipet 11.0 ml of 60% perchloric acid into a 1000 ml volumetric flask containing several hundred milliliters of glacial acetic acid. Add 36.0 ml of reagent grade acetic anhydride, mix, and dilute to volume with acetic acid. Bring the solution to room temperature before its standardization.

If 72% perchloric acid is available, the solution is prepared with 8.5 ml of 72% perchloric acid and 21.0 ml of acetic anhydride.

To standardize the solution, accurately weigh about 2 meq of dried primary standard potassium biphthalate into a dry Erlenmeyer flask and dissolve it, with mild heating, in 50 ml of glacial acetic acid. Cool to room temperature; add 6 drops of either *p*-naphtholbenzein or quinaldine red indicator solution, and titrate to the end point with the perchloric acid solution, using a 25 ml buret. Record the titrant temperature. Perform at least three such titrations, plus a blank titration, and calculate the mean normality and its standard deviation.

An excellent indicator for this titration is provided by using 1 drop of the *p*-naphtholbenzein and 6 drops of the quinaldine red solution; the color change is from pink to green.

p-Naphtholbenzein Indicator Solution. Dissolve 0.2 g of *p*-naphtholbenzein (α-naphtholbenzein) in 100 ml of acetic acid.

Quinaldine Red Indicator Solution. Prepare a saturated solution of quinaldine red in acetic acid.

Crystal Violet Indicator Solution. Dissolve 0.1 g of crystal violet (gentian violet) in 100 ml of acetic acid.

Mercuric Acetate Solution. Dissolve 3.2 g of mercuric acetate in enough glacial acetic acid to make 100 ml. This solution is 0.1 *M* (0.2 *N*).

pH Meter. Any commercial pH meter is satisfactory. A glass electrode is the indicator electrode; this should be stored in acetic acid. The reference electrode is a saturated calomel electrode, modified by replacing the aqueous potassium chloride in the salt bridge with a 0.1 *M* lithium perchlorate solution in glacial acetic acid. This will reduce electromotive force fluctuations caused by mixing of the titration solution and the salt bridge solution during the course of the titration. (See Chapter 6 for a treatment of potentiometric titrations.)

PROCEDURES

Equivalent Weight of a Base. Obtain a sample of a pure unknown base from your instructor. Accurately weigh about 2 meq into a dry Erlenmeyer flask and dissolve it in 40 ml of glacial acetic acid. Add 6 drops of *p*-naphtholbenzein solution and titrate with standard 0.1 *N* acetous perchloric acid. Carry out several titrations. Calculate the equivalent weight of your sample base. From a list of bases provided by your instructor, and including your sample, make a tentative identification of your compound. (Among the bases that are suitable are TRIS, sodium acetate, potassium acetate, glycine, chlorpheniramine maleate, nicotinamide, nikethamide, etc.)

Equivalent Weight of an Amine Hydrochloride. Obtain a sample of a pure unknown amine hydrochloride from your instructor. Accurately weigh about 2 meq and dissolve it, with mild heating if necessary, in 25 ml of glacial acetic acid plus 15 ml of 0.1 *M* mercuric acetate solution. Add 6 drops of *p*-naphtholbenzein solution and titrate with standard 0.1 *N* perchloric acid. Make several titrations, calculate the mean equivalent weight of your sample, and from a list of possible compounds (e.g., ammonium chloride, ephedrine hydrochloride, pyridoxine hydrochloride, tripellenamine hydrochloride, phenylpropanolamine hydrochloride) make a tentative identification of your compound.

Indicator Selection by Potentiometric Titration. Accurately weigh about 2 meq of pure anhydrous sodium acetate, transfer to a 250 ml beaker, and dissolve in 50 ml of glacial acetic acid. Add 2 drops of crystal violet solution. Immerse the glass and calomel electrodes in the solution and connect them to the pH meter. Titrate the solution with 0.1 *N* perchloric acid, adding the titrant in 1 ml increments until close to the end point; within 1–2 ml of the end point add the titrant in 0.1 ml increments. After each addition of titrant, mix the solution by swirling the flask, measure the electromotive force (emf) in millivolts, and record the indicator hue and intensity. Make a plot of emf (vertical axis) against volume of titrant, and draw a smooth curve through the experimental points. Indicate the observed indicator colors at the appropriate points on this titration curve. Select the color corresponding to the end point in this titration.

This experiment can be repeated with other bases and other indicators.

Experiment 2.2. Nonaqueous Titration of Acids

REAGENTS

0.1 N Alkali Methoxide. Rinse 2.3–2.6 g of freshly cut sodium or 0.7–1.0 g of lithium in absolute methanol. Add the metal to a mixture of 40 ml of absolute methanol and 50 ml of benzene. The reaction can be controlled by cooling the reaction flask in ice. When dissolution is complete, add methanol until the solution is homogeneous. Then add benzene until the solution is cloudy. Continue this alternate addition of methanol and benzene until the volume is 1 liter; the object is to form a clear solution while keeping the methanol content to a minimum. Store the solution in a Pyrex or polyethylene bottle and protect it from atmospheric carbon dioxide as much as possible.

Standardize the solution against benzoic acid. Accurately weigh 200–300 mg of benzoic acid into an Erlenmeyer flask. Add 25 ml of *N*,*N*-dimethylformamide (DMF) and 2 drops of thymol blue solution. Direct a stream of nitrogen into the flask. Titrate with the alkali methoxide solution to the blue color. Carry out a blank titration with the same volume of DMF and indicator. Subtract the blank titration volume from the sample titration volume, and calculate the normality of the alkali methoxide solution. It is advisable to make several titrations of both samples and blanks. Record the titrant temperature.

0.1 N Tetrabutylammonium Hydroxide. Tetrabutylammonium hydroxide is commercially available as a 25% solution in methanol. Dilute 60 ml of this solution to 500 ml with benzene. Standardize as described above for alkali methoxide.

Thymol Blue Indicator Solution. Dissolve 0.3 g of thymol blue in 100 ml of absolute methanol.

Azo Violet Indicator Solution. Prepare a saturated solution of *p*-nitrobenzeneazoresorcinol in benzene.

PROCEDURES

Equivalent Weight of an Acid. Obtain a sample of a pure unknown acid from your instructor. Accurately weigh about 2 meq into a dry Erlenmeyer flask, dissolve it in 25 ml of DMF, and add 2 drops of thymol blue solution. Pass a stream of nitrogen into the flask, and titrate with standard 0.1 *N* alkali methoxide or tetrabutylammonium hydroxide. Perform a blank titration, and calculate the equivalent weight of the sample acid. If the end point color change is not sharp with thymol blue, repeat the titration using azo violet as the indicator. From a list of possible substances provided by your instructor, make a tentative identification of your compound. Among the samples suitable for this titration are nicotinic acid, cinchophen, aspirin, salicylic acid, theophylline, salicylamide, and barbituric acid derivatives.

Analysis of Sulfathiazole Tablets. Obtain a sample of sulfathiazole tablets from your instructor. Accurately weigh 20 tablets and grind them to a fine powder in a mortar. Accurately weigh a portion of the powder equivalent to 1–2 meq of sulfathiazole, add 25 ml of DMF, and stir well to dissolve the drug; the tablet excipients may not dissolve. Add 2 drops of thymol blue solution and titrate with standard 0.1 *N* alkali methoxide or tetrabutylammonium hydroxide, playing a stream of nitrogen over the surface of the sample solution during the titration. Perform a blank titration. Make at least three determinations. Calculate the average weight of sulfathiazole per tablet.

References

1. Folin, O., and F. F. Flanders, *J. Am. Chem. Soc.*, **34,** 774 (1912).
2. Hall, N. F., and J. B. Conant, *J. Am. Chem. Soc.*, **49,** 3047 (1927).
3. Conant, J. B., and N. F. Hall, *J. Am. Chem. Soc.*, **49,** 3062 (1927).
4. Kolthoff, I. M., and S. Bruckenstein, Chap. 13 in *Treatise on Analytical Chemistry*, Part I, Vol. I, I. M. Kolthoff and P. J. Elving (eds.), Interscience, New York, 1959.
5. Bruckenstein, S., and I. M. Kolthoff, Chap. XIII in *Pharmaceutical Analysis*, T. Higuchi and E. Brochmann-Hanssen (eds.), Interscience, New York, 1961.
6. Higuchi, T., J. A. Feldman, and C. R. Rehm, *Anal. Chem.*, **28,** 1120 (1956).
7. Bruckenstein, S., and I. M. Kolthoff, *J. Am. Chem. Soc.*, **78,** 2974 (1956).
8. Higuchi, T., and K. A. Connors, *J. Phys. Chem.*, **64,** 179 (1960).
9. Sideri, C. N., and A. Osol, *J. Am. Pharm. Assoc.*, **42,** 586 (1953).
10. Levi, L., L. G. Chatten, and M. Pernarowski, *J. Am. Pharm. Assoc.*, **44,** 61 (1955).
11. Pifer, C. W., E. G. Wollish, and M. Schmall, *J. Am. Pharm. Assoc.*, **42,** 509 (1953).
12. Palit, S. R., *Ind. Eng. Chem. Anal. Ed.*, **18,** 246 (1946).
13. Chatten, L. G., *J. Pharm. Pharmacol.*, **7,** 586 (1955).
14. Paul, R. C., S. K. Vasisht, K. C. Malhotra, and S. S. Pahil, *Anal. Chem.*, **34,** 820 (1962).
15. Stock, J. T. and W. C. Purdy, *Chemist-Analyst*, **48,** 22, 50 (1959); **50,** 88 (1961).
16. Kucharsky, J. and L. Safarik, *Titrations in Nonaqueous Solvents*, Elsevier, Amsterdam, 1965.
17. Gyenes, I., *Titration in Nonaqueous Media*, D. Van Nostrand, Princeton, N.J., 1967.
18. Huber, W., *Titrations in Nonaqueous Solvents*, Academic Press, New York, 1967.
19. Pifer, C. W. and E. G. Wollish, *Anal. Chem.*, **24,** 300 (1952).

20. Harlow, G. A., C. M. Noble, and G. E. A. Wyld, *Anal. Chem.*, **28,** 787 (1956).
21. Cundiff, R. H., and P. C. Markunas, *Anal. Chem.*, **28,** 792 (1956).
22. Chatten, L. G. and C. A. Mainville, *J. Pharm. Sci.*, **52,** 146 (1963).

Problems

1. A perchloric acid solution is prepared by adding 17.0 ml of 72% (w/w) perchloric acid to enough glacial acetic acid to make 1000 ml. Calculate the volume of acetic anhydride required to react with all of the water added with the perchloric acid. The density of 72% perchloric acid is 1.60, and the density of acetic anhydride is 1.02.

2. An acetous perchloric acid solution was standardized when its temperature was 24°C, its strength being 0.4952 *N* at this temperature. Calculate the normality of this solution at 30°C.

3. 0.1560 g of pure benzoic acid was titrated to the thymol blue end point in DMF solution with sodium methoxide titrant, 8.53 ml being required. Calculate the normality of the titrant.

4. (*a*) Derive an equation for the hydrogen ion concentration as a function of the overall dissociation constant K_{HClO_4} and the formal concentration c_{HClO_4} in a solution of perchloric acid in glacial acetic acid. (Dissociation of the solvent, acetic acid, may be neglected.)

(*b*) By how many units will the pH of this solution change upon a tenfold dilution?

(*c*) If this were an aqueous solution of perchloric acid, by how many units would its pH change with a tenfold dilution?

(*d*) To what property of the solvent can the difference in behavior of $HClO_4$ in acetic acid and in water be ascribed?

5. Why does an amine that behaves as a weak base upon titration in aqueous solution behave as a strong base when titrated in glacial acetic acid?

6. One milliliter of exactly 0.1 *N* tetrabutylammonium hydroxide is equivalent to how many milligrams of diphenylhydantoin (structure **1**, $R_1 = R_2 = C_6H_5$)?

7. Twenty tablets of phenobarbital weighing a total of 6.025 g (structure **2**, $R_1 = C_2H_5$, $R_2 = C_6H_5$, MW 232.2) were powdered finely and a sample weighing 2.000 g was dissolved in DMF. It was titrated with 0.10 *N* lithium methoxide, 8.50 ml being consumed. Calculate the average weight of phenobarbital per tablet.

8. A sample of diphenhydramine hydrochloride, $(C_6H_5)_2CHOCH_2CH_2N(CH_3)_2 \cdot HCl$ (MW 291.8), weighing 0.6120 g, was dissolved in glacial acetic acid. Fifteen milliliters of 3.2% mercuric acetate solution was added and the mixture was titrated to the *p*-naphtholbenzein end point with 17.12 ml of 0.1145 *N* acetous perchloric acid. Calculate the percent purity of the sample.

9. A 0.5750 g sample of nicotinic acid (MW 123.1) was dissolved in glacial acetic acid to be titrated with perchloric acid. The analyst mistakenly overshot the end point, adding 35.00 ml of 0.115 *N* $HClO_4$. He therefore back-titrated with 0.085 *N* sodium acetate, but incompetently went past the end point again, adding 4.50 ml of this solution. Finally he completed the titration by adding 1.20 ml of the 0.115 *N* $HClO_4$ to the end point. Calculate the percent purity of the sample.

10. Referring to Table 2.3, suggest a reason for the variation in base strength in the series potassium, sodium, and lithium acetates.

3 PRECIPITATION TITRATIONS

3.1 Solubility of Slightly Soluble Salts

As a basis for titrimetric analysis a chemical reaction must occur "quantitatively"; that is, essentially it must proceed completely to form products. One type of reaction that may fit this requirement is the combination of two ionic species to form a very insoluble salt. Precipitation of this product then forces the reaction to completion. Titrations based on this kind of reaction are called precipitation titrations. The analysis of chloride by titration with silver ion is a familiar example.

The theoretical approach to precipitation titrations is made readily by considering the solubility of the product of the reaction, for it will be recognized that the titration reaction is simply the reverse of the dissolution of the salt. These considerations apply also to classical gravimetric analysis.

The Solution Process. The extent to which a compound dissolves is specified by its equilibrium molar solubility, which is the concentration of dissolved solute, in moles per liter, when the solution is in equilibrium with a solid solute. The solubility of a compound is dependent upon the solvent and the temperature, which must be specified.

In its solid state the solute is crystalline; that is, the solute molecules occupy space in accordance with a definite repeating pattern. The nature of this pattern depends upon the structure of the compound. Both ionic substances (for example, sodium chloride) and nonionic compounds (for example, benzoic acid) assume crystalline forms in the solid state. The crystal structure is formed and maintained by means of intermolecular forces of attraction. These may be purely electrostatic, as in a salt crystal, or they may involve other types of interaction, such as hydrogen bonding and dipole-dipole interactions.

For a solid to dissolve, the forces of attraction that hold molecules together in the crystal must be overcome. This is accomplished by the solvent. The solute-solute attraction within the crystal is replaced by a solute-solvent attraction and the substance dissolves. The molar solubility is determined by the relative strengths of the solute-solvent and solute-solute interactions.

Because of this competition between the solute-solute and the solute-solvent interactions, a solvent will be effective in dissolving a compound only if it can compete with the crystal forces. This often means that the solvent environment must be similar to that provided by the crystal structure in order for the solvent to be effective. Thus an ionic compound is apt to have a greater solubility in a polar solvent like water than in a nonpolar hydrocarbon solvent. This is the basis for the simple rule "like dissolves like"; that is, a solvent will most readily dissolve those substances that it resembles chemically. Although this rule is subject to many serious exceptions, it is a useful rough guide.

The phenomenon we have been considering is the equilibrium solubility. Another aspect of this problem is the rate of dissolution, or the velocity with which the equilibrium condition is established. This rate depends upon many factors besides the identities of the solute and solvent. Temperature is important, as is the rate of stirring the mixture. Probably the most important factor is the surface area of the solid phase, the rate of dissolution being increased by an increase in surface area of the solid. This observation can be useful in the laboratory, for solutions can be prepared more quickly if the solute is finely powdered; the smaller the particle size the greater is the surface area per gram of material.

The Solubility Product. Consider an aqueous solution of a slightly soluble salt BA in equilibrium with excess of the solid at constant temperature. The equilibrium can be represented by

$$\mathrm{BA}(s) \rightleftharpoons \mathrm{B}^+ + \mathrm{A}^- \tag{3.1}$$

where BA(s) represents the solid phase. In dilute aqueous solution essentially no undissociated BA will be present in the solution. Since the activity of the solid is constant, the equilibrium constant for Eq. 3.1 may be written

$$K_{sp} = [\mathrm{B}^+][\mathrm{A}^-] \tag{3.2}$$

K_{sp} is called the *solubility product;* some authors symbolize it S. The solubility product is a constant for a given solute, solvent, and temperature.

The stoichiometry of the reaction is reflected in the solubility product expression in the usual manner. For the general reaction

$$\mathrm{B}_m\mathrm{A}_n(s) \rightleftharpoons m\mathrm{B}^{n+} + n\mathrm{A}^{m-} \tag{3.3}$$

the solubility product is defined

$$K_{sp} = [\mathrm{B}^{n+}]^m[\mathrm{A}^{m-}]^n$$

The great value of the solubility product is that it permits the calculation of one of the ion concentrations if the other is known. In the pure saturated solution the situation is even simpler because the reaction stoichiometry provides a relationship between the ion concentrations. Thus in a solution of the salt BA, we can write $[B^+] = [A^-]$, because each molecule of BA that dissolves produces one B^+ ion and one A^- ion. For the general reaction 3.3, we find the corresponding relation $n[B^{n+}] = m[A^{m-}]$.

EXAMPLE 3.1. K_{sp} for silver chloride in water is 1×10^{-10}. What is the molar solubility of silver chloride?

By the argument of the preceding paragraph it is clear that $[Ag^+] = [Cl^-]$. Moreover, if we let s be the molar solubility, then $s = [Ag^+] = [Cl^-]$, since each mole of AgCl that dissolves yields one silver ion and one chloride ion. Therefore, $K_{sp} = [Ag^+][Cl^-] = s^2$, or $s = 1 \times 10^{-5}\ M$.

EXAMPLE 3.2. $pK_{sp} = 15.0$ for ferrous hydroxide. What is its molar solubility?

The reaction is

$$Fe(OH)_2(s) \rightleftharpoons Fe^{2+} + 2OH^-$$

Therefore $[OH^-] = 2[Fe^{2+}]$. Also, we can set the molar solubility s equal to the ferrous ion concentration by the argument of the preceding example: $s = [Fe^{2+}]$. Thus

$$K_{sp} = [Fe^{2+}][OH^-]^2 = (s)(2s)^2 = 4s^3$$

or

$$s = 6.3 \times 10^{-6}\ M$$

EXAMPLE 3.3. What is the silver ion concentration in a solution containing excess silver iodate ($pK_{sp} = 8$) plus 0.1 M sodium iodate?

$$AgIO_3(s) \rightleftharpoons Ag^+ + IO_3^-$$

If we let $x = [Ag^+]$ (thus maintaining a useful distinction between the solubility s in pure water and the solubility x in this different situation), then $[IO_3^-] = 0.1 + x$, since the iodate concentration is equal to that provided by the sodium iodate plus that available from dissolution of silver iodate. From the solubility product expression,

$$K_{sp} = [Ag^+][IO_3^-] = x(0.1 + x)$$

This quadratic equation can be solved for x. Let us assume, however, that x is negligible relative to 0.1, so the equation becomes $K_{sp} = 0.1x$, from which $x = 10^{-7}\ M$. Evidently the assumption introduced was a reasonable one.

Note that in water the silver ion concentration s would have been $10^{-4}\ M$; thus the addition of 0.1 M iodate has caused a thousandfold decrease in silver concentration (and therefore in the solubility of silver iodate). This is called the *common ion effect*. The solubility of any slightly soluble salt can be decreased by adding an excess of either of its ions. This behavior may be taken advantage of in gravimetric analysis, for by adding an excess of precipitating agent, the solute concentration can be driven far below its normal solubility level.

Effect of pH on Solubility of Salts. If the anion of a slightly soluble salt is the conjugate base of a weak acid, the solubility of the salt will be affected by the pH of the medium. Silver acetate is an example of such a salt. It is possible to relate the solubility of the salt to the hydrogen ion concentration of the solution. If BA represents the slightly soluble salt, at equilibrium this equation may be written

$$BA(s) \rightleftharpoons B^+ + A^- \tag{3.4}$$

Since A^- is the conjugate base of a weak acid, the acid-base equilibrium must be satisfied simultaneously.

$$HA \rightleftharpoons H^+ + A^-$$

The operation of this equilibrium increases the solubility of BA by drawing reaction 3.4 to the right. The molar solubility of BA is equal to the concentration of B^+, which is equal to the total concentration of A; that is,

$$s = [B^+] = [A^-] + [HA] \tag{3.5}$$

The equilibrium expressions are $K_{sp} = [B^+][A^-]$ and $K_a = [H^+][A^-]/[HA]$. Substituting these into Eq. 3.5 gives

$$[B^+] = \frac{K_{sp}}{[B^+]}\left(1 + \frac{[H^+]}{K_a}\right)$$

or

$$s = \sqrt{K_{sp}(1 + [H^+]/K_a)} \tag{3.6}$$

Equation 3.6 relates the molar solubility to K_{sp}, K_a, and the hydrogen ion concentration. Notice that when $[H^+]$ is very much smaller than K_a, the solubility approaches $K_{sp}^{1/2}$, which is the usual value for a slightly soluble salt whose component ions are not acids or bases. As the hydrogen ion concentration increases so does the solubility. In the special case when $[H^+] = K_a$ (that is, pH = pK_a), Eq. 3.6 becomes

$$s = 1.41 K_{sp}^{1/2}$$

That is, the equation predicts that when pH = pK_a, the solubility of BA is 41% greater than when the hydrogen ion concentration is negligible.

This is not the only type of salt whose solubility is pH dependent. A similar equation can be derived for a salt whose cation is the conjugate acid of a weak base; of course, the solubility will increase as the hydrogen ion concentration decreases for this kind of salt.

Fractional Precipitation. Suppose a solution containing the cation B^+ is added to a solution containing the anions A^- and C^-, where the salts BA and

BC are slightly soluble (for example, AgCl and AgI). It is of practical interest to be able to predict what will happen.

Let $K_{sp}{}^{A} = [B^+][A^-]$ and $K_{sp}{}^{C} = [B^+][C^-]$. Whenever the product of the ionic concentrations is larger than the corresponding K_{sp}, the salt will precipitate until the solubility product expression is satisfied. This means that the salt with the smaller of the two solubility products will precipitate first, thus keeping the B^+ concentration so low that the other salt cannot precipitate until nearly all of the first has reacted. Suppose enough B^+ is added so that solid phase of *both* BA and BC are present. Then the solubility product expressions apply. Since $[B^+]$ is the same for both, this being a single solution, we get

$$[B^+] = \frac{K_{sp}{}^{A}}{[A^-]} = \frac{K_{sp}{}^{C}}{[C^-]}$$

or

$$\frac{[A^-]}{[C^-]} = \frac{K_{sp}{}^{A}}{K_{sp}{}^{C}} \tag{3.7}$$

Thus the ratio of anion concentrations is equal to the ratio of solubility products when solid phase of both salts are present. Equation 3.7 permits us to calculate whether or not a titration can be quantitative for one ion in the presence of another.

EXAMPLE 3.4. Can the iodide in a solution containing 0.01 *M* NaI and 0.1 *M* NaCl be quantitatively titrated with silver nitrate?

$$pK_{sp}(AgCl) = 10 \qquad pK_{sp}(AgI) = 16$$

Since the iodide solubility product is very much smaller than the chloride product, silver iodide will first precipitate from the solution. When nearly all the iodide has been removed from solution, the silver ion concentration will rise, and then AgCl will begin to precipitate. At the end point of the titration, when the AgCl has just begun to precipitate, both solid phases are present so we can apply Eq. 3.7:

$$\frac{[Cl^-]}{[I^-]} = 10^6$$

In other words, at the end point the iodide concentration is one-millionth that of the chloride. If we suppose that in forming the first trace of solid AgCl a negligible amount of chloride ion was consumed, we can calculate the iodide ion concentration at the end point. (The volume change is ignored.)

$$[I^-] = \frac{[Cl^-]}{10^6} = \frac{0.1}{10^6} = 10^{-7}\ M$$

Thus at the end point 10^{-7} M iodide remains in solution of the original 10^{-2} M, or $(10^{-7}/10^{-2})$ 100 = 0.001% remains untitrated. This is certainly to be considered a quantitative titration.

An expression analogous to Eq. 3.7 can be derived for more complex systems in which one or more of the ions are polyvalent. For these systems the final result is not quite as simple as for univalent ions.

3.2 Precipitation Titrations

Calculation of Titration Curves. The course of a precipitation titration can be quantitatively predicted if the solubility product of the salt formed in the titration is known. The titration is represented graphically as a plot of pB (where pB = $-\log [B^+]$) or pA against the titrant volume. We shall consider the simplest kind of precipitation titration, in which a uni-univalent salt is formed.

EXAMPLE 3.5. Calculate the titration curve for the titration of 100 ml of 0.1 M NaCl with 0.2 M $AgNO_3$. pK_{sp} = 10 for silver chloride.

Before the titration begins, pCl = 1.00. The silver ion concentration is, of course, zero.

Upon the addition of 1.0 ml of titrant, the product $[Ag^+][Cl^-]$ is very much larger than K_{sp}, so solid AgCl immediately precipitates out. A simple calculation with the aid of K_{sp} will show that essentially all the silver added is precipitated as AgCl. (1)(0.2) = 0.2 meq of AgCl is therefore formed. There was (100)/(0.1) = 10.0 meq of chloride originally present; now there is 10.0 − 0.2 = 9.8 meq, which is contained in 101 ml. (Note that we can neglect the very small amount of chloride produced by dissolution of the AgCl.) The concentration of chloride is therefore 9.8/101 = 0.097 M, or pCl = 1.01.

From the relation $K_{sp} = [Ag^+][Cl^-]$, we find pK_{sp} = pAg + pCl; therefore, pAg = 8.99 at this point in the titration. The calculation is carried out similarly for other points prior to the end point.

At the end point the 10 meq of chloride has been reacted with 10 meq of silver. The only silver and chloride in solution arises from dissolution of solid AgCl, so $[Ag^+] = [Cl^-] = 10^{-5}$ M, or pAg = pCl = 5.00.

After the end point excess silver ion is present. Its concentration is known, so the chloride concentration is easily calculated with the K_{sp} relation. A few of the calculated points in the titration curve (ml of $AgNO_3$ followed by the corresponding pCl) are as follows: 0 ml, 1.00; 1 ml, 1.01; 10 ml, 1.14; 20 ml, 1.30; 30 ml, 1.51; 40 ml, 1.84; 50 ml, 5.00; and 60 ml, 8.10.

Notice that a very large change in pCl occurs in the vicinity of the end point. The sharper this change is, the more accurately the end point may be located.

Sharper end point changes are produced when the concentrations of the solutions being titrated are larger and when the solubility product is smaller.

The titration curve for the salt BA is symmetrical about the end point, but a similar calculation for a titration resulting in a salt B_2A will show that the curve is markedly asymmetrical.

Certain experimental limitations exist in some precipitation systems, and these may render impracticable quantitative calculations or accurate titrations. For example, in the titration of iodide with silver ion, calculation of pAg prior to the equivalence point is invalidated by formation of the soluble species AgI_2^-, whose presence is not taken into account in the computation. Some titrations that might seem feasible on the basis of K_{sp} values may not be practical because of slow precipitation or adsorption problems.

Visual Indicators. It is necessary to provide some means to signal the end point of the precipitation titration.* The simplest means of end point detection is with a visual indicator. Many indicators are available for this purpose, but it is not possible to give a general theory of their action as we did for acid-base indicators (Chapter 1), since most of the indicators are quite specific for certain titrations.

One of the mechanisms for indicator action in precipitation titrations involves formation of a colored substance by reaction of the indicator with excess titrant. The Mohr titration of chloride with silver ion is an example. Sodium chromate is incorporated as the indicator substance. First the silver chloride precipitates. After the equivalence point, when the silver ion concentration increases rapidly, formation of silver chromate, which is red, occurs to mark the end point. This is an example of an indicator that forms a colored precipitate at the end point ($pK_{sp} = 12.3$ for silver chromate).† Some indicators are known that function by forming a soluble colored compound with excess titrant. Thus, the end point in the titration of silver ion with thiocyanate, with ferric ion as indicator, is marked by the red-brown color imparted to the solution by ferric thiocyanate.

A different mechanism operates to produce a color change with certain substances known as adsorption indicators. An example will illustrate the phenomenon. If a solution of bromide is titrated with silver nitrate in the presence of the adsorption indicator eosin, a color change from reddish orange

* The distinction between the equivalence point and the end point should be kept in mind. The *equivalence point* is the point in the titration when equivalent amounts of titrant and sample have been contacted. The *end point* is the experimental estimate of the equivalence point, and may differ from it for many possible reasons, one of them being the inadequacy of the indicator for the particular titration.

† We usually expect that the salt with the smaller solubility product will precipitate first in order to satisfy the equilibrium conditions, but this is true only if both salts dissociate to yield the same number of ions. In the present case AgCl is less soluble than Ag_2CrO_4, even though its solubility product is larger.

to reddish violet will be observed in the region of the equivalence point. Close observation will show that the color change has occurred on the surface of the silver halide precipitate.

The color change appears to be associated with adsorption of the solution common ions to the precipitate. Before the equivalence point an excess of bromide ions is present. These are adsorbed, in a primary adsorption layer, to the silver bromide precipitate. Eosin, which exists as an anion under the usual titration conditions, has little tendency to be adsorbed or to displace the bromide ions from the negatively charged surface of the precipitate. After the equivalence point, however, the solution contains an excess of silver ions, which now form the primary adsorption layer. The anionic eosin is now adsorbed to the positively charged surface. The adsorption of the indicator apparently results in a change in its electronic structure, with the result that a color change occurs on the surface of the precipitate.

The application of adsorption indicators that exist as anions (that is, they are acidic dyes) is limited to systems in which the precipitate adsorbs its own cations strongly (as in the example just discussed). Basic indicators, which exist as cations, can be used with precipitates that adsorb their own anions. Most uses of adsorption indicators are in titrations with silver, lead, or mercurous mercury.

Experiment 3.1. Volhard Determination of Chloride

PRINCIPLE

In the Volhard titration, silver ion is titrated with thiocyanate in acid solution. Silver thiocyanate is precipitated. Ferric ion, present as the indicator, reacts with excess thiocyanate after the equivalence point to yield the reddish-brown ferric thiocyanate. The indicator is very sensitive, and the method is quite precise.

The most common application of the Volhard titration is in the determination of halide. A measured excess of standard silver nitrate is added, and the unreacted silver is back-titrated with thiocyanate. An advantage of this method is that an acid medium is used; most halide titrations require nonacidic conditions. Two sources of error must be guarded against. (1) In the titration of silver with thiocyanate some silver ions will be adsorbed by the precipitate, leading to a premature end point; this difficulty may be overcome simply by shaking the mixture vigorously, which helps to desorb the unreacted silver from the precipitate. (2) A more serious complication may occur when silver is back-titrated with thiocyanate in the presence of silver chloride. Silver thiocyanate is less soluble than silver chloride, so as soon as the silver has been titrated and an excess of thiocyanate is present, the equilibrium $AgCl + SCN^- \rightleftharpoons AgSCN + Cl^-$ occurs, consuming thiocyanate and leading to a significant overtitration. Many remedies have been suggested, of which the simplest is to add nitrobenzene to the mixture; the nitrobenzene seems to coat the silver chloride particles, making them inaccessible for reaction.

As the primary standard in this method we could use sodium chloride, silver nitrate, or potassium thiocyanate, and each of these has been employed. Since commercially available silver nitrate is of adequate purity for usual titrimetric studies, it has been adopted as the primary standard here.

REAGENTS

0.1 M Silver Nitrate. Accurately weigh about 17 g of dried reagent grade silver nitrate into a 1 liter volumetric flask. Dissolve the sample in water and dilute exactly to the mark. Calculate the molarity of the solution.

0.1 M Potassium Thiocyanate. Prepare 1 liter of approximately 0.1 *M* aqueous solution of reagent grade potassium thiocyanate. Standardize this solution against the silver nitrate solution as follows: deliver from a 50 ml buret an exactly known volume (in the range 30–45 ml) of standard 0.1 *M* $AgNO_3$ into a 250 ml Erlenmeyer flask. Add 5 ml of 1 : 1 nitric acid and 1 ml of ferric ammonium sulfate solution. Titrate with the potassium thiocyanate solution to the first slight reddish-brown color. Shake the flask vigorously and continue the titration until the color is permanent. Carry out a blank titration. Calculate the normality of the thiocyanate.

1 : 1 Nitric Acid. Add 25 ml of concentrated nitric acid to 25 ml of water, and boil the solution (in a hood) until it is colorless.

Ferric Ammonium Sulfate Solution. Prepare a saturated solution of ferric ammonium sulfate in 1 *M* nitric acid.

PROCEDURE

Known. Accurately weigh 0.1–0.25 g of sodium chloride into a 250 ml Erlenmeyer flask. Dissolve the sample in 25–50 ml of water. Add 5 ml of 1 : 1 nitric acid, then run in an accurately measured volume from a buret, in excess, of standard 0.1 *M* silver nitrate. (As the equivalence point is reached the precipitate will coagulate, indicating approximately the necessary volume.) Add 2 ml of nitrobenzene and shake the flask vigorously. Finally, add 1 ml of ferric ammonium sulfate solution and titrate with standard potassium thiocyanate to the permanent reddish-brown color. Calculate the purity of the sodium chloride.

Unknown. The preceding analysis will give you the experience needed to analyze an unknown sample. Obtain a sample of a chloride-containing substance from the instructor. This may be an inorganic chloride, like NaCl or NH_4Cl, or an organic salt, such as an amine hydrochloride or quaternary ammonium chloride. Accurately weigh samples equivalent to 2–4 meq of chloride. (Your instructor may indicate the approximate weight required.)

Analyze these samples as described in the preceding paragraph. Calculate the percent chloride (as Cl) in the sample. If requested, also report the percent purity of the sample compound, whose identity will be given.

FOR FURTHER READING

Kolthoff, I. M. and V. A. Stenger, *Volumetric Analysis*, 2nd ed., Interscience, New York, Vol. I, 1942, Chaps. II, III, V; Vol. II, 1947, Chap. VIII.

Coetzee, J. F., Chap. 19 in *Treatise on Analytical Chemistry*, Part I, Vol. I, I. M. Kolthoff and P. J. Elving (eds.), Interscience, New York, 1959.

Lewin, S., *The Solubility Product Principle*, Interscience, New York, 1960.

Problems

1. How many milligrams of lead chloride ($pK_{sp} = 5.0$) will dissolve in 100 ml of 0.1 *M* sodium chloride?

2. The pK_{sp} of ferric hydroxide is 37. Calculate its molar solubility.

3. Calculate the solubility of silver acetate ($pK_{sp} = 3$) at the following pH values: pH = 1, 2, 3, 4, 5, 6, 7, 8. Make a plot of solubility against pH.

4. 100 ml of solution containing 0.01 *M* NaCl and 0.01 *M* KIO_3 is titrated with 0.1 *M* $AgNO_3$. $pK_{sp}(AgCl) = 10$, $pK_{sp}(AgIO_3) = 8$.

(*a*) What is the ratio $[Cl^-]/[IO_3^-]$ at the end point?

(*b*) What is the silver ion concentration at the end point?

(*c*) What percentage of the chloride has been precipitated at the end point?

5. Barium can be determined gravimetrically by precipitation as the sulfate; $pK_{sp} = 9$.

(*a*) If 50 ml of 0.1 *M* Na_2SO_4 is added to 25 ml of 0.1 *M* $BaCl_2$ and the precipitate is removed by filtration and is dried, what weight of precipitate will be found?

(*b*) If the precipitate is removed by filtration and washed with 300 ml of water before drying, what is its final weight?

6. Derive an equation relating the solubility of the slightly soluble salt BA_2, where A^- is the anion of a weak acid, to the hydrogen ion concentration.

7. What is the solubility of barium fluoride in 0.10 *M* NaF? $pK_{sp}(BaF_2) = 5.0$.

8. pK_{sp} for magnesium hydroxide is 10.9. Calculate the solubility of magnesium hydroxide in (*a*) pure water, (*b*) 0.01 *M* magnesium sulfate, (*c*) pH 12 solution.

9. What final concentration of iodate (IO_3^-) is needed to precipitate quantitatively the barium ion in a solution initially containing 0.01 *M* Ba^{2+}? By a quantitative precipitation we will mean that 99.9% of the barium is precipitated. The K_{sp} of barium iodate is 1.5×10^{-9}.

10. Derive an equation relating molar solubility to K_{sp} for the slightly soluble salt AB_4.

11. At what pH will lead hydroxide begin to precipitate if alkali is added to a 0.001 *M* solution of lead ion? $pK_{sp} = 15$ for lead hydroxide.

12. Outline procedures for the quantitative analysis of each solute in these solutions.

(*a*) An aqueous solution of HCl and NaCl.

(*b*) An aqueous solution of $CaCl_2$ and acetic acid.

13. Give general expressions for s, the molar solubility, as a function of K_{sp} for each of these substances, calculate the molar solubilities, and arrange the substances in order of increasing solubility.

Salt	K_{sp}
Aluminum hydroxide	4×10^{-15}
Barium carbonate	8×10^{-9}
Calcium fluoride	4×10^{-11}
Silver bromide	8×10^{-13}
Zinc hydroxide	2×10^{-14}

4 COMPLEXOMETRIC TITRATIONS

4.1 EDTA Complexes

Introduction. It is difficult to give a satisfactory definition of a complex, but by sufficiently limiting the nature of the systems to be considered in this chapter a clear indication of the phenomenon of complexation can be given. All these complexes consist of one or more molecules bound to a central cation. (We exclude water as one of these complex-forming molecules because in aqueous solution probably every metal ion exists as the "aquo complex" anyway.) The molecule bound to the ion is called the *ligand*, and the maximum number of groups that can be bound to an ion is its *coordination number*. Ligands that are bound to the ion at only one point are called *unidentate* ("one-toothed"). Ammonia, for example, is a unidentate ligand capable of complexing with cupric ion according to these equations:

$$Cu^{2+} + NH_3 \rightleftharpoons Cu(NH_3)^{2+}$$
$$Cu(NH_3)^{2+} + NH_3 \rightleftharpoons Cu(NH_3)_2{}^{2+}$$
$$Cu(NH_3)_2{}^{2+} + NH_3 \rightleftharpoons Cu(NH_3)_3{}^{2+}$$
$$Cu(NH_3)_3{}^{2+} + NH_3 \rightleftharpoons Cu(NH_3)_4{}^{2+}$$

Many ligands are known that contain more than one group capable of bonding to the metal ion; such ligands are *multidentate*. Thus ethylenediamine, $H_2NCH_2CH_2NH_2$, is a bidentate ligand. A complex of a metal ion with two or more groups on a multidentate ligand evidently is a ring compound; this type of complex is often called a *chelate* (from the Greek for "claw"). Ligands that form chelates may be called chelating agents or chelons.

The most effective complexing groups in a ligand are amino and carboxylate groups. All the multidentate ligands important in analytical chemistry contain the structural component

$$-N\begin{matrix} \diagup CH_2COOH \\ \diagdown CH_2COOH \end{matrix}$$

The most widely used of these complexing agents is ethylenediaminetetraacetic acid (EDTA). EDTA possesses six groups—two amino and four carboxylate—

$$\begin{matrix} HOOC{-}CH_2 & & & & CH_2{-}COOH \\ & \diagdown & & \diagup & \\ & & N{-}CH_2CH_2{-}N & & \\ & \diagup & & \diagdown & \\ HOOC{-}CH_2 & & & & CH_2{-}COOH \end{matrix}$$

EDTA

capable of complexing with metal ions. It forms chelates with nearly all metal ions, and this reaction is the basis for a general analytical method for these ions by titration with a standard EDTA solution. Such titrations are called complexometric, chelatometric, or chelometric titrations.

Formation and Structure. Analysis of EDTA complexes has shown that the metal-ligand ratio is 1 : 1 and that the tetraanion of EDTA is the ligand species. The unusual effectiveness of EDTA as a chelating agent is a consequence of the formation of several five-membered rings, each of which contains the central metal ion. Figure 4.1 shows the structure of a metal-EDTA complex [1]; the solid lines represent the covalent bonds of the EDTA molecule and the dashed lines the bonds from the ion to the coordinating groups of the ligand. The location of charges, which has not been shown, will depend upon the identity of the metal ion.

Ethylenediaminetetraacetic acid is a tetrabasic acid and is often represented by the symbol H_4Y. The four dissociation equilibria then may be written:

$$H_4Y \overset{K_1}{\rightleftharpoons} H^+ + H_3Y^-$$

$$H_3Y^- \overset{K_2}{\rightleftharpoons} H^+ + H_2Y^{2-}$$

$$H_2Y^{2-} \overset{K_3}{\rightleftharpoons} H^+ + HY^{3-}$$

$$HY^{3-} \overset{K_4}{\rightleftharpoons} H^+ + Y^{4-}$$

The acid dissociation constants have the values $pK_1 = 2.0$, $pK_2 = 2.67$, $pK_3 = 6.16$, $pK_4 = 10.26$. Since Y^{4-} is the usual ligand species, evidently the complex formation equilibria will be affected by the pH of the medium.

Stability Constants. The complex formation equilibrium between a metal ion and EDTA can be represented as

$$M^{n+} + Y^{4-} \rightleftharpoons MY^{+n-4}$$

The equilibrium constant expression is

$$K = \frac{[MY^{+n-4}]}{[M^{n+}][Y^{4-}]} \tag{4.1}$$

The quantity K is called the ***stability constant***, or formation constant, of the complex. The reciprocal of K is the instability, or dissociation, constant. The stability constants for some metal-EDTA complexes are listed (as their

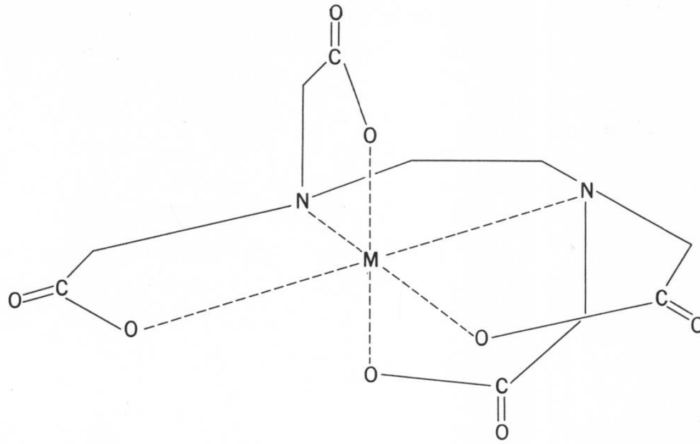

Fig. 4.1. Representation of the three-dimensional structure of an EDTA complex with a metal ion of coordination number six.

logarithms) in Table 4.1. The extremely large values of these constants should be noted.

Conditional Constants. The stability constant defined by Eq. 4.1 is a measure of the strength of the complex and permits calculation of the species concentrations in a system containing EDTA in the Y^{4-} form. In most practical analytical systems, however, the pH of the solution must be controlled at a level well below that needed to convert all the EDTA to the tetraanion. In general, the solution may contain several of the species H_4Y, H_3Y^-, H_2Y^{2-}, HY^{3-}, and Y^{4-}. Under such circumstances the stability constant K is not

TABLE 4.1
Stability Constants of Some Metal-EDTA Complexes[a,b]

Cation	log K	Cation	log K
Iron (III)	25.1	Cobalt	16.31
Thorium	23.2	Aluminum	16.13
Mercury	21.80	Cerium	15.98
Copper	18.80	Manganese	14.04
Nickel	18.62	Calcium	10.96
Lead	18.04	Magnesium	8.69
Zinc	16.50	Strontium	8.63
Cadmium	16.46	Barium	7.76

[a] At 20°C in 0.1 M KNO_3.

[b] From G. Schwarzenbach, R. Gut, and G. Anderegg, *Helv. Chim. Acta*, **37**, 937 (1954).

directly applicable to equilibrium calculations, and the presence of the several ionization states of the ligand molecule must be taken into account.

From the practical point of view, the analyst does not require detailed knowledge of the distribution of ionic species of the ligand; all he needs to know is the concentration of the product (the complex), the concentration of the free, unreacted ligand, and the concentration of the unbound metal. If we assume, for the present, that the only species in solution are M^{n+}, MY^{+n-4}, and the five possible forms of EDTA, then an equilibrium constant can be defined to describe the complex formation

$$K' = \frac{[MY^{+n-4}]}{[M^{n+}][Y']} \tag{4.2}$$

where $[Y']$ represents the formal concentration of free ligand regardless of ionic form; that is,

$$[Y'] = [H_4Y] + [H_3Y^-] + [H_2Y^{2-}] + [HY^{3-}] + [Y^{4-}] \tag{4.3}$$

K' is called the *conditional constant* (or sometimes the apparent or effective constant) because its value depends upon the conditions. If the pH is made very high so that essentially all of the EDTA is converted into Y^{4-}, then $[Y'] = [Y^{4-}]$ and $K' = K$. At all other pH's K' will be smaller than K. Since K' is the quantity that actually describes the equilibrium in a titration solution, whereas the K values are the ones available (as in Table 4.1), it is necessary to be able to estimate K' from K at any given pH value.

Let us define the quantity α_L by

$$\alpha_L = \frac{[Y']}{[Y^{4-}]} \tag{4.4}$$

An expression for α_L, which is a function of pH and of the four acid dissociation constants of H_4Y, is easily derived. For convenience the reciprocals of the acid dissociation constants will be used; thus if K_1 is the dissociation constant for the first protonic dissociation, $k_1 = 1/K_1$, $k_2 = 1/K_2$, etc., so that

$$k_1 = \frac{[H_4Y]}{[H^+][H_3Y^-]}$$

$$k_2 = \frac{[H_3Y^-]}{[H^+][H_2Y^{2-}]}$$

$$k_3 = \frac{[H_2Y^{2-}]}{[H^+][HY^{3-}]}$$

$$k_4 = \frac{[HY^{3-}]}{[H^+][Y^{4-}]}$$

These equilibrium constants may be combined with Eq. 4.3 to express all concentrations in terms of $[Y^{4-}]$.

$$[Y'] = [Y^{4-}](k_1k_2k_3k_4[H^+]^4 + k_2k_3k_4[H^+]^3 + k_3k_4[H^+]^2 + k_4[H^+] + 1) \tag{4.5}$$

By comparing Eq. 4.5 with 4.4,

$$\alpha_L = k_1k_2k_3k_4[H^+]^4 + k_2k_3k_4[H^+]^3 + k_3k_4[H^+]^2 + k_4[H^+] + 1 \tag{4.6}$$

Since the acid dissociation constants of EDTA are known, α_L can be calculated for any value of pH by means of Eq. 4.6. Equations 4.1, 4.2, and 4.4 lead to

$$K' = \frac{K}{\alpha_L} \tag{4.7}$$

which allows the conditional constant to be calculated at any pH if the stability constant K is known.

In this discussion we have assumed that the metal ion exists in either the bound form MY^{+n-4} or in the free form M^{n+}. Actually in many systems containing a third component capable of forming a complex with the metal (a solution of EDTA and Cu^{2+} in an ammonia buffer would be such a system) not all of the metal is free. Thus in the system just described the copper uncomplexed with EDTA is present as Cu^{2+}, $Cu(NH_3)^{2+}$, $Cu(NH_3)_2{}^{2+}$, $Cu(NH_3)_3{}^{2+}$, and $Cu(NH_3)_4{}^{2+}$. The stability constant K (Eq. 4.1) does not provide a practical measure of the extent of complexation in this system, and so again we define a conditional constant

$$K' = \frac{[MY^{+n-4}]}{[M'][Y^{4-}]}$$

where $[M']$ is the sum of concentrations of all species of metal other than MY^{+n-4}. By analogy with the case of the various species of ligand, we define α_M,

$$\alpha_M = \frac{[M']}{[M^{n+}]}$$

If the formation constants are known for the side reactions of M^{n+} with the extra solution component, α_M can be calculated and the conditional constant evaluated.

$$K' = \frac{K}{\alpha_M} \tag{4.8}$$

This treatment is in all respects analogous to that for estimating the pH effect on the ligand.

In a great many systems both effects will be operating, and it is necessary to evaluate both α_L (which is simple if EDTA is always employed as the ligand) and α_M (this quantity will be different for every metal and every extra component). The conditional constant that describes the relation between MY^{+m-4}, M′, and Y′ is then calculated;

$$K' = \frac{K}{\alpha_M \alpha_L} \tag{4.9}$$

Selectivity in EDTA titrations of mixtures of metals can often be achieved by adding to the solution a component that complexes strongly with one of the metals, thus decreasing its conditional constant with EDTA so that this metal is not titratable; then the second metal is available for titration without interference. This technique is called *masking*.

4.2 Titrations with EDTA

Titration Curves. In order for a chemical reaction to form the basis for an analytical procedure, the equilibrium constant must be large enough so that an appreciable "break" or change in concentration of one of the reaction components occurs near the equivalence point. Although many unidentate ligands form complexes with metal ions, and many of these reactions are characterized by large stability constants, very few of these systems are analytically useful. The reason lies in the stepwise nature of the reactions forming successively higher complexes. The coordination numbers of most cations are greater than one, so an unidentate ligand will form more than one complex. The copper-ammonia system, which was discussed in Section 4.1, is an example. Such a system could be represented by the equations

$$M + L \overset{K_1}{\rightleftharpoons} ML$$

$$ML + L \overset{K_2}{\rightleftharpoons} ML_2$$

$$ML_2 + L \overset{K_3}{\rightleftharpoons} ML_3$$

$$ML_3 + L \overset{K_4}{\rightleftharpoons} ML_4$$

The stability constants are defined in the usual way. It might seem that any of these reactions could provide the basis for an analysis of M by titration with a solution of the ligand L. In fact, however, if successive stability constants are not greatly different in magnitude, such a titration is difficult or impossible. This is because before one of these reactions (say, the formation of ML) is essentially complete, the next reaction (formation of ML_2) begins to consume a significant fraction of titrant L. Thus a sharp change in concentration of M is not observed.

This effect will be seen readily in a typical example. Assume a solution of metal M titrated with ligand L, the system being subject to the above equilibria,

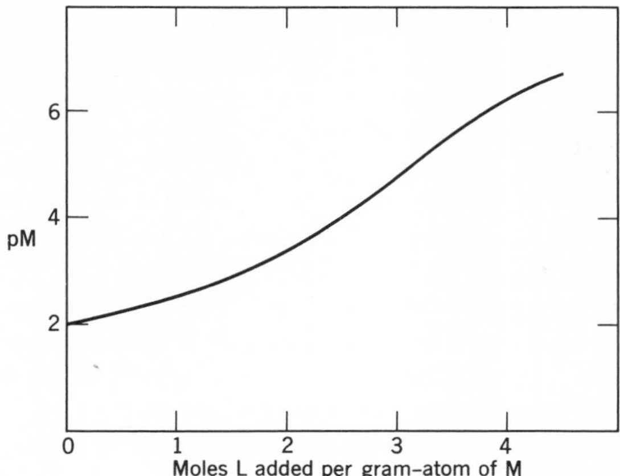

Fig. 4.2. Titration of 10^{-2} M metal ion (M) with unidentate ligand L; the stability constants are: $K_1 = 1 \times 10^4$, $K_2 = 3 \times 10^3$, $K_3 = 8 \times 10^2$, $K_4 = 1 \times 10^2$ (overall stability constant is 2.4×10^{12}).

and suppose the stability constants have the values $K_1 = 1 \times 10^4$, $K_2 = 3 \times 10^3$, $K_3 = 8 \times 10^2$, and $K_4 = 1 \times 10^2$. (These values are very close to those actually found for the copper-ammonia system.) The calculated titration curve* for a solution initially containing 10^{-2} g-atom/liter of M is shown in Fig. 4.2. Evidently no sharp change in pM is observed at any of the theoretical equivalence points. The system is not analytically useful, even though the equilibrium constant for the overall reaction

$$M + 4L \rightleftharpoons ML_4$$

is extremely large (2.4×10^{12} in this case).

* The calculation of a titration curve for such a complicated system may be of interest. The four complex formation constant expressions are combined with the mass balance equations

$$M_t = [M] + [ML] + [ML_2] + [ML_3] + [ML_4]$$

$$L_t = [L] + [ML] + 2[ML_2] + 3[ML_3] + 4[ML_4]$$

(where M_t and L_t are formal total concentrations of M and L) to give

$$M_t = [M](1 + K_1[L] + K_1K_2[L]^2 + K_1K_2K_3[L]^3 + K_1K_2K_3K_4[L]^4) \quad (4a)$$

$$L_t = [L] + [M](K_1[L] + 2K_1K_2[L]^2 + 3K_1K_2K_3[L]^3 + 4K_1K_2K_3K_4[L]^4) \quad (4b)$$

A value must be selected for M_t (in Fig. 4.2 $M_t = 10^{-2}$ M). Then the procedure is to assign a reasonable value to [L] and, with Eq. 4a, to calculate the corresponding value of [M]. This quantity is then inserted in Eq. 4b to calculate L_t. This gives all the necessary information, for from [M] the ordinate pM is calculated, whereas the abscissa (moles of L per gram-atom of M in Fig. 4.2) is given by the ratio L_t/M_t. The entire curve is constructed by altering the assumed value for [L] and repeating the calculation. The calculation is simplified by assuming that no volume change occurs during the titration.

The important difference between the unidentate and multidentate ligands is not in the magnitude of the overall stability constants with a particular cation (these are often very similar) but in the single-step nature of the multidentate complex formation as compared with the multistep nature of the unidentate reaction. Since one molecule of the multidentate ligand satisfies all bonding affinities of the metal ion, a 1 : 1 complex is necessarily formed in a single step. The resultant appearance of a titration curve of 10^{-2} *M* metal ion with a multidentate ligand (say, EDTA) is shown in Fig. 4.3; the conditional constant for the system was taken to be 2.4×10^{12}, the same as the overall constant for the titration system shown in Fig. 4.2. Notice the extremely sharp change in slope at the equivalence point. This graph, and this comparison, shows why EDTA is so useful as a titrant for cations.

The titration curve for an EDTA titration is readily calculated. First the conditional constant must be computed from a knowledge of the stability constant, the pH of the solution, and any side equilibria. The uncomplexed metal concentration is to be calculated as a function of the titrant volume.

Before the equivalence point is reached, the calculation is based upon essentially complete reaction between the metal and the ligand. Thus each mole of ligand added results in one mole of complex being formed, and the uncomplexed metal is obtained as the difference between the initial amount and the complexed amount.

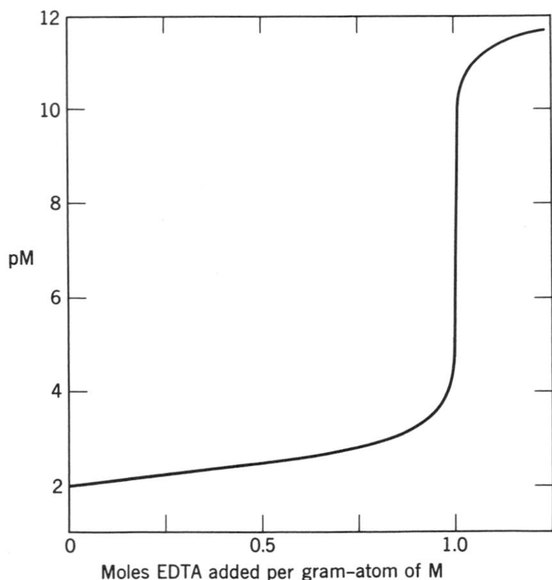

Fig. 4.3. Titration of 10^{-2} *M* metal ion (M) with EDTA; the conditional constant is 2.4×10^{12}.

At the equivalence point the concentration of free metal ion is controlled by the complexation equilibrium

$$M + Y' \rightleftharpoons MY$$

The concentrations [M] and [Y′] are equal at this point, since these species can be produced only by dissociation of the complex. The concentration of the complex is closely approximated by the formal concentration of metal. Thus from the equilibrium constant expression, the concentration [M] may be calculated.

After the equivalence point the calculation also utilizes the equilibrium constant. The unbound ligand Y′ is considered to be that added after the equivalence point and is therefore known. The amount of complex is unchanged from that present at the equivalence point. It is therefore possible to calculate the quantity [M].

EXAMPLE 4.1. 10.0 ml of 0.01 *M* Ca^{2+} is titrated with 0.01 *M* EDTA in a solution buffered to pH 10. Calculate the titration curve.

From the acid dissociation constants for EDTA (Section 4.1) and Eq. 4.6, α_L is calculated to be 2.8. The conditional constant for this system is therefore 3.3×10^{10}. (The stability constant is given in Table 4.1.)

Before any titrant is added to the sample solution, $[Ca^{2+}] = 10^{-2}\ M$, or pCa = 2.00. Now suppose 1.0 ml of titrant is added. This corresponds to the addition of (1.0)(0.01) = 0.01 mmole of ligand, and therefore to the formation of 0.01 mmole of complex. Since the sample initially contained (10.0)(0.01) = 0.01 mmole of calcium, evidently 0.09 mmole of calcium remains in a volume of 11.0 ml. Therefore $[Ca^{2+}] = 0.09/11 = 8.18 \times 10^{-3}\ M$, or pCa = 2.09.

The calculation is carried out similarly until near the equivalence point, which by definition is the point at which an amount of EDTA has been added that is equivalent to the calcium present. This corresponds to 10.0 ml in this case. At this point, 0.01 mmole of complex has been formed, and so [CaY] = 0.10/20, or $5.0 \times 10^{-3}\ M$. Since calcium and free EDTA can arise only by dissociation of complex, $[Ca^{2+}] = [Y']$. Therefore,

$$K' = \frac{[CaY]}{[Ca^{2+}]^2}$$

or

$$[Ca^{2+}] = 3.90 \times 10^{-7}\ M$$

and pCa = 6.41.

After the end point the solution still contains 0.10 mmole of complex.

Therefore, when 11.0 ml of titrant has been added,

$$[\mathrm{CaY}] = \frac{0.10}{21} = 4.76 \times 10^{-3}\ M$$

The uncomplexed ligand concentration

$$[\mathrm{Y'}] = 21/(1.0)(0.01) = 4.76 \times 10^{-4}\ M$$

Using the conditional constant, we therefore find

$$[\mathrm{Ca^{2+}}] = \frac{[\mathrm{CaY}]}{K'[\mathrm{Y'}]} = 3.04 \times 10^{-10}\ M$$

or pCa = 9.52. Table 4.2 gives the results of calculation over the entire course of the titration.

If the conditional constant is relatively small (less than 10^7), the approximations made in the previous treatment may not be valid, and an exact calculation must be used. Thus it was assumed that, before the equivalence point, the concentration of complex was equal to the concentration of added ligand. This is not strictly correct, and in the general case of the equilibrium

TABLE 4.2
Titration of 10.0 ml of 0.01 M Ca^{2+} with 0.01 M EDTA at pH 10

Volume EDTA (ml)	pCa
0	2.00
1	2.09
2	2.18
3	2.27
4	2.37
5	2.48
6	2.60
7	2.75
8	2.95
9	3.28
10	6.41
11	9.52
12	9.82

$M + L \rightleftharpoons ML$, the three simultaneous equations

$$K' = \frac{[ML]}{[M][L']}$$

$$M_t = [M] + [ML]$$

$$L_t = [L'] + [ML]$$

must be solved for [M]. (Here M_t and L_t are the formal concentrations of these substances.)

Metal Indicators. It is clear from the preceding discussion that many metal ions can be titrated with EDTA under conditions such that a sudden large change in metal ion concentration occurs near the equivalence point. In order for this phenomenon to be analytically useful some means must be available to indicate where this concentration change occurs. Many substances are known that function as visual indicators of these breaks in titration curves. These indicators form complexes with metal ions, the complexed and uncomplexed forms having different colors; such compounds are known as *metallochromic indicators.* The use of a metallochromic indicator to signal the end point in an EDTA titration is based on the reaction

$$MI + Y \rightleftharpoons MY + I$$

where I is the uncomplexed form of the indicator. The stability constant for the metal-indicator complex must be smaller than that for the metal-EDTA complex; on the other hand, the metal-indicator complex must be sufficiently stable so that essentially no free I is present before the end point. During the titration EDTA (Y) reacts with M to form the MY complex. When the equivalence point is reached, all free M has been consumed in reaction with Y, and addition of more Y displaces I from its complex with MI (only a trace of indicator is present). Since the free I has a different color from complexed I, a color change occurs.

The situation actually is somewhat more complicated than is implied by the preceding paragraph, since all metallochromic indicators are also acid-base indicators. For this reason it is important to control the pH in a titration solution so that the desired protonic species of the indicator is present.

A widely used metallochromic indicator is Eriochrome Black T. The two phenolic hydrogens are ionizable, the acid dissociation constants being $pK_1 = 6.3$ and $pK_2 = 11.55$. The acid-base indicator properties are represented as

$$\underset{\text{Wine red}}{H_2I^-} \overset{K_1}{\rightleftharpoons} \underset{\text{Blue}}{HI^{2-}} \overset{K_2}{\rightleftharpoons} \underset{\text{Orange}}{I^{3-}}$$

In the pH range 8–10 essentially only the form HI^{2-} is present, and this represents the uncomplexed form of the metallochromic indicator. The

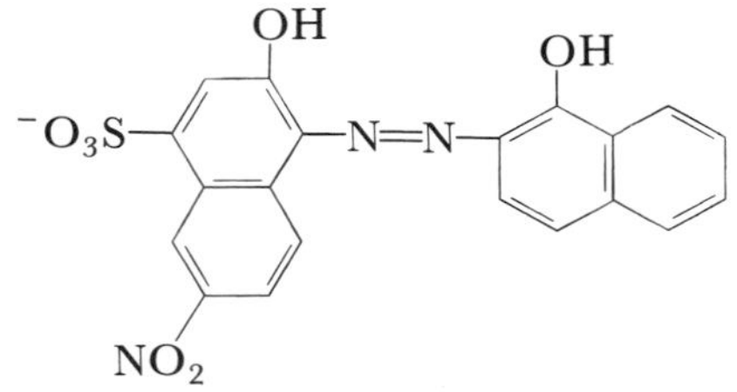

Eriochrome Black T

color change reaction with magnesium, for example, is written

$$\underset{}{Mg^{2+}} + \underset{\text{Blue}}{HI^{2-}} \rightleftharpoons \underset{\text{Wine red}}{MgI^{-}} + H^{+}$$

The titration of magnesium with EDTA at pH 10 in the presence of Eriochrome Black T is therefore marked by a red to blue color change at the end point.

An experimental difficulty occasionally encountered in complexometric titrations arises when the distilled water or other reagents contain traces of metal ions capable of forming strong complexes with the indicator. If such a complex is stronger than the EDTA complex of the trace metal, evidently the uncomplexed form of the indicator cannot be generated at the equivalence point and so no color change will occur. This phenomenon is known as blocking the indicator. Copper in distilled water is a frequent source of this trouble, which is avoided by removing trace cations by an ion-exchange method.

Although many other metallochromic indicators are known and used [2], their color changes can be accounted for in terms of equilibria similar to those described for Eriochrome Black T.

Methods and Applications. The simplest analytical method employing EDTA is the *direct titration* of a metal ion with a visual indicator used to signal the end point. The solution is buffered for reasons already considered.

Sometimes a direct titration with a solution of EDTA is not possible for one of several reasons: the metal ion may form an insoluble hydroxide because of the high pH required; it may not be possible to detect the end point accurately; or the rate of formation of the metal-EDTA complex may be too low. In these cases a successful analysis often may be made with a *back-titration* procedure. A measured excess of standard EDTA solution is added, and the excess is back-titrated with a standard solution of metal ion (usually magnesium or zinc).

Another technique is available if the end point of a titration is unsatisfactory. This may be illustrated with the determination of calcium. The direct titration of calcium with EDTA is not possible with Eriochrome Black T indicator because the calcium-indicator complex is very weak; thus the color change at the end point is vague. However, the magnesium-Eriochrome Black T complex is strong, and the end point for the titration of Mg^{2+} with EDTA is good. Moreover, the calcium-EDTA complex is stronger than the magnesium-EDTA complex. The determination is carried out by adding some Mg-EDTA complex to the calcium solution. This mixture is titrated with EDTA. The calcium complex of EDTA is formed, whereas the magnesium complex of the indicator maintains the typical red color. After all of the calcium has been titrated the EDTA displaces the indicator from the magnesium-Eriochrome Black T complex, and the color changes to blue. This is called a *replacement titration*. Note that no titrant is consumed by magnesium in this method, since Mg^{2+} is added as the EDTA complex.

Among the cations that can be determined by direct titration with EDTA are aluminum, ion (III), calcium, magnesium, zinc, cadmium, copper (II), nickel, cobalt, lead (II), barium, manganese, mercury, and many others. By the back-titration procedure it is possible to titrate lead (II), aluminum, mercury (II), and nickel; an advantage of this technique is its applicability to the titration of metals in the form of their insoluble salts; thus barium sulfate is dissolved in excess of ammoniacal EDTA and the back-titration is carried out with magnesium. The replacement method is useful for calcium, lead, mercury, and iron (III).

Experiment 4.1. Titration of Metals with EDTA

REAGENTS

Water. As noted earlier, indistinct end points may be caused by blocking of the indicator by trace impurities (especially copper) in the distilled water. The purity of the water may be tested [3]: Add 1 ml of pH 10 buffer to 50 ml of water and enough Eriochrome Black T indicator powder to give a faint color; the solution should be blue. If the color is violet or red, the solution contains impurities. To determine the source of these impurities, add a dilute EDTA solution (1 drop of 0.1 *M* EDTA plus 10 ml of water) drop by drop until the red color has disappeared. Add 50 ml more of the water. If the red color reappears, the impurities are in the water.

The troublesome impurities in the water may be removed by passing the water through an ion-exchange column, which removes the metal cations from the water and replaces them with hydrogen ions. Amberlite IR-120 or Dowex 50 (both sulfonic acid ion exchange resins) in the hydrogen form are satisfactory.

pH 10 Buffer. Dissolve 70 g of reagent grade ammonium chloride in 570 ml of concentrated ammonium hydroxide and dilute to 1 liter with water.

TRIS-Ammonia Buffer. Dissolve 13.1 g of tris(hydroxymethyl)aminomethane in 100 ml of water. Add 4.0 ml of concentrated hydrochloric acid and then 30 ml of concentrated ammonium hydroxide.

Eriochrome Black T Indicator Powder. Grind 100 mg of Eriochrome Black T with 10 g of sodium chloride to make a fine powder.

Hydroxy Naphthol Blue Indicator Powder. This commercially available indicator consists of 1-(2-naphtholazo-3,6-disulfonic acid)-2-naphthol-4-sulfonic acid disodium salt deposited on crystals of sodium chloride. In the pH range 12–13, its solutions are red to violet in the presence of calcium ion and clear blue in the presence of excess EDTA.

Arsenazo I Mixed Indicator. Dissolve 100 mg of Arsenazo I, 100 mg of Martius Yellow, 52.5 mg of Xylene Cyanole FF, and 1.0 g of TRIS in 10 ml of isopropanol. Slowly add 20 ml of water, transfer to a 100 ml volumetric flask, and dilute to volume with water. Arsenazo I is *o*-(1,8-dihydroxy-3,6-disulfo-2-naphthylazo)benzenearsonic acid.

0.01 M EDTA. Primary standard grade disodium EDTA is commercially available. The formula is $Na_2H_2Y \cdot 2H_2O$, and the ordinary product contains 0.3% adsorbed moisture [3], which is taken into account. Without drying the product, accurately weigh 3.729 g, transfer to a 1000 ml volumetric flask, and dilute to volume with water. This solution is 0.0100 *M*.

If it is desired to standardize this solution, proceed as follows. Accurately weigh about 1 g of primary standard grade calcium carbonate, previously dried at 110°C for 2 h, transfer quantitatively to a 1000 ml volumetric flask with the aid of water, and add, dropwise, just enough 10% HCl (prepared by diluting 225 ml of concentrated HCl to 1 liter) to dissolve the $CaCO_3$. Dilute to volume with water.

Pipet 20.0 ml of the $CaCO_3$ solution into an Erlenmeyer flask, add 30 ml of water, 6 ml of 1 *N* NaOH, and enough Hydroxy Naphthol Blue powder (about 300 mg) to give a distinct color. Titrate with the 0.01 *M* EDTA, from a 25 ml buret, to the clear blue color. Calculate the molarity of the solution.

PROCEDURES

Determination of Calcium in Ringer's Solution. Give your instructor a clean dry flask and obtain a sample of Ringer's solution (a solution of the chlorides of sodium, potassium, and calcium). Pipet 50.0 ml of the sample into an Erlenmeyer flask, add 6 ml of 1 *N* NaOH and enough Hydroxy Naphthol Blue to give a distinct color, and titrate with standard 0.01 *M* EDTA to the clear blue color. Calculate the result as milligrams of calcium per 100 ml of solution, and compare your analytical result with the official requirement.

Assay of Zinc Chloride. Accurately weigh 1.0–1.3 g of zinc chloride, weighing rapidly to minimize absorption of water from the atmosphere. Transfer it quantitatively to a 1000 ml volumetric flask with the aid of water, add about 2 g of ammonium chloride to produce a clear solution, and dilute to volume with water.

Pipet 25.0 ml of the zinc chloride solution into an Erlenmeyer flask, add

5 ml of pH 10 buffer and enough Eriochrome Black T powder (40–50 mg) to give a strong color. Titrate with standard 0.01 *M* EDTA to the clear blue color. Calculate the percent purity of the zinc chloride.

Determination of Total Hardness in Water [4]. Typical samples are municipal water or well water. Pipet 25.0 ml of the sample water into an Erlenmeyer flask. Add 25 ml of distilled water, 2 ml of TRIS-ammonia buffer, and 2 drops of Arsenazo I mixed indicator. Titrate with standard 0.01 *M* EDTA to the clear yellow color. Calculate the total hardness as calcium carbonate, expressing the result both as mg% (that is, the number of milligrams of $CaCO_3$ per 100 ml of water) and as parts per million (ppm, the number of grams of $CaCO_3$ per 10^6 ml of water).

Complete the titration within 5 min of the time the buffer is added. A 10 ml buret should be used. The end point color change, while certainly not dramatic, is quite sharp, but its detection requires close attention. Observe the color against a white background under fluorescent lighting, shielded from direct window illumination.

References

1. Martell, A. E., *J. Chem. Educ.*, **29,** 270 (1952).
2. West, T. S., *Complexometry with EDTA and Related Reagents*, BDH Chemicals, Ltd., Poole, England, 1969.
3. Flaschka, H. A., *EDTA Titrations: An Introduction to Theory and Practice*, Pergamon Press, New York, 1959.
4. Fritz, J. S., J. P. Sickafoose, and M. A. Schmitt, *Anal. Chem.*, **41,** 1954 (1969).

Problems

1. Suppose a metal M forms complexes in two steps with the ligand L:

$$M + L \overset{K_1}{\rightleftharpoons} ML$$

$$ML + L \overset{K_2}{\rightleftharpoons} ML_2$$

(*a*) Derive an expression relating the stability constants K_1 and K_2 to the overall stability constant K for the reaction

$$M + 2L \overset{K}{\rightleftharpoons} ML_2$$

(*b*) If $K_1 = 2 \times 10^5$ and $K_2 = 4 \times 10^2$, what is the value of K?

2. What is the concentration of zinc ion at the end point of the titration of 50 ml of 0.02 *M* zinc with 0.02 *M* EDTA at pH 10?

3. 40.00 ml of 0.02 *M* zinc chloride is titrated with 0.04 *M* EDTA under conditions such that the conditional constant is 10^{15}. Calculate pZn when the following volumes

of titrant have been added:

(*a*) 0.00 ml;
(*b*) 15.00 ml;
(*c*) 20.00 ml;
(*d*) 30.00 ml.

4. 35.00 ml of 0.055 *M* EDTA (an excess) is added to 20.00 ml of a magnesium chloride solution. The excess EDTA is back-titrated with 12.50 ml of 0.048 *M* zinc chloride. Calculate the concentration of magnesium chloride in the sample solution.

5. Propose methods with which you could quantitatively determine the concentration of each substance in the following mixtures.

(*a*) An aqueous solution of NaCl, HCl, and $MgCl_2$.
(*b*) Benzoic acid and ethylenediaminetetraacetic acid.

6. Calculate and plot the titration curve for the titration of 20 ml of 0.02 *M* metal ion with 0.05 *M* EDTA, if the conditional constant is 10^{12}.

7. Calculate α_L (with Eq. 4.6) for EDTA at pH = 8, 9, 10, 11, 12, 13. Plot α_L against pH. This graph can subsequently be used to estimate α_L at any value of pH within the range 8–13.

8. Dihydroxyaluminum aminoacetate, NF, $NH_2CH_2COOAl(OH)_2{\cdot}xH_2O$, is analyzed in terms of the equivalent amount of aluminum oxide. The assay procedure follows.

Transfer about 2.5 g of dihydroxyaluminum aminoacetate, accurately weighed, to a beaker, add 15 ml of hydrochloric acid, and warm to dissolve the sample. Transfer the solution quantitatively to a 500 ml volumetric flask, dilute to volume with water, and mix. Pipet 20.0 ml of this solution into a beaker, add 25.0 ml of 0.05 *M* EDTA and 20 ml of acetic acid-ammonium acetate buffer, and heat for 5 min. Cool, add 50 ml of alcohol, and dithizone (indicator). Titrate with 0.05 *M* zinc sulfate.

(*a*) What dilution factor must be used to calculate from the final titration value back to the sample taken?

(*b*) Each ml of 0.05 *M* EDTA consumed is equivalent to how many mg of Al_2O_3?

9. 10.0 ml of 0.02 *M* $MgCl_2$ is titrated with 0.015 *M* EDTA. Under the conditions of the titration the conditional constant is 1×10^8. Calculate pMg at these points:

(*a*) Before any titrant has been added
(*b*) When 5.0 ml of titrant has been added
(*c*) At the end point
(*d*) When 15.0 ml of titrant has been added

10. Sketch resonance structures that might account for the acid-base indicator properties of Eriochrome Black T.

5 OXIDATION–REDUCTION TITRATIONS

5.1 Oxidation–Reduction Reactions

Half-Reactions. From Chapter 1 we are familiar with acid-base reactions in which an acid is defined as a proton donor and a base as a proton acceptor, each related acid-base couple being called a conjugate pair. The acid-base properties of a conjugate pair are not manifested in the absence of a second conjugate pair. Thus the net result of an acid-base reaction is the transfer of a proton from one conjugate pair to another. This familiar situation has a close parallel in another important type of analytical reaction: oxidation-reduction (*redox*) reactions. Here also two half-reactions must be involved; each half-reaction includes a redox conjugate pair, and the net process of the overall reaction is the transfer of one or more electrons from one pair to the other.

We can represent a general redox half-reaction by the equation

$$\text{red} \underset{\text{reduction}}{\overset{\text{oxidation}}{\rightleftharpoons}} \text{ox} + ne \tag{5.1}$$

where red represents the reduced form (also called the reductant or reducing agent), ox the oxidized form (oxidant, oxidizing agent), n is the number of electrons transferred, and e represents the electron. It is not possible to observe a redox half-reaction; two half reactions are required, one to furnish electrons and the other to consume them. Equation 5.1 shows that oxidation is the process in which a substance loses electrons, and reduction is the process in which a substance gains electrons.

Some simple examples of redox half-reactions are

$$Fe^{2+} \rightleftharpoons Fe^{3+} + e$$
$$H_2 \rightleftharpoons 2H^+ + 2e$$
$$Cu \rightleftharpoons Cu^{2+} + 2e$$
$$2I^- \rightleftharpoons I_2 + 2e$$

More complicated half-reactions, in which the reduced form of the atom appears in a different combination from the oxidized form, may be encountered. Thus the oxidizing agent MnO_4^- is reduced to Mn^{2+}, and $Cr_2O_7^{2-}$ is reduced to Cr^{3+}.

Balancing Equations. In order to make analytical calculations, which are based upon reaction stoichiometry, it is necessary to balance the reaction equation. The method of balancing redox equations, which is a systematic one, will be illustrated with the oxidation of hydrogen peroxide by permanganate in acid solution.

STEP I. Balance each half-reaction both chemically and electrically.

The permanganate half-reaction (unbalanced) is: $MnO_4^- \rightleftharpoons Mn^{2+}$. This is first balanced chemically (by suitable addition of water and hydrogen ions) to give

$$MnO_4^- + 8H^+ \rightleftharpoons Mn^{2+} + 4H_2O$$

By adding an appropriate number of electrons, this half-reaction is balanced electrically.

$$MnO_4^- + 8H^+ + 5e \rightleftharpoons Mn^{2+} + 4H_2O$$

The oxidation half-reaction, when balanced chemically and electrically, is

$$H_2O_2 \rightleftharpoons O_2 + 2H^+ + 2e$$

STEP II. Equate the electron yield in the oxidation to the electron consumption in the reaction.

Since $5e$ were consumed in the balanced reduction half-reaction, whereas only $2e$ were produced by the oxidation of peroxide, the second half-reaction must be multiplied through by $\frac{5}{2}$ in order to yield five electrons.

$$\tfrac{5}{2}H_2O_2 \rightleftharpoons \tfrac{5}{2}O_2 + 5H^+ + 5e$$

STEP III. Add the half-reactions, canceling electrons.

$$MnO_4^- + 3H^+ + \tfrac{5}{2}H_2O_2 \rightleftharpoons Mn^{2+} + 4H_2O + \tfrac{5}{2}O_2$$

STEP IV. Reduce the coefficients to whole numbers and, if desired, express the equation in molecular form.

$$2MnO_4^- + 6H^+ + 5H_2O_2 \rightleftharpoons 2Mn^{2+} + 8H_2O + 5O_2$$

or, supposing that potassium permanganate was the oxidant and sulfuric acid the source of hydrogen ion,

$$2KMnO_4 + 3H_2SO_4 + 5H_2O_2 \rightleftharpoons 2MnSO_4 + 8H_2O + 5O_2 + K_2SO_4$$

A final check should show that the equation is balanced both chemically and electrically, and that it contains no free electrons.

Redox Equivalent Weights. As in calculation of acid-base titration results, it is convenient in redox analyses to employ the concept of equivalents in expressing concentrations. The equivalent in a redox reaction is that part of a mole that corresponds to the loss or gain of one "mole" of electrons. The simplest definition based upon this concept is this: the equivalent weight of a substance is equal to the molecular weight divided by the number of electrons that one molecule gains or loses in the reaction.

When the half-reaction is known, the equivalent weight is readily calculated. Thus for the reduction of permanganate (that is, the employment of permanganate as an oxidizing agent) in acid solution, the half-reaction is written

$$MnO_4^- + 8H^+ + 5e \rightleftharpoons Mn^{2+} + 4H_2O$$

Therefore the equivalent weight of $KMnO_4$ is MW/5 under these conditions.

The equivalent weight of a substance depends upon the reaction in which it is involved. In acid solution, EW = MW/5 for potassium permanganate, but in basic solution, where the half-reaction is written

$$MnO_4^- + 4H^+ + 3e \rightleftharpoons MnO_2 + 2H_2O$$

EW = MW/3 for this substance. The normality of a redox titrant may therefore be an ambiguous quantity unless the reaction is specified.

If an analytical method utilizes two or more redox reactions, the calculations of equivalent weight will be affected. Suppose the sample is reacted with another substance and then a reaction product is determined by redox titration. Then the equivalent weight of the sample is determined by the equation describing the final titration. For example, iodate in acid solution reacts with iodide.*

$$IO_3^- + 5I^- + 6H^+ \rightleftharpoons 3I_2 + 3H_2O \qquad (5.2)$$

According to the half-reaction

$$2IO_3^- + 12H^+ + 10e \rightleftharpoons I_2 + 6H_2O$$

the equivalent weight of iodate is MW/5, which it would be if reaction 5.2 actually described the way in which this analysis is carried out. Usually, however, the iodine produced in reaction 5.2 is titrated with thiosulfate

$$2S_2O_3^{2-} + I_2 \rightarrow S_4O_6^{2-} + 2I^- \qquad (5.3)$$

to complete the analysis. From the half-reaction $2e + I_2 \rightleftharpoons 2I^-$, we see that the equivalent weight of iodine in the final reaction is MW/2; therefore,

* This is an unusual reaction in that both the oxidant (IO_3^-) and the reductant (I^-) yield the same substance (I_2).

according to Eq. 5.2, each mole of iodate produces six equivalents of iodine, so the equivalent weight of iodate in this analysis is MW/6.

EXAMPLE 5.1. A sample of pure arsenious oxide weighing 0.2015 g was titrated in acid medium with potassium permanganate solution, with 39.80 ml being required. When a 0.3420 g sample of sodium oxalate was titrated with the same potassium permanganate solution, 40.15 ml was consumed. What is the purity of the sodium oxalate sample?

The first titration is a standardization. Arsenious oxide is dissolved in water to give arsenious acid,

$$As_2O_3 + 3H_2O \rightarrow 2H_3AsO_3$$

which is titrated with permanganate, the half-reaction being

$$H_3AsO_3 + H_2O \rightarrow H_3AsO_4 + 2H^+ + 2e$$

The equivalent weight of As_2O_3 is therefore MW/4, each mole of As_2O_3 yielding four equivalents of H_3AsO_3. In this case, 0.2015/49.45 equivalents, or 4.079 meq, of arsenious oxide was titrated. The normality of the potassium permanganate is $4.079/39.80 = 0.1024$.

The titration of oxalate showed that the sample contained (40.15) $(0.1024) = 4.111$ meq of sodium oxalate. Since according to the reactions

$$C_2O_4{}^{2-} + 2H^+ \rightleftharpoons H_2C_2O_4$$
$$H_2C_2O_4 \rightarrow 2CO_2 + 2H^+ + 2e$$

the equivalent weight of sodium oxalate is MW/2, there are $(0.004111) \times (67.00) = 0.2754$ g of sodium oxalate, so the sample purity is

$$\frac{(0.2754)(100)}{0.3420} = 80.53\%$$

5.2 Oxidation–Reduction Titrimetry

Introduction. In treating acid-base, precipitation, and complexation reactions we described titration behavior with the aid of equilibrium constants. Redox titration reactions may be similarly described; it is, however, conventional to utilize the electrical potential associated with the electron transfer process as a measure of the tendency for a reaction to occur, rather than the corresponding equilibrium constant. A titration curve for a redox titration is represented as a plot of potential (in volts) against volume of titrant. The theory of these systems is treated in Chapter 6. This section is a practical discussion of some known redox analytical methods, with theoretical accounts used only where necessary to avoid arbitrariness.

Titrations with Permanganate. For more than a century potassium permanganate has been used as a valuable oxidizing agent in redox titrimetry. Most of these analyses are conducted in acid solution, the half-reaction being written (as was seen in Section 5.1)

$$MnO_4^- + 8H^+ + 5e \rightleftharpoons Mn^{2+} + 4H_2O$$

Since solutions of manganous ions are colorless, and permanganate is intensely colored, the titrant serves as its own indicator.

It is apparent from the preceding equation that oxidations with permanganate are greatly affected by the pH of the solution. This factor is also important in determining the stability of standard solutions of permanganate, and maximum stability is obtained with a neutral solution. It has been observed also that manganese dioxide accelerates the decomposition of permanganate with the formation of even more manganese dioxide, which promotes the decomposition at an increased rate. Manganous ions react similarly by reacting with permanganate to form manganous dioxide. Since manganous ions are formed by the reduction of permanganate in acid medium, whereas manganese dioxide results from the reduction of permanganate in neutral or alkaline solution, it is important that neither reaction be permitted to take place in the standard solution of permanganate; otherwise a progressive decrease in its strength will occur. This is the reason for the heating and filtration steps (Experiment 5.1) in the preparation of permanganate solution; any oxidizable impurities in the water are reacted completely by heating the solution, and the precipitated MnO_2 is removed by filtration.

Potassium permanganate is not available in primary standard grade, so its solutions must be standardized against a pure reducing agent. The best substance for this purpose is arsenic trioxide, As_2O_3. (The reactions and calculations were discussed in Example 5.1.) Individual samples may be weighed out, or a standard solution may be accurately prepared and aliquots withdrawn for titration. In the latter procedure the solution should be essentially neutral, for it is found that acidic or basic solutions of arsenious oxide are not stable.

The oxidation of arsenious oxide by permanganate does not proceed rapidly at room temperature. In the presence of iodide, iodate, or iodine monochloride as a catalyst, the reaction occurs quickly and titration is possible at room temperature. The end point is detected by the appearance of the pink permanganate color. A more sensitive indication, especially for titrations with dilute permanganate solutions, is given by the redox indicator* *o*-phenanthroline-ferrous sulfate (ferroin); the color change is from pink to very faint blue.

* A redox indicator is a substance whose oxidized and reduced forms have different colors. Indicators may be characterized by their transition potentials and selected so that the transition potential coincides with the end point potential in the redox titration.

Permanganate oxidimetry is the basis for numerous analytical methods. The determination of *arsenic trioxide*, which is used in the standardization as discussed in the preceding paragraph, is commonly carried out by permanganate titration. *Iodide* is quantitatively oxidized to iodine by permanganate. Since iodine is also colored, a simple visual titration is not possible. This problem has been solved by adding hydrocyanic acid to the titration mixture; the oxidation by permanganate then occurs to give iodine cyanide:

$$I^- + HCN \rightleftharpoons ICN + H^+ + 2e$$

which is colorless. The end point is usually detected with ferroin. This titration is sometimes used to standardize permanganate solutions because of the availability of very pure potassium iodide. Another common primary standard is *sodium oxalate*. The stoichiometric relationship has been shown in Example 5.1, although the mechanism of the reaction is extremely complicated. The reaction is catalyzed by manganous ions, and it is therefore very slow at the beginning of the titration when there are no manganous ions. The reaction is carried out at an elevated temperature near the end point to ensure that the reaction occurs rapidly enough for an accurate location of the end point. Besides its use for the standardization of permanganate, this method is employed for the analysis of *oxalic acid* and its salts. Any metal that forms an insoluble oxalate may be assayed in this way, and until the development of EDTA titrimetry (see Chapter 4), a preferred method for the analysis of *calcium* involved its precipitation as calcium oxalate, filtration and solution of the precipitate in dilute sulfuric acid, and titration of the oxalic acid with permanganate. *Magnesium*, *zinc*, *barium*, *lead*, and *silver* can be determined similarly. Of course, this method is subject to interference by any associated metal that forms an insoluble oxalate.

The determination of *iron* is widely accomplished by permanganate titrimetry. Iron (II) is quantitatively oxidized to ferric ion. When this titration is carried out in sulfuric acid solution, the end point change is somewhat obscured by the yellow color produced by ferric sulfate, which turns the first pink permanganate color to orange. This difficulty is overcome by adding phosphoric acid, which forms a colorless complex with ferric ion. A more serious difficulty is presented by chloride ion in the presence of ferrous ion. Under certain conditions of acidity and speed of titration, a consumption of permanganate by chloride occurs, leading to positive errors in ferrous titrations. This error can be eliminated by adding manganous ions to the mixture. It is now usual to employ a solution (known as Reinhardt-Zimmermann solution, after the analysts who introduced it) composed of manganous sulfate, phosphoric acid, and sulfuric acid as the solvent for titrations of iron (II).

Many indirect analyses for oxidizing agents utilize this titration as the final step. For example, *persulfate* is reduced by ferrous iron to sulfate:

$$S_2O_8^{2-} + 2Fe^{2+} \rightarrow 2SO_4^{2-} + 2Fe^{3+}$$

A known excess of ferrous iron is reacted with the sample of persulfate, and then the excess of Fe^{2+} is back-titrated with standard permanganate. The method is applicable to the determination of *chlorate*, *perchlorate*, *nitrate*, *vanadium*, and *chromium*. *Permanganate* can itself be assayed in this way.

Ferric ion may be quantitatively reduced to ferrous ion, which is then titrated with permanganate. The reduction may be carried out with numerous reducing agents. Stannous chloride is suitable. Since the solution contains chloride after reduction, it is necessary to add Reinhardt-Zimmermann solution before titration with permanganate. Metals may be used as reducing agents in the ferric iron determination. A column of granules of amalgamated zinc (this is known as a Jones reductor), through which the ferric solution is passed, effects quantitative conversion of Fe^{3+} to Fe^{2+}, which is titrated with permanganate.

Hydrogen peroxide is oxidized by permanganate; the equation for this reaction is discussed in Section 5.1. This titration (Experiment 5.1) is used as the USP assay of hydrogen peroxide solution.

Iodometric Titrations. Iodine is reduced according to the half-reaotion

$$I_2 + 2e \rightleftharpoons 2I^-$$

Iodine is a nıld oxidizing agent. Few substances can be determined by *direct titration* with iodine, but two of these, the titrations of arsenite and of thiosulfate, are of great importance. Many substances are capable of oxidizing iodide to iodine, and these substances can therefore be analyzed by titrating the liberated iodine with thiosulfate; this is the *indirect titration* method.

Standard solutions of iodine may be prepared by accurately weighing the pure reagent. It is simpler to make up the solution from a reagent grade product and then to standardize it. Iodine is slightly soluble in water, but it forms a soluble triiodide ion in solutions of iodide.

$$I_2 + I^- \rightleftharpoons I_3^-$$

The equilibrium constant for this reaction is 768. The use of iodide in the solution both increases the solubility of iodine and decreases its volatility, thus contributing to the stability of iodine solutions.

Arsenic trioxide is the best primary standard substance for iodine solutions. This substance (which is present in aqueous solution as arsenious acid, H_3AsO_3) is oxidized by iodine according to the equation

$$H_3AsO_3 + I_2 + H_2O \rightleftharpoons HAsO_4^{2-} + 4H^+ + 2I^-$$

from which it is seen that the position of the equilibrium depends upon the pH.

A further pH dependence is imposed by the possibility of ionization of the arsenious acid. For the quantitative titration of arsenious acid with iodine at a convenient speed, it has been found that the pH should be in the approximate range 6–9; a lower pH is permissible if the titration is carried out slowly, whereas a higher pH is satisfactory if the solution contains iodide [1].

All indirect iodometric methods utilize the thiosulfate titration of iodine, so the reaction between these substances is of great importance. The stoichiometric equation is

$$2S_2O_3^{2-} + I_2 \rightleftharpoons S_4O_6^{2-} + 2I^-$$

If the titration mixture is alkaline, the oxidation to tetrathionate is not quantitative, the side reaction

$$S_2O_3^{2-} + 4I_2 + 10OH^- \rightleftharpoons 2SO_4^{2-} + 8I^- + 5H_2O$$

occurring with the production of sulfate. To eliminate this undesirable side reaction, titrations of iodine with thiosulfate are carried out in acidic or neutral solution.

Standard solutions of thiosulfate, on the other hand, are not stable at an acid pH. A pH of 9–10 gives the best stability. Oxygen may promote decomposition of thiosulfate, and this decomposition is catalyzed by copper impurities in the water. The purity of the water is therefore important. Microbial action is a major factor in the instability of thiosulfate solutions. Bacteria capable of utilizing thiosulfate as a source of sulfur cause rapid decomposition of standard solutions. By boiling the water and adding a preservative, thiosulfate solutions may be rendered fairly stable, but they should be restandardized frequently.

The standardization of thiosulfate is conveniently carried out against a standard iodine solution, although a disadvantage of this procedure is that the iodine is a secondary standard. Potassium iodate is a good primary standard; an exactly known amount of iodate is reacted with excess iodide in acid medium, with an equivalent amount of iodine being liberated by oxidation of the iodide:

$$IO_3^- + 5I^- + 6H^+ \rightarrow 3I_2 + 3H_2O$$

The iodine is titrated with the thiosulfate.

In the indirect iodometric method, exemplified by the titration of iodate as described in the preceding paragraph, a source of error is oxidation of iodide by atmospheric oxygen. Obviously such a side reaction will lead to a positive error, for iodine is produced and is titrated along with that from the sample reaction.

$$4I^- + O_2 + 4H^+ \rightarrow 2I_2 + 2H_2O$$

Copper catalyzes this reaction. It is also accelerated by strong light, so solutions containing iodide should be kept in dark bottles. Titrations should not be performed in direct sunlight.

The end point in iodometric titrations can be detected by means of the characteristic iodine color; about 5×10^{-5} N iodine, seen through 8 cm of solution, will produce a visible color. The sensitivity can be increased about twofold by the use of starch as an indicator. In the presence of iodide, iodine is adsorbed by starch to give a characteristic blue color. In the absence of iodide, no color is produced. The sensitivity of the indicator is increased by acid, and it is decreased by organic substances and by heat.

A different end point detection method in iodometric titrations utilizes a water-immiscible organic solvent, especially chloroform or carbon tetrachloride, into which iodine is preferentially partitioned and therefore concentrated. After each addition of titrant, the mixture is shaken well, the end point being marked by the first or last tinge of violet (depending upon whether a direct or indirect titration is being performed) in the organic phase. The violet color is due to a complex between the iodine and the organic solvent molecules.

Because of the simplicity and accuracy of the iodometric method, analytical chemists have exercised great ingenuity in designing assay schemes that include an iodometric titration as their final quantitative step. A few of the most important of these methods will be described briefly.

Iodide may be oxidized to iodine with excess iodate; the liberated iodine is titrated with thiosulfate. This reaction was discussed previously as the basis for the standardization of thiosulfate solutions. *Bromide* ion can be analyzed by an indirect procedure involving oxidation to bromate by sodium hypochlorite; the excess hypochlorite is destroyed with sodium formate, excess potassium iodide is added, and the liberated iodine, which is produced by reaction with bromate, is titrated with thiosulfate. *Hypochlorite* oxidizes iodide, in acid solutions, according to the reaction

$$OCl^- + 2I^- + 2H^+ \rightarrow Cl^- + I_2 + H_2O$$

The iodine is titrated with thiosulfate. A direct titration of hypochlorite is based upon the oxidation of a standard arsenite solution; the excess arsenite is titrated with standard iodine. The indirect determination of iodate by oxidation of iodide has already been discussed.

A method for *oxygen* dissolved in water is based upon the quantitative oxidation of manganous hydroxide by the oxygen. The solution is acidified and, in the presence of excess iodide, an equivalent amount of iodine is released and titrated with thiosulfate [2]. These are the reactions:

$$2Mn(OH)_2 + O_2 \rightleftharpoons 2H_2MnO_3$$

$$H_2MnO_3 + 4H^+ + 2I^- \rightleftharpoons I_2 + Mn^{2+} + 3H_2O$$

This technique is known as the Winkler method. *Hydrogen peroxide* oxidizes iodide to iodine, which is titrated with thiosulfate; the reaction is rather slow unless ammonium molybdate is added as a catalyst. *Hydrogen sulfide* may be oxidized to sulfate in an alkaline iodate solution; excess KI is added, and the liberated iodine, which is equivalent to the iodate unconsumed by sulfide, is titrated with thiosulfate. *Thiosulfate* is determined by adding excess standard iodine and back-titrating with standard thiosulfate; this reaction was discussed earlier. *Trivalent arsenic* is determined by direct titration with iodine as described for the standardization of iodine. *Dichromate* oxidizes iodide in acid medium:

$$Cr_2O_7^{2-} + 6I^- + 14H^+ \rightleftharpoons 2Cr^{3+} + 3I_2 + 7H_2O$$

The liberated iodine is titrated with thiosulfate. This reaction is sometimes employed in the standardization of thiosulfate, since potassium dichromate is readily obtainable in pure form. *Chromate* is also determined in this way, because in acidic solution chromate is converted to dichromate:

$$2CrO_4^{2-} + 2H^+ \rightleftharpoons Cr_2O_7^{2-} + H_2O$$

Metals such as *barium*, *strontium*, and *lead*, which form insoluble chromates, may be analyzed by precipitation as the chromate, filtration, dissolution of the salt in acid, addition of excess iodide, and titration of the liberated iodine with thiosulfate. *Ferric iron* oxidizes iodide and can be determined by indirect iodometric titration. *Cupric ion* is reduced by iodide to yield cuprous iodide:

$$2Cu^{2+} + 4I^- \rightarrow 2CuI + I_2$$

The iodine produced is titrated with thiosulfate. This procedure has been used for the standardization of thiosulfate, because very pure copper metal is easily obtained; this is dissolved in nitric acid and analyzed as described.

Many organic compounds may be analyzed iodometrically. *Thiols* are oxidized to disulfides by iodine:

$$2RSH + I_2 \rightarrow R—S—S—R + 2HI$$

The excess iodine is titrated with thiosulfate. *Hydroquinone* is oxidized to quinone under suitable conditions:

$$C_6H_4(OH)_2 + I_2 \rightleftharpoons C_6H_4O_2 + 2I^- + 2H^+$$

An excess of standard iodine is added and the back-titration is made with thiosulfate.

Titrations with Ceric Salts. In acidic medium ceric cerium is a strong oxidizing agent:

$$Ce^{4+} + e \rightleftharpoons Ce^{3+}$$

The simple one-electron reaction is an advantage of this system over others, such as permanganate, because the complications due to unstable intermediates are eliminated. Additional advantages are that hydrochloric acid does not interfere in analytical applications and that standard ceric solutions are extremely stable. The oxidizing power of tetravalent cerium depends upon the concentration and identity of the strong acid incorporated in the titration solution; this dependence results from complex formation between Ce^{4+} and the anions of the acids. Some specificity of oxidizing ability is attainable by proper selection of the acid.

Among the ceric salts available for preparation of standard solutions are ceric ammonium nitrate, $(NH_4)_2Ce(NO_3)_6$, ceric hydroxide, and ceric sulfate. The ceric titrant in dilute sulfuric acid is usually standardized against arsenic trioxide [3]. The oxidation of arsenic trioxide by ceric ion is extremely slow unless a catalyst is present, and osmium tetroxide commonly is employed for this purpose. Sodium oxalate is also a good standard substance; it is titrated with ceric sulfate in the presence of iodine chloride as a catalyst. Ferrous ion is another primary standard; it is obtained by dissolving pure iron metal in acid.

Redox indicators are usually employed to detect the end point in oxidimetric titrations with ceric sulfate. The most satisfactory indicator is ferrous *o*-phenanthroline (ferroin), whose reduced form is red and oxidized form pale blue.

Arsenic compounds can be analyzed by ceric titration. As in the standardization procedure, trivalent arsenic is titrated directly with ceric sulfate. Trivalent or pentavalent arsenic is determinable by reduction to elemental arsenic with hypophosphite, oxidation to pentavalent arsenic by excess standard ceric sulfate, and back-titration with standard arsenite. *Azides* are oxidized to nitrogen by tetravalent cerium:

$$2N_3^- + 2Ce^{4+} \rightarrow 3N_2 + 2Ce^{3+}$$

An excess of standard ceric titrant is added to the azide sample, and the excess is back-titrated with standard ferrous sulfate, using ferroin as the indicator. *Hydroxylamine* is quantitatively oxidized by Ce^{4+}.

$$2NH_2OH + 4Ce^{4+} \rightarrow N_2O + 4Ce^{3+} + H_2O + 4H^+$$

A back-titration procedure is used because the reaction is too slow for successful direct titration. The titration of *hydrogen peroxide* is feasible with ceric sulfate, even in the presence of organic substances. *Iron (II)*, preferably in a sulfuric acid medium, although hydrochloric acid is permissible, is directly titratable with ceric sulfate; this assay is employed for the analysis of many ferrous compounds of pharmaceutical importance. *Iron (III)*, after reduction to ferrous with silver or zinc, may be determined in the same way. *Oxalates* are analyzed by titration with ceric sulfate, as in the standardization against sodium oxalate; the procedure may be used to determine *calcium* after precipitation as the oxalate. Many other *organic acids*, including formic, tartaric, malonic, malic, benzoic, phthalic, and salicylic, are oxidized stoichiometrically to carbon dioxide and water by excess ceric sulfate in strongly acid medium; prolonged heating is required. The excess ceric is back-titrated. *Hydroxy compounds* can be oxidized quantitatively with Ce^{4+}, with formic acid the product under the recommended conditions. The reaction of glycerol is illustrative:

$$HO{-}CH_2CH(OH)CH_2{-}OH + 8Ce^{4+} + 3H_2O \rightarrow 3HCOOH + 8Ce^{3+} + 8H^+$$

Experiment 5.1. Titrations with Potassium Permanganate

REAGENTS

0.1 N Potassium Permanganate. Dissolve about 3.2 g of reagent grade potassium permanganate in 1 liter of distilled water. Boil the solution for 10–15 min and allow it to cool and stand overnight. Filter through a fine porosity sintered-glass funnel to remove any precipitated manganese dioxide. If a brown precipitate of MnO_2 is observed subsequently, the solution must be refiltered and restandardized. Store the solution in a glass-stoppered bottle previously cleaned with chromic acid cleaning solution* and well rinsed with distilled water.

The solution is standardized against arsenic trioxide. Accurately weigh about 0.2 g of dried primary standard As_2O_3 into a 250 ml flask. Dissolve the solid in 10 ml of 6 *N* sodium hydroxide. Dilute the solution to about 100 ml with water; add 10 ml of concentrated hydrochloric acid and 1 drop of 0.002 *M* potassium iodide or iodate. Titrate with the permanganate solution until the appearance of the first persistent faint pink color. Perform at least three titrations. Calculate the mean normality and its standard deviation.

PROCEDURES

Analysis of Hydrogen Peroxide Solution. Accurately pipet 2.0 ml of hydrogen peroxide solution USP into 20 ml of water in an Erlenmeyer flask. Add 20 ml of 10% sulfuric acid, and titrate to the first pink color with 0.1 *N* potassium permanganate. Calculate the weight of hydrogen peroxide in the sample, and calculate the weight/volume percentage of H_2O_2 in the sample solution.

Blank titrations should be carried out for every determination.

Analysis of Soluble Oxalate. Obtain a sample of oxalate from your instructor. Dry at 105°C and cool in a desiccator. Accurately weigh a portion equivalent to about 0.2 g of sodium oxalate into a 250 ml flask, and dissolve it in about 75 ml of 1.5 *N* sulfuric acid. Heat the solution to 75–85°C, and titrate with standard 0.1 *N* potassium permanganate. Near the end point add titrant drop

* Prepared by slowly adding 1500 ml of concentrated sulfuric acid to a solution of 200 g of sodium dichromate in 100 ml of water.

by drop until a pink color persists for 30 sec. The temperature at the end point should be about 60°C. Perform three analyses, and calculate the percent of sodium oxalate in the sample.

Analysis of Ferrous Sulfate. Ferrous sulfate occurs as the heptahydrate, $FeSO_4 \cdot 7H_2O$, and as dried ferrous sulfate, $FeSO_4$. Do not dry the sample. Accurately weigh about 1 g of $FeSO_4 \cdot 7H_2O$ or 0.8 g of $FeSO_4$, dissolve in 50 ml of 5% sulfuric acid (prepared by diluting 28 ml of concentrated sulfuric acid to 1000 ml with water), and titrate with standard 0.1 *N* potassium permanganate to the first permanent pink color. Calculate the purity of the sample as $FeSO_4 \cdot 7H_2O$ and as $FeSO_4$.

Experiment 5.2. Iodometric Titrations

REAGENTS

0.1 N Iodine. Dissolve about 40 g of iodate-free* potassium iodide in 20 ml of water. Dissolve about 12.7 g of iodine in this solution and dilute to 1 liter with water.

Standardize the solution against As_2O_3. Accurately weigh about 0.2 g of dried primary standard arsenious oxide into a 250 ml Erlenmeyer flask. Dissolve in 10 ml of 1 *N* sodium hydroxide, warming if necessary. Add 50 ml of water, 2 drops of methyl orange indicator, and 1 *N* hydrochloric acid until the color changes to pink. Dissolve 2 g of sodium bicarbonate in the solution, and add 50 ml of water. Add 5 ml of starch indicator solution, and titrate with the iodine solution until a permanent blue color appears. Calculate the normality of the iodine solution.

0.1 N Sodium Thiosulfate. Dissolve about 25 g of sodium thiosulfate pentahydrate in enough freshly boiled and cooled water to make 1 liter.

This solution may be standardized against potassium iodate. Accurately weigh about 0.15 g of dried primary standard potassium iodate into a 250 ml Erlenmeyer flask and dissolve in 25 ml of water. Add 2 g of iodate-free potassium iodide. Add 10 ml of 1 *N* hydrochloric acid and immediately titrate the liberated iodine with the thiosulfate solution, adding 3 ml of starch indicator solution near the end point. Calculate the normality of the thiosulfate solution.

The thiosulfate may also be standardized by titration of the standard iodine solution, using starch as the indicator.

Starch Indicator Solution. Make a smooth paste of 2 g of soluble starch and 10 mg of mercuric iodide by triturating with 30 ml of water. Add this paste to

* Test for iodate: add 1 ml of 5 *N* H_2SO_4 to 10 ml of a 10% solution of the potassium iodide; if a yellow color does not appear immediately, the product is free of iodate.

1 liter of boiling water and boil, if necessary, until a clear solution is obtained. Cool and store in a glass bottle.

The mercuric iodide is added as a preservative.

PROCEDURES

Analysis of Sodium Hypochlorite Solution. Deliver 3 ml of sodium hypochlorite solution (such as commercial household bleach) into a weighed glass-stoppered flask, and weigh accurately. Add 2 g of potassium iodide and 15 ml of 4 *N* sulfuric acid, and titrate the liberated iodine with standard 0.1 *N* sodium thiosulfate, using starch solution as the indicator. Calculate the percent of NaOCl (w/w) in the sample solution.

Analysis of Ascorbic Acid. Accurately weigh about 400 mg of ascorbic acid (vitamin C) into a 250 ml Erlenmeyer flask and dissolve it in 25 ml of 10% sulfuric acid plus 100 ml of water. Immediately titrate with standard 0.1 *N* iodine, adding starch solution as an indicator when the end point is approached. Calculate the percent purity of the ascorbic acid. (The equivalent weight of ascorbic acid is one-half its molecular weight in this reaction.)

References

1. Kolthoff, I. M. and R. Belcher, *Volumetric Analysis*, Vol. III, Interscience, New York, 1957.
2. Treadwell, F. P. and W. T. Hall, *Analytical Chemistry*, Vol. II, 9th ed., John Wiley and Sons, New York, 1942.
3. Schlitt, R. C. and K. Simpson, *Anal. Chem.*, **41,** 1722 (1969).

Problems

1. Balance these equations:

(*a*) $Cr_2O_7^{2-} + Fe^{2+} = Cr^{3+} + Fe^{3+}$

(*b*) $ClO_3^- + Sn^{2+} = Cl^- + Sn^{4+}$

(*c*) $MnO_4^- + H_2C_2O_4 = Mn^{2+} + CO_2$

(*d*) $PbO_2 + I^- = I_2 + Pb^{2+}$

(*e*) $Cr_2O_7^{2-} + V^{3+} = VO^{2+} + Cr^{3+}$

(*f*) $OBr^- + NH_3 = Br^- + N_2$

(*g*) $KIO_3 + N_2H_4 + HCl = ICl + N_2$

(*h*) $H_2O_2 + I^- = I_2 + H_2O$

2. Calculate the weight of arsenic trioxide, As_2O_3, required to make 1 liter of 0.1000 *N* arsenious acid, H_3AsO_3.

3. 0.2800 g of pure copper metal was dissolved in acid. After appropriate adjustment of the solution conditions, an excess of potassium iodide was added, and the liberated

iodine was titrated with 0.1050 *N* thiosulfate. How many milliliters of titrant were consumed?

4. Devise a practical method for the quantitative analysis of each substance in these mixtures. You may use more than one portion of sample if necessary. (*a*) An aqueous solution of sulfuric acid and oxalic acid. (*b*) Ferrous sulfate and ferric sulfate.

5. One milliliter of 0.1000 *N* potassium permanganate (used in acidic medium) is equivalent to how many milligrams of the following substances? (*a*) hydrogen peroxide; (*b*) sodium iodide; (*c*) ferrous sulfate; (*d*) arsenic trioxide; (*e*) calcium oxalate.

Summary: Part One

The student may actually enjoy, at this point in the book, browsing through the *National Formulary* and the *United States Pharmacopeia* and reading the assay specifications. Simple titrations account for a surprisingly large number of these assay methods, and these first five chapters provide a basis for understanding most of them. It is not very important that a particular indicator, titrant, or sample in a USP or NF assay may not have been mentioned in Chapters 1–5; it *is* important, however, that in most of these instances the basis of the analysis (type of reaction, nature of end point detection, choice of conditions) should now be clear to the student.

In many assay procedures a titration serves as the final step, being preceded by other chemical reactions, separation techniques, or other manipulations. These operations are treated in later chapters, but it may be noted here that titrimetry is a widely applicable approach for quantitative analysis, and is often coupled with other methods.*

One of the advantages of titrimetry as an analytical approach is that it is an absolute method of analysis. The meaning of this statement will not be fully clear until we have studied methods lacking this attribute, but it simply means that, by titrimetric analysis, the purity of a sample compound can be determined without reference to a separate specimen of that same compound (whose purity might itself be in doubt). For example, a sodium hydroxide solution can be standardized against primary standard grade potassium biphthalate, and then the purity of, say, a sample of acetic acid can be determined by titration with the NaOH solution. Thus the purity of the acetic acid has been obtained without making any assumptions about acetic acid (that is, without using acetic acid as a primary standard). Such assumptions were of course made about the potassium biphthalate, and independent evidence must be available to support them.

* A valuable collection of titrimetric methods and applications has been compiled by M. R. F. Ashworth in *Titrimetric Organic Analysis*, Parts I and II, Interscience, New York, 1964–1965.

A titration is feasible when (1) the titration reaction is rapid compared with the speed of titration; (2) its equilibrium constant is large enough to give a sharp "break" at the end point; (3) a method of end point detection is available. Whether or not the titration should be used for a particular analysis will depend upon many factors, including the sensitivity required, possible interfering substances that would also be titrated, and alternative methods of analysis.

Part Two: Physical and Instrumental Methods

This part of the book introduces analytical methods based upon measurements of physical properties and measurements with instruments. Separation of the properties of matter into physical and chemical properties is arbitrary but often convenient. A physical property can be defined as a quality of matter that is manifested without the occurrence of chemical reactions. The arbitrariness enters when we define chemical reactions. Solubility, for example, can be thought of as either a chemical or a physical property.

The next 10 chapters describe methods that find daily use in analytical laboratories. Many other physical techniques are available, although these are of more limited applicability in pharmaceutical analysis. Some of these additional methods are described briefly in the summary of this part following Chapter 15.

6 POTENTIOMETRY

6.1 Electromotive Force of Chemical Cells

Chemical Cells. A chemical cell (galvanic cell) is a system in which chemical energy is transformed into electrical energy. The chemical reaction involved is an oxidation-reduction reaction, and as we have seen in Chapter 5, a redox reaction is an electron-transfer process. It is the transfer of electrons from one redox half-reaction to the second half-reaction that is manifested as available electrical energy.

Consider the chemical cell composed of a piece of zinc metal partly immersed in a solution of zinc sulfate and a piece of copper in a cupric sulfate solution, with the two solutions in electrical contact (but not mixed) and the electrodes connected externally by an electric conductor (Fig. 6.1). The voltmeter *V* will indicate that a difference in electric potential exists between the two pieces of metal (the electrodes). The half-reactions in this cell (which is called the Daniell cell) are

$$Zn \rightleftharpoons Zn^{2+} + 2e$$

$$2e + Cu^{2+} \rightleftharpoons Cu$$

If the concentrations of zinc ion and cupric ion are each about 1 *M*, these reactions will proceed in the directions written. That is, the zinc electrode is oxidized (it dissolves), providing electrons to the external circuit. Copper ions are reduced to copper (which is deposited on the copper electrode), thus consuming the electrons provided by the oxidation of zinc. These reactions are the source of the electric potential difference (or, synonymously, *electromotive force*, emf), which results from the charge difference between the two electrodes.

Chemical cells are represented schematically by chemical symbols, with physical states and chemical compositions often specified; the Daniell cell, for example, is written

$$Zn \mid ZnSO_4\ (c_1) \parallel CuSO_4\ (c_2) \mid Cu$$

A single vertical line represents a phase boundary across which a potential

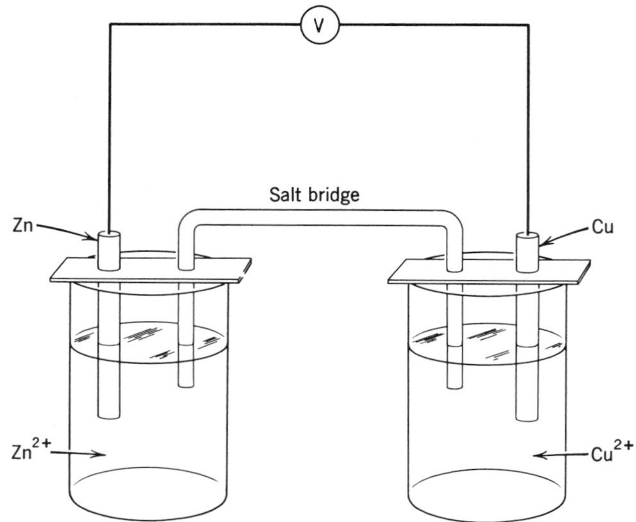

Fig. 6.1. The Daniell cell. The salt bridge is a gel containing an electrolyte; it permits the passage of current, but prevents mixing of the solutions.

difference exists; this potential difference is called an *electrode potential.* A double vertical line signifies a boundary between two solutions of different composition (a "salt bridge") across which a potential difference exists; this is a *liquid-junction potential.* The rest of this section is concerned mainly with the description of electrode potentials, which is upon a sound theoretical basis. Liquid-junction potentials, on the other hand, are undesirable phenomena to the electrochemist, because they are not directly related to the cell reaction. The source of the liquid-junction potential is recognized, however. Consider the solution interface HCl (0.1 *M*)‖ HCl (0.01 *M*). Both hydrogen ions and chloride ions will tend to diffuse from the more concentrated into the less concentrated solution. However, hydrogen ions diffuse much more rapidly than do chloride ions, with the result that the right-hand side of the boundary develops a net positive charge. This charge difference across the solution boundary is the source of the liquid-junction potential. Since, in the relatively simple example given here, the liquid-junction potential depends only upon the relative mobilities of the cation and anion diffusing across the boundary, this potential could evidently be reduced by incorporating a high concentration of a salt with its cation and anion of the same ionic mobility; most of the current would thus be carried by this salt, and the potential developed by the charge separation would be reduced. Potassium ion and chloride ion have nearly the same mobility, so KCl is usually used in salt bridges in order to minimize the liquid-junction potential. Typical liquid-junction potentials are in the range 1–20 mV [1].

Concentration and Activity. Many of the quantitative relationships describing solution behavior are relatively simple functions of concentration terms. The equilibrium constant is an important example. For the general reaction

$$aA + bB \rightleftharpoons mM + nN \tag{6.1}$$

the quantity K_c is defined as

$$K_c = \frac{c_M{}^m c_N{}^n}{c_A{}^a c_B{}^b} \tag{6.2}$$

where c_A represents (usually) the equilibrium molar concentration of A, etc. We expect K_c to be a constant independent of the equilibrium concentrations. In practice, however, it is observed that this "constant" varies somewhat with alterations in the concentrations. Because the form of Eq. 6.2 is so conveniently simple, this variability of K_c has been circumvented by inventing the concept of *activity* (which may be crudely thought of as an effective, or corrected, concentration), and by retaining the usual equation with activities replacing concentrations.

$$K = \frac{a_M{}^m a_N{}^n}{a_A{}^a a_B{}^b} \tag{6.3}$$

This quantity K is a true constant (at constant temperature and pressure) because the activities have been defined to make it so. The activity and concentration of a solute are linearly related as

$$a = fc \tag{6.4}$$

where f is a proportionality constant called the *activity coefficient*. The most frequently employed convention is to define, arbitrarily, the value of the activity coefficient to be unity in the infinitely dilute solution.* Thus in the infinitely dilute solution the activity of a solute is equal to its concentration, whereas at higher concentrations the activity and concentration usually differ.

As suggested previously, the numerical value of the activity coefficient depends upon an arbitrary assignment of a standard state, which may be chosen for convenience. The conventions we shall employ (which are the usual ones) lead to these estimates of activity.

1. The activity of a solute in the infinitely dilute solution is equal to the molar concentration of the solute. At finite concentrations the activity is different from the concentration.

* For most work a solution 10^{-4} M may be considered infinitely dilute. The activity coefficient of a solute may depend not only upon its own concentration but also upon the concentrations of other solutes.

2. The activity of the solvent is equal to its mole fraction N, where N is the ratio of the number of moles of solvent to the total number of moles. The mole fraction of pure solvent is one. This is why the "concentration" of water does not explicitly appear in Eqs. 1.4 and 1.5 of Chapter 1.

3. The activity of a gas is equal to its partial pressure in atmospheres.

4. The activity of a solid is equal to one. This is the reason that the "concentration" of the solid phase does not appear in the solubility product expression (Chapter 3).

The Nernst Equation. A chemical system such as the general reaction represented by Eq. 6.1 tends to assume an equilibrium configuration characteristic of the components, the temperature, and the pressure. In its progress toward equilibrium, the system can yield work. The maximum net work obtainable from a process at constant temperature and pressure is called the free energy change of the process. The free energy change of a process is symbolized ΔG. (Free energy is also referred to as Gibbs free energy, after J. Willard Gibbs, an American physicist who provided much of the theoretical development of thermodynamics.) The condition for a spontaneous process is that ΔG be negative for the process. Since a system at equilibrium is incapable of doing work on its surroundings, the condition for equilibrium is that $\Delta G = 0$.

It is a fundamental result of thermodynamics [2] that the molar free energy G_i of any substance i is given by

$$G_i = G_i^{0} + RT \ln a_i \tag{6.5}$$

where R is the gas constant (8.314 V-C/deg), T is the absolute temperature, a_i is the activity of the substance, and G_i^{0} is its free energy in the standard state. The free energy change of reaction 6.1 is given by

$$\Delta G = G \text{ (products)} - G \text{ (reactants)}$$

or

$$\Delta G = mG_M + nG_N - aG_A - bG_B \tag{6.6}$$

Combining Eqs. 6.5 and 6.6 leads to

$$\Delta G = \Delta G^0 + RT \ln \left(\frac{a_M{}^m a_N{}^n}{a_A{}^a a_B{}^b} \right) \tag{6.7}$$

where $\Delta G^0 = mG_M{}^0 + nG_N{}^0 - aG_A{}^0 - bG_B{}^0$. Equation 6.7, which is called the reaction isotherm, relates the free energy change of a reaction to the activities of the system components. It is important to note that *the activities specified in Eq. 6.7 do not necessarily refer to equilibrium conditions.*

A useful relationship may now be obtained by letting the activities in Eq. 6.7 assume their values at equilibrium. Then the ratio within parentheses in Eq. 6.7 may be replaced by K, the equilibrium constant (Eq. 6.3); moreover, as we noted above, $\Delta G = 0$ for a process at equilibrium. Thus Eq. 6.7 leads to

$$\Delta G^0 = -RT \ln K \tag{6.8}$$

which relates the equilibrium constant to the standard free energy change ΔG^0, which is the change in free energy when the reactants and products are in their standard states. ΔG^0 is usually expressed in calories per mole, so in using Eq. 6.8 the appropriate value of R is 1.987 cal/deg · mole.

One of the kinds of work that a chemical system can do is electrical work; we began this chapter with a description of systems, called chemical cells, that convert chemical energy to electrical energy. If such a cell operates under reversible conditions,* all the work will be manifested as electrical work, and this must therefore be equivalent to the free energy change of the system, which is the maximum work (exclusive of work of expansion) that can be performed. If the emf of the cell is E V, and the number of equivalents of electricity transferred in the cell reaction is n, then the free energy change is

$$\Delta G = -n\mathbf{F}E \tag{6.9}$$

where $\mathbf{F}$ is the Faraday, or an equivalent of electricity; $\mathbf{F} = 96{,}493$ C. The negative sign is introduced to achieve agreement between the conventions that a spontaneous reaction is associated with a negative ΔG and a positive E. Sign conventions will be considered in detail later.

Equations 6.7 and 6.9 are combined to yield

$$E = E^0 - \frac{RT}{n\mathbf{F}} \ln L \tag{6.10}$$

where $E^0 = -\Delta G^0/n\mathbf{F}$, and $L = (a_M{}^m a_N{}^n / a_A{}^a a_B{}^b)$. Equation 6.10 is the *Nernst equation.* It relates the potential of a chemical cell to the activities of the reactants and products. Equation 6.8 leads to a relationship between the equilibrium constant and E^0, the potential of the cell when $L = 1$:

$$E^0 = \frac{RT}{n\mathbf{F}} \ln K \tag{6.11}$$

At 25°C the Nernst equation takes the form

$$E = E^0 - \frac{0.059}{n} \log L \tag{6.12}$$

where the final term has been converted from natural logarithms to base 10 logarithms.

* Reversible operation requires that an infinitesimal amount of reaction occur, so that the system is always very close to equilibrium. The reversible emf of a cell must be determined with zero or infinitesimal current flowing through the cell.

Electrochemical Conventions. An isolated redox half-reaction cannot be observed, and so the potential of a single electrode cannot be measured. A complete electrical circuit is required, and this means that two electrodes are involved in every emf measurement. Every chemical cell is composed of at least two electrodes. Although it is impossible to determine the potential of a single electrode, it is convenient to employ this concept in calculations, and so we consider a cell emf to be equal to the sum of its electrode potentials. Thus for the Daniell cell,

$$Zn \mid Zn^{2+} \| Cu^{2+} \mid Cu$$

the cell potential is written

$$E_{cell} = E_{Zn,Zn^{2+}} + E_{Cu^{2+},Cu} \tag{6.13}$$

It is important to notice how the order of the subscripts indicates whether the half-reaction is a reduction or an oxidation. Each cell is composed of one reduction and one oxidation.

It becomes necessary at this point to consider the sign of a potential. Two entirely distinct concepts are involved in describing sign conventions of electrochemical systems [3].

1. *The potential of the physical electrode.* Since it is possible to measure only the potential of a cell, that is, the potential difference between two electrodes, whereas for theoretical manipulations single electrode potentials would be convenient, it has been universally agreed to assign an arbitrary emf to one electrode; then by forming a cell of this reference electrode with any other electrode, the potential of the second electrode can be measured. By international agreement the reference electrode is the standard hydrogen electrode, S.H.E. (also called the normal hydrogen electrode, N.H.E.) represented as Pt, H_2 (1 atm) $\mid H^+$ ($a = 1$); the electrode reaction is $H_2 \rightleftharpoons 2H^+ + 2e$. The potential of the standard hydrogen electrode is defined to be 0 V at all temperatures.

If a cell of the S.H.E. and a second electrode is now formed, the measured cell emf can be ascribed to the second electrode. But in addition to its magnitude, this electrode potential must be characterized by sign. Consider the cell

$$Zn \mid Zn^{2+} \ (a = 1) \| H^+ \ (a = 1) \mid H_2 \ (1 \text{ atm}), Pt$$

The cell reaction is

$$Zn + 2H^+ \rightleftharpoons Zn^{2+} + H_2$$

Zinc is oxidized, releasing electrons at the zinc electrode. This means that the zinc electrode is negative relative to the standard hydrogen electrode, simply because we have decided (with Benjamin Franklin) to call the charge of an electron negative. No matter in what direction on the paper we write the cell, or how it is oriented on the laboratory bench, the zinc electrode will be negative relative to the S.H.E. The sign of an electrode potential depends solely upon whether the electrode furnishes electrons to or consumes electrons from the S.H.E. If neither of the electrodes is the S.H.E., the same general considerations apply; one of the electrodes (that at which oxidation occurs) is negative relative to the other. The electrode at which oxidation occurs is the anode; the electrode where reduction takes place is the cathode.

2. *The potential of a half-reaction.* This concept has nothing whatever to do with the potential of an electrode as described in the preceding two paragraphs. A convenient place to start is with the free energy change and with Eq. 6.9. If we accept Eq. 6.9 and the thermodynamic conclusion that a negative value of ΔG means that the reaction is spontaneous, then it follows that E for the spontaneous reaction must be positive. If the reaction is written in the opposite direction, it is nonspontaneous, so ΔG must be positive and E must be negative. The emf of a reaction changes its sign when the written reaction is reversed. The potential of the reaction

$$Zn \rightleftharpoons Zn^{2+} + 2e$$

is written $E_{Zn,Zn^{2+}}$, whereas that of the reverse action

$$Zn^{2+} + 2e \rightleftharpoons Zn$$

is $-E_{Zn,Zn^{2+}} = E_{Zn^{2+},Zn}$. This illustrates the convenience of the subscript order in helping to reduce confusion. We now can see that an equivalent form of Eq. 6.13 is

$$E_{cell} = E_{Zn,Zn^{2+}} - E_{Cu,Cu^{2+}}$$

The electrode that appears on the left-hand side of a chemical cell representation is arbitrarily considered to be the one at which oxidation occurs. Thus for the cell

$$\text{Pt, H}_2\ (1\ \text{atm})\ |\ \text{H}^+\ (a = 1) \|\ \text{Zn}^{2+}\ (a = 1)\ |\ \text{Zn} \tag{6.14}$$

the cell reaction is

$$H_2 + Zn^{2+} \rightleftharpoons 2H^+ + Zn$$

If the cell reaction as written is spontaneous, then

(*a*) The cell potential is (+), by convention 2.

(*b*) The left-hand electrode, at which oxidation is occurring, is negative, by convention 1.

(*c*) The current flow in the external circuit is from left to right.

(*d*) Positive ions flow from left to right in the cell, and negative ions flow from right to left.

These conclusions apply to *any* cell whose cell reaction, written as previously specified, is spontaneous. The cell reaction of cell 6.14 happens to be nonspontaneous as written, so the relations (*a*) to (*d*) are reversed.

Anson [4] has given a particularly clear discussion of the electro-chemical conventions. He has pointed out that much of the confusion associated with sign conventions is caused by the application of the same words—positive and negative—to the totally different concepts discussed above, and he suggests that if Benjamin Franklin had named the opposite kinds of electric charge black and white instead of negative and positive, much subsequent confusion might have been avoided. The potential of an electrode could then be labeled black or white E volts, while the potential of a half-reaction could be positive or negative, and there would be no confusing the two concepts.

Standard Potentials and Their Applications. We have agreed to adopt as the standard half-reaction $H_2 \rightleftharpoons 2H^+ + 2e$, as noted earlier, and to define its potential, when $p_{H_2} = 1$ atm and $a_{H^+} = 1$, to be 0 V at all temperatures. From the Nernst equation for this reaction

$$E = E^0_{H_2,H^+} - \frac{0.059}{2} \log \frac{a_{H^+}{}^2}{p_{H_2}}$$

it follows that $E^0_{H_2,H^+} = 0$ for the hydrogen electrode. If we combine the S.H.E. with any other electrode, it is evident that the measured cell potential is to be ascribed entirely to the second electrode. For the cell

$$\text{Pt, } H_2 \text{ (1 atm)} \mid H^+ \ (a = 1),\ Zn^{2+} \ (a = 1) \mid Zn$$

the cell potential is $E_{\text{cell}} = E_{H_2,H^+} + E_{Zn^{2+},Zn}$. Since $E_{H_2,H^+} = 0$ for the S.H.E., then $E_{\text{cell}} = E_{Zn^{2+},Zn}$. Applying the Nernst equation (at 25°C):

$$E_{Zn^{2+},Zn} = E^0_{Zn^{2+},Zn} - \frac{0.059}{2} \log \frac{a_{Zn}}{a_{Zn^{2+}}}$$

By our earlier definition of the standard state of solids, $a_{Zn} = 1$; therefore the final term is equal to zero, and $E_{Zn^{2+},Zn} = E^0_{Zn^{2+},Zn}$. This quantity, $E^0_{Zn^{2+},Zn}$, is called the *standard potential* of the zinc electrode. It is the reduction potential of the zinc couple when all reactants are in their standard states of unit activity (or more generally when $L = 1$ in the Nernst equation for the half-reaction). The standard potential is always the potential of the reduction half-reaction. The sign conventions for the emf of a half-reaction apply to standard potentials. Thus for the zinc electrode

$$E^0_{Zn^{2+},Zn} = -E^0_{Zn,Zn^{2+}}$$

Only $E^0_{Zn^{2+},Zn}$ should be referred to as the standard potential. This quantity has been determined to be -0.76 V. (This negative sign is a manifestation of the sign of the actual physical electrode, relative to the S.H.E.; see p. 114.)

TABLE 6.1
Standard Potentials at 25°C[a]

Half-reaction	E^0 (V)
$Zn^{2+} + 2e = Zn$	−0.76
$2CO_2 + 2H^+ + 2e = H_2C_2O_4$	−0.49
$Fe^{2+} + 2e = Fe$	−0.44
$Cd^{2+} + 2e = Cd$	−0.40
$AgI + e = Ag + I^-$	−0.15
$Sn^{2+} + 2e = Sn$	−0.14
$Pb^{2+} + 2e = Pb$	−0.13
$2H^+ + 2e = H_2$	0
$S_4O_6{}^{2-} + 2e = 2S_2O_3{}^{2-}$	+0.08
$AgBr + e = Ag + Br^-$	+0.10
$Sn^{4+} + 2e = Sn^{2+}$	+0.15
$AgCl + e = Ag + Cl^-$	+0.22
$Cu^{2+} + 2e = Cu$	+0.34
$I_3{}^- + 2e = 3I^-$	+0.54
$H_3AsO_4 + 2H^+ + 2e = H_2AsO_3 + H_2O$	+0.56
$Fe^{3+} + e = Fe^{2+}$	+0.77
$Ag^+ + e = Ag$	+0.80
$Cu^{2+} + I^- + e = CuI$	+0.86
$IO_3{}^- + 6H^+ + 5e = \frac{1}{2}I_2 + 3H_2O$	+1.20
$Cr_2O_7{}^{2-} + 14H^+ + 6e = 2Cr^{3+} + 7H_2O$	+1.33
$Cl_2 + 2e = 2Cl^-$	+1.36
$MnO_4{}^- + 8H^+ + 5e = Mn^{2+} + 4H_2O$	+1.51
$MnO_4{}^- + 4H^+ + 3e = MnO_2 + 2H_2O$	+1.70

[a] From Ref. 3 and W. M. Latimer, *Oxidation States of the Elements and Their Potentials in Aqueous Solutions*, 2nd ed., Prentice-Hall, Englewood Cliffs, N.J. 1952

The quantity $E^0_{Zn,Zn^{2+}}$ is then +0.76 V. (This sign change is a manifestation of the sign conventions governing the potential of the half-reaction, p. 115.)

Table 6.1 gives some half-reactions and their standard potentials. The quantity E^0_{cell} for an overall reaction is computed by combining the standard electrode potentials bearing in mind the conventions for the emf of a half-reaction. For the cell Zn | Zn^{2+}, Cl^-, AgCl | Ag the overall reaction is

$$Zn + 2AgCl \rightleftharpoons Zn^{2+} + 2Ag + 2Cl^-$$

and $E^0_{cell} = E^0_{Zn,Zn^{2+}} + E^0_{AgCl,Ag} = 0.76 + 0.22 = +0.98$ V. It is only because the electrons cancel exactly in a net reaction (that is, the amount of oxidation is equivalent to the amount of reduction) that this simple addition gives the proper quantity. In calculating E^0_{cell} no account should be taken of the numbers of electrons involved in the half-reactions. If two half-reactions are added together to give a third *half-reaction*, then the standard potential of the third half-reaction can be obtained by weighting the potentials according to the number of electrons contributed [3]. The simplest way to do this is by converting potentials to free energy changes (from the equation $\Delta G^0 = -n\mathbf{F}E^0$), which are directly additive; after addition, the resultant free energy change is converted back to a potential (see Example 6.3).

We are now in a position to understand much of the practical chemistry described in Chapter 5. According to the convention determining the sign of an electrode, which is reflected in the signs of the potentials in Table 6.1, the more negative electrode is the one at which oxidation is occurring. If then any two of the half-cells represented in Table 6.1 are combined to form a cell with all reaction components in their standard states, the half-reaction that is more negative will represent the oxidation. Thus we predict that permanganate ($E^0 = +1.51$ V) will oxidize arsenious acid ($E^0 = +0.56$ V). Iodine ($E^0 = +0.54$ V) oxidizes (is reduced by) thiosulfate ($E^0 = +0.08$ V). The more positive the standard potential, the greater the oxidizing power. Iodine is therefore considered to be a mild oxidizing agent, whereas permanganate is a powerful oxidant.

The situation is actually more complicated than is indicated in the preceding paragraph, because the standard potentials are strictly applicable only when activities, not concentrations, appear in the Nernst equation. In fact, in most practical work the concentrations of reactants and other solution components may be quite high, and their activities may differ markedly from their concentrations. A further complication is the operation of factors such as acid-base equilibria and complex formation, which may alter the concentrations of the electroactive species, and the usual presence of a liquid-junction potential of unknown magnitude. To overcome these complications a sort of practical standard potential has been introduced. This is called the *formal potential.* The formal potential of an electrode (often symbolized $E^{0\prime}$) is the observed potential versus the S.H.E. when the formal concentrations of the oxidized and reduced substances are equal; the concentrations of other substances must be specified. For example, the standard potential of the Fe^{3+},Fe^{2+} couple is $+0.77$ V (Table 6.1), whereas the formal potential of the Fe^{3+},Fe^{2+} couple in 0.5 M H_3PO_4 – 1 M H_2SO_4 is $+0.61$ V. This alteration occurs because phosphoric acid forms a complex with ferric ion, in effect displacing the equilibrium $Fe^{3+} + e = Fe^{2+}$ to the left, and rendering ferric ion a less powerful oxidizing agent. The oxidizing power of Ce (IV) is subject to the same type of effect, with the formal potential of the reaction $Ce^{4+} + e = Ce^{3+}$ being $+1.70$ V in 1 M $HClO_4$, $+1.61$ volts in 1 M HNO_3, and $+1.44$ V in 1 M H_2SO_4. It is often possible to take advantage of these changes in formal potentials to permit some selectivity and control in redox analysis. An example is the reaction

$$2Fe^{3+} + 2I^- \rightleftharpoons 2Fe^{2+} + I_2 \tag{6.15}$$

which can be used for the determination of iron, since ferric ion oxidizes iodide quantitatively. If fluoride is added, a stable complex is formed between ferric ion and fluoride, altering the potential of the ferric-ferrous couple so that oxidation of iodide does not occur. This behavior is taken advantage of to eliminate interference by iron in the iodometric analysis of other substances [5]. Reaction 6.15 can even be made to reverse its direction by adding EDTA; then ferrous ion can be titrated with iodine.

EXAMPLE 6.1. Calculate the potential of the following Daniell cell at 25°C. Assume activities equal concentrations, and ignore the liquid-junction potential.

$$\text{Zn} \mid \text{Zn}^{2+}\ (0.15\ M) \| \text{Cu}^{2+}\ (0.01\ M) \mid \text{Cu}$$

The cell reaction is

$$\text{Zn} + \text{Cu}^{2+} \rightleftharpoons \text{Zn}^{2+} + \text{Cu}$$

so the cell emf is given by

$$E_{\text{cell}} = E^0_{\text{cell}} - \frac{0.059}{n} \log \frac{a_{\text{Cu}} a_{\text{Zn}^{2+}}}{a_{\text{Cu}^{2+}} a_{\text{Zn}}}$$

Since $E^0_{\text{cell}} = E^0_{\text{Zn,Zn}^{2+}} + E^0_{\text{Cu}^{2+},\text{Cu}} = +0.76\text{ V} + 0.34\text{ V} = +1.10\text{ V}, n = 2$, and the activities of the metals are unity, this becomes

$$E_{\text{cell}} = +1.10 - 0.03 \log \frac{0.15}{0.01}$$

$$E_{\text{cell}} = +1.10 - 0.05 = +1.05\text{ V}$$

The cell reaction is spontaneous as written because the cell potential is positive. You should satisfy yourself that, even if the cell had been written in the reverse direction, the correct conclusion would have been reached concerning the direction of the overall reaction; that is, that zinc metal is oxidized and cupric ion is reduced.

EXAMPLE 6.2. What is the equilibrium constant at 25°C of the following reaction?

$$\text{Sn}^{2+} + 2\text{Fe}^{3+} \rightleftharpoons \text{Sn}^{4+} + 2\text{Fe}^{2+}$$

From Table 6.1 the cell emf E^0 is calculated as $E^0 = E^0_{\text{Sn}^{2+},\text{Sn}^{4+}} + E^0_{\text{Fe}^{3+},\text{Fe}^{2+}} = -0.15\text{ V} + 0.77\text{ V} = +0.62\text{ V}$. Applying Eq. 6.11,

$$\log K = \frac{nE^0}{0.059} = \frac{+1.24}{0.059}$$

$$\log K = 21.0$$

$$K = 10^{21}$$

EXAMPLE 6.3. What is the standard potential for the following half-reaction?

$$Fe^{3+} + 3e = Fe$$

Let us first treat this in a general way. Consider two half-reactions that, when added, give the desired half-reaction.

Half-reaction	E^0	ΔG^0
$ox_1 + n_1 e = red_1$	$E_1{}^0$	$-n_1 \mathbf{F} E_1{}^0$
$ox_2 + n_2 e = red_2$	$E_2{}^0$	$-n_2 \mathbf{F} E_2{}^0$
$ox_1 + (n_1 + n_2)e = red_2$	$E_3{}^0$	$-\mathbf{F}(n_1 E_1{}^0 + n_2 E_2{}^0)$

where the half-reactions have been selected so that $ox_2 \equiv red_1$. Since the free energy changes are additive, the standard potential $E_3{}^0$ is given by

$$E_3{}^0 = \frac{n_1 E_1{}^0 + n_2 E_2{}^0}{n_1 + n_2}$$

The appropriate half-reactions for this problem are found in Table 6.1.

$$\begin{aligned} Fe^{3+} + e &= Fe^{2+} \qquad & E^0_{Fe^{3+},Fe^{2+}} &= +0.77 \\ Fe^{2+} + 2e &= Fe \qquad & E^0_{Fe^{2+},Fe} &= -0.44 \\ \hline Fe^{3+} + 3e &= Fe \end{aligned}$$

$$E^0_{Fe^{3+},Fe} = \frac{+0.77 - 2(0.44)}{3} = -0.04 \text{ V}$$

EXAMPLE 6.4. What is the solubility product of silver iodide?

The solubility product is simply the equilibrium constant of the reaction

$$AgI \rightleftharpoons Ag^+ + I^-$$

This can be regarded as the overall reaction composed of the two half-reactions

$$\begin{aligned} AgI + e &\rightleftharpoons Ag + I^- \\ Ag &\rightleftharpoons Ag^+ + e \\ \hline AgI &\rightleftharpoons Ag^+ + I^- \end{aligned}$$

The cell potential E^0 for the overall reaction is readily calculated from data in Table 6.1.

$$E^0_{cell} = E^0_{AgI,Ag} + E^0_{Ag,Ag^+} = -0.15 \text{ V} - 0.80 \text{ V}$$

$$E^0_{cell} = -0.95 \text{ V}$$

As in Example 6.2, the equilibrium constant is given by Eq. 6.11.

$$\log K_{sp} = \frac{-0.95}{0.059} = -16.1$$

$$\mathrm{p}K_{sp} = 16.1$$

or

$$K_{sp} = 7.9 \times 10^{-17}$$

6.2 Electrometric Determination of pH

Relationship between pH and Electromotive Force. The electrical measurement of pH is probably the most frequently applied physical measurement (other than "weighings" with a balance) in the modern laboratory. This measurement is possible because the emf of certain chemical cells varies with the hydrogen ion concentration of the solution in the cell. This means that if the other variables in the cell are controlled, the emf of the cell can be correlated with the pH, and this correlation is the basis of potentiometric measurements of pH. We can establish the form of the correlation by applying the Nernst equation to one of these cells whose emf is responsive to pH.

Consider the cell

$$\mathrm{Pt},\ H_2(p)\,|\,H^+(a)\,|\ \text{reference electrode}$$

where the left-hand electrode is the hydrogen electrode and the right-hand electrode is one whose potential is not affected by the pH. The cell potential is given by

$$E_{\mathrm{cell}} = E_{\mathrm{H_2,H^+}} + E_{\mathrm{ref}}$$

or

$$E_{\mathrm{cell}} = E_{\mathrm{ref}} + E^0_{\mathrm{H_2,H^+}} - \frac{\mathrm{RT}}{n\mathbf{F}} \ln\left(\frac{a_{\mathrm{H^+}}{}^2}{p_{\mathrm{H_2}}}\right)$$

By definition $E^0_{\mathrm{H_2,H^+}} = 0$ and $\mathrm{pH} = -\log a_{\mathrm{H^+}}$; moreover it is possible experimentally to set $p_{\mathrm{H_2}}$ equal to 1 atm or at least to correct the data to this basis, so the equation simplifies at 25°C to

$$E_{\mathrm{cell}} - E_{\mathrm{ref}} = 0.059\ \mathrm{pH} \qquad (6.16)$$

The potential of the reference electrode can be independently determined, so by measuring the cell potential the pH of the solution can be calculated. Notice that a change of 1 pH unit corresponds to a change of 59 mV (millivolts) in the cell potential at 25°C (mathematically, $\Delta E/\Delta\mathrm{pH} = 59$ mV). This is the theoretical response of a pH indicator electrode. The hydrogen electrode obeys Eq. 6.16, and this electrode is regarded as the standard with which all others are compared.

The interpretation of electrometrically determined pH values deserves some consideration. Sørensen's original definition of pH made in 1909 was

$$\mathrm{pH} = -\log [\mathrm{H}^+]$$

where $[\mathrm{H}^+]$ signifies the concentration of hydrogen ion in gram-ions per liter. It was later recognized that the pH measurement reflects the activity rather than the concentration of hydrogen ion, so the conventional interpretation now is

$$\mathrm{pH} = -\log a_{\mathrm{H}^+} \tag{6.17}$$

or, by Eq. 6.4,

$$\mathrm{pH} = -\log f_{\mathrm{H}^+}[\mathrm{H}^+]$$

Measurement of pH. We have seen that the pH of an aqueous solution can be measured with a cell composed of the hydrogen electrode and a reference electrode immersed in the solution. Many reference electrodes are available for this measurement, but of these only one, the *saturated calomel electrode* (S.C.E.), is widely used. The saturated calomel electrode may be represented KCl (sat), Hg_2Cl_2 (sat) | Hg. The electrode consists of a saturated solution of potassium chloride that is also saturated with respect to mercurous chloride (calomel), the solution being in contact with mercury metal. The half-cell reaction is $Hg_2Cl_2 + 2e = 2Hg + 2Cl^-$. The formal potential of the S.C.E. at 25°C is +0.244 V [6], and its potential is not affected by pH. Because the electrode potential is sensitive to the potassium chloride concentration, which must not be diluted by the sample solution, it is necessary to interpose a salt bridge between the two half-cells. The cell composed of a hydrogen electrode and a S.C.E. may then be diagrammed

$$\mathrm{Pt}, \mathrm{H_2}(p)\,|\,\mathrm{H}^+(a)\,\|\,\mathrm{KCl}\ (\mathrm{sat}), \mathrm{Hg_2Cl_2}\ (\mathrm{sat})\,|\,\mathrm{Hg}$$

The potential of this cell is related to the pH by Eq. 6.18, which is very similar to Eq. 6.16.

$$E_{\mathrm{cell}} - (E_{\mathrm{ref}} + E_{\mathrm{l.j.}}) = 0.059\ \mathrm{pH} \tag{6.18}$$

Here $E_{\mathrm{l.j.}}$ is the liquid-junction potential, which is usually an unknown, small quantity (see p. 110). The uncertain magnitude of $E_{\mathrm{l.j.}}$ introduces some ambiguity into the pH definition. This is overcome largely by utilizing Eq. 6.18 to measure *differences* in pH between two solutions. Suppose E represents the cell potential when the cell solution has a certain pH, and E_s is the potential of the same cell when the cell solution has the corresponding pH_s. Writing Eq. 6.18 for both measurements, and assuming that the liquid-junction potential is the same in both cells (which is probably a good assumption if pH and pH_s are fairly close), then we find, on subtracting these equations:

$$\mathrm{pH} = \mathrm{pH}_s + \frac{E - E_s}{2.303\,RT/\mathbf{F}} \tag{6.19}$$

where the equation is valid at all temperatures. Equation 6.19 is the operational definition of pH. Evidently if the pH_s of a standard solution is known, the determination of any unknown pH is accomplished simply by measuring the difference in cell emf when the standard and unknown solutions are placed in the cell, and then utilizing Eq. 6.19 to calculate the unknown pH. The success of this method depends upon the constancy of $E_{l.j.}$ in the two measurements, and upon the accuracy with which pH_s is known.

The assignment of pH_s values to standard buffer solutions has been accomplished largely through the careful work of Bates and his colleagues at the National Bureau of Standards. These assignments were made with the aid of cells without liquid junctions. At the present time, seven primary standard solutions are available to cover the approximate pH range 3.5–10.0, with secondary standards at pH 1.7 (potassium tetroxalate), 8.1 (TRIS), and 12.5 (calcium hydroxide); a wide temperature range is covered [7–10]. Table 6.2 gives the compositions of the seven primary standard buffer solutions, and their recommended pH_s values are tabulated in Table 6.3.

As mentioned earlier, it is advisable to "standardize" the cell with one of the standard solutions whose pH_s is close to the estimated pH of the sample solution. This precaution helps to ensure constancy of the liquid-junction potential, since major contributors to the liquid-junction potential are the highly mobile hydrogen and hydroxide ions. It is also good practice to measure the pH of a second standard solution after standardization against the first one; in effect, this measurement checks the adherence of the cell to

TABLE 6.2
Compositions of Standard Buffer Solutions[a]

Solution		Substance	Weight (g)[b]	pH_s at 25°C
Tartrate	~0.034 *m*	$KHC_4H_4O_6$	Saturated at 25°C	3.557
Citrate	0.05 *m*	$KH_2C_6H_5O_7$	11.41	3.776
Phthalate	0.05 *m*	$KHC_8H_4O_4$	10.12	4.008
Phosphate	0.025 *m*	KH_2PO_4	3.39	6.865
(1:1)	0.025 *m*	Na_2HPO_4	3.53	
Phosphate	0.008695 *m*	KH_2PO_4	1.179	7.413
(1:3.5)	0.03043 *m*	Na_2HPO_4	4.30	
Borax	0.01 *m*	$Na_2B_4O_7 \cdot 10H_2O$	3.80	9.180
Carbonate	0.025 *m*	$NaHCO_3$	2.092	10.012
	0.025 *m*	Na_2CO_3	2.640	

[a] From Refs. 8 and 9.

[b] Weight of substance (in air near sea level) per liter of solution, prepared with carbonate-free distilled water.

TABLE 6.3
Standard pH_s Values[a,b]

t (°C)	Tartrate	Citrate	Phthalate	Phosphate (1:1)	Phosphate (1:3.5)	Borax	Carbonate
0	—	3.864	4.003	6.984	7.534	9.464	10.321
5	—	3.839	3.999	6.951	7.500	9.395	10.243
10	—	3.819	3.998	6.923	7.472	9.332	10.178
15	—	3.802	3.999	6.900	7.448	9.276	10.116
20	—	3.788	4.002	6.881	7.429	9.225	10.060
25	3.557	3.776	4.008	6.865	7.413	9.180	10.012
30	3.552	3.767	4.015	6.853	7.400	9.139	9.968
35	3.549	3.759	4.024	6.844	7.389	9.102	9.928
38	3.548	—	4.030	6.840	7.384	9.081	—
40	3.547	3.754	4.035	6.838	7.380	9.068	9.892
45	3.547	3.750	4.047	6.834	7.373	9.038	9.856
50	3.549	3.749	4.060	6.833	7.367	9.011	9.825
55	3.554	—	4.075	6.834	—	8.985	—
60	3.560	—	4.091	6.836	—	8.962	—
70	3.580	—	4.126	6.845	—	8.921	—
80	3.609	—	4.164	6.859	—	8.885	—
90	3.650	—	4.205	6.877	—	8.850	—
95	3.674	—	4.227	6.886	—	8.833	—

[a] From Refs. 8 and 9.
[b] Solution compositions are given in Table 6.2.

the theoretical behavior predicted by the Nernst equation.

The discussion has so far considered the hydrogen electrode as the pH indicator electrode. Many other pH indicator electrodes are known, and some of these are more practical than the hydrogen electrode, which requires a flow of hydrogen gas through the test solution. The most extensively used pH indicator electrode is the *glass electrode*, which is a thin membrane of glass that, when placed in contact with a solution, develops a potential the magnitude of which is related to the pH of the solution. In fact, the response of the glass electrode follows the theoretical relationship, Eq. 6.16. It is, of course, necessary to make an electrical contact with the glass membrane, and this is done by adding another electrode on the side of the glass membrane opposite to the test solution. Usually this contact is made through a silver-silver chloride electrode. The complete cell used for pH measurements is then represented schematically by

$$\text{Ag} \mid \text{AgCl (sat), HCl} \mid \text{glass} \mid \text{unknown solution} \parallel \text{reference electrode}$$

in which the reference electrode is usually the S.C.E. This cell has five sources of potential [11]:

1. The potential of the silver-silver chloride electrode.
2. The reference electrode potential.
3. The liquid-junction potential at the salt bridge.
4. The potential at the glass-HCl solution boundary.
5. The potential at the glass-unknown solution boundary.

The first four of these potentials are constant for a series of measurements conducted as recommended above for the hydrogen electrode. The pH response of this cell therefore is described by an equation of the same form as 6.18, and so the operational definition of pH, Eq. 6.19, applies to the glass electrode as well as to the hydrogen electrode.

The convenience of the glass electrode accounts for its popularity as a pH indicator electrode. It possesses another advantage worth noting, which is its insensitivity to oxidation-reduction reactions, the occurrence of which could vitiate pH measurements made with the hydrogen electrode. The glass electrode does have limitations that restrict its application, however. These are results of the mechanism of the electrode response. It appears that the glass membrane acts as a cation exchanger toward hydrogen ions. The difference in activities of hydrogen ion in the solution and within the glass itself gives rise to the potential that is measured. Water may also be able to penetrate the membrane, and if the activity of water in the solution is greatly different from unity, the observed pH will be in error; presumably this deviation from the theoretical response results from a difference in the water activity between the solution and the glass. The activity of water is reduced by large concentrations of electrolytes and nonaqueous solvents, so pH values determined with the glass electrode under these conditions may be in error.

A more serious limitation of the glass electrode is encountered in strongly alkaline solutions. When the concentrations of alkali metal ions become large, these ions seem to permeate the membrane, resulting in significant errors in the measured pH. With the so-called general-purpose glass electrodes, which contain a high percentage of sodium in the special glass used to construct the membrane, the error caused by sodium ion in alkaline solutions can be quite large. These electrodes perform well up to pH 9, but above this limit a negative error (the "alkaline error") in pH is observed. New glasses rich in lithium have been introduced; these give fairly reliable results in the presence of sodium ion up to about pH 13.

The potential of most chemical cells can be measured with a simple instrument called a potentiometer. Figure 6.2 shows the basic potentiometer circuit. D is a battery whose emf is larger than that of the cell to be measured.

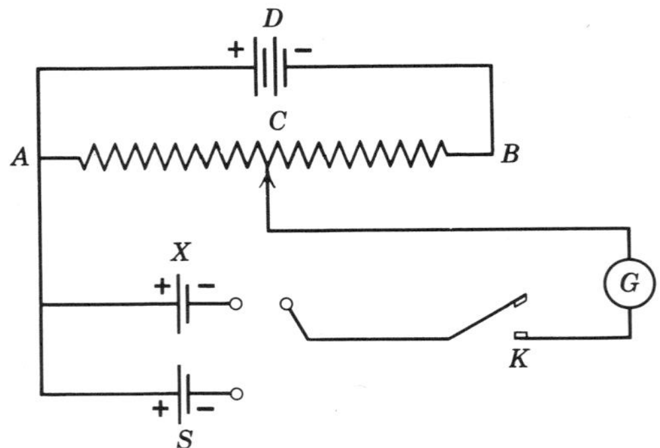

Fig. 6.2. A potentiometer circuit.

AB is a slide wire of uniform resistance, so that resistance is directly proportional to length. G is a galvanometer and K is a tapping key. X is the cell of unknown potential and S is a standard cell, that is, a cell whose potential is precisely known.

The unknown cell X is first placed in the circuit. The sliding contact C is adjusted until the galvanometer needle does not deflect when the key K is closed momentarily. It is essential that no current be drawn through the cell, for such behavior would cause electrode reactions to occur, changing the concentrations of the cell reactants. This phenomenon was briefly mentioned earlier, when it was noted that the cell must function reversibly if the maximum emf is to be delivered. When the galvanometer needle shows no deflection, there is no current passing through the cell circuit. Then the potential of cell X, E_X, is exactly opposed by the potential drop across AC, which by Ohm's law is proportional to the resistance.

$$E_X = k(AC)$$

Next the standard cell is placed in the circuit and the contact is adjusted to position C' such that no current flows through the cell. Then

$$E_S = k(AC')$$

Combining these equations gives an expression for the unknown potential

$$E_X = E_S \frac{AC}{AC'}$$

Cell potentials can be measured easily with a sensitivity of 0.1 mV on such a simple instrument.

Perhaps the most important cell in analytical practice is the glass-S.C.E. cell for pH measurements. The resistance of a glass electrode is extremely large (of the order 100 MΩ), so the currents involved are too small to permit the use of a galvanometer as a null point detector. One solution is to amplify the current with a suitable electronic circuit, and all commercial instruments for pH determination utilize electronic amplification of current with the glass-S.C.E. cell. These instruments are called pH meters. The procedure followed in their use is identical with that outlined earlier; the meter is "standardized" with a standard solution; then the unknown solution is measured. The dial of the pH meter is calibrated in millivolts and also directly in pH units, so Eq. 6.19 does not have to be solved explicitly for the unknown pH.

All pH meters include a temperature compensation adjustment. This is an electronic adjustment that controls the value of the function $\Delta E/\Delta \text{pH}$ within the instrument; recall (from p. 121) that this quantity is 59 mV at 25°, but it varies with temperature. Therefore, this temperature compensator calculates the quantity $RT/\mathbf{F}$ required for the correct conversion of emf to pH.

6.3 Determination of Acid-Base Dissociation Constants

Apparent Constants. In Chapter 1 we defined acid-base dissociation constants in terms of molar concentrations of participating species, and we noted that this procedure was not entirely correct. We may now introduce the rigorous definitions in terms of activities. For a weak acid HA,

$$K_a = \frac{a_{\mathrm{H^+}} a_{\mathrm{A^-}}}{a_{\mathrm{HA}}} \tag{6.20}$$

for a weak base B,

$$K_b = \frac{a_{\mathrm{OH^-}} a_{\mathrm{BH^+}}}{a_{\mathrm{B}}} \tag{6.21}$$

and for water,

$$K_w = a_{\mathrm{H^+}} a_{\mathrm{OH^-}} \tag{6.22}$$

These constants are called *thermodynamic constants;* they are true constants, dependent only upon temperature. The constants dealt with in Chapter 1 were concentration constants; for the acid HA, for example

$$K_c = \frac{[\mathrm{H^+}][\mathrm{A^-}]}{[\mathrm{HA}]}$$

This relation can be combined with 6.20, making use of Eq. 6.4, to give

$$K_a = K_c\left(\frac{f_{\mathrm{H^+}} f_{\mathrm{A^-}}}{f_{\mathrm{HA}}}\right) \tag{6.23}$$

Since we have selected the infinitely dilute solution as the state in which the activity coefficients assume the value of unity, Eq. 6.23 implies that in very dilute solution the concentration constant K_c approaches the thermodynamic constant K_a.

The potentiometric determination of dissociation constants involves a measurement of pH with a glass electrode-S.C.E. cell. The concentrations of the conjugate acid and base are established from knowledge of the appropriate volumes and concentrations of reactants, as will be described in detail later. Since the pH is a measure of activity, these experimental measurements lead to the evaluation of a quantity that is neither K_a nor K_c. It is instead a composite quantity, called the apparent constant K'_a or the mixed constant K_m [12], and defined by

$$K'_a = \frac{a_{H^+}[A^-]}{[HA]} \tag{6.24}$$

For many purposes K'_a is sufficiently close to K_a. The deviation one is willing to tolerate depends partly upon the accuracy with which the pH can be measured. An uncertainty in pH of 0.01–0.02 unit is common. Evidently, if K'_a and K_a do not differ by more than this amount, it is unnecessary to correct the K'_a value. The greatest accuracy requires cells without liquid junction, but for ordinary purposes the results obtainable with a glass-S.C.E. cell are adequate.

The procedure for the potentiometric determination of K'_a is really a titration. Let us consider the weak acid HA. A solution of this acid is prepared in carbonate-free water. A glass electrode-S.C.E. combination, which has been previously standardized as discussed in Section 6.2, is immersed in the solution. Next a standard solution of sodium or potassium hydroxide is added from a buret, in about 10 equal portions, until the acid is completely titrated. After each addition of alkali the solution is stirred well and its pH is recorded. The apparent constant is then calculated with the logarithmic form of Eq. 6.24:

$$pK'_a = pH - \log \frac{[A^-]}{[HA]} \tag{6.25}$$

The ratio $[A^-]/[HA]$ is evaluated as follows: let c be the formal concentration of solute. (This is not the same as the initial concentration because of dilution by the titrant, although if the titrant is very concentrated it may be permissible to take c as a constant equal to the initial concentration.) Then

$$c = [A^-] + [HA]$$

By the electroneutrality rule, which states that the number of positive charges must equal the number of negative charges in a solution, we may write

$$[Na^+] + [H^+] = [A^-] + [OH^-]$$

where we suppose that sodium hydroxide is the titrant. Letting b equal the stoichiometric concentration of conjugate base formed from reaction between HA and the titrant (which is evidently equal to the concentration of sodium ion provided by the titrant), we find

$$[A^-] = b + [H^+] - [OH^-] \tag{6.26}$$

$$[HA] = c - b - [H^+] + [OH^-] \tag{6.27}$$

It is important to note the difference between $[A^-]$, which is the equilibrium concentration of A^-, and b, which is the stoichiometric concentration. Usually c and b will be of the order 10^{-2}; then if the pH of the solution is in the range 4–10, neither $[H^+]$ nor $[OH^-]$ will be significant relative to b or $c - b$, and Eq. 6.25 becomes

$$pK'_a = pH - \log \frac{b}{c - b} \tag{6.28}$$

If, however, the pH is less than about 4, the hydrogen ion concentration is no longer negligible. Equation 6.25 is then combined with 6.26 and 6.27 to give

$$pK'_a = pH - \log \frac{b + [H^+]}{c - b - [H^+]} \tag{6.29}$$

The quantity $[H^+]$ is calculated from the known pH; since it amounts to a small correction factor, the difference between $[H^+]$ and a_{H^+} is not important in this connection.

If the pH is greater than 10, then the hydroxide ion concentration must be taken into account, and the applicable form of Eq. 6.25 is

$$pK'_a = pH - \log \frac{b - [OH^-]}{c - b + [OH^-]} \tag{6.30}$$

Equations 6.28–6.30 apply to the titration of any weak acid with strong base; the acid may be neutral (such as acetic acid), positive (for example, ammonium chloride), or negative (for example, monosodium phosphate).

Now consider the determination of K'_a when the sample is a base B. (It may be neutral, positive, or negative.) The titration may be carried out with standard hydrochloric acid. A development analogous to that given previously leads to Eqs. 6.31 and 6.32 for the equilibrium concentrations of the solute species.

$$[B] = c - a - [OH^-] + [H^+] \tag{6.31}$$

$$[BH^+] = a + [OH^-] - [H^+] \tag{6.32}$$

where c is the formal solute concentration and a is the concentration of chloride ion provided by the HCl titrant. By arguments like those used for the weak acid example, the expression for pK_a for a base becomes, if the pH is 4–10,

$$pK_a' = pH - \log \frac{c - a}{a} \tag{6.33}$$

If the pH is less than 4,

$$pK_a' = pH - \log \frac{c - a + [H^+]}{a - [H^+]} \tag{6.34}$$

If the pH is greater than 10,

$$pK_a' = pH - \log \frac{c - a - [OH^-]}{a + [OH^-]} \tag{6.35}$$

The same value for pK_a' should be obtained for a substance whether we start with the conjugate acid (for example, benzoic acid) and titrate with base, or start with the conjugate base (sodium benzoate) and titrate with acid.

According to Eq. 6.24, $pK_a' = pH$ when $[A^-] = [HA]$. This condition holds, to a good approximation, at the midpoint of the titration, that is, when one-half of the sample has been titrated. A common procedure is to carry out a potentiometric pH titration and to take the pH at the half-titration point as the pK_a'. This practice does not yield as reliable a value as the technique outlined above because it does not utilize the available data to the fullest extent. It does, however, give a very rapid estimate of pK_a' (see Fig. 1.5).

The estimation of pK values for polyfunctional acids and bases is similar to the treatment given for monofunctional compounds if the successive pK values are separated by at least three units. For such substances the separate functions are titrated separately, without significant simultaneous reaction at two sites. If the pK values are more closely spaced, however, the titration of the first group will not be completed before the second group begins to consume titrant. The simple calculational treatment will then fail, and more sophisticated methods are required [12].

In Chapter 1 we noted that K_a (or pK_a) values are usually tabulated, even for bases. The reason is now evident. Since pH is the quantity measured, even in alkaline solutions, it is the acid dissociation constant that is determined directly for both acids and bases, and so this value is the one reported. The corresponding K_b can be calculated with the relation $K_w = K_a K_b$.

Thermodynamic Constants. The deviation of an activity coefficient from unity is associated with the ionic atmosphere of the medium. The electrostatic forces of attraction and repulsion between ions are the source of this effect; thus in the immediate neighborhood of a negative ion there is a greater accumulation of positive charge than would be expected on the basis of a uniform distribution of the charge. The ionic character of an electrolyte solution is most usefully expressed as its *ionic strength I*.

$$I = \tfrac{1}{2} \sum c_i Z_i^2 \tag{6.36}$$

where c_i is the molar concentration of ion i, and Z_i is its valence. The ionic strength of a solution of a univalent-univalent strong electrolyte, like NaCl, is equal to its molarity.

The problem of correcting the mixed constant K'_a to the thermodynamic constant K_a resolves itself into one of estimating an activity coefficient. At moderate values of the ionic strength the activity of a neutral species may be taken equal to its concentration, so K'_a (for HA) may be written $K'_a = a_{H^+}[A^-]/a_{HA}$, whereas K_a is written $K_a = a_{H^+}a_{A^-}/a_{HA} = a_{H^+}[A^-]f_{A^-}/a_{HA}$; therefore $K_a = K'_a f_{A^-}$, or

$$pK_a = pK'_a - \log f_{A^-} \tag{6.37}$$

The activity coefficient of an ion may be estimated by the Debye-Hückel equation [10, 11]

$$-\log f_i = \frac{AZ_i^2\sqrt{I}}{1 + aB\sqrt{I}} \tag{6.38}$$

where Z_i is the valence of ion i, a is a quantity that may be roughly considered the radius of the ion in angstrom units, and A and B are constants dependent upon the temperature and dielectric constant of the medium. For aqueous solutions at 25°C with a taken as 3 Å (a reasonable figure), this equation becomes

$$-\log f_i = \frac{0.509Z_i^2\sqrt{I}}{1 + \sqrt{I}} \tag{6.39}$$

Equation 6.39 is often valid at ionic strengths up to about 0.1 M, but in more concentrated solutions it may fail. When the ionic strength is very small, Eq. 6.39 may be written

$$-\log f_i = 0.509Z_i^2\sqrt{I} \tag{6.40}$$

which is known as the Debye-Hückel limiting law.

It is now possible to combine Eqs. 6.37 and 6.39:

$$pK_a = pK'_a + \frac{0.509\sqrt{I}}{1 + \sqrt{I}} \tag{6.41}$$

This expression may be used to correct K'_a to K_a for neutral acids (and therefore for negatively charged bases) at 25°C. The ionic strength is calculated from knowledge of the appropriate normalities and volumes. If the correction term is less than 0.02 unit, it may be ignored if the pH measurements were uncertain by this amount.

For a positively charged acid (or a neutral base) the activity coefficient appears in the denominator of the dissociation constant expression, so $pK_a = pK'_a + \log f_{BH^+}$, and

$$pK_a = pK'_a - \frac{0.509\sqrt{I}}{1 + \sqrt{I}} \tag{6.42}$$

EXAMPLE 6.5. What is the ionic strength of (1) 0.1 M Na_2SO_4; (2) a solution 0.02 M in Na_3PO_4 and 0.1 M in NaCl?

(1) Evidently, $[Na^+] = 0.2\ M$, $Z_{Na} = 1$, $[SO_4^{2-}] = 0.1\ M$, $Z_{SO_4} = 2$. Substituting into Eq. 6.36,

$$I = \tfrac{1}{2}(0.2 \times 1 + 0.1 \times 4) = 0.3\ M$$

(2) $[Na^+] = 0.16\ M$, $[PO_4^{3-}] = 0.02\ M$, $[Cl^-] = 0.1\ M$. From Eq. 6.36,

$$I = \tfrac{1}{2}(0.16 \times 1 + 0.02 \times 9 + 0.1 \times 1) = 0.22\ M$$

EXAMPLE 6.6. 1.50 ml of 0.100 N KOH was added to 47.5 ml of 0.010 M boric acid. The pH of this solution was 8.90. Calculate pK'_a for boric acid.

The formal concentration c is corrected for dilution by the titrant: $c = (0.01)(47.5)/(49.0) = 0.00970\ M$. The concentration b, which may be regarded as the stoichiometric concentration of the borate ion, is equal to the potassium ion concentration.

$$b = \frac{(0.1)(1.5)}{(49.0)} = 0.00306\ M$$

Then from Eq. 6.28

$$pK'_a = 8.90 - \log 0.461 = 8.90 + 0.34 = 9.24$$

EXAMPLE 6.7. 0.40 ml of 1 N HCl was added to 50 ml of 0.01 M p-chloroaniline; the pH of the solution was 3.43. What is pK'_a?

Proceeding as previously, $c = (0.01)(50)/(50.4) = 0.00993\ M$; $a = (1)(0.40)/(50.4) = 0.00794\ M$. Since pH is less than 4, it is necessary to use Eq. 6.34, with $[H^+] = 0.00037\ M$. Therefore,

$$pK'_a = 3.43 - \log \tfrac{236}{757} = 3.94$$

If the titrant is very concentrated, as in this example, the volume change caused by addition of titrant usually may be neglected. If we do so, we find $c = 0.01$ and $a = 0.008$; the final result is again $pK'_a = 3.94$.

EXAMPLE 6.8. 10.0 ml of a solution 0.1 M with respect to both acetic acid and sodium chloride was mixed with 10.0 ml of 0.05 M sodium hydroxide.

The pH of this solution was 4.64. What is the thermodynamic pK_a of acetic acid?

First find pK'_a in the usual way. $c = 0.05\ M$ and $b = 0.025\ M$. By Eq. 6.28, then, $pK'_a = 4.64$.

The ionic strength is a function of the NaCl concentration (0.05 M) and the sodium acetate (0.025 M), with $I = 0.075\ M$. Using Eq. 6.41,

$$pK_a = 4.63 + \frac{(0.509)(0.274)}{1.274}$$

$$pK_a = 4.75$$

EXAMPLE 6.9. Calculate the standard free energy change for the ionization of acetic acid at 25°C.

From Eq. 6.8 we have $\Delta G^0 = -RT \ln K_a$; moreover $pK_a = -\log K_a$, so $\Delta G^0 = 4.576\ T\, pK_a$, where the units of ΔG^0 are calories per mole. At $T =$ 298.16°C with $pK_a = 4.75$ for acetic acid, $\Delta G^0 = 6481$ cal/mole or 6.48 kcal/mole. This problem shows that ΔG^0 is directly proportional to pK_a, which is why pK values can appear as sums and differences.

6.4 Ion–Selective Membrane Electrodes

Theory of Membrane Electrode Response. Consider a cell that is formally diagrammed as

$$\text{Internal ref} \mid a_{\text{int}} \mid \text{Membrane} \mid a_{\text{ext}} \parallel \text{External ref} \qquad (6.43)$$

The membrane, whose nature will be examined later, has the property that it functions as an ion exchanger for the ion whose activity is to be measured. A fixed activity of this ion, a_{int}, is established on the inside of the membrane. The activity of the ion in the sample solution is a_{ext}. Internal and external reference electrodes complete the cell. The glass pH electrode is a special (though very important) example of this type of cell, and this section will describe recent extensions to the measurement of many other ionic activities.

The potential of cell 6.43 is given by

$$E_{\text{cell}} = E_{\text{int ref}} + E_{\text{ext ref}} + E_{\text{l.j.}} + E_{\text{membrane}} \qquad (6.44)$$

The membrane potential is formally a consequence of the sum of two symmetrical half-reactions, namely, for ion M^{n+},

$$M_{\text{int}} \rightleftharpoons M^{n+}_{\text{int}} + ne$$
$$ne + M^{n+}_{\text{ext}} \rightleftharpoons M_{\text{ext}}$$

$$\text{Sum:} \qquad M^{n+}_{\text{ext}} \rightleftharpoons M^{n+}_{\text{int}}$$

To each half-reaction the Nernst equation can be applied.

$$E_{\text{membrane}} = E^{\text{int}}_{\text{M,M}^{n+}} + E^{\text{ext}}_{\text{M}^{n+},\text{M}} = E^{\text{ext}}_{\text{M}^{n+},\text{M}} - E^{\text{int}}_{\text{M}^{n+},\text{M}}$$

$$E_{\text{membrane}} = -\frac{RT}{n\mathbf{F}}\ln\frac{1}{a_{\text{ext}}} - \left(-\frac{RT}{n\mathbf{F}}\ln\frac{1}{a_{\text{int}}}\right) \tag{6.45}$$

where the standard potential for the M^{n+},M couple vanishes because it is identical for the two half-reactions. Equation 6.45 leads to

$$E_{\text{membrane}} = \frac{RT}{n\mathbf{F}}\ln\frac{a_{\text{ext}}}{a_{\text{int}}} \tag{6.46}$$

which can also be obtained by direct application of the Nernst equation to the net cell reaction. Combining Eqs. 6.44 and 6.46,

$$E_{\text{cell}} = \text{constant} + \frac{RT}{n\mathbf{F}}\ln a_{\text{ext}} \tag{6.47}$$

or, at 25°C,

$$E_{\text{cell}} = \text{constant} + \frac{0.059}{n}\log a_{\text{ext}} \tag{6.48}$$

Membrane electrodes in which the ion-exchange process is equilibrium controlled, so that the Nernst equation is applicable, therefore give a response of $59/n$ mV per unit change in log a_{ext} at 25°C.

Types of Membrane Electrodes. The origin of the membrane potential is in the ion-exchange properties of the membrane. Three general types of ion-selective membrane electrodes have been devised.

(*a*) Solid ion-exchange membranes. The most common examples of this class are glass membrane electrodes, of which the pH electrode has been in longest use. Glass is a mixture of SiO_2 with oxides of trivalent elements plus oxides of monovalent or divalent elements; typical electrode glasses contain SiO_2, Al_2O_3, and Na_2O [13]. In the solid state only the cations are mobile. When placed in contact with an ionic solution, cations of the glass surface can exchange with cations of the solution. Glass is therefore a cation exchanger. The composition of the glass determines which cations are preferentially exchanged.

A single crystal can also serve as a solid membrane, which in this case acts as an ion exchanger for both its cation and its anion. Because of the difficulty in obtaining and mounting single crystals, an alternative arrangement is to embed small particles of solid ion exchanger in a solid matrix, such as a silicone rubber.

(*b*) Liquid ion-exchange membranes. Consider a liquid composed of a hydrophobic electrolyte such as a long-chain fatty acid. Its hydrophobic nature ensures that it will be immiscible with water, and therefore it will form a separate phase (the membrane) when in contact with water. The anion portion (say, R—COO^-), because of the long-chain R group, remains within the membrane phase. The cation, however, is mobile and exchangeable with cations of the contiguous aqueous phase. Thus this system acts as a liquid cation-exchange membrane. By using hydrophobic cations such as long-chain quaternary ammonium compounds R_4N^+, liquid anion-exchange membranes can be formulated. The exchanger molecule can also be dissolved in another organic solvent to form the membrane.

(*c*) Neutral sequestering agents. Macrocyclic molecules are known that form inclusion complexes with metal ions and other ions by sequestering them within a molecular cavity. The antibiotic valinomycin is such a molecule. Much research is being devoted to a series of polycyclic ethers known as crown ethers [14], one of which is shown below. The external surface of these

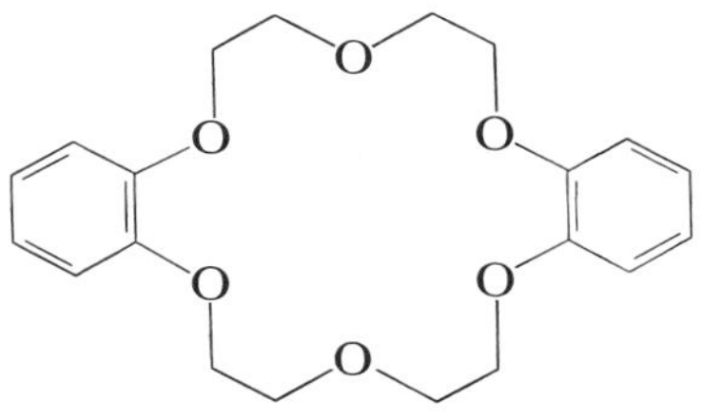

Dibenzo-18-crown-6

molecules is largely hydrophobic, as revealed by molecular models, and they are soluble in organic solvents even when complexed with a metal ion. They therefore have the capability of transferring metal ions from water to an organic phase. For electrode purposes, the polycyclic ether is dissolved in an organic solvent. Distribution of ions into this organic membrane phase occurs via inclusion in the molecular cavity. A deviation from electroneutrality, and therefore development of a potential, results from this distribution.

The capability of these membrane phases for developing potentials is a consequence of their selective permeability to the ion of interest. When the electrode is immersed in the sample solution, a concentration gradient is established, with a transient movement of ions from the direction of higher to lower activity. This ionic displacement develops an electric potential that opposes further ionic migration, so an equilibrium is established. The thinner the membrane phase, the more rapidly this equilibrium can be attained, and the more quickly steady electrode potentials can be determined. Figure 6.3 shows two designs for liquid membrane electrodes [15]. In Fig. 6.3*a* a configuration with long response time is shown. The internal reference electrode is a silver-silver chloride electrode. The liquid ion-exchange

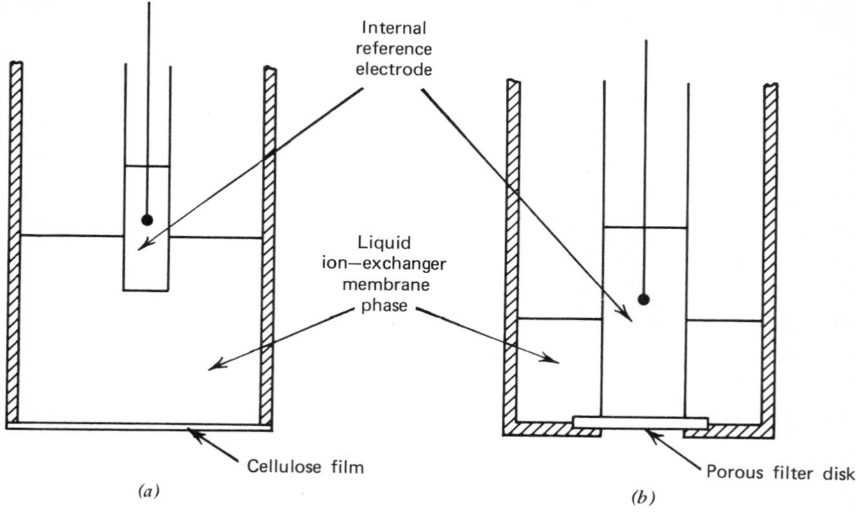

Fig. 6.3. Schematic diagrams of liquid ion-selective membrane electrodes (after Ross [15]).

membrane phase is held in a glass tube, separated from the sample solution by a cellulose film acting as a physical barrier to mixing; however, ions can pass through this film. The design in Fig. 6.3*b* produces a very thin liquid membrane phase, and therefore a short response time, by separating the sample solution from the internal reference electrode by an inert porous filter disk saturated, from the adjacent reservoir solution, with the liquid ion-exchange phase.

Electrode Selectivity. The total membrane potential can be divided into these three components: (1) the interfacial potential developed by ion-exchange equilibria at the membrane-internal solution interface; (2) the interfacial potential developed by ion-exchange equilibria at the membrane-external solution interface; and (3) the diffusion potential developed by the charge gradient within the membrane. The last of these is rate-controlled and is determined by the mobilities of ions in the membrane phase. The first two are equilibrium properties that lead to selectivity on the basis of differing affinities of ions for the membrane ion-exchange sites. The selectivity of an electrode for ion A^{n_A+} in the presence of ion B^{n_B+} is empirically expressed by

$$E = \text{constant} + \frac{2.3\,RT}{n\mathbf{F}} \log \left(a_A + k_{AB} a_B^{n_B/n_A}\right) \tag{6.49}$$

The parameter k_{AB} is the selectivity coefficient for interfering ion B relative to

TABLE 6.4
Liquid Membrane Systems and Selectivity Coefficients

Ion Measured (A)	Exchange Site	Selectivity Coefficients: Ion B	k_{AB}
Ca^{2+}	$(RO)_2PO_2^-$	Zn^{2+}	3.2
		Fe^{2+}	0.80
		Mg^{2+}	0.01
		Ba^{2+}	0.01
		Na^+	0.0016
Pb^{2+}	$RSCH_2COO^-$	Cu^{2+}	2.6
		Zn^{2+}	0.003
		Ni^{2+}	0.007
Cl^-	R_4N^+	I^-	17
		Br^-	1.6
		OH^-	1.0
		SO_4^{2-}	0.14
		F^-	0.10
NO_3^-	$\left[\text{Ni}\,(\text{N},\text{N}\text{–R})\right]_3^{2+}$	Cl^-	0.006
		OAc^-	0.006
		F^-	0.0009
		PO_4^{3-}	0.0003
		SO_4^{2-}	0.0006

sample ion A. If k_{AB} is less than one, then the electrode is more responsive to A than to B, and if k_{AB} is very small the activity of ion A can be determined in the presence of B with an extent of interference that can be roughly estimated. For example, $k_{Ca,Ba} = 0.01$ in a liquid membrane using $(RO)_2PO_2^-$ as the exchange site; thus at equal concentrations, Ba^{2+} will introduce about 1% error into a Ca^{2+} determination with this electrode. Table 6.4 gives selectivity constants for some practical liquid membrane electrodes [15].

A large number of ions can now be detected with ion-selective membrane electrodes. Most of the present applications are for inorganic cations and anions, but electrodes have also been designed for organic ions. Since many drug molecules are acids or bases, and can therefore be transformed into ions, it can be anticipated that membrane electrodes selective for particular drugs will be developed into practical analytical devices.

6.5 Potentiometric Titrations

Location of the End Point. Potentiometry is used in two ways in analytical work. (1) From the potential of a cell the activity of a cell component is calculated according to the Nernst equation (or via an empirical calibration); this technique is used for the determination of pH (see Sections 6.2 and 6.3) and, more recently, of many other ions, as described in Section 6.4. (2) The potential of a cell is measured throughout the course of a titration, the variation in potential being used to locate the end point. This second technique is called potentiometric titration.

The location of the end point can be accomplished graphically or analytically. We find, both theoretically and experimentally, that a more or less abrupt change in the slope of a plot of potential (or pH) versus titrant volume coincides with the equivalence point of the titration. (See Figs. 1.5, 2.1, 2.2, and 4.3.) If the electrode reaction is reversible and the titration reaction is symmetrical (that is, one molecule or ion of titrant reacts with one molecule or ion of sample), the potentiometric titration curve will be symmetrical with a typical sigmoid shape. For such a curve the equivalence point corresponds to the inflection point, which can be determined by inspection of the titration plot, as for example in Fig. 6.4*a*, which is the curve for titration of tris(hydroxymethyl)aminomethane with hydrochloric acid. This end point detection method is rapid but subjective.

A less subjective method is available. If the end point coincides with the inflection point in the titration curve, it must also coincide with the maximum in the first derivative, $d\text{pH}/dV$ or dE/dV; some analysts evaluate $\Delta\text{pH}/\Delta V$ or $\Delta E/\Delta V$ and plot this against V to locate this maximum. Another method utilizes the fact that the second derivative, which may be approximated by $\Delta^2\text{pH}/\Delta V^2$ or $\Delta^2 E/\Delta V^2$, is equal to zero at the volume corresponding to the inflection point in the curve. The evaluation of these quantities is made easily if equal increments of titrant are added in the vicinity of the end point. A typical calculation is illustrated in Table 6.5. The point at which the function $\Delta^2\text{pH}/\Delta V^2$ is equal to zero is found by linear interpolation between the two points on either side of zero. The second derivative method does not require plotting nor is it subjective. Figure 6.4 illustrates the interrelationship of the plots of pH, $\Delta\text{pH}/\Delta V$, and $\Delta^2\text{pH}/\Delta V^2$ against V.

Another technique for locating end points is becoming increasingly popular. Consider the titration of V_0 ml of strong acid of initial concentration C_0 with strong base of normality N; let V be the volume of titrant added at any point and $V_{\text{e.p.}}$ be the end point volume. Then

$$a_{\text{H}^+} = \frac{\text{meq of acid}}{\text{volume in ml}} = \frac{C_0 V_0 - NV}{V_0 + V} \qquad (6.50)$$

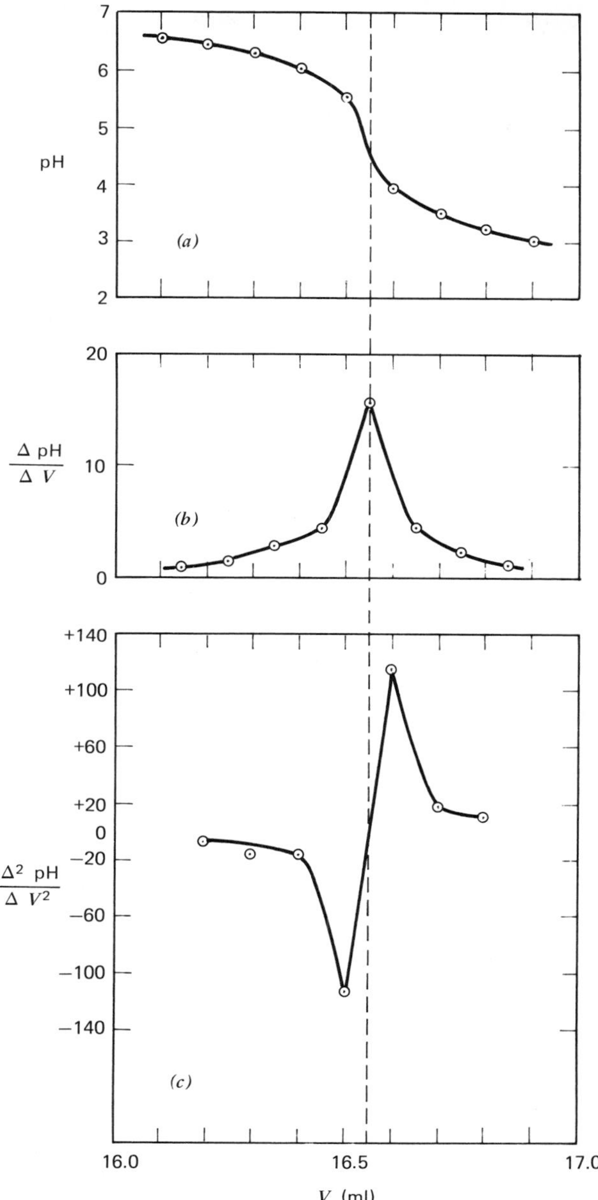

Fig. 6.4. (*a*) Potentiometric titration plot of data in Table 6.5; (*b*) first derivative of the titration curve; (*c*) second derivative of the titration curve.

TABLE 6.5
Calculation of the End Point by the Second Derivative Method[a]

V (ml)	pH	$\Delta pH/\Delta V$ (ml^{-1})	$\Delta^2 pH/\Delta V^2$ (ml^{-2})
16.10	6.58		
		1.0	
16.20	6.48		−6
		1.6	
16.30	6.32		−14
		3.0	
16.40	6.02		−15
		4.5	
16.50	5.57		−114
		15.9	
16.60	3.98		+114
		4.5	
16.70	3.53		+19
		2.6	
16.80	3.27		+12
		1.4	
16.90	3.13		

$$V_{e.p.} = 16.50 + 0.1\left(\frac{114}{114 + 114}\right) = 16.55 \text{ ml}$$

[a] Titration of 1.816 meq of TRIS with HCl at 20°C.

where the distinction between activity and concentration is being ignored; it can, if desired, be taken into account. Since $C_0V_0 = NV_{e.p.}$, Eq. 6.50 can be rearranged to

$$a_{H^+}(V_0 + V) = N(V_{e.p.} - V) \tag{6.51}$$

According to Eq. 6.51, a plot of $a_{H^+}(V_0 + V)$ against V should be a straight line intersecting the latter axis at $V = V_{e.p.}$. After the end point the development is based on

$$a_{OH} = \frac{\text{meq of base}}{\text{volume in ml}} = \frac{N(V - V_{e.p.})}{V_0 + V} \tag{6.52}$$

Using the expression $K_w = a_{H^+}a_{OH^-}$ gives

$$\frac{V_0 + V}{a_{H^+}} = \frac{N(V - V_{e.p.})}{K_w} \tag{6.53}$$

A plot of $(V_0 + V)/a_{H^+}$ against V also will extrapolate to the end point volume. A similar development can be carried out for titrations of strong bases with strong acids. These linear extrapolation methods of potentiometric titration data are known as Gran plots [16, 17].

Let us treat in the analogous manner the titration of V_0 ml of weak base B having initial concentration C_0 with strong acid of normality N; V is the volume of titrant added. The pH is controlled by the conjugate acid-base ratio according to

$$K_a = \frac{a_{H^+}[B]}{[BH^+]}$$

Since $C_0V_0 = NV_{e.p.}$, this can be transformed to

$$a_{H^+} = \frac{K_aV}{V_{e.p.} - V} \tag{6.54}$$

A plot of V/a_{H^+} against V should be linear, the intercept giving $V_{e.p.}$. After the end point, a development similar to that given earlier shows that $a_{H^+}(V_0 + V)$ should be plotted against V.

Figure 6.5 is a Gran plot for the same titration described in Fig. 6.4 and Table 6.5. The data and calculations are given in Table 6.6. Curvature in Gran plots can be caused by activity coefficient changes during the course of the titration or by interfering substances (for example, carbonate in a titration of hydroxide). These plots can be used for potentiometric acid-base titrations, as shown, as well as other types of potentiometric titrations, such as those using ion-selective membrane electrodes.

Sometimes a potentiometric titration is carried out simply by titrating to a predetermined potential or pH. This technique is similar to the use of a visual indicator. It is very rapid, because no potentials are measured during the titration, but it requires knowledge of the potential or pH at the end point.

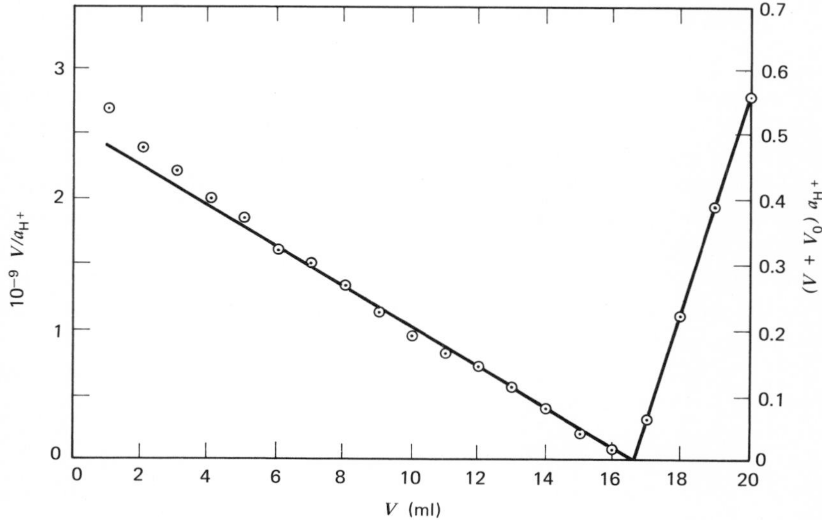

Fig. 6.5. Gran plot of titration data in Table 6.6.

TABLE 6.6
Gran Plot Calculations[a]

V (ml)	pH	a_{H^+}	$10^{-9} V/a_{H^+}$	$a_{H^+}(V_0 + V)$
1	9.43	3.72×10^{-10}	2.69	—
2	9.08	8.32×10^{-10}	2.40	—
3	8.87	1.35×10^{-9}	2.22	—
4	8.70	2.00×10^{-9}	2.00	—
5	8.57	2.69×10^{-9}	1.86	—
6	8.43	3.72×10^{-9}	1.61	—
7	8.33	4.68×10^{-9}	1.50	—
8	8.22	6.03×10^{-9}	1.33	—
9	8.10	7.94×10^{-9}	1.13	—
10	7.98	1.05×10^{-8}	0.95	—
11	7.87	1.35×10^{-8}	0.82	—
12	7.78	1.66×10^{-8}	0.72	—
13	7.63	2.34×10^{-8}	0.56	—
14	7.45	3.55×10^{-8}	0.39	—
15	7.16	6.92×10^{-8}	0.21	—
16	6.69	2.04×10^{-7}	0.008	—
17	2.97	1.07×10^{-3}	—	0.061
18	2.42	3.80×10^{-3}	—	0.220
19	2.18	6.61×10^{-3}	—	0.390
20	2.03	9.33×10^{-3}	—	0.560

[a] $V_0 = 40$ ml; other conditions as given in Table 6.5.

This method, incidentally, is the only one that requires accurate knowledge of the potential or pH as defined by the concepts given earlier in this chapter. The graphical and analytical techniques described earlier in this section are based only upon *changes* in potential; it is not essential that the magnitudes of the measured potentials be "correct" in order to apply the potentiometric titration method.

Acid-Base Titrations. Acid-base titrations solve many analytical problems. Visual location of the end point with an acid-base indicator is simple and convenient, but if the sample solution is colored, if the sample substance is very weakly acidic or basic, if its strength is unknown, or if the sample contains a mixture of acids or bases, a visual titration will not be possible. Then the analysis may still be conducted with potentiometric detection of the end point.

Acid-base titrations in nonaqueous solutions are perfectly feasible (see Chapter 2), but the meaning of pH in these systems may not be clear. It is possible to define a pH scale for any solvent that dissociates to yield a proton.

In order to define an operational pH scale in a solvent, it is necessary to know the autoprotolysis constant K_s and the acid dissociation constant for an acid in the solvent. Then a standard buffer solution can be specified. pH scales have been defined for water, methanol, ethanol, acetic acid, and some alcohol-water mixtures. As we noted previously, however, absolute values of pH are not necessary in a potentiometric titration, and for analytical applications it is sufficient merely to record potentials in any nonaqueous titration. Figures 2.1 and 2.2 are examples of this practice. It is always advisable to obtain correct pH values in fully aqueous systems, however, because the titration data then yield the acid dissociation constant, in addition to the end point of the titration.

Precipitation and Complexometric Titrations. The potentiometric titration method is a powerful adjunct to the precipitation and complexometric titration procedures, because often a suitable visual indicator cannot be found. Both types of reaction usually involve a metal ion as either the titrant or the sample species. An indicator electrode for this kind of system often consists of the corresponding metal. Thus for titrations with silver nitrate, the indicator electrode could be a piece of silver wire. For precipitation titrations an electrode may be used whose potential is affected by the anion concentration.

Reilley [18] has developed the mercury electrode into a general indicator electrode for potentiometric chelometric titrations. The electrode consists of mercury metal in contact with a solution containing the metal ion M^{n+} being titrated, the metal-EDTA complex MY^{+n-4}, and some added mercury (II)-EDTA complex HgY^{2-}. The electrode reaction is

$$2e + Hg^{2+} \rightleftharpoons Hg$$

and the corresponding Nernst equation, at 25°C, is

$$E = E^0_{Hg^{2+},Hg} + \frac{0.059}{2} \log a_{Hg^{2+}} \tag{6.55}$$

The complex stability constants K_{MY} for MY^{+n-4} and K_{HgY} for HgY^{2-} are defined in the usual way. Combining these expressions with Eq. 6.55 gives

$$E = E^0_{Hg^{2+},Hg} + \frac{0.059}{2} \log \frac{[M^{n+}][HgY^{2-}]K_{MY}}{[MY^{2-}]K_{HgY}} \tag{6.56}$$

Since $[HgY^{2-}]$ is constant throughout a titration, the cell potential is a linear function of log ($[M^{n+}]/[MY^{2-}]$), which changes during the titration.

Ion-selective membrane electrodes are finding increasing use as indicator electrodes for precipitation and complexometric titrations.

Oxidation-Reduction Titrations. The indicator electrode in redox titrations usually is a noble metal that, ideally, serves merely as a locus of electron transfer from the solution to the external circuit. Platinum is usually used.

A reference electrode, often the S.C.E., completes the cell. The potential of this cell varies according to the concentrations of the titration reaction components. A source of some confusion in understanding the behavior of this system is the presence of two redox half-reactions in the titration solution plus another half-reaction at the reference electrode. The two titration half-reactions are not to be considered as a cell, however. The titrant is added to the sample, and equilibrium is almost instantaneously established between these two redox couples. Since they are in equilibrium, their potentials are identical, and it is this potential that is measured relative to the reference electrode.

Let us consider the titration of ferrous ion by ceric ion in 1 *M* nitric acid. The half-reactions are

$$Fe^{2+} \rightleftharpoons Fe^{3+} + e \qquad E^0_{Fe^{2+},Fe^{3+}} = -0.77\ V$$

$$Ce^{4+} + e \rightleftharpoons Ce^{3+} \qquad E^0_{Ce^{4+},Ce^{3+}} = +1.61\ V$$

We may use a platinum wire as an indicator electrode, and a S.C.E. will serve as the reference electrode. Before any titrant has been added, the potential is undefined, but as soon as some ceric ion is added to the solution it forms an equivalent amount of ferrous ion and is itself reduced to cerous. As we noted previously, after each addition of titrant equilibrium is attained, so the potential of the iron couple must equal the potential of the cerium couple:

$$E_{Fe^{3+},Fe^{2+}} = E_{Ce^{4+},Ce^{3+}}$$

and each of these is given by the Nernst equation,

$$E_{Fe^{3+},Fe^{2+}} = E^0_{Fe^{3+},Fe^{2+}} - 0.059 \log \frac{[Fe^{2+}]}{[Fe^{3+}]}$$

$$E_{Ce^{4+},Ce^{3+}} = E^0_{Ce^{4+},Ce^{3+}} - 0.059 \log \frac{[Ce^{3+}]}{[Ce^{4+}]}$$

where the potential is expressed relative to the S.H.E. Before the equivalence point the equation based upon the iron couple is easier to use because the requisite concentrations can be calculated from the titration data. Suppose 3 ml of 0.1 *N* ceric ion has been added to 10 ml of 0.1 *N* ferrous ion. The concentration of ferrous ion is now $[(10)(0.1) - (3)(0.1)]/13$, whereas the ferric ion concentration is $(3)(0.1)/13$. The standard potential is $+0.77$ V. The iron couple potential, relative to the S.H.E., is therefore

$$E_{Fe^{3+},Fe^{2+}} = +0.77 - 0.059 \log \left(\tfrac{7}{3}\right) = +0.75\ V$$

Since the potential of the S.C.E. is itself $+0.24$ V versus the S.H.E., the potential of the platinum electrode is $+0.51$ V versus the S.C.E. In this manner the observed potential can be calculated until very close to the equivalence point.

At the equivalence point the equality $[Fe^{3+}] = [Ce^{3+}]$ holds by definition of the equivalence point. The concentrations of ferrous and ceric ions, although very small, are finite, and the equilibrium

$$Fe^{2+} + Ce^{4+} \rightleftharpoons Fe^{3+} + Ce^{3+}$$

ensures that $[Fe^{2+}] = [Ce^{4+}]$. Adding the equations for the potential of the indicator electrode (and letting $E = E_{Fe^{3+},Fe^{2+}} = E_{Ce^{4+},Ce^{3+}}$)

$$2E = E^0_{Fe^{3+},Fe^{2+}} + E^0_{Ce^{4+},C^{3+}} + 0.059 \log \frac{[Fe^{3+}][Ce^{4+}]}{[Fe^{2+}][Ce^{3+}]}$$

Because of the equalities noted, the final term goes to zero, and at the equivalence point the indicator electrode potential versus S.H.E. is

$$E = \frac{E^0_{Fe^{3+},Fe^{2+}} + E^0_{Ce^{4+},Ce^{3+}}}{2}$$

$$E = \frac{+0.77 + 1.61}{2} = +1.19 \text{ V versus S.H.E.}$$

so the equivalence point potential is +0.95 V versus S.C.E. This figure may be used to select a redox indicator for the titration. For this titration ferroin, with a transition potential of +1.06 V versus S.H.E., would be a suitable visual indicator.

After the end point, the potential may be calculated with the equation expressing the ceric-cerous concentration dependence.

Experiment 6.1. Potentiometric Acid-Base Titrations

APPARATUS AND REAGENTS

pH Meter. Any commercial pH meter allowing readings to be estimated at the 0.01 unit level is satisfactory. Follow the manufacturer's instructions concerning electrical grounding of the meter, and use electrodes recommended for the meter. *Glass electrodes* should be soaked in distilled water overnight before their first use, and then stored in water. *Saturated calomel electrodes* should be stored in a saturated solution of KCl. Commercial saturated calomel electrodes consist of the electrode proper plus the salt bridge, all built into a single glass-enclosed unit. (Combination electrodes, in which a single unit incorporates both the glass and S.C.E., are also available.) Electrical contact between the sample solution and the salt bridge is through a small hole in the tip of the glass tube; loss of KCl solution through this hole is reduced by a fiber filling or a covering glass sleeve. Nevertheless, the level of saturated KCl solution in the salt bridge may fall, and solution should be added as necessary.

0.1 N Sodium Hydroxide. Prepare and standardize as in Experiment 1.1.

0.1 N Hydrochloric Acid. Prepare and standardize as in Experiment 1.2.

Standard Phthalate Buffer. Dissolve 1.012 g of reagent grade potassium biphthalate in enough water to make 100.0 ml.

Standard Borate Buffer. Dissolve 0.380 g of sodium borate decahydrate in enough water to make 100.0 ml.

PROCEDURES

Standardization of pH Meter. Connect the glass electrode and S.C.E. to the meter, and place it in operation as directed by your laboratory instructor. Rinse the electrodes with water and carefully dry them. Immerse the electrodes in the standard biphthalate buffer and standardize the meter by bringing the meter needle to indicate the pH appropriate to the solution temperature (pH 4.01 at 25°C (—see Table 6.3). Check the performance of the meter and electrodes by measuring the pH of the borate buffer; the measured pH should be within 0.02 unit of 9.18 at 25°C. Always rinse and dry the electrodes before placing them in a solution.

Measurement of Unknown pH. Obtain from the instructor a sample of a buffer solution. Measure and report its pH.

Potentiometric Titration of Soda Ash. Obtain a sample of soda ash (crude sodium carbonate). Accurately weigh a portion of soda ash equivalent to 150–250 mg of Na_2CO_3 (your instructor will tell you a suitable sample weight range). Transfer the sample to a 250 ml beaker and dissolve it in about 75 ml of freshly boiled water. Immerse the standardized glass-S.C.E. electrode pair in the solution and promptly titrate with standard 0.1 *N* HCl, carrying the titration to about pH 2. Stirring may be accomplished manually by swirling the beaker after each addition of titrant, or it may be done with a magnetic stirrer. Add titrant in 1.0 ml portions except in the vicinity of the two end points, where it should be added in smaller (0.1 or 0.2 ml) increments. After each addition stir the solution and read the pH; record both the volume and the pH.

It is interesting to add some phenolphthalein indicator solution at the beginning of the titration and to observe its color change in relation to the potentiometric titration curve; after the phenolphthalein end point, methyl orange indicator can be added to detect the second end point.

Plot the potentiometric titration data (pH on the vertical axis, titrant volume on the horizontal axis). Draw a smooth curve through the points. Estimate the two end points from the titration curve. Calculate the weight of Na_2CO_3 contained in the sample taken for the titration, and report the percent purity of the soda ash. From the potentiometric titration curve estimate pK_1 and pK_2 for carbonic acid, and compare your experimental values with values found in the literature.

Analysis of Phenobarbital. Obtain from the instructor a sample of phenobarbital, which may be impure. Accurately weigh about 500 mg into a beaker, dissolve it in 40 ml of alcohol, and add 20 ml of water. Immerse glass and saturated calomel electrodes and titrate potentiometrically with standard 0.1 *N* NaOH. Determine the end point by the second derivative method, and calculate the percent purity of the phenobarbital.

Determination of pK'_a *for an Acid.* Choose a weak monobasic acid from a selection provided by your instructor. Accurately weigh about 0.5 mmole of the acid into a 250 ml beaker, and dissolve it in 50.0 ml of water. Heat may be used to effect solution, if necessary, but the solution should be brought back to room temperature before proceeding.

Immerse the glass electrode and S.C.E. in the solution and record the pH. Add standard 0.1 *N* NaOH, from a 10 ml buret, in increments of 0.5 ml, until 5 ml has been added. After each addition stir the solution well and measure the pH. Record the temperature of the solution.

Calculate the acid dissociation constant of your acid as described in Section 6.3. The easiest way to arrange your data and results is to construct a table with eight column headings: (1) volume of titrant; (2) pH; (3) b; (4) $c - b$; (5) $[H^+]$ or $[OH^-]$; (6) $[A^-]/[HA]$; (7) $\log [A^-]/[HA]$; and (8) pK'_a. If the measured pH is in the range 4–10, column 5 is unnecessary as discussed earlier, and Eq. 6.28 is used to calculate pK'_a. Otherwise, either Eq. 6.29 or 6.30 may be necessary.

Determination of Equivalent Weight of a Base. A sample of a pure base of unknown identity will be provided. Accurately weigh a portion corresponding to 2–4 meq, dissolve it in 75 ml of water, and titrate potentiometrically with standard 0.1 *N* HCl, using a glass-S.C.E. system and adding titrant in 1.0 ml increments. Determine the end point from a Gran plot, as described in Section 6.5. Calculate the equivalent weight of the base and estimate its pK'_a from the potentiometric titration curve. (With the EW, the pK'_a, and its physical appearance, you may be able to make a tentative identification of the compound.)

Note: Experiment 2.1 describes nonaqueous potentiometric acid-base titrations.

References

1. Meites, L. and H. C. Thomas, *Advanced Analytical Chemistry*, McGraw-Hill, New York, 1958, Chap. 3.
2. Glasstone, S., *Thermodynamics for Chemists*, D. Van Nostrand Co., Princeton, N.J., 1947, Chap. XIII.
3. Lingane, J. J., *Electroanalytical Chemistry*, 2nd ed., Interscience, New York, 1958, Chap. III.
4. Anson, F. C., *J. Chem. Educ.*, **36**, 394 (1959).

5. Kolthoff, I. M. and R. Belcher, *Volumetric Analysis*, Vol. III, Interscience, New York, 1957, p. 200.
6. Bates, R. G., Chap. 10 in *Treatise on Analytical Chemistry*, Part I, Vol. I, I. M. Kolthoff and P. J. Elving (eds.), Interscience, New York, 1959.
7. Bates, R. G. and E. A. Guggenheim, *Pure Appl. Chem.*, **1,** 163 (1960).
8. Bates, R. G., *J. Res. Natl. Bur. Stand.*, **66A,** 179 (1962).
9. Staples, B. R. and R. G. Bates, *J. Res. Natl. Bur. Stand.*, **73A,** 37 (1969).
10. Bates, R. G. and R. A. Robinson, *Anal. Chem.*, **45,** 420 (1973).
11. Ref. 1, Chap. 4.
12. Albert, A. and E. P. Serjeant, *Ionization Constants of Acids and Bases*, Methuen, London, 1962.
13. Eisenman, G., *Advan. Anal. Chem. Instrum.*, **4,** 213 (1965).
14. Pedersen, C. J., *J. Am. Chem. Soc.*, **89,** 7017 (1967).
15. Ross, J. W., Jr., *Ion-Selective Electrodes*, Natl. Bur. Stand. Spec. Pub. 314, R. A. Durst (ed.), Washington, D.C., 1969, Chap. 2.
16. Gran, G., *Analyst*, **77,** 661 (1952).
17. Rossotti, F. J. C. and H. Rossotti, *J. Chem. Educ.*, **42,** 375 (1965).
18. Reilley, C. N. and R. W. Schmid, *Anal. Chem.*, **30,** 947 (1958).

FOR FURTHER READING

Buck, R. P., "Potentiometry: pH Measurements and Ion-Selective Electrodes," *Techniques of Chemistry*, Vol. I, Part IIA, A. Weissberger and B. W. Rossiter (eds.), Wiley-Interscience, New York, 1971, Chap. II.

Adams, R. N., "Applications of Modern Electroanalytical Techniques to Pharmaceutical Chemistry," *J. Pharm. Sci.*, **58,** 1171 (1969).

Cookson, R. F., "The Determination of Acidity Constants," *Chem. Rev.*, **74,** 5 (1974).

Problems

1. (*a*) Calculate the normality of the hydrochloric acid used in the titration described in Table 6.5.

(*b*) Estimate the pK'_a of TRIS from the titration data given in Tables 6.5 and 6.6.

2. What is the ionic strength of these solutions?

(*a*) 0.2 *M* sodium iodide

(*b*) 0.1 *M* sodium sulfate

(*c*) 0.1 *M* ferric chloride

(*d*) A solution prepared by mixing 100 ml 0.1 *M* acetic acid, 50 ml 0.1 *N* NaOH, and 50 ml 0.1 *M* NaCl.

3. One milliliter of 0.100 *N* KOH was added to 9.0 ml 0.030 *M* acetic acid. The pH of this solution was 4.480 at 25°C. Calculate the constant pK'_a and the thermodynamic constant pK_a for acetic acid.

4. The emf of a solution consisting of 50 ml of 0.115 *N* HCl was measured in a glass-S.C.E. system. Then 5.0 ml of 0.080 *N* NaOH was added, and the emf of the new solution was measured. What was the change in emf?

5. (*a*) Suppose 50.0 ml of 0.05 *M* stannous ion is titrated with 0.10 *M* ferric ion. Calculate the volume of titrant needed to reach the end point.

(*b*) For the titration in part (*a*), calculate the molar concentrations of all four species at the end point.

6. Calculate the standard free energy change and the equilibrium constant for the reaction

$$2Ag^+ + Sn^{2+} \rightleftharpoons Sn^{4+} + 2Ag$$

7. Given the cell

$$\text{Ag, AgX} \mid \text{KX } (0.05\ M) \parallel \text{KCl } (1\ M) \mid \text{Hg}_2\text{Cl}_2\text{, Hg}$$

If the standard potential of the calomel electrode is $E^0_{\text{Hg}_2\text{Cl}_2,\text{Hg}} = +0.28$ V and the cell potential is $+0.30$ V, what is the standard potential $E^0_{\text{AgX,Ag}}$?

8. For the cell

$$\text{Pb, PbBr}_2 \mid \text{Br}^- \ (0.01\ M) \parallel \text{Ce}^{4+} \ (0.01\ M),\ \text{Ce}^{3+} \ (0.1\ M) \mid \text{Pt}$$

(*a*) Write the balanced cell reaction.
(*b*) Calculate the cell potential.
(*c*) Does the reaction proceed spontaneously as you have written it?
The standard potentials are

$$E^0_{\text{PbBr}_2,\text{Pb}} = -0.28 \text{ V},\ E^0_{\text{Ce}^{4+},\text{Ce}^{3+}} = +1.61 \text{ V}$$

9. Consider this cell (this is known as a concentration cell, because the two half-cells are identical except for reactant concentrations):

$$\text{Ni} \mid \text{Ni}^{2+} \ (0.15\ M) \parallel \text{Ni}^{2+} \ (0.015\ M) \mid \text{Ni}$$

(*a*) What is the overall reaction?
(*b*) What is the emf of the cell at 25°C?
(*c*) Is the reaction spontaneous as you have written it?

10. These are standard potentials for the reactions

$$\text{Mg(OH)}_2 + 2e \rightleftharpoons \text{Mg} + 2\text{OH}^- \qquad E^0_{\text{Mg(OH)}_2,\text{Mg}} = -2.69 \text{ V}$$
$$\text{Mg}^{2+} + 2e \rightleftharpoons \text{Mg} \qquad E^0_{\text{Mg}^{2+},\text{Mg}} = -2.37 \text{ V}$$

Calculate the solubility product of magnesium hydroxide.

11. The emf of this cell is -0.116 V. Calculate the pH of the weak acid solution and the $\text{p}K'_a$ of acid HA.

$$\text{Pt} \mid \text{H}_2 \ (p = 1 \text{ atm}),\ \text{H}^+ \ (0.20\ M) \parallel \text{HA } (0.04\ M),\ \text{H}_2 \ (p = 1 \text{ atm}) \mid \text{Pt}$$

12. (*a*) Calculate the standard cell potential and the equilibrium constant for this reaction.

$$5\text{Fe}^{2+} + 8\text{H}^+ + \text{MnO}_4^- \rightleftharpoons \text{Mn}^{2+} + 5\text{Fe}^{3+} + 4\text{H}_2\text{O}$$

(*b*) If 1 mmole of Fe^{2+} is mixed with an equivalent amount of permanganate in a final volume of 100 ml, at pH = 0, calculate the concentration of Fe^{2+} remaining at equilibrium.

13. Calculate the potential of this cell at 25°C. The $\text{p}K_a$ of benzoic acid is 4.20 and the standard potential of the S.C.E. is $+0.24$ V.

$$\text{Pt, H}_2 \ (p = 1 \text{ atm}) \mid \text{benzoic acid } (0.10\ M) \parallel \text{S.C.E.}$$

14. Outline procedures that could be used to analyze for each component in the following mixtures.
(*a*) Acetic acid and hydrochloric acid.
(*b*) Aminopyrine, aspirin, and sodium bromide.
(*c*) Calcium lactate and lactic acid.

7 VOLTAMMETRY

7.1 Polarography

Current-Potential Curves. When a chemical cell is operated under reversible conditions (that is, at essentially zero current), the potential of the cell is given by the Nernst equation, as we saw in Section 6.1. Now suppose that an external emf is applied to the cell (for example, by placing a battery in the external circuit), thus changing the potential between the electrodes; then in order for the Nernst equation to be satisfied at the new potential, it is necessary that the ratio of concentrations of the cell reactants also change. This can occur if the cell reaction takes place, and occurrence of the cell reaction necessarily produces a current in the cell.

The interpretation of this kind of experiment is simpler if the reactant concentrations of one of the electrodes are quite high, or if this electrode possesses a relatively large area, so that the current density (current per unit area) is small at this electrode. Its potential will then be essentially constant and unaffected by the applied emf. This is the reference electrode. The indicator electrode, on the other hand, is designed to have a small area, with the result that the potential of this electrode (relative to the reference electrode) may be taken equal to the applied emf.

Let us consider the cell composed of a S.C.E. reference electrode and a small platinum indicator electrode, with the platinum electrode immersed in a dilute *unstirred* solution of chromic ions. A battery and voltage divider are incorporated into the external circuit so that any desired voltage (up to about 2 V) may be applied to the cell such that the platinum electrode is given a negative potential relative to the reference electrode. A current-measuring device is included in the circuit. The experiment is conducted by applying increasingly larger (more negative) potentials to the cell. After each alteration in the applied emf (E), the current (i) through the cell is measured. A plot of these data reveals the characteristic shape illustrated in Fig. 7.1; such a plot is a *current-potential curve.*

This curve may be accounted for on the simple basis presented in the first paragraph. The formal potential of the S.C.E. is $+0.24$ V, and the standard potential of the chromic-chromous couple is -0.41 V, or -0.65 V versus

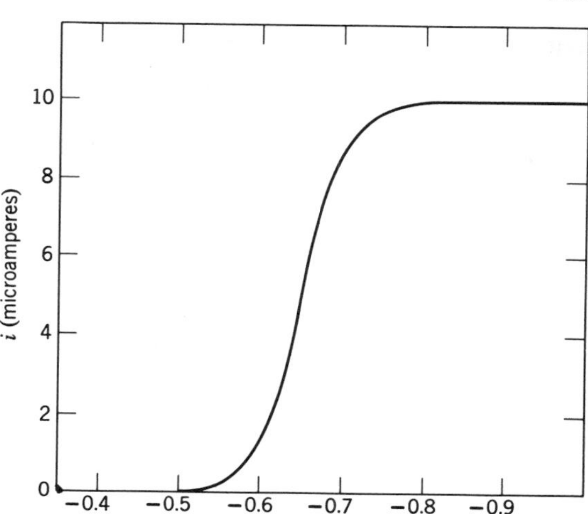

Fig. 7.1. A hypothetical current-potential curve for the reduction of chromic ion to chromous ion.

S.C.E. If, for the initial point on the current-potential curve, the circuit is simply shorted so that no external emf is applied, the potential of the indicator electrode will be 0 V versus S.C.E. Applying the Nernst equation,

$$0 = -0.65 - 0.059 \log \frac{[Cr^{2+}]}{[Cr^{3+}]}$$

or the ratio $[Cr^{2+}]/[Cr^{3+}]$ must be, at the electrode surface, about 10^{-11}; in other words, at this potential essentially no reduction of chromic ion occurs, and so no current is observed. As the applied emf is made more negative relative to the S.C.E., application of the Nernst equation shows that the ratio $[Cr^{2+}]/[Cr^{3+}]$ becomes progressively larger, accounting for the rise shown in Fig. 7.1.

As the applied emf becomes more negative than the standard potential of the chromic-chromous couple, practically every chromic ion that reaches the surface of the electrode is immediately reduced. The solution adjacent to the electrode therefore becomes depleted of chromic ions, but more ions diffuse toward the electrode surface from the bulk solution. At very negative potentials a steady state is established in which the current is limited by the rate at which reducible ions can reach the electrode surface, and beyond this point an increasingly negative potential cannot cause an increase in current. This mass transport-controlled process gives rise to the plateau region of the current-potential curve.

The study of current-potential curves is known as *voltammetry*. The next pages explore the properties of these curves.

We can now see that the subject matter treated in Chapter 6 is a special case of voltammetry: potentiometry is voltammetry at zero current.* In potentiometry we measure one point on the current-potential curve—the potential corresponding to zero current—as a function of the reactant concentrations. In the present, more general case we measure current as a function of potential while holding the reactant concentrations constant. It is important to realize that, because of the small size of the indicator electrode in the voltammetric experiment, the total amount of ion reacted is practically undetectable, so the bulk concentration is constant throughout the experiment.

The Dropping Mercury Electrode. The experiment described in the preceding paragraphs does not yield results as simple as implied in the interpretation. The difficulty is with the platinum indicator electrode. As the potential is made very negative (reducing), a rise in current is observed that is due to the reduction of hydrogen ions in the solution.

$$2H^{+} + 2e \rightleftharpoons H_2$$

This current tends to obscure currents resulting from the reduction of solute species. Fortunately, the potential at which this reaction occurs depends upon the metal of which the electrode is composed. It is found that the hydrogen ion reduction occurs at a potential 0.8 V more negative at a mercury electrode than at platinum [1]. This is an example of *overpotential* (overvoltage), which is the difference between the observed potential of an electrode and the theoretical potential as calculated with the Nernst equation. The overpotential of hydrogen ion at the mercury electrode (which may be caused by slowness in one or more of the reaction steps) is of great practical importance, for it extends the potential range available for reductions at the indicator electrode. The *dropping mercury electrode* (D.M.E.) is used widely as the indicator electrode in current-potential studies. The current-potential curve obtained with the dropping mercury electrode is known as a *polarogram*, and the study of these curves is *polarography*.

The D.M.E. consists simply of a reservoir of mercury culminating in a fine capillary tube that dips into the solution. The mercury falls in small drops from the capillary tip. Electrical connection to the external circuit is through a wire placed in the mercury reservoir. A great advantage of the D.M.E. is the periodic re-formation of a fresh electrode surface as each new drop forms (the life of a drop is usually 3–6 sec). Surface contamination is not a problem with the D.M.E.

A current-potential curve obtained with the dropping mercury electrode has the same shape as that in Fig. 7.1. Most polarographic measurements are

* A more general definition states that potentiometry is voltammetry at constant current. Successful potentiometric titrations can be made at constant, nonzero current.

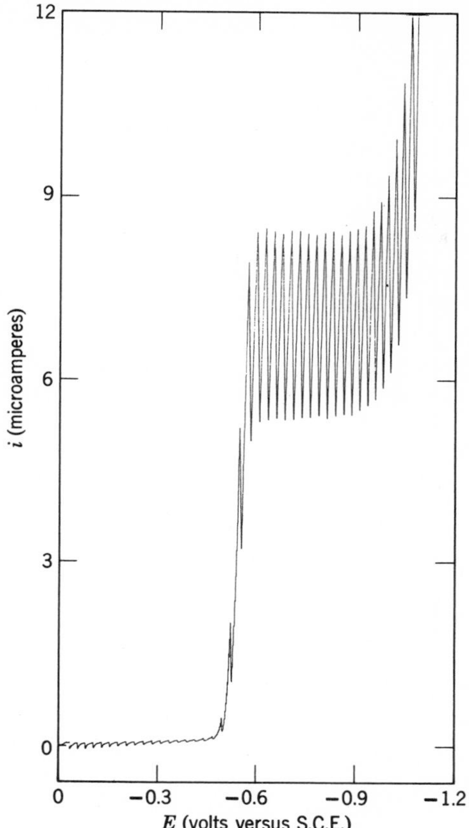

Fig. 7.2. A polarogram of 10^{-3} M cadmium ion at the dropping mercury electrode.

now made with automatic recording equipment that traces the current as a function of the continuously varying applied emf. Since the polarographic current is related to the electrode surface area, the current measured at the D.M.E. varies in a complicated way during the life of each drop, finally falling to zero as the drop falls. A galvanometer with a long period tends to smooth out these fluctuations, but they are apparent on recorded polarograms (see Fig. 7.2). By current we shall mean the average current, which is easily estimated from the polarogram.

The rising portion of the current-potential curve is called the polarographic wave. The flat plateau region gives the *limiting current*, to which the principal contributor is the *diffusion current*, i_d; the diffusion current is the diffusion-controlled current caused by the reduction of the solute species. A minor contributor to the limiting current is the *residual current*, which is largely caused by reducible impurities in the solution; the residual current is estimated by extrapolation of the small current observed before the wave. The value of the applied emf at the point where the current is equal to one-half the diffusion current is the *half-wave potential*, $E_{1/2}$.

The half-wave potential is characteristic of the identity of a substance, so it is useful as an aid in qualitative analysis. The diffusion current is proportional to the bulk concentration of the electroactive species, and this relationship is the basis of quantitative polarographic analysis.

Most reactions at the dropping mercury electrode are reductions, that is, the D.M.E. is the cathode. Oxidations can also be studied, with the D.M.E. acting as the anode.

The Diffusion Process. The residual current, which is caused mainly by the reduction of impurities in the reagents, can be estimated by extrapolation or by carrying out a "blank" determination in which the sample is omitted. In the unstirred solution the limiting current (corrected for the residual current) is the result of a steady-state condition in which the chemical reaction at the cathode is a fast step and the slow (rate determining) step is the supply of reducible species to the electrode surface. In the absence of transfer by convection, only two ways are available for the transfer of reducible ions to the D.M.E. One of these is called migration. A potential gradient exists between the electrodes, with the D.M.E. negative relative to the S.C.E. Cations will therefore migrate toward the D.M.E. under the influence of this potential, and their reduction gives rise to the *migration current.* This current will depend upon the applied emf, and its elimination is desirable. Current is carried through a solution by all the ions present. The fraction of current carried by any given species depends primarily upon its relative concentration. Therefore, to reduce the current carried by the reducible ion, a large concentration of a non-reducible electrolyte is added to the solution. This substance, the *indifferent electrolyte* (or supporting electrolyte), then carries essentially all the current, and the migration current is eliminated.

The only remaining transfer process is diffusion. The residual current-corrected limiting current is therefore the diffusion current. The factors important in the diffusion process can be revealed by studying a type of diffusion amenable to simple mathematical treatment. In order to obtain an insight into mass transfer by diffusion, let us consider the diffusion of an ion to an idealized planar electrode in two-dimensional space. The model is pictured in Fig. 7.3. The electrode reaction is assumed to be very fast, so that diffusion is the rate-determining (and current-determining) step. The rate of diffusion of the reducible species to the electrode surface is given by

$$\frac{dN}{dt} = AD\frac{dC}{dx} \tag{7.1}$$

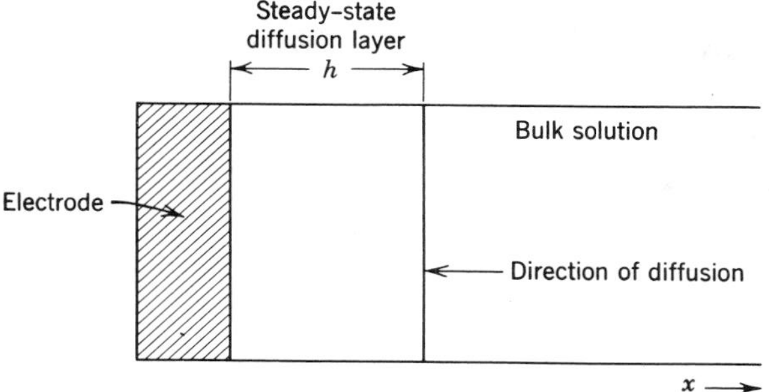

Fig. 7.3. Linear diffusion to a planar electrode.

where dN/dt is the rate of diffusion in terms of the number of moles per unit time, A is the cross-sectional area of the electrode, D is a proportionality constant called the diffusion coefficient (with dimensions of length squared divided by time), and dC/dx is the concentration gradient. Equation 7.1 is known as Fick's first law.

This equation will hold at any time. However, when steady-state conditions prevail, the concentration gradient becomes a constant. At steady state the diffusion layer, which is the layer of solution from the electrode surface to the point where the concentration is essentially that of the bulk solution, is of constant thickness denoted by h in Fig. 7.3; that is, $dx = h$. Moreover, the differential $dC = C - C_0$, where C is the bulk concentration and C_0 is the concentration at the electrode surface. C_0 is essentially zero. Equation 7.1 then becomes

$$\frac{dN}{dt} = \frac{ADC}{h} \tag{7.2}$$

Now the quantity of electricity produced by the reduction of the ions is equal to the product of the current and the time:

$$dQ = i\,dt$$

This quantity is also equal to the product of the number of electrons n involved in the electrode reaction, the Faraday $\mathbf{F}$ (quantity of electricity corresponding to one equivalent), and the number of moles undergoing reaction, dR:

$$dQ = i\,dt = n\mathbf{F}\,dR$$

$$\frac{dR}{dt} = \frac{i}{n\mathbf{F}} \tag{7.3}$$

At steady state every ion that reaches the electrode surface is immediately reduced, so that $dR/dt = dN/dt$, or, equating Eqs. 7.2 and 7.3,

$$i_d = \frac{n\mathbf{F}ADC}{h} \tag{7.4}$$

where i_d is written to indicate that the current is diffusion-controlled. Equation 7.4 demonstrates several important dependencies: the diffusion current is directly proportional to the number of electrons involved in the reaction, to the area of the electrode surface, to the diffusion coefficient of the reducible species, to the bulk concentration of the reducible species, and it is inversely proportional to the thickness of the diffusion layer.

The Ilkovic Equation. The dropping mercury electrode is an expanding spherical electrode. Diffusion to the D.M.E. is therefore a much more complicated process to describe theoretically than is the analogous situation with a planar electrode, but the same factors are important. The equation for the diffusion current at the D.M.E. is

$$i_d = 607\ nD^{1/2}Cm^{2/3}t^{1/6} \tag{7.5}$$

where i_d is the average diffusion current (in microamperes), n is the number of electrons in the reduction reaction, D is the diffusion coefficient (cm^2/sec), C is the bulk concentration (mmole/liter), m is the rate of flow of mercury from the D.M.E. (mg/sec), t is the lifetime of a drop of mercury (sec), and 607 is a combination of some numerical constants, including the faraday. Equation 7.5 is called the *Ilkovic equation*. It was derived with arguments similar to those we used for the simple planar electrode [2], and it exhibits some of the same dependencies. Of particular analytical importance is the direct proportionality between diffusion current and concentration of the reducible species. The Ilkovic equation may be written $i_d = kC$, where $k = 607\ nD^{1/2}m^{2/3}t^{1/6}$. k obviously depends upon the particular reducible species (through n and D). It also depends upon the particular capillary used, through m and t. Analytically useful diffusion currents are routinely obtained with concentrations in the range 0.01–50 mM.

Diffusion current measurements are sometimes complicated by the presence of a pronounced maximum in the current-potential curve as a continuation of the rising portion of the wave. These polarographic maxima are believed to be caused by streaming phenomena that bring more reducible ions into contact with the electrode surface than can reach it by diffusion alone. The addition of trace amounts of *maximum suppressors* will eliminate maxima. Gelatin is often used for this purpose. Surface-active agents, some anions, amines, and methyl red are sometimes effective.

The Half-Wave Potential. An equation can be derived relating the potential of the D.M.E. to the current in a polarographic reduction. Consider the reduction of a metal ion to form a metal-mercury solution (amalgam):

$$M^{n+} + ne + Hg = M(Hg)$$

The potential of this couple at the D.M.E. is given by the Nernst equation

$$E_{\text{D.M.E.}} = \mathbf{E}^{0'}_{M^{n+},M(Hg)} - \frac{0.059}{n} \log \frac{[M(Hg)]}{[M^{n+}]_s} \tag{7.6}$$

where the potential $E_{\text{D.M.E.}}$ and the formal potential $\mathbf{E}^{0'}_{M^{n+},M(Hg)}$ are, for convenience, considered to be expressed relative to the S.C.E. $[M(Hg)]$ is the concentration of the amalgam in the electrode surface and $[M^{n+}]_s$ is the concentration of ion in the solution at the electrode surface.

Since ions are supplied to the electrode only by diffusion, the current at any point in the polarogram is directly proportional to the difference in ion concentration at the electrode and in the bulk solution.

$$i = k_{\text{ox}}([M^{n+}] - [M^{n+}]_s) \tag{7.7}$$

When the current reaches its maximum value i_d, the concentration of ions at the electrode surface is negligible, and Eq. 7.7 becomes

$$i_d = k_{\text{ox}}[M^{n+}] \tag{7.8}$$

It is apparent from a comparison of Eqs. 7.8 and 7.5 that

$$k_{\text{ox}} = 607\ nD_{\text{ox}}^{1/2}m^{2/3}t^{1/6}$$

with D_{ox} being the diffusion coefficient of the ion in the solution. Combining 7.7 and 7.8 gives for the concentration of ion at the electrode surface

$$[M^{n+}]_s = \frac{i_d - i}{k_{\text{ox}}} \tag{7.9}$$

Because the electrode reaction is reversible, the current may also be expressed in terms of the reverse reaction, or

$$i = k_{\text{red}}[M(Hg)] \tag{7.10}$$

where $k_{\text{red}} = 607\ nD_{\text{red}}^{1/2}m^{2/3}t^{1/6}$, and D_{red} is the diffusion coefficient for the reduced species in the mercury electrode. Substituting Eqs. 7.9 and 7.10 into 7.6,

$$E_{\text{D.M.E.}} = E^{0'}_{M^{n+},M(Hg)} - \frac{0.059}{n} \log \frac{k_{\text{ox}}}{k_{\text{red}}} - \frac{0.059}{n} \log \frac{i}{(i_d - i)} \tag{7.11}$$

Making the definition $E_{1/2} = E^{0'}_{M^{n+},M(Hg)} - \frac{0.059}{n} \log \frac{k_{\text{ox}}}{k_{\text{red}}}$ allows Eq. 7.11 to be written

$$E_{\text{D.M.E.}} = E_{1/2} - \frac{0.059}{n} \log \left(\frac{i}{i_d - i}\right) \tag{7.12}$$

$E_{1/2}$ is the half-wave potential; it is evidently equal to the potential of the D.M.E. when $i = i_d/2$. The half-wave potential is seen from its definition to be closely related to the formal potential for the couple, differing from $E^{0\prime}$ only by the ratio k_{ox}/k_{red}, which in turn is governed only by the ratio $D_{ox}^{1/2}/D_{red}^{1/2}$.

Equation 7.12 describes the entire current-potential curve. Adherence to Eq. 7.12 is usually accepted as the criterion of polarographic reversibility of a reaction. This is demonstrated most easily by making a plot of $E_{\text{D.M.E.}}$ versus $\log i/(i_d - i)$; if the reaction is reversible, a straight line should be obtained with slope equal to $0.059/n$ (or its reciprocal, depending upon the choice of axes). The $E_{1/2}$ is read from this graph as the potential of the D.M.E. when the logarithmic term is equal to zero.

The most notable characteristic of the half-wave potential is its independence of the concentration of the reducible ion. It is therefore of value for purposes of qualitative analysis. It may be markedly affected by the kind and concentration of indifferent electrolytes, however, and these must be controlled and specified.

If a metal ion forms a complex with a component of the solution, a change in $E_{1/2}$ usually occurs. In general, a complex is more difficult to reduce than is the corresponding simple ion, and so the $E_{1/2}$ shifts to a more negative value. Advantage may be taken of complex formation to permit polarographic determination of certain mixtures. If the sample contains two ions whose half-wave potentials are within a few tenths of a volt, it is not possible to resolve the current-potential curve into two distinct waves. If an agent is added that complexes with only one of these ions, thus changing its $E_{1/2}$, it may be possible to distinguish the separate waves and to make an analysis of the two ions. For example, in acid solution both lead and thallium are reduced at the D.M.E. with identical half-wave potentials of −0.5 V. If EDTA is added to the solution, the thallium half-wave potential remains at −0.5 V, whereas the lead half-wave potential is shifted to −0.9 V; a polarogram of the mixture then shows two well-defined waves, permitting the analysis of both metals.

Because of the large overpotential of hydrogen on mercury, reduction of hydrogen ion at the D.M.E. does not interfere with most reductions. In fact, usually the reduction of the indifferent electrolyte (often potassium chloride) determines the most reducing potential attainable. Another complication is reduction of dissolved oxygen:

$$\tfrac{1}{2}O_2 + H_2O + 2e \rightleftharpoons 2OH^-$$

All oxygen is removed by flushing the solution with nitrogen before the polarogram is recorded.

7.2 Related Techniques

Amperometric Titrations. Imagine a polarographic experiment in which the polarographic wave of a reducible ion is recorded in the usual manner; then a

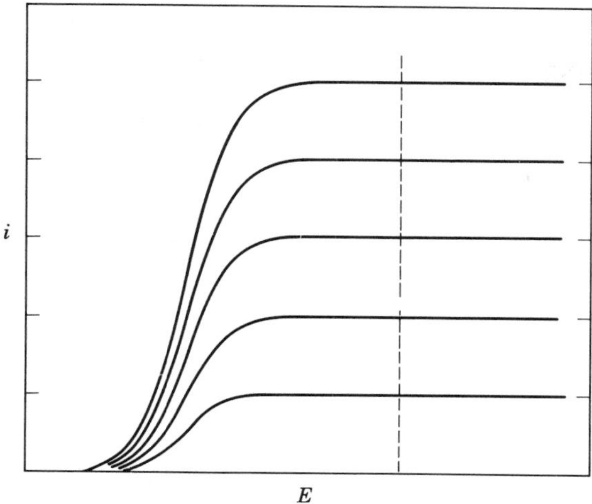

Fig. 7.4. Successive polarograms (from top to bottom) obtained during the titration of a reducible species with a nonreducible precipitating agent.

small amount of a precipitating agent is added and the polarogram is recorded again. This procedure, which is clearly a titration, is repeated until a stoichiometric excess of titrant has been added. The set of polarograms will look like Fig. 7.4, if the titrant is itself not reducible at the D.M.E.

If, now, the current at a selected potential (for example, at the dashed line in Fig. 7.4) is plotted against volume of titrant, Fig. 7.5 is obtained. The end point of the titration is marked by the intersection of the straight-line segments. This technique is called *amperometric titration*. It is not necessary to record the entire polarogram, but merely to set the applied emf in the plateau region and read i_d.

The amperometric titration plot may take several shapes. The one shown in Fig. 7.5 is obtained when the sample is reducible and the titrant is not. An example is the titration of lead ion with sulfate. If the titrant is reducible but the sample is not, the current will remain at zero until the end point, and after that it will rise; the titration of halides with silver ion gives this plot. If both the sample and the titrant are reducible, a V-shaped plot is observed.

Most amperometric titrations are based upon precipitate formation. The larger the equilibrium constant for the formation of the insoluble compound (that is, the smaller its solubility product), the more abrupt the change in slope at the end point in the titration plot. Usually some curvature is apparent and the end point is located by extrapolation from points taken well before and after the end point.

Although the D.M.E. is frequently used as the indicator electrode in amperometric titrations, a platinum electrode is more convenient and is equally

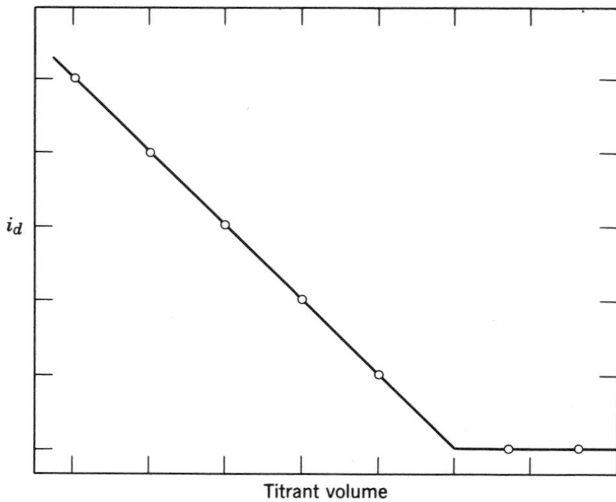

Fig. 7.5. Amperometric titration plot of the polarographic data in Fig. 7.4.

satisfactory. In a quiescent solution several minutes are required for the establishment of a steady-state current at the platinum electrode, but in a stirred solution the steady state is achieved rapidly. The best results seem to be obtained with a rotating platinum electrode. The rest of the instrumentation is similar to that used for polarography (see Section 7.3). The constant potential may be applied by means of a battery and a voltage divider, but high accuracy in the selection and measurement of the applied emf is not necessary because the diffusion current is practically independent of minor changes in potential. Some amperometric titrations can be carried out with no external applied emf if the potential of the reference electrode is sufficiently negative to effect reduction of the sample or titrant species. Titrations with silver ion are illustrative. If the S.C.E. is the reference electrode, and no external emf is applied, then when the indicator electrode is connected to the S.C.E., its potential becomes 0 V versus S.C.E. Since the formal potential of the S.C.E. is +0.24 V, this is also the potential of the indicator electrode. This is very much more negative (more reducing) than the standard potential of the Ag^+, Ag couple, so silver ion is reduced at the indicator electrode. This use of the reference electrode as the source of emf simplifies the instrumentation.

The current measurement in an amperometric titration should be accurate, but absolute values are not required, because the end point is located by the change in current rather than the current itself. It is sufficient merely to record galvanometer scale readings, which are proportional to current. Usually the titrant is made much more concentrated than the sample solution in order to circumvent large volume change effects. If deviations from linearity are noted before or after the end point, it may be necessary to make a correction for the volume change. The diffusion current is directly proportional to concentration, but the concentration of the reducible species does not change linearly because of the volume change. This effect can be compensated for by multiplying each galvanometer reading by $(V + v)/V$, where V is the initial volume of the sample solution and v is the volume of titrant added.

Amperometric titration is voltammetry at constant potential; the current is measured as a function of reactant concentration while holding the potential constant. This description can be compared with the earlier ones (Section 7.1) for potentiometry and polarography; see Table 7.1.

Modified Polarographic Methods. Many modifications of polarography have been devised. The goals of these studies have been to increase analytical sensitivity, to improve the resolution of species with similar half-wave potentials, and to investigate the mechanisms of electrode reactions. The approaches taken have been mainly instrumental in nature, with the manner of varying the electrode potential as a function of time being the principal experimental manipulation. These modifications have been dependent upon the more recent availability of highly sophisticated electronic technology.

A relatively simple modification is *derivative polarography*, in which the first derivative di/dE of the current-potential curve is plotted against the applied potential E. This derivative plot shows a peak with its maximum at the half-wave potential; the peak height is proportional to concentration. The main advantage of derivative polarography is its greater resolution of closely spaced polarographic waves.

The saw-toothed appearance of the conventional current-potential curve (see Fig. 7.2) can be eliminated by electronically "sampling" each mercury drop at only one point in its lifetime. The current-potential plot then is a smooth wave, with one point per drop. This technique, called *Tast polarography* (Tast is German for touch; in this method each drop is physically dislodged at a preselected time), yields a maximum sensitivity of about 5×10^{-7} M in the

TABLE 7.1
Comparison of Voltammetric Analytical Methods

Technique	Dependent Variable (Property Measured)	Independent Variable (Property Varied)	Constant Factor
Polarography	i	E	Concentration
Potentiometry	E	Concentration	i
Amperometry	i	Concentration	E

reducible species, compared with 1×10^{-5} *M* for conventional polarography. In Tast polarography the potential is applied as a continuously increasing function of time, and the current is measured during a brief time period in the life of each drop. In *pulse polarography* the potential is applied only once during the life of the drop, for about 50 msec, during which period the drop is not significantly changing in size. The current is measured during the later portion of this pulse period. Pulse polarography is capable of sensitivity at the 1×10^{-8} *M* level. A combined method, *derivative pulse polarography*, has given a sensitivity of 5×10^{-9} *M*.

All these methods use a series of drops, with the potential being applied and current being measured according to various time schedules. In *single-sweep polarography* (also called peak polarography and oscillographic polarography) the entire current-potential curve is recorded during the life of a single drop. The resulting curve does not have the appearance of Fig. 7.1, but instead shows a peak in the region of $E_{1/2}$. The peak results because diffusion from the bulk solution to the electrode surface is not fast enough to keep up with the rapidly scanning potential. A maximal sensitivity of 3×10^{-7} *M* is possible.

A technique related to peak polarography achieves great sensitivity by using a preconcentration step. The metal ion to be determined is subjected to a reducing potential in the presence of a hanging mercury drop or other stationary electrode. The metal plates onto the electrode or forms an amalgam in the mercury surface. After several minutes of deposition in a stirred solution, the metal concentration at the electrode surface is adequate for the subsequent analysis. A single-sweep anodic potential scan is now made, oxidizing the metal from the electrode, and the current peak is measured. This technique is called *stripping voltammetry;* a maximum sensitivity of about 10^{-11} *M* has been claimed. Sensitivities of this level are difficult to achieve routinely, at least in part because of the introduction of interferences as impurities in reagents.

7.3 Analytical Application

Instrumentation. The principle of polarographic instrumentation is illustrated with the very simple circuit of Fig. 7.6. The battery need deliver no more than about 2.7 V, so two 1.5 V dry cells will suffice. The voltmeter *V* measures the potential supplied by the battery. *AB* is a precision linear resistance with which any known fraction of the battery potential may be tapped by means of the sliding contact *C*. This known, variable potential is applied across the polarographic cell. The resulting current is read with a damped microammeter *M*. A somewhat more sophisticated circuit for a manual polarograph has been described [3]; in this instrument the current is determined by measuring the

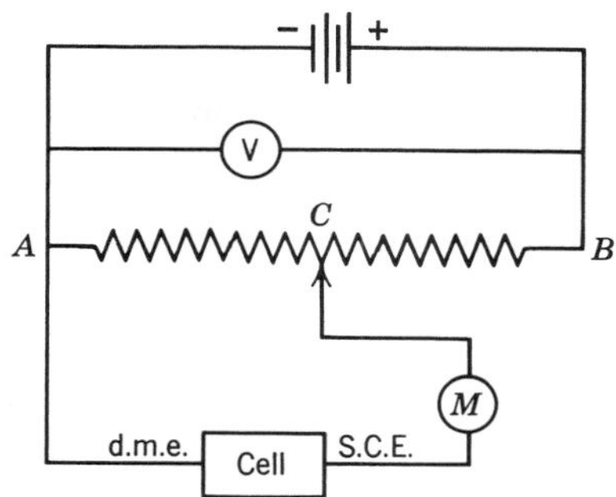

Fig. 7.6. A simple manual polarograph circuit.

iR drop across a precision fixed resistor* in series with the cell. This circuit permits very accurate measurements to be made. Manual determination of a current-potential curve is very time-consuming and tedious, however, and automatic recording instruments are almost universally used. Although the circuitry of these instruments is very complex, it accomplishes the same task as the simple device of Fig. 7.6—measurement of the applied potential and the resulting current. The polarogram in Fig. 7.2 was recorded automatically.

The polarographic cell is a glass vessel with provisions for the capillary tip of the dropping mercury electrode, inlet and outlet tubes for flushing oxygen from the solution, temperature control, and electrical connection through a salt bridge to the reference electrode.

Amperometric titrations may be conducted with the same instrumentation used for polarography. (When the D.M.E. is used, amperometric titrations are sometimes called polarometric titrations.) Often the rotating platinum electrode is employed as the indicator electrode. This electrode is simply a piece of platinum wire fused into the end of a length of glass tubing. The tubing is bent at a right angle about $\frac{1}{2}$ in. from the end. Electrical contact is made by pouring mercury into the tubing, where it contacts the platinum wire; the external circuit lead is immersed in the mercury. The electrode is grasped by the chuck of an electric motor. The rotating platinum electrode is described in greater detail in Experiment 7.1.

Analytical Methods. Quantitative polarographic analysis is based upon the Ilkovic equation, which predicts that the diffusion current is directly proportional to the concentration of electroactive substance. This expectation is usually realized in practice; that is, the equation $i_d = kC$ is obeyed, where k is a constant characteristic of the substance, the capillary, and the experimental

* By Ohm's law, $E = iR$; if the resistance of the resistor is accurately known, measurement of the potential drop across the resistor (with a potentiometer, Fig. 6.2) permits calculation of the current through the cell.

conditions (Eq. 7.5). Several general techniques are based upon the linear relationship between diffusion current and concentration.

In the "standard solution" method several solutions of the substance to be determined are prepared with known concentrations. The polarograms of these solutions are recorded, and the ratio $i_d/C = k$ is calculated for each solution. Then the sample solution of unknown concentration is subjected to the same experimental conditions (same temperature, indifferent electrolyte, and capillary), and its diffusion current is measured. Then from the relationship $C = i_d/k$ and the predetermined value of k the unknown concentration is calculated. This analytical approach may be replaced by a graphical one, a plot being made of i_d versus C for the standard solutions, and the unknown concentration is then read from the graph. The graphical method works even if the direct proportionality between i_d and C should fail.

The principal disadvantage of the standard solution method is the requirement that all conditions be the same for the known solutions and the unknown. This is not always convenient.

The "diffusion current constant" method is developed by rearranging the Ilkovic equation (Eq. 7.5) to

$$607nD^{1/2} = \frac{i_d}{Cm^{2/3}t^{1/6}} = I$$

where I is the diffusion current constant. This constant, which is characteristic of a given reaction with a particular set of conditions, is calculated from a polarogram of a solution of known concentration, since i_d, m, and t are all easily measured. Once I has been evaluated for a given substance (at specified temperature and electrolyte concentration), it provides a simple means to analyze any unknown solution of that substance under the same conditions, since the relationship can be solved for C.

$$C = \frac{i_d}{Im^{2/3}t^{1/6}}$$

It is only necessary to determine i_d, m, and t, since I is available from earlier work. A notable advantage of this approach is that different capillaries can be used for the known and unknown samples, since the procedure involves measuring and accounting for m and t. However, this method is generally less accurate than the others available.

The "pilot ion" method [4] eliminates the need to measure the capillary characteristics. To the unknown solution is added a known concentration of a second substance whose half-wave potential is well-separated from the first. The polarogram of the mixture is determined, from which the diffusion currents of the individual substances can be measured. Suppose copper ($E_{1/2} = -0.5$ V) is to be determined. A known concentration of zinc ($E_{1/2} = -1.4$ V) may be added. Then the diffusion currents caused by the reduction of these ions may be written

$$(i_d)_{\mathrm{Cu}} = k_{\mathrm{Cu}} C_{\mathrm{Cu}}$$

$$(i_d)_{\mathrm{Zn}} = k_{\mathrm{Zn}} C_{\mathrm{Zn}}$$

Dividing these and solving for the unknown concentration

$$C_{\mathrm{Cu}} = C_{\mathrm{Zn}} \left[\frac{(i_d)_{\mathrm{Cu}}}{(i_d)_{\mathrm{Zn}}} \right] \frac{k_{\mathrm{Zn}}}{k_{\mathrm{Cu}}} \tag{7.13}$$

The ratio $k_{\mathrm{Zn}}/k_{\mathrm{Cu}}$ is determined from an independent measurement on a solution containing known concentrations of zinc and copper. Since the experimental quantities in Eq. 7.13 appear only as ratios, and a change in experimental conditions that changes one diffusion current changes the other one by the same amount, this equation is applicable even if conditions vary from those under which the ratio $k_{\mathrm{Zn}}/k_{\mathrm{Cu}}$ was originally evaluated.

The "method of standard increments" is a simple method that combines some of the features of the standard solution and pilot ion methods. The polarogram of the unknown solution is recorded. Then a known amount of the *same* substance is added to the solution, and the current-potential curve is again recorded. The ratio of the diffusion currents before and after the addition of the known amount of material is equal to the ratio of the concentrations before and after the addition. This method eliminates the effects of most variables because the two measurements are made at practically the same time.

An accuracy of 1–2% can be expected in routine polarographic analysis. The optimum range of concentration of the electroactive species is 0.01–1 mM, with a volume of 1–10 ml being easily handled; much smaller volumes can be analyzed if necessary. Amperometric titrations can be carried out with similar samples, often with even better accuracy.

The analysis of many inorganics is particularly simple by polarography. The sample may be brought into solution by very drastic treatment if necessary. The solution conditions (pH, indifferent electrolyte, complexing agents) are adjusted, and the polarographic wave is recorded. The quantitative analysis is performed by one of the techniques just discussed. The half-wave potential is a criterion of identity and may aid in qualitative analysis. For most substances the electrode reaction is a reduction (the D.M.E. functions as a cathode). Among the easiest substances to analyze at the D.M.E. are the ions of lead, thallium, copper, cadmium, zinc, manganese, iron, cobalt, and nickel. Some anions—bromate, iodate, nitrate—can be reduced at the D.M.E. Dilute solutions of oxygen may be analyzed polarographically by reduction.

Very many organic compounds are polarographically reducible, although these reactions are reversible in only a few cases. The irreversibility of the reaction does not prevent development of practical analytical methods. The product of the electrode reaction is not known for most reactions. Organic halogen compounds are reducible, and polarography is applicable to the analysis of chloroform, iodoform, and halogenated insecticides. Aldehydes are reduced to alcohols; polarographic analysis of aldehydes in fermentation mixtures is practical. Nitro compounds give well-defined waves at the D.M.E. Many other functional groups are electroactive. Anodic waves (waves resulting from oxidations) find limited analytical use. The monograph by Brezina and Zuman [5] is a rich source of applications of polarography in pharmacy.

Most precipitation titrations that can be carried out with visual detection of the end point (Chapter 3) can also be carried out as amperometric titrations. Organic compounds may be titrated with suitable reagents [6]. Nitrogen bases, for example, may be titrated with silicotungstic acid or with other heteropoly acids; the base forms a precipitate with the titrant, and after the end point the reduction of excess precipitating agent produces a current. Mercury salts have been used as titrants for barbituric acid derivatives. Alkaloids have been analyzed by titration with Reinecke's salt (ammonium tetrathiocyanodiammonochromate), which is an effective precipitant for nitrogen bases.

Experiment 7.1. Amperometric Titration of Halides with Silver

PRINCIPLE

Silver forms very insoluble salts with the halides. This common precipitation reaction forms the basis of an amperometric titration of bromide and chloride, singly and in mixture. It is observed [7] that silver chloride is reduced at the rotating platinum electrode, but when the particles of AgCl are coated with gelatin their reduction is no longer possible. This behavior permits the analysis to be carried out very simply. The mixture of halides, acidified with nitric acid, is titrated with silver nitrate. Silver bromide forms first because its solubility product is smaller than that of silver chloride. After the bromide end point, silver chloride forms, but a rise in current is observed because of the fortuitous reduction of silver chloride. Thus the bromide end point is located. Next gelatin is added to the solution, the current drops to a low value, and the titration of chloride is continued. The diffusion current after the chloride end point is caused by the reduction of silver ions.

The rotating platinum electrode is short-circuited through a galvanometer to a S.C.E. of large area; the emf provided by the S.C.E. is sufficiently negative to reduce silver but not to cause the reduction of oxygen, so the solution need not be deaerated.

This method is suitable for the analysis of halides in pharmaceuticals [8]. The accuracy is 1–3% on samples 0.001–0.01 N in halide.

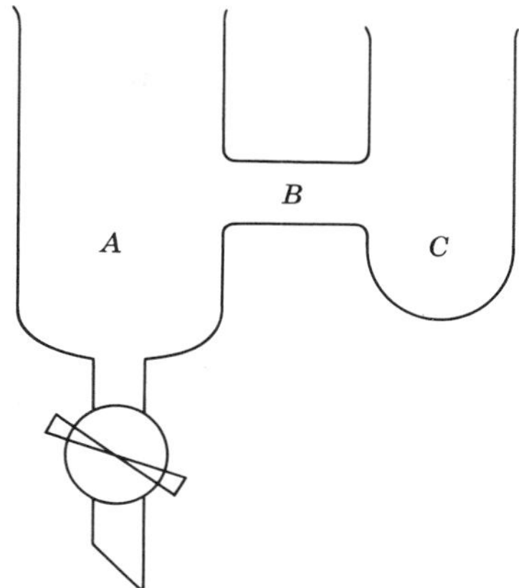

Fig. 7.7. H-cell for amperometric titrations [8]. *A*, titration chamber; *B*, salt bridge; *C*, reference electrode chamber.

APPARATUS AND REAGENTS

H-cell. A glass titration cell suitable for amperometric titrations is shown in Fig. 7.7. The capacity of the titration chamber is about 100 ml. Chamber *C* contains the S.C.E., which is described in the next paragraph. The two chambers are connected by a salt bridge, filled with an agar-KNO_3 gel as follows. Prepare a solution by gently heating 3 g of agar, 20 g of potassium nitrate, and 100 ml of water. Close one end of the salt bridge with a cork and run the warm agar solution into the bridge. After the gel has solidified, remove the cork and fill its space with agar solution.

Saturated Calomel Electrode. Place a few milliliters of clean mercury in the electrode arm of the H-cell. Make electrical contact with the external circuit by means of a copper wire, contained in a glass tube, dipping below the surface of the mercury. Prepare a paste by triturating mercurous chloride (calomel), mercury, and a small amount of saturated potassium chloride solution in a mortar. Transfer this paste to the surface of the mercury pool in the electrode arm. Place a few crystals of potassium chloride on top of the calomel paste. Fill the chamber to above the level of the salt bridge with saturated potassium chloride solution. The potential of this S.C.E. will not be immediately stable; for best results wait several days before using it. This equilibration period is not essential, however.

Rotating Platinum Electrode. Seal a piece of No. 18 platinum wire into the end of a length of 6 mm soft glass tubing to give an exposed electrode 5–10 mm long. The platinum must also extend inside the tube. Bend the tubing at a right angle to the main tube about 2 cm from the end. The tip and wire should trail in the direction opposite to the direction of rotation. Place a few drops of mercury within the tubing to make an electrical contact between the platinum wire and a copper wire leading to the external circuit.

Variable Speed Motor. A cone drive electric motor with a hollow chuck is convenient to hold the platinum electrode, since the wire can be passed through it without an elaborate contact system.

Galvanometer or Microammeter. Preferably with variable sensitivity. The currents will be in the range 0–200 μA.

0.1 N Silver Nitrate. See Experiment 3.1.

0.1 N Sodium Chloride and *0.1 N Sodium Bromide.* Prepare these accurately.

1% Gelatin Solution. This solution is prepared with halide-free gelatin.

PROCEDURES

Titration of Chloride. Pipet 5.0 ml of 0.1 *N* sodium chloride into the titration cell. Add 2 ml of concentrated nitric acid, 5 ml of 1% gelatin, and enough water to make about 50 ml. Lower the platinum electrode into the titration cell, and make a complete circuit from the platinum electrode to the galvanometer to the S.C.E. Set the platinum electrode in motion. The higher the rate of rotation, the greater the sensitivity; it is therefore necessary to keep the rate of rotation constant throughout a titration. Titrate the solution with standard 0.1 *N* $AgNO_3$, recording two or three values of the current before the end point and three to five values after it. Plot current (vertical axis) against volume and locate the end point. Calculate the percent recovery.

Titration of Bromide. Prepare a solution of sodium bromide and nitric acid as described in the preceding paragraph; gelatin is not necessary. Titrate amperometrically with standard 0.1 *N* $AgNO_3$ and calculate the percent recovery.

The titration cell is cleaned by washing from a wash bottle with the wash water being removed through the stopcock. The platinum electrode can be cleaned by dipping it in an ammonia solution.

Titration of a Bromide-Chloride Mixture. Prepare a solution with 5.0 ml of 0.1 *N* NaCl, 5.0 ml of 0.1 *N* NaBr, 2 ml of concentrated nitric acid, and enough water to make about 50 ml. Titrate amperometrically with 0.1 *N* silver nitrate until the first end point has been located. Add 5 ml of gelatin and titrate until the second end point is determined. Use the lowest practicable galvanometer sensitivity. Plot the titration curve and calculate the recoveries.

Analyze the unknown solutions of chloride, bromide, and chloride-bromide mixture provided by your instructor.

Deviations from linearity well beyond the end point may be removed by applying a volume change correction as described on p. 161.

References

1. Lingane, J. J., *Electroanalytical Chemistry*, 2nd ed., Interscience, New York, 1958, Chap. X.
2. Kolthoff, I. M. and J. J. Lingane, *Polarography*, Vol. I, 2nd ed., Interscience, New York, 1952, Chap. II.

3. Lingane, J. J., *Anal. Chem.*, **21,** 47 (1949).
4. Meites, L. and H. C. Thomas, *Advanced Analytical Chemistry*, McGraw-Hill, New York, 1958, p. 170.
5. Brezina, M. and P. Zuman, *Polarography in Medicine, Biochemistry, and Pharmacy*, Interscience, New York, 1958.
6. Berka, A. J., J. Dolezal, and J. Zyka, *Chemist-Analyst*, **53,** 122 (1964).
7. Laitinen, H. A., W. P. Jennings, and T. D. Parks, *Ind. Eng. Chem. Anal. Ed.*, **18,** 355, 358 (1946).
8. Mader, W. J. and H. A. Frediana, *J. Am. Pharm. Assoc.*, **45,** 24 (1951).

FOR FURTHER READING

Stock, J. T., *Amperometric Titrations*, Interscience, New York, 1965.
Purdy, W. C., *Electroanalytical Methods in Biochemistry*, McGraw-Hill, New York, 1965.
Zuman, P., *Organic Polarographic Analysis*, Macmillan, New York, 1964.
Adams, R. N., "Applications of Modern Electroanalytical Techniques to Pharmaceutical Chemistry," *J. Pharm. Sci.*, **58,** 1171 (1969).
Müller, O. H., "Polarography," *Techniques of Chemistry*, Vol. I, Part IIA, A. Weissberger and B. W. Rossiter (eds.), Wiley-Interscience, New York, 1971.

Problems

1. For the reaction

$$Hg + Cd^{2+} + 2e \rightleftharpoons Cd(Hg)$$

at the D.M.E., the following data were recorded:

$C = 0.1847$ mmole/liter
$t = 2.47$ sec
$m = 3.299$ mg/sec
$i_d = 1.700\ \mu A$

(*a*) Calculate the diffusion current constant, *I*.
(*b*) What is the diffusion coefficient of cadmium ion?
(*c*) What value of the diffusion current would be observed if the concentration of cadmium ion were 4.22 mmole/liter?

2. Thirty milliliters of a solution of lead ion was titrated amperometrically with 0.015 *M* sulfate, the following titration data being obtained.

Milliliters of Titrant	Galvanometer Scale Reading
1	9.45
2	7.80
3	5.79
4	4.05
5	2.37
6	1.50
7	1.23
8	1.22
9	1.21
10	1.22

What was the concentration of the lead solution?

3. How could you quantitatively determine each component in an aqueous solution of hydrochloric acid, lead chloride, sodium chloride, and acetic acid?

4. Sketch the polarogram of a mixture of Pb^{2+} and Zn^{2+} polarographed at the dropping mercury electrode versus S.C.E. (Any arbitrary values may be selected for the diffusion currents.) $E_{1/2}$(lead) = -0.40 V, $E_{1/2}$(zinc) = -1.0 V, both versus S.C.E.

5. Estimate the half-wave potential of cadmium from Fig. 7.2.

6. Make a rough estimate of the time required to record the polarogram shown in Fig. 7.2.

7. Why is KNO_3 (rather than KCl) used as the salt bridge electrolyte in Experiment 7.1?

8. Show that the peak maximum in derivative polarography occurs at the half-wave potential and that the peak height is proportional to concentration. (Suggestion: start with Eq. 7.12, finding the value of di/dE at its maximum.)

8 ABSORPTION SPECTROSCOPY

8.1 The Origin of Absorption Spectra

All atoms and molecules are capable of absorbing energy in accordance with certain restrictions, these limitations depending upon the structure of the substance. Energy may be furnished in the form of electromagnetic radiation ("light"). The kind and amount of radiation absorbed by a molecule depend upon the structure of the molecule; the amount of radiation absorbed also depends upon the number of molecules interacting with the radiation. The study of these dependencies is called *absorption spectroscopy.*

Absorption spectroscopy is undoubtedly one of the most valuable analytical techniques yet invented. It will probably remain a useful tool, despite further advances in analytical chemistry, because of its several overwhelming advantages for the solution of many problems. These advantages include speed, simplicity, specificity, and sensitivity. In this chapter we explore the principle of absorption spectroscopy, its capabilities for qualitative and quantitative analysis, its practice, and its limitations.

Electromagnetic Radiation. Electromagnetic radiation, of which visible light is one type, may be regarded as energy propagated in a wave form. Several terms and relations are used to describe the wave. The *wavelength* is the linear distance from any point on one wave to the corresponding point on the adjacent wave (see Fig. 8.1). The dimension of wavelength is length (L). It can be expressed in centimeters (cm) or, more commonly, in the following units:

1 angstrom (Å) $= 10^{-8}$ cm $= 10^{-10}$ m
1 nanometer (nm) $= 10^{-9}$ m $= 10^{-7}$ cm $=$ 1 millimicron (mμ) $=$ 10 Å.
1 micrometer (μm) $= 10^{-6}$ m $= 10^{-4}$ cm $=$ 1 micron (μ)

The term nanometer is now preferred to the older unit millimicron. The Greek letter lambda (λ) is a common symbol for wavelength.

Frequency is the number of waves passing a given point in unit time. The dimension of frequency is reciprocal time (T^{-1}), and the usual unit is $\sec^{-1}$, which may also be denoted cycles per second (cps) or hertz (Hz). Frequency is usually symbolized by the Greek letter nu (ν). *Wave number* is the reciprocal

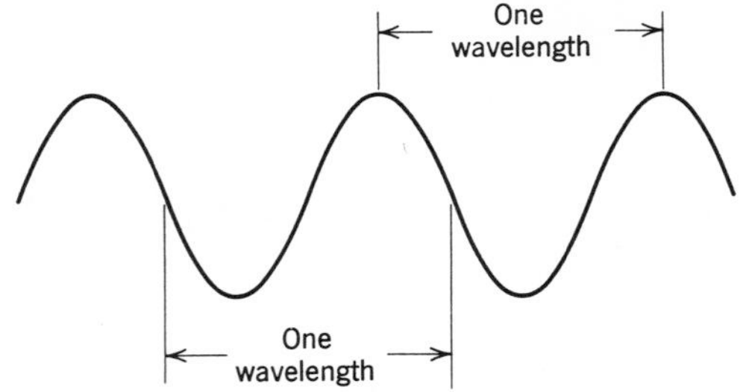

Fig. 8.1. A wavelength is the distance in the direction of propagation between corresponding points on adjacent waves.

of wavelength (when wavelength is expressed in centimeters). Its dimension is therefore reciprocal length, and its unit is cm^{-1}. (Wave number may be expressed in kaysers, where 1 kayser $= 1\ cm^{-1}$.)

Evidently the product of the number of waves to pass a point in 1 sec and the wavelength of a single wave is equal to the distance traversed by the radiation per second, which is its velocity:

$$v = \lambda \nu \tag{8.1}$$

The frequency of electromagnetic radiation is unaffected by the medium through which the wave passes. The wavelength, however, does vary with the medium. This means that the velocity of radiation depends upon the medium of propagation. In vacuum all electromagnetic radiation travels with the same velocity c. This quantity (the speed of light in vacuo) has the value 3.00×10^{10} cm/sec; it is a fundamental constant of nature. The velocity of light in air may for most purposes be taken as equal to c.

TABLE 8.1
The Electromagnetic Spectrum

Approximate Wavelength Range (cm)[a]	Region of Spectrum
10^{-12}–10^{-11}	Cosmic rays
10^{-11}–10^{-8}	Gamma rays
10^{-8}–10^{-6}	X rays
10^{-6}–10^{-5}	Ultraviolet
10^{-5}–10^{-4}	Visible
10^{-4}–10^{-2}	Infrared
10^{-2}–10	Microwave
10–10^{8}	Radio frequency

[a] Rounded to orders of magnitude

TABLE 8.2
Correlation of Color with Wavelength of Visible Light[a]

Wavelength (nm)	Color	Complement
400–450	Violet	Yellow-green
450–480	Blue	Yellow
480–490	Green-blue	Orange
490–500	Blue-green	Red
500–560	Green	Purple
560–575	Yellow-green	Violet
575–590	Yellow	Blue
590–625	Orange	Green-blue
625–750	Red	Blue-green

[a] Note that below 400 nm the color gradually becomes invisible as it passes into the ultraviolet; above 750 nm it passes into the infrared.

Frequency is a more fundamental property of radiation than is wavelength, for reasons to be considered later. Wave number, which is proportional to frequency, shares its significance. The wavelength, however, is the quantity that analysts usually use to describe radiation of spectroscopic interest, and this will be the practice in this chapter. It should be remembered that the nature of radiation can be specified in terms of its frequency or its wavelength, and that these quantities are related inversely (that is, $\nu = c/\lambda$).

All electromagnetic radiation is fundamentally similar, regardless of its wavelength, but names have become attached to radiation of different frequency ranges. The entire range of radiations is called the electromagnetic spectrum, and it is conventionally categorized as shown in Table 8.1. The ranges of spectroscopic interest may be more finely defined as the following:

Region	Wavelength Range
Far ultraviolet	100–200 nm
Ultraviolet	200–400 nm
Visible	400–750 nm
Near infrared	0.75– 4 μm
Infrared	4– 25 μm

The color of visible light can be correlated with its wavelength. White light contains radiation of all wavelengths within the visible region. Light of a single wavelength (*monochromatic* radiation) can be selected from white light (for example by means of a prism). The colors associated with wavelengths are listed in Table 8.2. In the third column of the table are listed the color complements, which have this significance: if white light is deprived of one of its colors (usually by absorption), the resulting light will appear as the complement of that color. Thus if blue light (450 to 480 nm) is removed from white light, the resulting radiation will be yellow.

We have thus far treated electromagnetic radiation as a wave phenomenon. Some aspects of radiation are more successfully described if the light is thought of as a stream of particles. Each particle (*photon*) has a definite amount of energy associated with it. The energy of a photon depends only upon its frequency, as shown by

$$E = h\nu \tag{8.2}$$

where E is the energy (in ergs) of one photon, ν is the frequency of the monochromatic radiation, and h is a universal constant called Planck's constant; $h = 6.625 \times 10^{-27}$ erg-sec. According to Eq. 8.2, the energy of radiation is directly proportional to its frequency and, combining 8.1 with 8.2 to give $E = hc/\lambda$ (where v is taken equal to c), the energy is inversely proportional to wavelength. Therefore ultraviolet (uv) light has more energy per photon than does visible light, which in turn has higher energy than infrared (ir) light. An equivalent of photons (that is, 6.023×10^{23} photons) is called an einstein. The energy of an einstein obviously depends upon the frequency of the radiation.

EXAMPLE 8.1. Calculate the following quantities for radiation of wavelength 400 nm:

(*a*) wavelength in angstroms and in cm; (*b*) wave number; (*c*) frequency; (*d*) energy in erg/photon; (*e*) energy in kcal/einstein. The results are:

(*a*) $\lambda = 4000$ Å or 4.00×10^{-5} cm.

(*b*) wave number $= 1/(4 \times 10^{-5}\ \text{cm}) = 2.50 \times 10^{4}\ \text{cm}^{-1}$.

(*c*) $\nu = c/\lambda = 3 \times 10^{10}\ \text{cm/sec}/4 \times 10^{-5}\ \text{cm} = 7.5 \times 10^{14}$ Hz.

(*d*) $E = h\nu = 4.97 \times 10^{-12}$ erg.

(*e*) Energy $= (6.023 \times 10^{23}\ \text{photon/einstein})\ (4.97 \times 10^{-12}\ \text{erg/photon})$
$= 2.99 \times 10^{12}$ erg/einstein.

Since 1 joule (J) $= 10^{7}$ erg and 1 kcal $= 4.184 \times 10^{3}$ J,

Energy $= 2.99 \times 10^{5}\ \text{J/einstein}/4.184 \times 10^{3}\ \text{J/kcal}$
$= 71.5$ kcal/einstein.

Absorption of Radiation by Molecules. All molecules possess energy, which may be ascribed to several phenomena. (1) The molecule as a whole may move; this is called *translation*, and the associated energy is the translational energy, E_{trans}. (2) The parts of the molecule, that is, the atoms or groups of atoms, may move with respect to each other. This motion is called *vibration*, and a vibrational energy, E_{vib}, is associated with it. (3) The molecule may rotate about an axis, and such *rotation* is characterized by the rotational energy, E_{rot}. (4) Besides these modes of movement, the molecule possesses an *electronic* configuration, and the electronic energy E_{elec} depends upon the electronic state of the molecule.

The energy of a molecule consists of the sum of its translational, vibrational rotational, and electronic energy components.

$$E = E_{trans} + E_{vib} + E_{rot} + E_{elec}$$

It is an important result of quantum mechanics that the vibrational, rotational, and electronic energy components (the internal energy) may assume only certain values for a given molecule; these energies are said to be quantized. The permitted levels of E_{vib}, E_{rot}, and E_{elec} will obviously be intimately related to the structure of the molecule, and we may expect that no two kinds of molecule will possess identical rotational, vibrational, and electronic energy levels. A reasonable corollary is that a close similarity of molecular structure may lead to a similarity in the allowed energy levels. The energy states of the molecule reflect the energy levels of its rotational, vibrational, and electronic components.

If the molecule passes from one of its allowed energy levels to a lower one, some energy must be released. This energy may be lost as radiation, and emission of radiation is then said to have occurred. If a molecule is allowed to encounter electromagnetic radiation of a proper frequency such that the energy of the molecule is raised from one level to a higher one, we say that absorption of radiation has taken place. Because of the limitation on the permissible energy levels of the rotational, vibrational, and electronic components, the amount of energy absorbed by a molecule in this process is severely restricted. In order for absorption to occur, the energy difference between the two energy levels must be equal to the energy of the photon absorbed. Mathematically this may be expressed

$$E_2 - E_1 = h\nu \tag{8.3}$$

where E_1 is the energy of the lower level, E_2 the energy of the upper level, and ν is the frequency of the absorbed photon. A graphical representation of this process is shown in Fig. 8.2. This energy jump from one level to another is known as a *transition*, and the energy component involved in the absorption process may be specified by speaking of rotational, vibrational, and electronic transitions.

It is experimentally a simple matter to measure the extent of absorption of radiation by a molecule (actually by a large number of molecules) as a function of the frequency of the radiation. A graph of the extent of light absorption against the frequency (or wavelength) of the light is an *absorption spectrum* (plural *spectra*). As we noted above, the allowed transitions are different for molecules of different structure, so their absorption spectra should be different. Spectra are therefore useful for the identification of compounds, and this

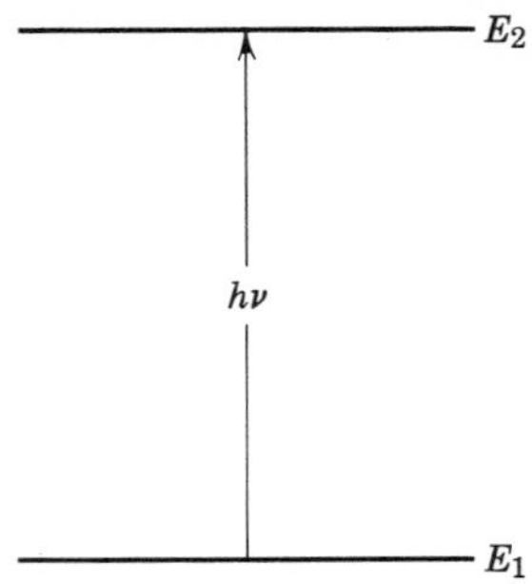

Fig. 8.2. Absorption of radiation of frequency ν causing a transition from energy level 1 to level 2: $E_2 - E_1 = h\nu$.

application is considered in Sections 8.3 and 8.4. The amount of light absorbed (at a given frequency) should be related to the number of molecules absorbing the radiation, so absorption spectra are also useful as a means of quantitative analysis (Section 8.2).

It appears that the amount of energy required for rotational transitions can be supplied by radiation in the far infrared. The far infrared absorption spectrum is therefore called the rotational spectrum. This spectrum is not important analytically. Vibrational transitions can occur with the absorption of infrared radiation. Associated with each vibrational transition is a number of rotational transitions; thus instead of a sharp peak in the absorption spectrum corresponding to the frequency of the vibrational transition, a broadened band is observed, which can be ascribed to the rotational transitions superimposed on the vibrational transition. Infrared spectra are sometimes called vibrational-rotational spectra.

Visible and ultraviolet light provides enough energy for electronic transitions. Visible and ultraviolet spectra are therefore called electronic spectra. The lowest energy state of a molecule is the ground state. Electronic transitions raise the molecular energy from that of the ground state to one of several "excited" electronic states. Many vibrational transitions are associated with each electronic transition, so the electronic spectrum consists of relatively broad absorption bands, or envelopes, that mask the fine structure of the individual transitions. Examples of absorption spectra will be shown later.

A molecule raised to a higher energy level by absorption of radiation quickly returns to the ground state. Energy must be lost in this process. The usual route is by collisional processes that transform the internal energy into thermal energy, which is dissipated. The excited molecule may undergo fragmentation (dissociation into uncharged radicals) or ionization (loss of an electron), or it may enter into a chemical reaction (this would be a photochemical reaction). Molecules in which the excited state is prevented from returning to the ground state via the usual thermal dissipation mechanism may lose their energy by emitting it as radiation, which is known as fluorescence; this phenomenon is discussed in Chapter 9.

8.2 Quantitative Uses of Absorption Spectra

Beer's Law. Quantitative spectroscopic analysis is based upon a relationship between the amount of light absorbed and the amount of absorbing substance. This relationship, which can be theoretically demonstrated, is observed experimentally in most practical analytical situations. Let us consider a dilute solution of a substance capable of absorbing light of the wavelength selected for the experiment, the solvent being nonabsorbing (transparent) to light of this wavelength. It is noted that if monochromatic light is passed through a layer of solution of thickness db, the decrease in light intensity dI, as a result of passing through the solution, is directly proportional to the intensity I of the radiation, to the concentration c of the absorbing species, and to the thickness db of the solution layer.

$$-dI = kIc\,db$$

This equation can be rearranged and integrated between the limits of I_0 (the intensity of the incident light) and I, the intensity of the light after passing through the thickness b of solution.

$$-\int_{I_0}^{I} \frac{dI}{I} = k\int_0^b c\,db$$

$$-\ln \frac{I}{I_0} = kbc$$

$$I = I_0 e^{-kbc}$$

Changing to logarithms to the base 10:

$$I = I_0 10^{-abc} \tag{8.4}$$

where $a = k/2.303$. Equation 8.4 can be written in the equivalent forms

$$\log \frac{I_0}{I} = abc \tag{8.5}$$

$$A = abc \tag{8.6}$$

Equations 8.4–8.6 are representations of *Beer's law*, which is the relationship referred to in the opening sentence of this section. The spectroscopic quantities that are measured are the *transmittance* T, where $T = I/I_0$, and the *absorbance* A, where $A = \log(1/T)$. Beer's law is most usefully expressed as Eq. 8.6, which states that the absorbance A of a solution is directly proportional to the concentration c of the absorbing solute. (The names of Bouguer and Lambert are often associated with the dependence of absorbance on the path length b of the light through the solution, and Eq. 8.6 is sometimes called the Beer-Lambert equation.) The absorptivity a is a proportionality constant that is independent of concentration, path length, and intensity of incident radiation. The absorptivity depends upon the temperature, solvent, molecular structure, and the wavelength of the radiation. The units of a are determined by those of b and c. When b is in centimeters and c is in grams per liter, the absorptivity has the units liters per gram-centimeter. If c is a molar concentration, the absorptivity is called the molar absorptivity, it is labeled ϵ, and its units are liters per mole-centimeter. When c is expressed in weight/volume percent (g/100 ml), the absorptivity may be written $A_{1\,\text{cm}}^{1\%}$. The absorptivity may be interpreted as the absorbance (of a given substance at a specified wavelength) of a solution of unit concentration.

The nomenclature of absorption spectroscopy can be a source of confusion because of the considerable number of synonymous terms. The preferred spectroscopic terms and symbols [1] are listed in Table 8.3. It is necessary to understand the older nomenclature also, because it is employed in so much of the analytical literature, and these terms are also given in the table.

An absorption spectrum is determined by measuring the absorbance or transmittance of a solution as a function of wavelength or frequency of the light. Infrared spectra are usually plotted as percent transmittance versus wavelength (the wavelength scale being linear). Visible and ultraviolet spectra are more often presented as plots of absorbance (ordinate axis) versus wavelength. Figure 8.3 shows a typical absorption spectrum. It is characterized

TABLE 8.3
Spectroscopic Nomenclature

Term	Symbol	Older Terms
Transmittance	T	Transmission
Percent transmittance	$\%T = 100\ T$	Percent transmission
Absorbance	A	Extinction E, density D, optical density OD, absorbancy
Absorptivity	a	Extinction coefficient, absorbancy index, specific extinction $E_{1\,\text{cm}}^{1\%}$
Molar absorptivity	ϵ	Molar extinction coefficient
Path length	b	l, d
Concentration	c	

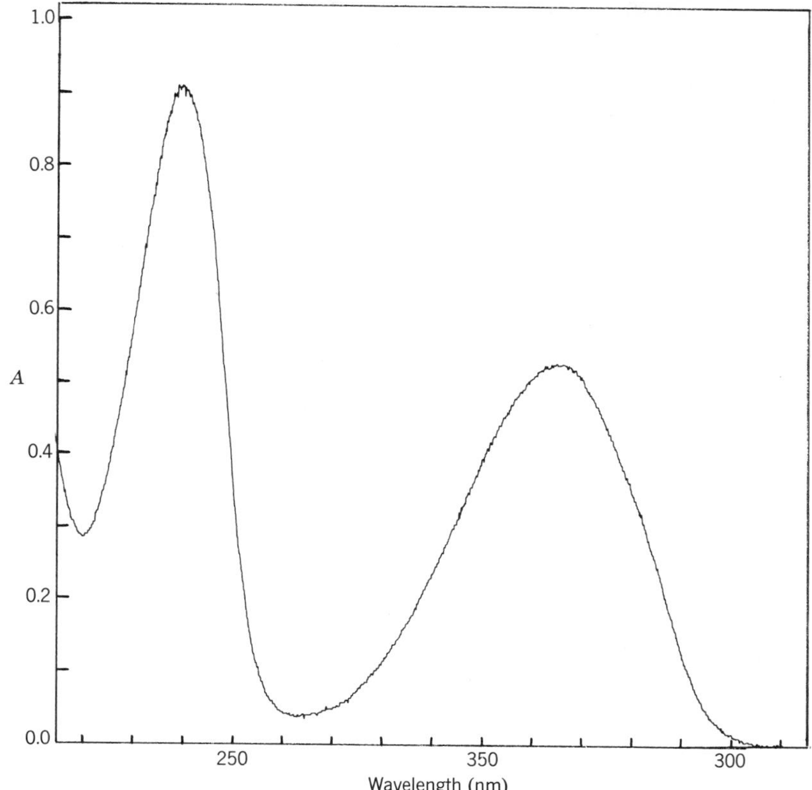

Fig. 8.3. Ultraviolet absorption spectrum of tripelennamine hydrochloride in 0.25 *N* HCl; $b = 1$ cm, $c = 1.94$ mg/100 ml.

by rather broad absorption bands. The wavelengths corresponding to maxima and minima in the absorbance-wavelength plot are symbolized λ_{max} and λ_{min}.

From the definition of absorbance, $A = \log (1/T)$, it is seen that a decrease in the amount of light transmitted by the solution corresponds to a decrease in transmittance and an increase in absorbance. The absorbance is logarithmically related to the transmittance. Thus when $T = 1.00$, $A = 0.00$; when $T = 0.10$, $A = 1.00$; when $T = 0.01$, $A = 2.00$, etc.

Single-Component Analysis. If the absorbance of each of a series of solutions of the same substance is measured at the same wavelength, temperature, and solvent conditions, and the absorbance of each solution is plotted against its concentration, a straight line passing through the origin will usually be observed, in accordance with Eq. 8.6. This graph is called a Beer's law plot, and if the line is straight Beer's law is said to be obeyed over the concentration range investigated. Figure 8.4 shows a Beer's law study of theophylline, and Fig. 8.5 is the Beer's law plot of the data in Fig. 8.4. The slope of the line is equal to ab and, since b is known (b is the internal path length of the sample cell), the absorptivity a can be calculated. An alternative treatment of these spectral data involves calculation of the absorptivity for each pair of absorbance-concentration data; $a = A/bc$. If a is constant, Beer's law is obeyed.

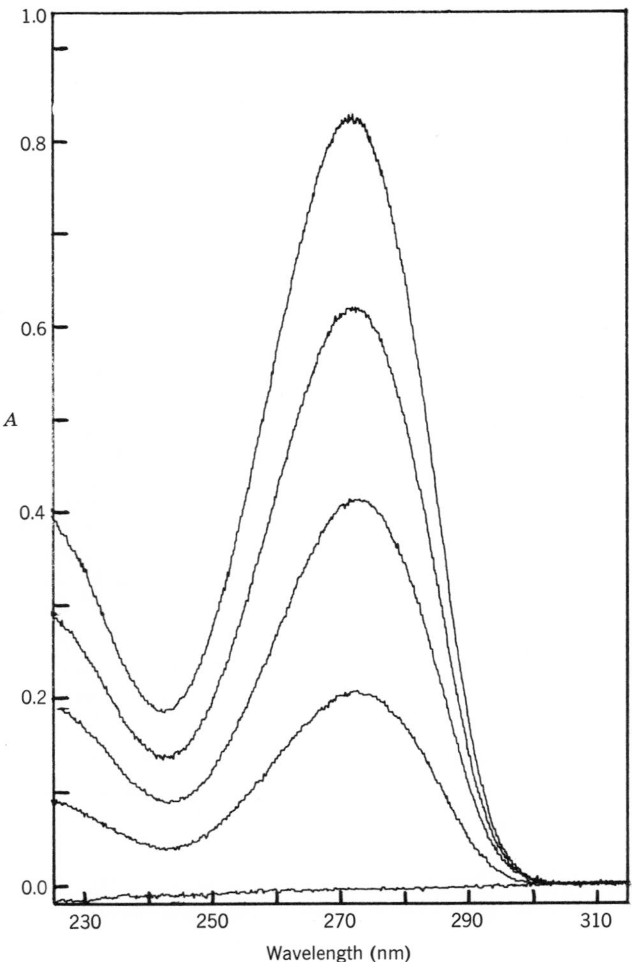

Fig. 8.4. Absorption spectra of four solutions of theophylline in water; b = 1 cm. The concentrations are given in Table 8.4. (The bottommost line is a reference "base line," determined by placing solvent alone in the sample cell.)

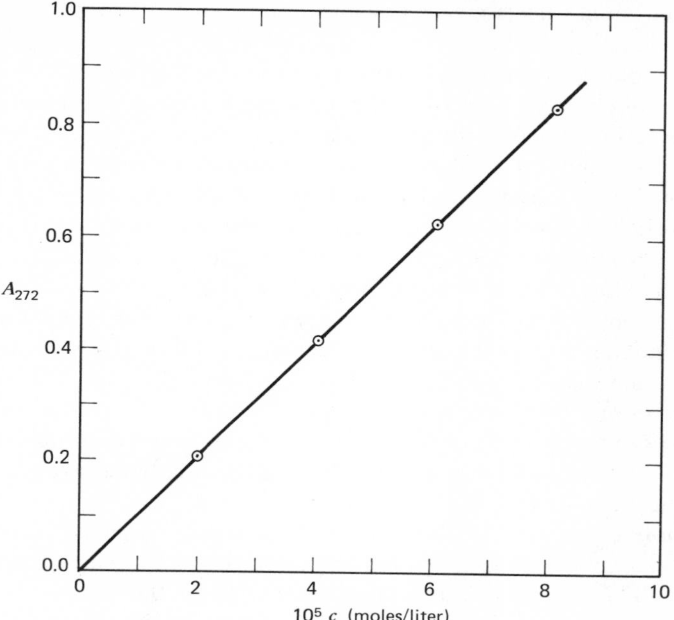

Fig. 8.5. Beer's law plot for theophylline in aqueous solution; data from Fig. 8.4 and Table 8.4.

Table 8.4 gives the data with which Fig. 8.5 was plotted, and the table includes the molar absorptivities calculated for each solution. Evidently Beer's law is obeyed by this system. The precision of these results is typical of that attainable with electronic spectral studies.

The wavelength selected for the absorptivity determination is usually λ_{max}, for two reasons: (1) maximum sensitivity is achieved by working at the

TABLE 8.4
Ultraviolet Absorption Data for Theophylline in Water[a]

$10^5 c$ (M)	A_{272}	$10^{-4}\epsilon_{272}$
2.04	0.209	1.025
4.08	0.414	1.015
6.12	0.621	1.015
8.16	0.827	1.013
	$\epsilon_{272} = 1.02 \times 10^4$ liter/mole-cm	

[a] At the absorption maximum, 272 nm; data from Fig. 8.4.

band maximum, since a given concentration produces the strongest signal at this wavelength; (2) the change of absorbance with small change in wavelength is minimal at the band maximum (unless the band is extremely sharp); therefore minor errors in setting the instrument wavelength selector dial do not cause serious errors in the absorbance measurement.

The absorptivity of a substance (at a specified wavelength) having been determined, the analysis of unknown samples of this same substance is readily accomplished. A solution of the substance is prepared in the same solvent used for the known samples; the estimated concentration of this solution should fall within the extremes used in the Beer's law study. The absorbance of the unknown sample is measured at the analytical wavelength. Then from Beer's law the unknown concentration is calculated. Alternatively the unknown concentration may be read directly from the Beer's law plot. This method is successful even if Beer's law is not obeyed. In order for these simple analytical techniques to be successful it is imperative that no interfering substance (that is, a substance capable of absorbing light of the analytical wavelength) be present in the sample.

A simplified version of these methods uses a "one-point" concomitant measurement of the sample solution and a solution prepared with a reference standard. This standard is the same compound as the sample, but it is a specimen whose purity is known. The standard and the sample are carried through exactly the same procedure, and Beer's law is written for each solution:

$$A^s = abc^s$$

$$A^r = abc^r$$

where the superscript s refers to the sample and r to the reference standard. Dividing these equations and solving for the unknown c^s, we obtain

$$c^s = c^r \frac{A^s}{A^r}$$

All the quantities on the right are known. This procedure is used widely in analyses involving the formation of colored substances of uncertain and poorly reproducible composition, since the absorptivity of these substances cannot be determined accurately. Spectrophotometric assay procedures in the USP and NF usually specify this method of analysis, and the final equation may include a numerical factor accounting for dilution of the sample.

Although the implication up to this point has been that the absorptivity of a substance at specified conditions is a physical constant that, once determined, need not again be measured, this is nevertheless an oversimplification. The accurate determination of absorptivities is difficult because of certain instrumental problems (Section 8.5). The reproducibility within a single series of measurements is usually 0.5–2%, as indicated by the data of Table 8.4.

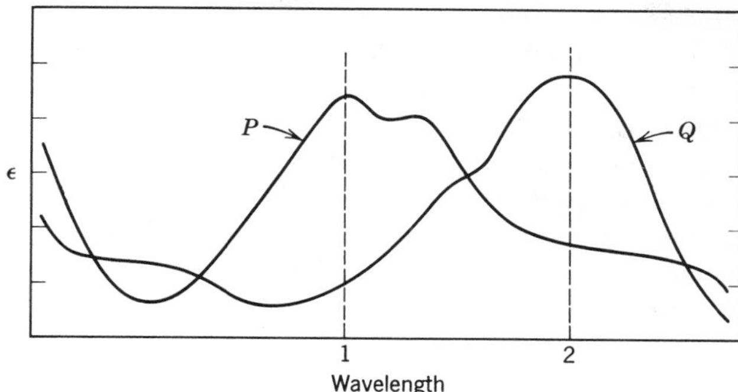

Fig. 8.6. Superimposition of absorption spectra of substances *P* and *Q* preparatory to conducting an analysis of their mixture. Suitable analytical wavelengths are indicated by dashed lines.

The absorptivity can be reproduced fairly closely on subsequent measurements *on the same instrument*, but agreement between measurements on different instruments is less satisfactory. It is therefore recommended that absorptivities be determined on the same instrument to be used in the actual analytical measurement, and for highest accuracy the absorptivity should be measured at the same time as the sample measurement. If prior work has shown that Beer's law is obeyed by the system, the reference standard method outlined in the preceding paragraph is particularly convenient.

Multicomponent Analysis. Up to this point we have considered only systems containing a single absorbing species. Now suppose that we have a mixture of two substances (in a transparent solvent), each of which absorbs light. If the absorption spectra of the two components are so different that two wavelengths can be found at which each substance absorbs light without interference from the other, the problem reduces to that of single-component analysis, since neither component interferes with the analysis of the other. In the more general case both substances will absorb light at the same wavelengths, but if their absorption spectra are markedly different, the mixture can still be analyzed.

It is first necessary to determine the absorption spectra of the two pure compounds. These spectra are compared by converting absorbance values to a common basis as molar absorptivities, and superimposing the spectra as shown in Fig. 8.6. Two analytical wavelengths, indicated by 1 and 2 in Fig. 8.6, are selected such that the difference in absorption by the compounds is maximal at these wavelengths, with the absorptivity for compound *P* being greater than that for *Q* at one wavelength and less at the other. (In general, it is necessary to select as many analytical wavelengths as there are components in the mixture.)

The next step in the analysis is to make Beer's law plots, using solutions of the pure substances, for each compound at each wavelength. This gives four Beer's law plots from which are calculated four absorptivities, which may be symbolized a_1^P, a_2^P, a_1^Q, a_2^Q, with the superscript indicating the compound and the subscript the wavelength.

Now any solution containing compounds P and Q can be analyzed. The absorbance of the solution is measured at wavelengths 1 and 2. It will be assumed that the absorbance of a mixture is equal to the sum of the absorbances of the components of the mixture. Therefore, if A_1 and A_2 are the absorbances of the mixture at wavelengths 1 and 2,

$$A_1 = A_1^P + A_1^Q \tag{8.7}$$

$$A_2 = A_2^P + A_2^Q \tag{8.8}$$

The absorbances on the right sides of Eqs. 8.7 and 8.8 can be replaced by the corresponding Beer's law expressions; thus $A_1^P = a_1^P bc^P$, etc.

$$A_1 = a_1^P bc^P + a_1^Q bc^Q \tag{8.9}$$

$$A_2 = a_2^P bc^P + a_2^Q bc^Q \tag{8.10}$$

Equations 8.9 and 8.10 are two independent relations in the two unknowns c^P and c^Q, and the equations are readily solved for the concentrations. This approach to mixture analysis can be extended to mixtures of more than two components if the absorption spectra are suitably different. The solution of the equations (an n-component mixture requires n equations) becomes cumbersome for these complex problems, and more efficient methods have been developed [2].

Measurement of Equilibrium Constants. The determination of an equilibrium constant requires the estimation of the equilibrium concentrations of the reactants by direct analysis or by analysis combined with knowledge of the reaction stoichiometry. If the absorption spectra of the species involved in the reaction are sufficiently different, evidently a spectrophotometric determination of the equilibrium constant is possible. As in all methods of quantitative spectrophotometric analysis, this technique is an application of Beer's law. It will be illustrated with an acid-base equilibrium, but the principle is applicable to any equilibrium.

Consider the dissociation of the weak acid HA in aqueous solution.

$$HA \rightleftharpoons H^+ + A^-$$

The thermodynamic equilibrium constant of this reaction is the conventional acid dissociation constant, K_a (see Chapter 1). At finite ionic strength the experimentally accessible quantity is the apparent constant, K_a' (Eq. 6.24).

$$K_a' = a_{H^+} \frac{[A^-]}{[HA]}$$

The logarithmic form of this equation is

$$\mathrm{pK}'_a = \mathrm{pH} - \log \frac{c_{\mathrm{A}^-}}{c_{\mathrm{HA}}} \tag{8.11}$$

where c_{HA} and c_{A^-} are written for $[\mathrm{HA}]$ and $[\mathrm{A}^-]$ to be consistent with the symbolism in the earlier parts of this section. The pH of the solution can be measured potentiometrically (see Chapter 6) and the ratio $c_{\mathrm{A}^-}/c_{\mathrm{HA}}$ can be determined spectrophotometrically if the absorption spectra of A^- and HA are different. Because of the great sensitivity of spectral analysis, very low concentrations of the acid and conjugate base are used. The pH is controlled with an added buffer, and it is the contribution of this buffer to the ionic strength that may lead to activity coefficients different from unity.

Suppose that A^- and HA have significantly different absorption spectra, and that an analytical wavelength is selected at which the absorptivities of these two species are different. We shall suppose that Beer's law is obeyed by each species. Then

$$A_{\mathrm{HA}} = a_{\mathrm{HA}} b c_{\mathrm{HA}}$$

$$A_{\mathrm{A}^-} = a_{\mathrm{A}^-} b c_{\mathrm{A}^-}$$

where these equations refer to the same wavelength. A_{HA} is the absorbance due to HA in the solution, and A_{A^-} is due to A^-. The observed absorbance of any solution containing both HA and A^- is given by

$$A_{\mathrm{obs}} = A_{\mathrm{HA}} + A_{\mathrm{A}^-} = b(a_{\mathrm{HA}} c_{\mathrm{HA}} + a_{\mathrm{A}^-} c_{\mathrm{A}^-}) \tag{8.12}$$

It is possible to define an "apparent" absorptivity a_{obs} of the mixture of species according to

$$A_{\mathrm{obs}} = a_{\mathrm{obs}} b c \tag{8.13}$$

where c is the formal concentration of the acid; that is,

$$c = c_{\mathrm{HA}} + c_{\mathrm{A}^-} \tag{8.14}$$

Since the absorbance given by Eq. 8.12 is identical with that of 8.13, they can be set equal, and combined with 8.14 to give

$$a_{\mathrm{obs}}(c_{\mathrm{HA}} + c_{\mathrm{A}^-}) = a_{\mathrm{HA}} c_{\mathrm{HA}} + a_{\mathrm{A}^-} c_{\mathrm{A}^-}$$

which is rearranged to

$$\frac{c_{\mathrm{A}^-}}{c_{\mathrm{HA}}} = \frac{a_{\mathrm{obs}} - a_{\mathrm{HA}}}{a_{\mathrm{A}^-} - a_{\mathrm{obs}}} \tag{8.15}$$

for the case in which $a_{\mathrm{A}^-} > a_{\mathrm{HA}}$. If $a_{\mathrm{HA}} > a_{\mathrm{A}^-}$, the equivalent form is

$$\frac{c_{\mathrm{A}^-}}{c_{\mathrm{HA}}} = \frac{a_{\mathrm{HA}} - a_{\mathrm{obs}}}{a_{\mathrm{obs}} - a_{\mathrm{A}^-}} \tag{8.16}$$

Combining Eq. 8.15 or 8.16 with 8.11,

$$\mathrm{pK}'_a = \mathrm{pH} - \log \frac{a_{\mathrm{obs}} - a_{\mathrm{HA}}}{a_{\mathrm{A^-}} - a_{\mathrm{obs}}} \tag{8.17}$$

Equation 8.17 provides the basis for the spectrophotometric determination of dissociation constants. The absorptivities of the conjugate acid and base forms are measured in solutions of high acidity and alkalinity, respectively, that is, at least 2 pH units removed from the pK'_a. The substance is then incorporated in a buffer solution of known pH (within about 1 unit of the pK'_a) and the apparent absorptivity of the equilibrium mixture is measured. If the total concentration c of the solute is held constant in all these measurements, the absorbances A_{HA}, $A_{\mathrm{A^-}}$, and A_{obs} may be substituted for the absorptivities a_{HA}, $a_{\mathrm{A^-}}$, and a_{obs} in Eq. 8.17. This technique is used in Experiment 8.3.

The thermodynamic pK_a can be estimated from pK'_a and the ionic strength as described in Chapter 6.

We can now describe indicator behavior more precisely than was possible in Part I. An acid-base indicator is a substance whose conjugate acid and base forms have different absorption spectra.* The spectral behavior of methyl orange is shown in Fig. 8.7. This definition includes as acid-base indicators substances that are not colored at all—that is, whose acid and base forms do not absorb visible light—and therefore cannot be utilized as visual indicators. These substances may still be useful indicators, but their "color" changes must be observed instrumentally.

If the absorption spectra of the pure acid and pure base forms of a substance cross, the absorptivities of the two forms must be equal at the crossing point. The apparent absorptivity of any mixture of the two forms must, therefore, also pass through this point. This point through which all spectra pass is called an *isosbestic point;* Fig. 8.7 shows an isosbestic point for methyl orange. The wavelength corresponding to the isosbestic point of an equilibrium is characteristic of the two species contributing to the spectrum and therefore is useful as an aid to identification. This wavelength also is a suitable analytical wavelength for the determination of the total concentration of the two species, since the absorptivity is unaffected by the distribution of species at the isosbestic point.

Measurement of Rate Constants. It is often of interest to measure the rate of a reaction, for example, when assessing the stability of a drug in a dosage form. If the reactant molecule has a different absorption spectrum from its product, then a spectral change will occur as the reaction proceeds, and spectrophotometry is a convenient analytical method for studying the rate of such a reaction.

* Even this definition can be made more general, to include any property of the substance. Thus an acid-base smell indicator is a substance whose acid and base forms have different odors [3]. Pyridine is an example.

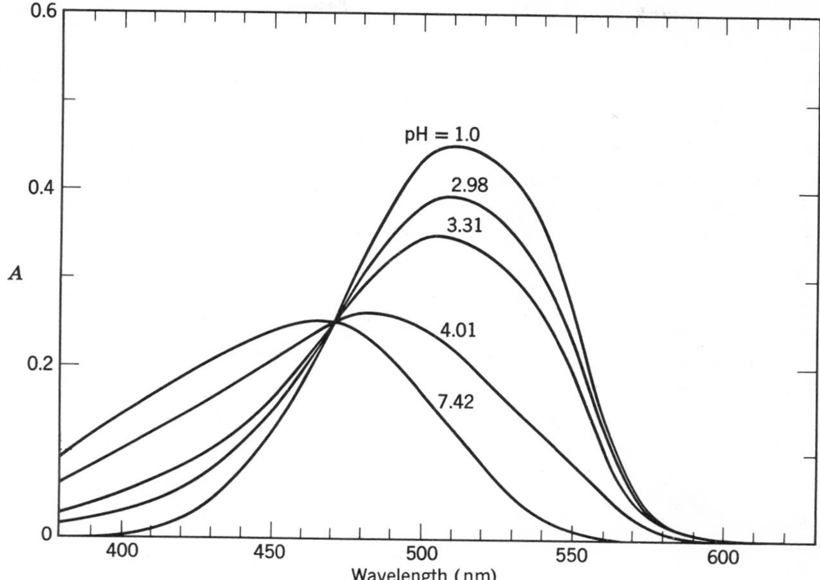

Fig. 8.7. Absorption spectra of methyl orange in aqueous solutions; $b = 1$ cm, $c \approx 2.5 \times 10^{-5}$ *M*. The pH of each solution is indicated on the appropriate spectrum. The extreme spectra are those of the pure conjugate acid and base forms of the indicator. An isosbestic point occurs at 470 nm.

We will examine this application of absorption spectroscopy to chemical kinetics for a simple but very important class of reactions. Suppose the reactant molecule R undergoes reaction to give product P in an irreversible reaction as follows.

$$R \rightarrow P$$

The rate of this reaction is found to be described by Eq. 8.18, which is called a rate equation.

$$-\frac{dc_R}{dt} = kc_R \tag{8.18}$$

This can be rearranged and integrated between the limits of $c_R = c_R^\circ$ at $t = 0$ (that is, at the beginning of the reaction) and $c_R = c_R$ at time t:

$$\int_{c_R^\circ}^{c_R} \frac{dc_R}{c_R} = -k\int_0^t t$$

$$\ln \frac{c_R}{c_R^\circ} = -kt$$

Transforming to base 10 logarithms,

$$\log \frac{c_{\mathbf{R}}}{c_{\mathbf{R}}^{\circ}} = -\frac{kt}{2.303} \tag{8.19}$$

The experimental goal is to evaluate k, the *rate constant* for the reaction. Since the concentration $c_{\mathbf{R}}$ appears in the rate equation to the first power, k is said to be a first-order rate constant. Its dimension is time^{-1} and its usual unit is sec^{-1}. More complicated rate equations are often encountered, but the first-order rate equation is extremely important.

Now suppose that the absorption spectrum of R is significantly different from that of P. Then a wavelength can be selected at which the absorbance of the reaction solution undergoes a change from its initial value A_0 at $t = 0$ to its final value A_∞ at $t = \infty$ (that is, when the reaction is essentially complete). We assume that Beer's law is obeyed by both R and P at this wavelength. At $t = 0$ we have $c_{\mathbf{R}} = c_{\mathbf{R}}^{\circ}$ and $c_{\mathbf{P}} = 0$. Let A_t be the absorbance at any time t, and $\epsilon_{\mathbf{R}}$ and $\epsilon_{\mathbf{P}}$ the molar absorptivities of R and P at the selected wavelength. Then Eq. 8.20 can be written for $t = 0$,

$$A_0 = \epsilon_{\mathbf{R}} b c_{\mathbf{R}}^{\circ} \tag{8.20}$$

and Eq. 8.21 applies at $t = \infty$, since $c_{\mathbf{P}}^{\infty} = c_{\mathbf{R}}^{\circ}$:

$$A_\infty = \epsilon_{\mathbf{P}} b c_{\mathbf{R}}^{\circ} \tag{8.21}$$

At any intermediate time the system is described by

$$A_t = \epsilon_{\mathbf{R}} b c_{\mathbf{R}} + \epsilon_{\mathbf{P}} b c_{\mathbf{P}} \tag{8.22}$$

Combining these three equations with the mass balance relationship $c_{\mathbf{R}}^{\circ} = c_{\mathbf{R}} + c_{\mathbf{P}}$ leads to Eq. 8.23, which relates the concentration ratio to observable spectral quantities.

$$\frac{c_{\mathbf{R}}}{c_{\mathbf{R}}^{\circ}} = \frac{A_t - A_\infty}{A_0 - A_\infty} \tag{8.23}$$

Combining Eqs. 8.19 and 8.23,

$$\log \frac{A_t - A_\infty}{A_0 - A_\infty} = -\frac{kt}{2.303} \tag{8.24}$$

By measuring A_0, A_∞, and A_t at time t, the rate constant k can be calculated. Another way to use the equation is to measure A_t at various times t, and then to plot $\log (A_t - A_\infty)$ against t; the slope of the resulting straight line will be equal to $-k/2.303$. (The quantity $A_t - A_\infty$ is positive if $\epsilon_{\mathbf{R}} > \epsilon_{\mathbf{P}}$; for the reverse condition one uses $A_\infty - A_t$.)

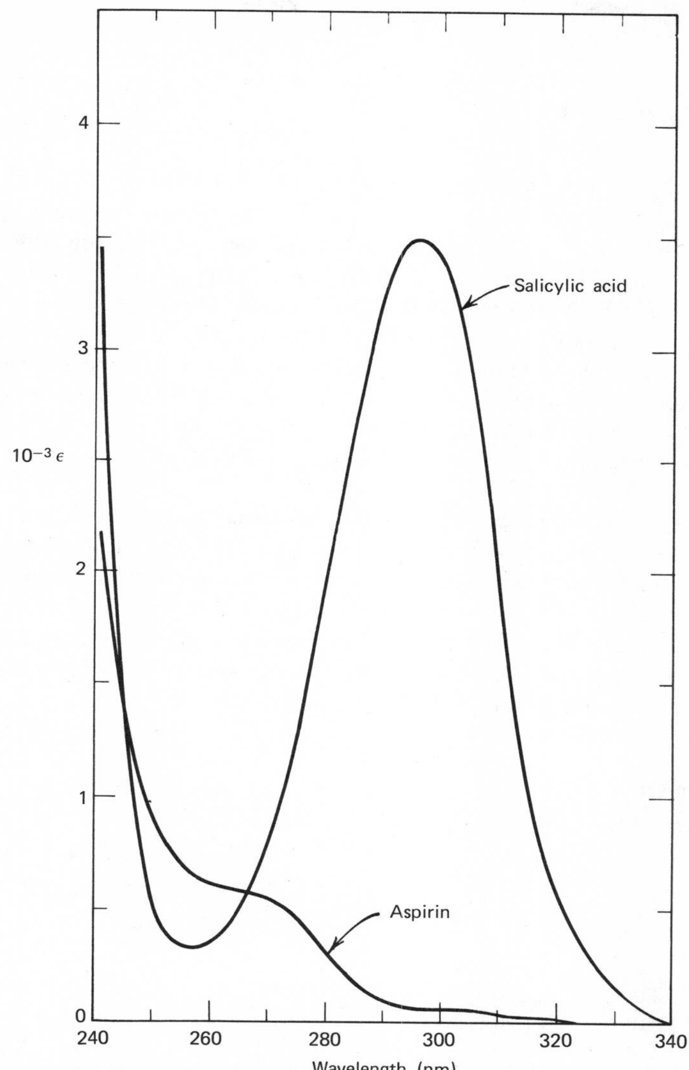

Fig. 8.8. Absorption spectra of aspirin and salicylic acid in pH 5.0 acetate buffer.

The hydrolysis of aspirin (acetylsalicylic acid) is a reaction of pharmaceutical and chemical interest. Figure 8.8 shows the ultraviolet absorption spectra of aspirin and salicylic acid. Since these spectra have been presented in molar absorptivities, they are on an equivalent basis, and they show that the hydrolysis of aspirin will be accompanied by a substantial increase in absorbance due to the appearance of salicylic acid. By measuring the absorbance as a

$$C_6H_4(COO^-)(OCOCH_3) + H_2O \longrightarrow C_6H_4(COO^-)(OH) + CH_3COOH$$

function of time, therefore, the rate constant for the hydrolysis of aspirin can be determined. Table 8.5 shows such a determination, in which 296 nm, corresponding to λ_{max} for salicylic acid, was selected for the absorbance measurements. (This reaction can be treated as a first-order reaction, despite the presence of water as a second reactant, because the concentration of water is essentially constant during the course of the reaction.)

Rate constants have many uses, including stability prediction and the study of reaction mechanisms. The rate constant of a given reaction is a function of the reaction medium (solvent and ionic strength) and of the temperature. Most rate constants increase by a factor of 2–3 with a temperature increase of 10°C.

Beer's Law Deviations of Chemical Origin. Usually the Beer's law plot of absorbance against concentration is linear and the line passes through the origin, as in Fig. 8.5. Occasionally it happens that curvature is observed in the Beer's law plot, when it is said that Beer's law has failed. This failure is apparent rather than real when it is caused by the operation of chemical equilibrium. A simple example will illustrate the effect. Suppose a Beer's law study is to be made of a substance M, and that this substance is involved in the unsuspected

TABLE 8.5
Rate Study of the Hydrolysis of Aspirin[a]

t (sec)	A_t	$\frac{A_\infty - A_t}{A_\infty - A_0}$	$10^3 k$ (sec^{-1})[b]
0	0.007	1.000	—
360	0.273	0.640	1.24
540	0.383	0.491	1.32
720	0.470	0.373	1.37
900	0.525	0.298	1.35
1200	0.602	0.194	1.37
1500	0.650	0.129	1.37
∞	0.745	0.000	—
Mean value: $k = 1.34 \times 10^{-3}$ sec^{-1}			

[a] At 98°C in pH 5.01 acetate buffer.
[b] Calculated with Eq. 8.24.

equilibrium

$$2M \rightleftharpoons D$$

where D is a dimeric form of M. The absorbance will be measured at a wavelength where M absorbs strongly but (for simplicity) D does not absorb at all. Then the observed absorbance will be interpreted according to the equation

$$A_{obs} = a_{obs}bc$$

where c is the formal (total) concentration of M. In actuality, the absorbance is controlled by the real concentration of M:

$$A_{obs} = a_M b c_M$$

Combining these equations gives

$$a_{obs} = \frac{a_M c_M}{c}$$

and, since $c = 2c_D + c_M$, whereas $K = c_D/c_M{}^2$, this may be transformed to

$$a_{obs} = \frac{a_M}{2Kc_M + 1}$$

According to this result, the Beer's law plot of A_{obs} versus c would display curvature toward the concentration axis, since a_{obs} is clearly not a constant, but decreases as c is increased.

Association and dissociation equilibria are the usual chemical causes of Beer's law failures. These systems may still be accurately analyzed spectrophotometrically, however, by preparing the Beer's law plot (the "standard curve") with a sufficient number of points to define the curve accurately. An unknown concentration is then determined graphically from the curve.

Applications. Most quantitative spectrophotometric analyses utilize measurements made in the ultraviolet and visible regions of the electromagnetic spectrum. Besides the basic requirement that the sample compound, or its derivative, must exhibit absorption of sufficient intensity to be analytically useful, it is also necessary that the sample not be contaminated with substances capable of interfering through their own absorption. One of the advantages of absorption spectroscopy is its specificity, or freedom from interference. Even when absorption bands partially overlap, a quantitative analysis may be possible with the approach described as multicomponent analysis. The possibility of interfering absorbers must always be kept in mind when designing spectrophotometric analyses.

One way to overcome spectral interference is to cause the absorption spectrum of the sample compound to be shifted to a wavelength range free of interfering bands. Sometimes this is accomplished simply by raising or lowering the pH of the medium; as noted earlier, the spectra of acids and bases may alter significantly with changes in pH. Another way to shift a compound's absorption spectrum is to convert it into a derivative; the structural change will usually result in a spectral change. Many thousands of analyses have been worked out upon this basis. Usually the analysis is designed to produce absorption in the visible region, the compound being converted from a colorless substance to a derivative that is strongly colored. The usual principles of spectrophotometric analysis are then applied to the colored solution. This technique is called *colorimetric analysis*. Experiments 8.1, 20.2, and 23.2 are examples of colorimetric analyses.

Sometimes the colored derivative is of known structure and its solutions show highly reproducible spectral properties. Often it happens that the structure of the colored product is not known, and the intensity of absorption is dependent upon many factors, including temperature, pH, and time of reaction. Under such circumstances an absorptivity is of no quantitative value, and it is essential to prepare a standard Beer's law plot, or to use the reference standard method, at the same time as the unknown determination is made in order to render negligible the effects of variations in the reaction conditions. Many reviews of colorimetric analyses are available [4–7].

Most organic pharmaceuticals absorb intensely in the ultraviolet region and can be analyzed spectrophotometrically. The United States Pharmacopeia and the National Formulary include many such assays. The sensitivity of the method is high. The intensity of an absorption band, which is measured by the absorptivity at the band maximum, is determined by the probability of the transition. The theoretical prediction of absorption intensity is not practical, but an approximate value of the absorptivity may often be estimated by analogy with spectral data for closely related compounds. Many examples of such data are given in Section 8.3. Very extensive compilations of electronic spectral data are available [8].

A rough classification of compounds according to the intensity of their absorption will indicate the ranges of concentration within which spectrophotometric analysis is usually possible (Table 8.6). The absorbance should,

TABLE 8.6
Intensity of Electronic Absorption Bands

Type of Absorption	ϵ_{max}
Very weak	1–10
Weak	$10–10^2$
Moderate	$10^2–10^3$
Strong	$10^3–10^4$
Very strong	$10^4–10^5$

for most instruments, be within the range 0.2–2 for best performance. If a 1 cm cell is assumed, and an absorbance of 1.0 is taken as optimum, Beer's law gives the approximate molar concentrations required to yield good spectrophotometric results. Thus for a fairly strong absorber with $\epsilon_{max} = 5 \times 10^3$, the molar concentration should be about 2×10^{-4}. The lower concentration limit for spectrophotometric analysis, without modification of the instrument, is about 1×10^{-6} M; this concentration would give an absorbance of 0.1 in a 1 cm cell if $\epsilon = 10^5$.

8.3 Molecular Structure and Electronic Spectra

Electronic Transitions and Electronic Spectra. Electrons in molecules conventionally are pictured as occupants of orbitals, which are really mathematical constructions that represent the probable location of the electrons. It is necessary to postulate several kinds of orbitals, and it is customary to speak of the types of electrons occupying these orbitals. Four kinds of electrons are important in organic molecules. (1) Closed-shell electrons not involved in bonding have very high excitation energies and they do not contribute to absorption in the ultraviolet or visible regions. (2) Electrons in covalent single bonds occupy σ orbitals and are called σ electrons. Their excitation energy is high, and absorption due to transitions involving σ electrons may be observed in the far ultraviolet. (3) Nonbonding, paired, outer-shell electrons such as those in oxygen, sulfur, nitrogen, and the halogens, which are designated n electrons, can lead to absorption in the ultraviolet region. (4) Electrons in π orbitals, as in double and triple bonds, are responsible for much of the absorption in the ultraviolet and visible regions.

A molecule possesses unoccupied orbitals (antibonding orbitals) in addition to the occupied orbitals. In terms of the description given in Section 8.1, an antibonding orbital corresponds to an excited state energy level. An electronic transition is, in orbital description, a removal of an electron from an occupied orbital to a higher-energy antibonding orbital.

The lowest unoccupied orbital in a molecule is usually a π orbital, and the highest occupied orbitals are n and π orbitals. Figure 8.9 schematically indicates this relationship, the vertical dimension representing energy. The most common electronic transitions are from n and π orbitals to antibonding π^* orbitals; these are symbolized as $n \rightarrow \pi^*$ and $\pi \rightarrow \pi^*$ transitions. They account for most of the absorption in the ultraviolet and visible regions. At very low wavelengths $n \rightarrow \sigma^*$ transitions may also occur. (Recall that the energy of a photon is inversely proportional to wavelength according to $E = h\nu = hc/\lambda$.)

Electronic transitions can be very roughly visualized with valence bond

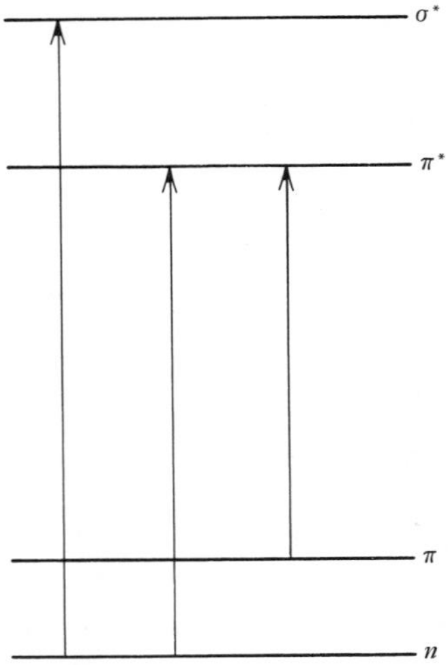

Fig. 8.9. Schematic illustration of electronic transitions; no quantitative significance should be attached to vertical distances. The diagram indicates (from left to right) $n \rightarrow \sigma^*$, $n \rightarrow \pi^*$, and $\pi \rightarrow \pi^*$ transitions.

structures, though oversimplification is introduced. A ketone, for example, is capable of undergoing both $\pi \rightarrow \pi^*$ and $n \rightarrow \pi^*$ transitions, which are indicated below.

$R_1R_2C{=}O \qquad R_1R_2\overset{+}{C}{-}\overset{-}{O}$

$\pi \rightarrow \pi^*$ transition

$R_1R_2C{=}O \qquad R_1R_2\overset{-}{C}{\equiv}\overset{+}{O}$

$n \rightarrow \pi^*$ transition

These structures attempt to depict the electronic redistribution that occurs when the transition takes place.

The wavelength of absorption, as we have seen, is determined by the energy gap between the ground and excited state energy levels for the transition. The intensity of absorption, however, is determined by the probability of the transition. Both theory and experiment indicate that the probability of the $\pi \rightarrow \pi^*$ transition is greater than that of the $n \rightarrow \pi^*$ transition, and this is reflected in the intensities of the absorption bands produced by the two transitions. The $\pi \rightarrow \pi^*$ transitions can yield bands with ϵ_{max} in the range 10^3–10^5, whereas the $n \rightarrow \pi^*$ transitions produce bands with ϵ_{max} less than 10^3.

Spectra of Isolated Chromophores. A vast amount of experimental work has established the absorption characteristics of most types of functional groups and classes of molecules. The most useful piece of information to be obtained from the absorption spectrum is the positions of band maxima; the intensity of absorption, usually expressed as the molar absorptivity at the band maximum, may also be helpful. Such spectral information can be used to help identify a compound by establishing the presence or absence of functional groups and their relative positions in the molecule.

Some specialized terminology has been developed to describe structure-spectra relationships. A *chromophore* is a group responsible for light absorption by a molecule; most chromophores therefore contain one or more multiple bonds. The carbonyl group in acetone is a chromophore; so is the benzene ring in toluene. An *auxochrome* is a group that does not possess notable absorption properties of its own, but that enhances absorption by a chromophore situated elsewhere in the molecule. All auxochromes contain atoms with unshared electron pairs, and they function by entering into electronic interaction with a nearby chromophore. Hydroxy and amino groups act as auxochromes. A *bathochromic shift* is a displacement of a band maximum to a longer wavelength by a change in medium or molecular structure. A bathochromic shift is also called a "red shift" because λ_{max} is shifted toward the infrared portion of the electromagnetic spectrum. A *hypsochromic shift* ("blue shift") is a displacement of λ_{max} toward shorter wavelengths. *Hyperchromism* is an increase in ϵ_{max} caused by a structural or medium change, and *hypochromism* is a decrease in ϵ_{max}.

Table 8.7 gives the characteristic positions of absorption bands for many isolated chromophores. If more than one band is produced, the band appearing at the longest wavelength usually has been tabulated. Some compounds exhibit spectra with multiple peaks; this fine structure has been indicated in the table.

The explanation given earlier for electronic transitions in terms of the local electronic configuration in the region of a multiple bond leads to the prediction that the spectral effects of two isolated chromophores (that is, chromophores separated by two or more single bonds) should be independent. For some substances this prediction is reasonably successful. Thus for ethyl isothiocyanate, C_2H_5NCS, $\lambda_{max} = 245$ nm and $\epsilon_{max} = 800$, whereas for $SCNCH_2$-CH_2CH_2NCS, $\lambda_{max} = 247$ nm and $\epsilon_{max} = 2000$; the spectrum of the latter

TABLE 8.7
Positions and Intensities of Absorption by Single Chromophores[a]

Chromophore	Typical Compound	λ_{max} (nm)[b]	log ϵ_{max}
—HC=CH—	1-Butene	181 (*f*)	4.2
—C≡C—	1-Butyne	172	3.7
—CHO	Acetaldehyde	278	0.9
—CO— (ketone)	Acetone	265	1.3
—OH (alcohol)	Ethanol	185	2.5
—COOH	Acetic acid	203	1.6
$—NH_2$	Methylamine	215 (*f*)	2.8
$—CONH_2$	Acetamide	205	2.2
—COCl	Acetyl chloride	220	2.0
—COOR	Ethyl acetate	209	1.9
—SH	Ethane thiol	230	2.2
—O— (ether)	Diethyl ether	188	3.3
—S— (sulfide)	Dimethyl sulfide	210	3.0
—S—S— (disulfide)	Dimethyl disulfide	255	2.5
—C≡N (nitrile)	Acetonitrile	none	—
$—NO_2$ (nitro)	1-Nitropropane	270	1.6
—ONO (nitrite)	*n*-Butyl nitrite	356 (*f*)	1.9
$—ONO_2$ (nitrate)	Ethyl nitrate	260	1.1
$—N_2$ (diazo)	Diazomethane	435	0.5
$—N_3$ (azide)	Azidoethane	290	1.5
$—C_6H_5$ (phenyl)	Benzene	255 (*f*)	2.5

[a] From Ref. 8.
[b] (*f*) signifies fine structure present.

compound is essentially equivalent to that of the former, with ϵ multiplied by 2. If this simple additivity is not observed, it may be inferred that an interaction between the chromophores is perturbing their electronic energy levels and altering the spectrum.

A second prediction is that the electronic absorption band caused by a transition within an isolated multiple bond should not be markedly altered by minor structural changes elsewhere in the molecule. This is because the electronic transition is mainly a local effect, and alterations in the molecule's electronic structure at points distant from the multiple bond should not change the local energy levels. For example, acetone, CH_3COCH_3, has λ_{max} 269 nm, ϵ_{max} 15, and 2-butanone, $CH_3COCH_2CH_3$, has λ_{max} 272, ϵ_{max} 18. If the structural alteration is very close to the chromophore or if it is a major alteration, then spectral changes can be expected; in fact a new chromophore may be created. See, for example, the spectral character (Table 8.7) of the acyl group R—C=O and how it is affected by the remaining bond to the carbon atom; compare acetaldehyde, acetone, acetic acid, etc.

Since compounds of similar structure may have similar absorption spectra, the important conclusion is reached that two samples are not proved to be identical just because their electronic absorption spectra appear to be identical.

Conjugated Chromophores and Aromatic Molecules. Conjugated multiple bonds, and multiple bonds in conjugation with nonbonding electrons, do not behave as isolated groups, but interact with each other in accordance with the postulates of the resonance theory of organic chemistry. The result of conjugation is to shift the band maxima to longer wavelengths (lower frequencies), which means that the energy differences between the ground and excited states must be decreased relative to the differences when the groups are not conjugated. This effect can be understood in terms of the orbital picture adopted earlier [9]. It appears that the larger the orbitals in a molecule, the smaller is the energy difference between orbitals. The π orbitals characteristic of double and triple bonds are much larger than the σ orbitals of a single bond. When two or more multiple bonds are conjugated, the π orbitals merge, increasing the volume of the orbital and decreasing the energy gap between adjacent orbitals. A longer conjugation path results in a larger orbital volume, smaller energy differences between the ground and excited states, and therefore absorption at longer wavelengths. Aromatic molecules display this effect also. In these compounds nearly the entire aromatic ring may be considered to have π orbital character, and band maxima are observed at long wavelengths. In a very naive way this relationship between orbital volume and transition energy can be seen as a result of the π electrons being less firmly held in a larger bonding orbital, and therefore more readily translated to an antibonding orbital.

Conjugated chromophores exhibit bathochromic shifts when compared with the isolated chromophores. Table 8.8 shows the extent of this effect for some systems containing two chromophores in conjugation. Comparison of the band maxima with those for the corresponding single chromophores shows that in each case a bathochromic shift has occurred. The effect is enhanced when additional double bonds are placed in conjugation, and in Table 8.9

TABLE 8.8
Absorption Data for Two Conjugated Chromophores

Conjugated System	Example	λ_{max} (nm)	log ϵ_{max}
—HC=CH—CH=CH—	1,3-Butadiene	217	4.3
—HC=CH—C≡C—	1-Buten-3-yne	208–241 (*f*)	
—HC=CH—CH=O	Crotonaldehyde	220, 322	4.2, 1.5
—HC=CH—C≡N	Acrylonitrile	216	1.7

TABLE 8.9
Bathochromic Shift Caused by Conjugation of Double Bonds

Compound	Number of Double Bonds	λ_{max} (nm)
Ethylene	1	174
1,3-Butadiene	2	217
1,3,5-Hexatriene	3	267
Vitamin A	5	325

the bathochromic shift produced by several conjugated olefinic bonds is very evident.

Aromatic compounds exhibit more complex spectra than do aliphatic substances. Benzene has a very high intensity absorption near 200 nm and lower intensity bands between 230 and 270 nm. This lower intensity absorption is resolved into four strong peaks with superimposed fine structure (see Fig. 8.10). The introduction of substituents on the benzene ring alters the spectrum, usually with a smoothing out of the fine structure. Figure 8.11 shows this effect (compare with Fig. 8.10) for ephedrine, structure **1**. Hydroxy, methoxy, or amino substituents on an aromatic ring act as auxochromes, with the absorption intensity being increased by a factor of about 10.

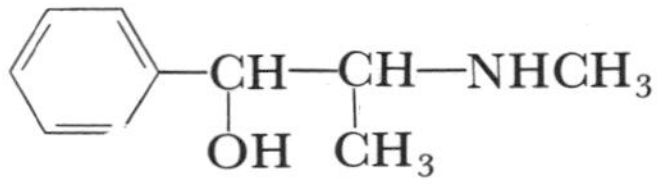

C_6H_5—CH(OH)—CH(CH_3)—$NHCH_3$

1

The polycyclic fused ring aromatics are extended orbital systems and may be expected to show absorption at relatively long wavelengths. This behavior is observed (Table 8.10); in fact, absorption is extended to such long wavelengths that solutions of naphthacene are yellow and solutions of pentacene blue. The utility of the resonance theory in rationalizing spectral data is demonstrated by the polyphenyl compounds. These aromatics can be linked either *para* or *meta*. The *p*-polyphenyls with the general structure

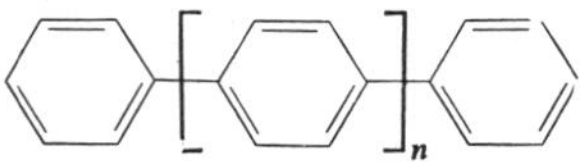

$C_6H_5[C_6H_4]_nC_6H_5$

are capable of resonance interactions involving the entire system of conjugated bonds, with contributing structures of the type

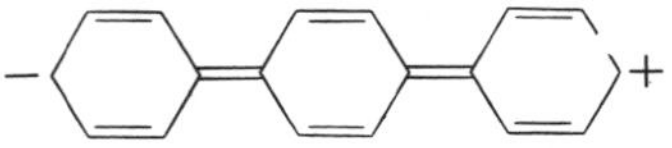

$^{-}$ (quinoid polyphenyl structure) $^{+}$

The greater the number of *para*-linked rings, then, the longer should be the wavelength of maximum absorption. Table 8.11 shows that this behavior is observed [10]. The intensity of absorption also increases as n increases.

The *m*-polyphenyls, which have the structure

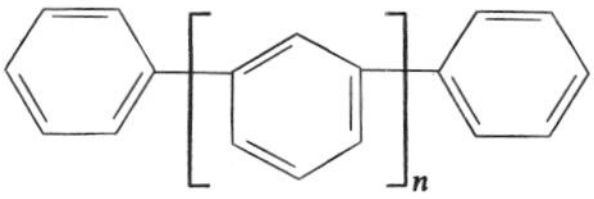

are not capable of entering into extended resonance interaction involving the entire molecule. The band maximum remains essentially unmoved at 252–255 nm as n varies from 0 to 16 in these compounds [10]. The molar absorptivity, meanwhile, increases in a regular manner consistent with an additive effect, as described for noninteracting chromophores.

It should now be clear why dyes and acid-base indicators are usually large molecules with extensive conjugation and possibilities for resonance delocalization; these features cause large bathochromic shifts with resultant absorption in the visible region. The loss or addition of a proton markedly changes the electron distribution and therefore the color.

It is not possible to identify a compound unambiguously on the basis of its electronic absorption spectrum. Spectral data can tell a great deal about the types of functional groups present, however, and are useful in demonstrating the absence of chromophores. Spectra of similar compounds and a spectrum of an authentic sample, if available, will be found useful for comparisons. The wavelengths of maximum absorption are not the only data of importance; the intensities of absorption, expressed as absorptivities, are also valuable. The ratio of intensities at two wavelengths is often useful as a criterion of identity or purity.

By combining wavelength and intensity data with dosage information, many drugs can be tentatively identified by uv spectroscopy [11]. Steroids with an α,β-unsaturated ketone function in the A ring (such as hydrocortisone **2**) show a single absorption band with λ_{max} at 240 nm. A large number of

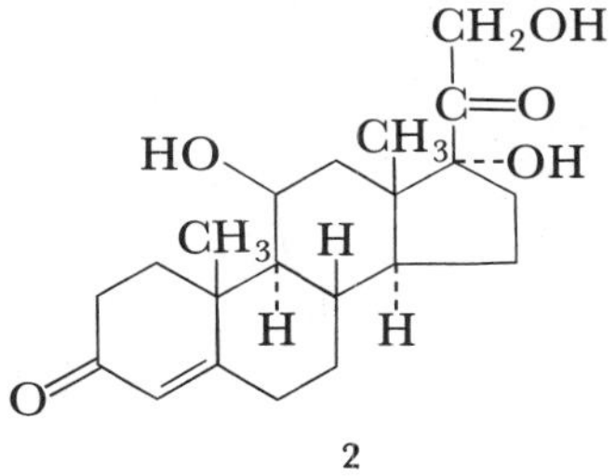

2

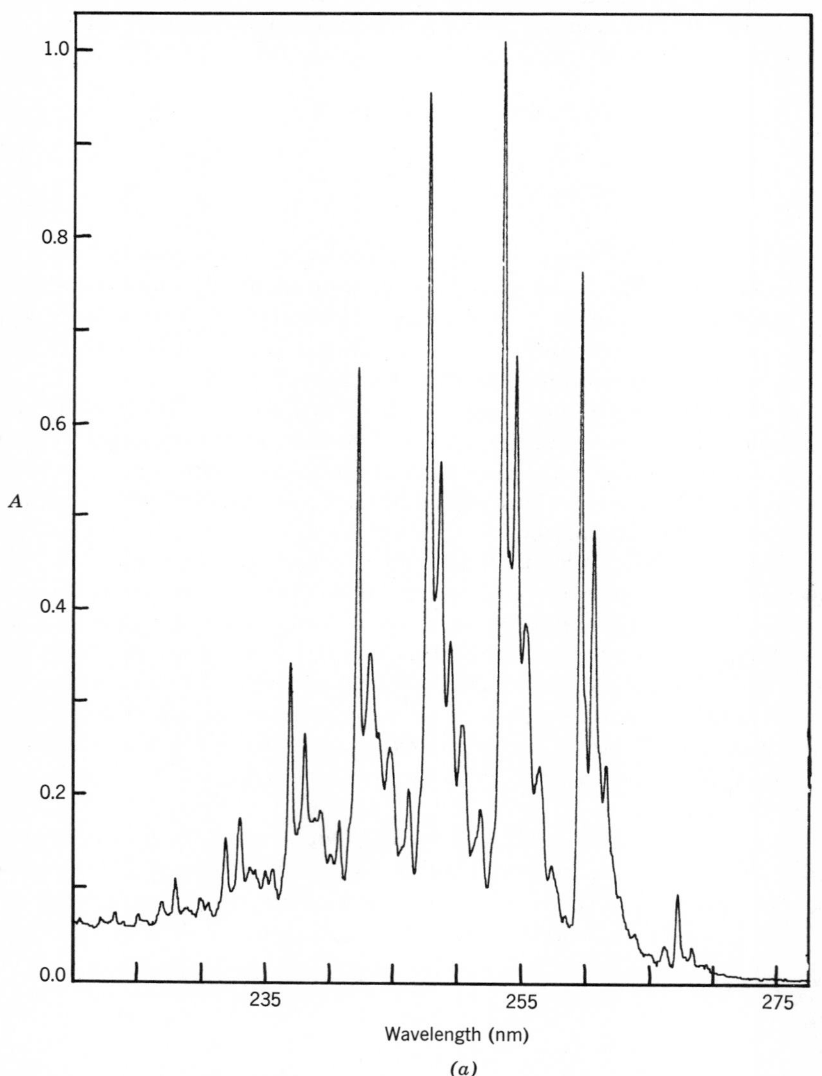

Fig. 8.10. Electronic absorption spectrum of benzene: (*a*) benzene vapor; (*b*) benzene in ethanol solution.

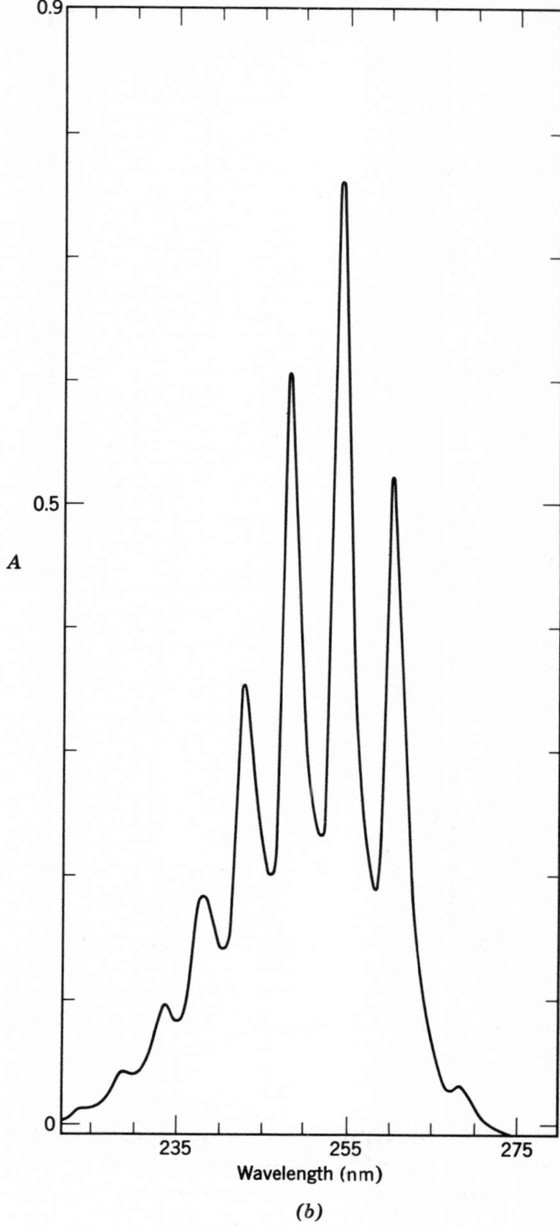

(b)

Fig. 8.10. *(Cont'd.)*

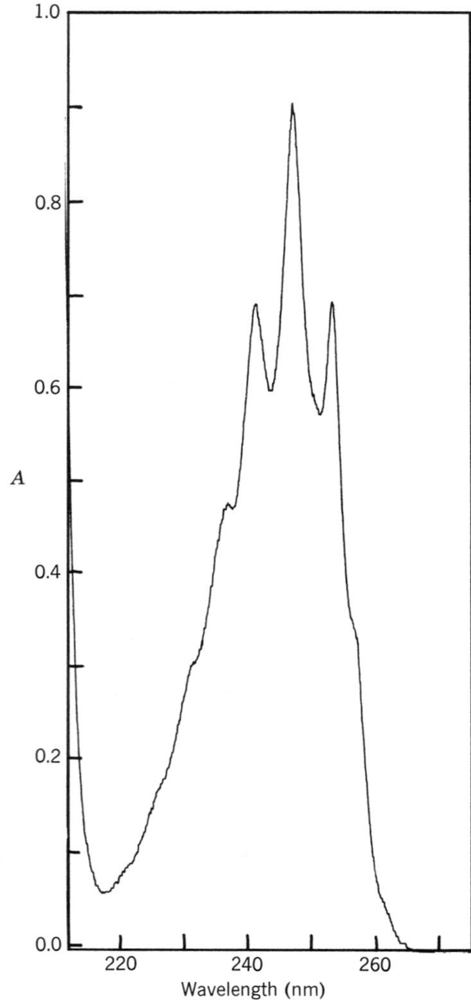

Fig. 8.11. Absorption spectrum of ephedrine hydrochloride in water; $b = 1$ cm, $c = 0.09614$ g/100 ml.

drugs have benzenoid absorption with λ_{max} at 257 nm. Since their usual therapeutic doses may be widely dissimilar, the absorbance produced by dissolving the drug from a single dosage form (tablet, capsule, etc.) in a given volume of solvent is a function of both ϵ_{max} and the dosage, thus narrowing the possible compounds to a very few. Another group of benzenoid drugs absorbs with λ_{max} at 262–268 nm [11].

TABLE 8.10
Absorption Band Maxima for Fused Ring Aromatics

Compound	Number of Rings	λ_{max}[a] (nm)
Benzene	1	261
Naphthalene	2	312
Anthracene	3	375
Naphthacene	4	471
Pentacene	5	575

[a] Maximum of the band appearing at longest wavelength.

Medium Effects. When a substance is in the gaseous state its absorption spectrum is essentially that of the isolated molecules, and it is possible to observe individual electronic transitions and even their associated vibrational and rotational transitions. Figure 8.10*a*, the vapor-phase spectrum of benzene, shows this fine structure. When a solute is dissolved in a liquid solvent, solute-solvent interactions (dispersion and dipole-dipole interactions) prevent free rotation and also change the possible vibrational transitions. The usual result is extensive loss of fine structure in the spectrum, as seen for a benzene solution in Fig. 8.10*b*. The more polar the solvent, the greater is the extent of solute-solvent interaction and the less the vibrational structure revealed in the spectrum. Hydrocarbon solvents therefore give greater spectral detail than do polar solvents like alcohols and water.

Aside from loss of fine structure on passing from nonpolar to polar solvents, it is observed that the wavelength of maximum absorption may change. Whether this is a bathochromic (red) shift or a hypsochromic (blue) shift depends upon the nature of the transition and of the solute-solvent interactions. Consider as an example the carbonyl function, which can undergo $n \rightarrow \pi^*$ and

TABLE 8.11
Band Maxima of Para Polyphenyls [10]

Compound	n	λ_{max} (nm)
Diphenyl	0	252
Terphenyl	1	280
Quaterphenyl	2	300
Quinquiphenyl	3	310
Sexiphenyl	4	318

$\pi \rightarrow \pi^*$ transitions as indicated earlier. In its ground state the electronic distribution of the carbonyl group can be represented as in **3**, resulting in a dipole moment with its negative pole oriented toward the oxygen.

$$\delta^+ \rangle C{=}O\delta^-$$

3

In solution this molecule will be solvated, its dipole moment tending to orient solvent molecules in its vicinity so as to yield the most stable solute-solvent system. Upon electronic excitation, the electronic distribution will change, and it is well accepted that during the time required for this electronic redistribution to occur, the atomic nuclei, which are much more massive than electrons, will not change their locations. (This principle is called the Franck-Condon effect.) Therefore the excited state will not be optimally stabilized by solvation, since the time for the necessary reorientation of solvent molecules is not available. The actual effect of the solvent on the energy of the excited state will therefore depend upon whether the excited state is electronically similar to the ground state, or dissimilar. More precisely, it depends upon whether the dipole moment increases or decreases upon excitation. Table 8.12 summarizes the argument for the carbonyl group. These predictions are successful; thus on passing from hexane to ethanol as solvents, acetone undergoes a blue shift of its low-intensity $n \rightarrow \pi^*$ transition and a red shift of its high-intensity $\pi \rightarrow \pi^*$ transition.

Very dramatic solvent effects can be seen in the spectra of acids and bases when the pH of the medium is changed. These effects were used in Section 8.2 to measure pK_a values spectrophotometrically. Acid-base indicator color changes illustrate the phenomenon; see Fig. 8.7. An important pharmaceutical

TABLE 8.12
Prediction of Solvent Effects on Carbonyl Absorption Bands

Transition	Excited State Representation	Dipole Moment	Effect of More Polar Solvent on Excited State	Energy Gap	Wavelength Shift
$\pi \rightarrow \pi^*$	$\rangle \overset{+}{C}—\overset{-}{O}$	Increases	Stabilizes	Decreases	Bathochromic
$n \rightarrow \pi^*$	$\rangle \overset{-}{C}—\overset{+}{O}$	Decreases	Destabilizes	Increases	Hypsochromic

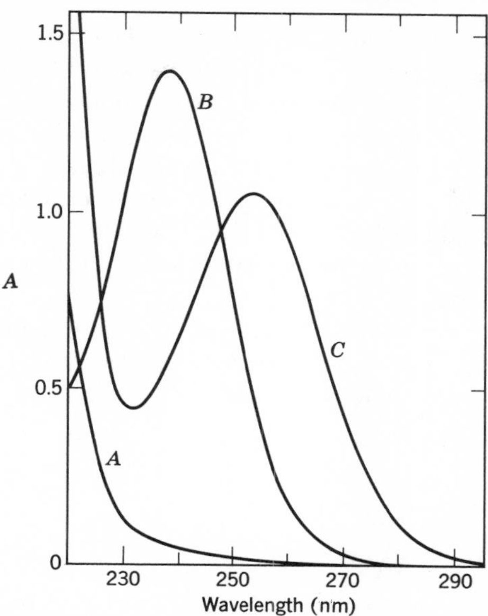

Fig. 8.12. Ultraviolet absorption spectra of barbital. *A*, in 0.1 *N* sulfuric acid (un-ionized form); *B*, in pH 9.9 buffer (singly ionized form); *C*, in 1 *N* sodium hydroxide (doubly ionized form). $b = 1$ cm, $c = 0.0250$ g/liter.

example is provided by the barbituric acid derivatives, which undergo ionization with pK_1 values about 8 and pK_2 values about 12, as follows:

Figure 8.12 shows the spectra of barbital at three pH's, corresponding to the un-ionized, single ionized, and doubly ionized forms. This behavior is very characteristic of the barbiturates. The spectral shifts of many other drugs upon pH change have been described; these can be very helpful for identification [11]. The direction of the shift can usually be rationalized in terms of the extent of conjugation.

8.4 Molecular Structure and Infrared Spectra

Vibrational Transitions. The chemical bond between two atoms in a molecule may be idealized as a tiny spring connecting two point masses. A molecule is then an arrangement in space of masses (atoms) connected by springs (bonds). Different kinds of bonds are represented by springs of different lengths and "stiffness." If energy is imparted to such a model, the masses will vibrate. This motion is analogous to the vibrations of atoms and groups in real molecules. In the molecular system the energy is furnished as electromagnetic radiation of infrared frequency, and the energy absorption process results in a vibrational transition, or change in vibrational energy level. (The molecule remains in its ground electronic state during this vibrational transition.) The infrared absorption spectrum is a record of the frequencies of radiation capable of exciting vibrational transitions.

Let us consider the possible ways in which a simple linear molecule, say, carbon dioxide, can vibrate (its vibrational modes). Only three independent modes exist; these are shown as structures **4** (symmetric stretching mode), **5** (antisymmetric stretching mode), and **6** (bending mode). Stretching

$$\overleftarrow{O}=C=\overrightarrow{O} \qquad \overrightarrow{O}=C=\overrightarrow{O} \qquad \overset{\uparrow}{O}=\underset{\downarrow}{C}=\overset{\uparrow}{O}$$

4 **5** **6**

vibrations correspond to changes in bond lengths, and bending vibrations to changes in bond angles. It is a result of quantum mechanics that infrared absorption will take place only if the vibrational mode is accompanied by a change in dipole moment. Since the stretching vibration **4** is symmetrical, it results in no change in dipole moment and therefore does not absorb radiation; it is said to be inactive in the infrared. The two other modes give rise to absorption at what are called the fundamental frequencies of CO_2*.

The many fundamental frequencies ($\nu_1, \nu_2, \ldots$) possessed by complex molecules give rise to intense absorption bands. Besides these bands, absorption may also be observed at multiples of the fundamentals (that is, at $2\nu_1$, $2\nu_2$, etc.); these bands, which are relatively weak, are called overtones. Combination tones also may occur at frequencies corresponding to sums of fundamental frequencies, for example, $\nu_1 + \nu_2$. Infrared spectra are therefore very complex, and theoretical interpretation is difficult and seldom attempted for complex molecules.

Frequency-Structure Correlations. The characteristic vibrational frequency of the bond between atoms or groups of atoms is not markedly altered by changes in the molecular environment. For example, the carbonyl group C=O absorbs at a frequency of about 1700 cm^{-1} for all aldehydes and ketones, thus providing a convenient indication of the presence of this group in a molecule. Minor shifts of absorption frequency can be associated with

* For a linear molecule containing N atoms, there are $3N - 5$ fundamental modes; in CO_2 one of these (**4**) is inactive, and mode **6** has another identical mode at right angles to it. For a nonlinear molecule there are $3N - 6$ vibrational modes.

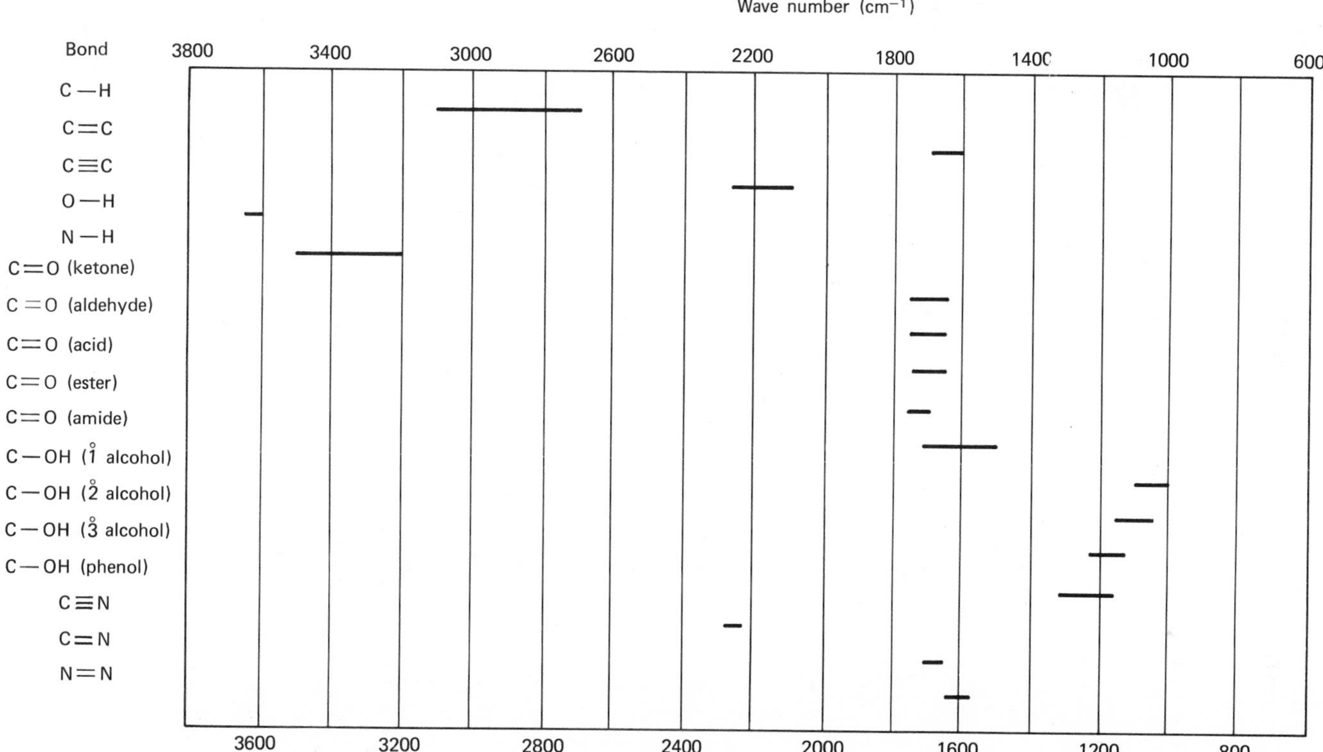

Fig. 8.13. Correlation chart for infrared absorption frequencies of some common bond types.

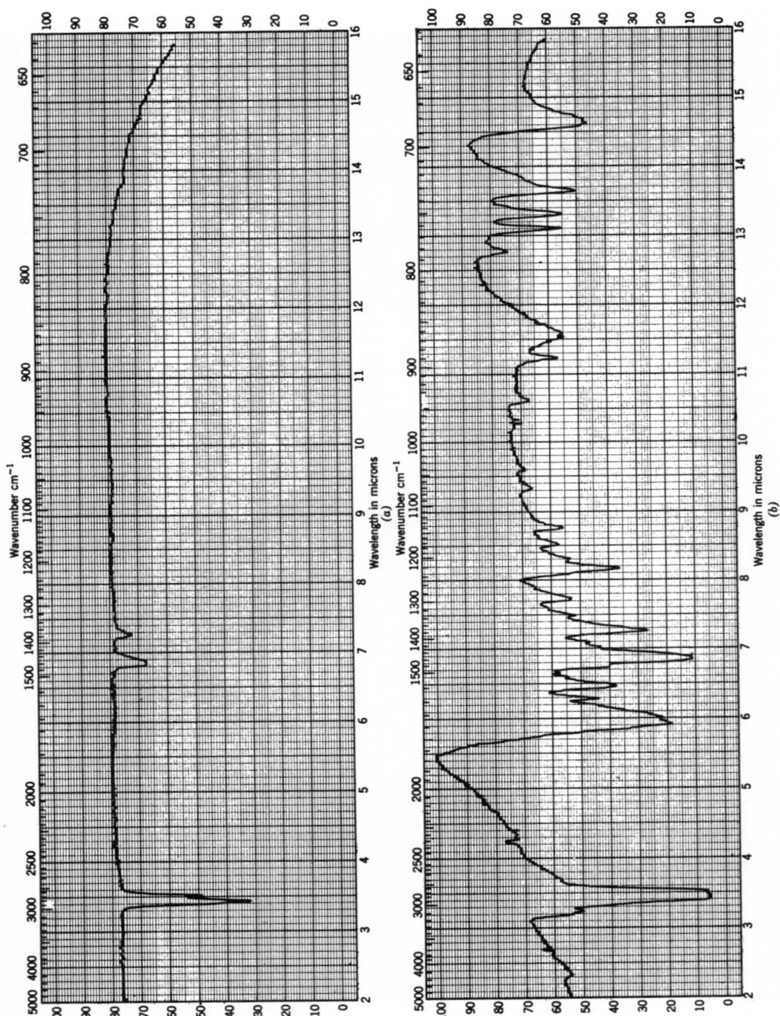
Wavenumber cm⁻¹
Wavelength in microns
(a)
Wavenumber cm⁻¹
Wavelength in microns
(b)

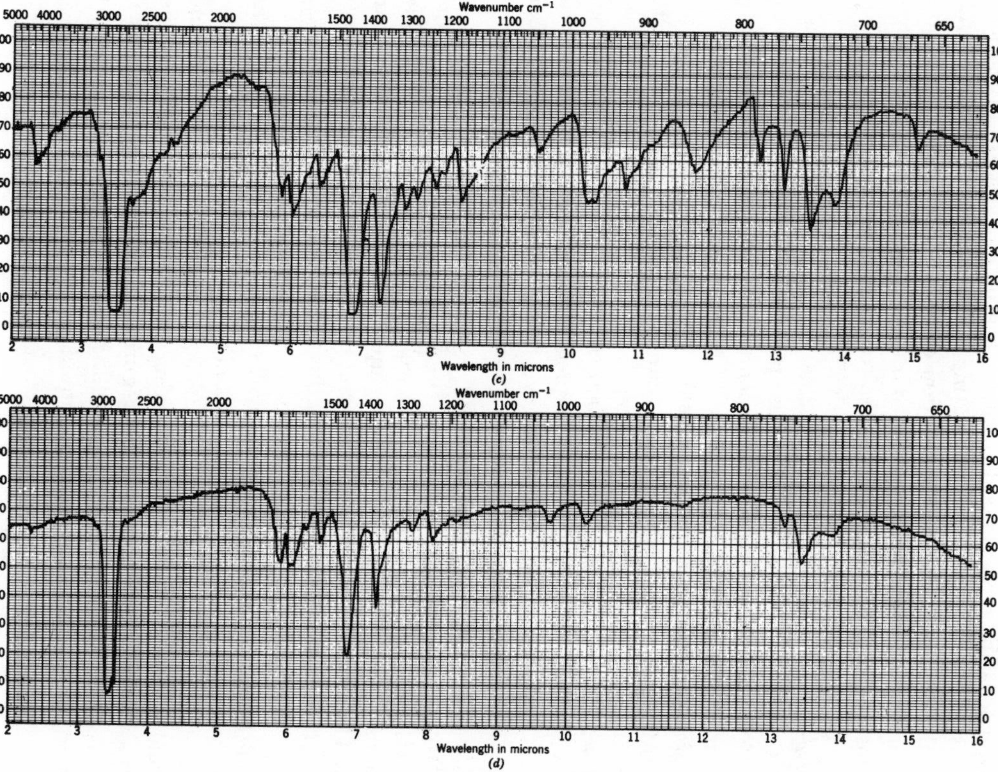

Fig. 8.14. Infrared spectra of xanthines. (*a*) Spectrum of the medium, liquid petrolatum (Nujol). (*b*) Spectrum of theobromine in Nujol. (*c*) Spectrum of theophylline in nujol. (*d*) Spectrum of caffeine in nujol.

structural changes, however, and so additional information may be obtained about the group, such as the presence of aromatic or aliphatic substituents, or its proximity to other groups. Tens of thousands of ir spectra have been recorded, and empirical correlations have been established between absorption frequencies and types of bonds or chemical groups. These group frequency correlations are of great value in elucidating the structures of new compounds. A very abbreviated frequency correlation chart is shown in Fig. 8.13. It is found that the ir spectrum can be divided into several regions depending upon the atoms or groups whose vibrations are responsible for absorption.

1. *Hydrogen Stretching Region* (3700–2500 cm^{-1}). Stretching vibrations of C—H, O—H, N—H, and S—H bonds are responsible for absorption in this region. The absorption frequency depends upon the atom to which the hydrogen is bonded.

2. *Triple Bond Stretching Region* (2500–2000 cm^{-1}). Carbon-carbon and carbon-nitrogen triple bonds, as well as cumulated double bonds (that is, the system C=C=C), absorb in this region.

3. *Double Bond Stretching Region* (2000–1600 cm^{-1}). C=C, C=O, and C=N vibrations are excited in this frequency range. The type of group can often be determined by the frequency; thus carbonyls absorb at about 1700 cm^{-1}, for esters and acids the frequency is higher, and for amides it is lower. Conjugation also lowers the frequency.

4. *Single Bond Stretch and Bend Region* (1500–700 cm^{-1}). Bending vibrations of C—H bonds occur in this region, as well as both bending and stretching vibrations of single bonds connecting groups such as methylene, methyl, and amino. This region is called the fingerprint region because of the specificity of the structure-spectrum relationships in this portion of the ir spectrum.

The principal value of infrared spectra to the pharmaceutical analyst is as a tool to establish the identity of a compound whose structure is known. If the ir spectra of the sample and the authentic specimen are identical, the substances are usually identical, although supporting data should always be obtained. This is a very powerful method [12]. Figure 8.14 shows the ir spectra for the three xanthines, theobromine, theophylline, and caffeine (in the solid form, the substance being suspended in liquid petrolatum). Despite the close

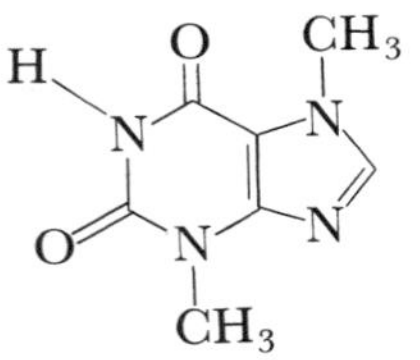

Theobromine

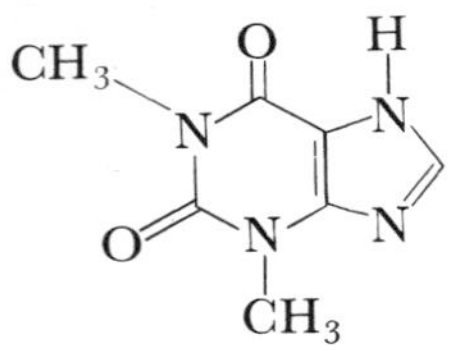

Theophylline

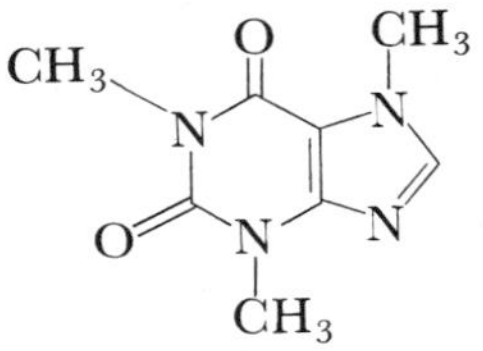

Caffeine

structural similarities, the infrared spectra of these compounds are quite different, and it would be a simple matter to distinguish between the compounds if spectra of the three are available for comparison. In contrast to the uniqueness of the ir spectra, the ultraviolet spectra of these compounds are practically identical.

Quantitative analysis can be carried out in the ir region, and, although not as sensitive as spectrophotometric analysis in the uv, it can be quite specific because of the large number of ir transitions. Multicomponent analysis of mixtures is often quite successful in the ir.

Infrared spectrophotometers record percent transmittance, so that absorption maxima appear as transmittance minima. The frequency axis may be linear in wavelength, as in Fig. 8.14, or in frequency, which is given in cm^{-1} (the wave number).

8.5 Measurement of Absorption Spectra

Spectrophotometers. Any instrument used to measure a spectrum is called a spectroscope or a spectrometer. If the light passing through the sample is detected with a photographic film or plate, the spectrometer is a spectrograph; the instrument is a spectrophotometer if the light intensity is measured with a photoelectric cell. Most instruments presently used are spectrophotometers. A spectrometer designed to make absorption measurements solely in the visible region may be called a colorimeter.

All spectrophotometers contain the components shown in Fig. 8.15. (The order in which these parts are arranged may vary slightly from that in the figure.) The materials and details of construction depend upon the wavelength range to be studied, and two general types of instrument are necessary: electronic spectra are measured with an ultraviolet spectrophotometer (which can be used for both the uv and visible regions), and an infrared spectrophotometer is necessary for the spectral range beyond about 1 μm. The near-infrared is accessible to some ultraviolet spectrophotometers especially designed to measure near-ir spectra. A brief description of the basic parts of a spectrophotometer will indicate the similarities and differences between instruments.

1. *Light Source.* For the visible region an ordinary tungsten lamp is a good source of radiation. In the uv region the usual energy source is a hydrogen

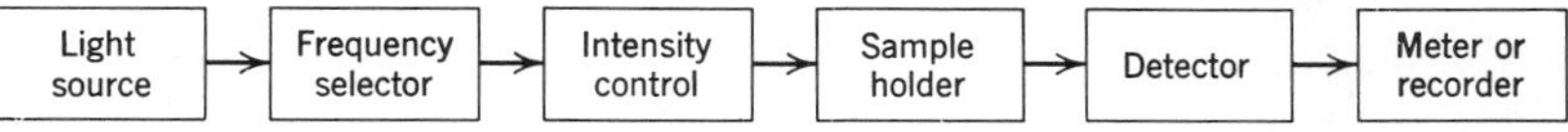

Fig. 8.15. Schematic organization of a spectrophotometer.

discharge lamp, which emits radiation of nearly constant intensity over the entire ultraviolet range. Infrared light sources are considerably different. A widely used ir source consists of a silicon carbide rod heated to 1200°C electrically.

2. *Frequency Selector.* The determination of an absorption spectrum requires the measurement of absorbance or transmittance as a function of wavelength. It is therefore necessary to be able to choose the wavelength (or frequency) of the radiation at will. In some very inexpensive instruments designed for colorimetric analyses the selection of wavelength is accomplished by passing the light through colored glass filters that remove all radiation from the beam except that of the desired wavelength. Actually this relatively crude method cannot isolate a single wavelength; the filter actually transmits a wide band of wavelengths. A filter colorimeter cannot, therefore, be employed to determine an absorption spectrum, although it may yield satisfactory analytical results for a given band of wavelengths if the absorption peak of the absorbing compound is very broad.

A prism is usually the dispersing element (that is, the unit that spreads the light into its component wavelengths) in a spectrophotometer. For visible light, glass is a good prism material, but ultraviolet light, which is absorbed by glass, must be dispersed with a prism constructed of silica (SiO_2). Sodium chloride (rock salt) is the usual prism material in infrared spectrophotometers.

The light is thus resolved by the prism into its component wavelengths, or rather into narrow bands containing very few wavelengths. By rotating the prism different bands are brought to focus on a slit that admits the light to the next stage of the instrument. This light is obviously not monochromatic (of a single wavelength), but in a good spectrophotometer it includes very little light other than that of the desired wavelength. The prism, with associated optics, is called the monochromator.

Some spectrophotometers use a diffraction grating as the dispersing element. A grating is a flat surface engraved with thousands of small grooves per centimeter. This microscopically serrated surface reflects light and disperses it by a diffraction mechanism.

3. *Intensity Control.* It is not sufficient merely to pass light of the selected wavelength through the sample—enough light must pass through the sample to elicit a measurable response from the detector. The amount of light required will depend upon its wavelength (because the detector response varies with wavelength) and upon the nature of the sample (that is, on what fraction of the incident light is transmitted by the sample). Because these are variables, most spectrophotometers include one or more mechanical slits, operated manually or automatically, whose width can be varied, thus controlling the intensity of light reaching the sample.

4. *Sample Holder.* All spectral studies in the uv and visible regions are

carried out on dilute solutions. The cells (cuvettes) holding the sample must be transparent to the light, so glass cells are used in the visible region and silica cells in the ultraviolet. The glass cells (Pyrex, Vycor, Corex) may be employed for measurements down to about 325 nm; below this wavelength absorption by the glass is excessive. Cells are available with internal path lengths of 0.1, 1, 2, 5, and 10 cm.

Infrared spectra may be determined for samples in solution, the cell being composed of sodium chloride or other halides. Very satisfactory ir spectra can be obtained from crystalline samples, which are finely dispersed in liquid petrolatum or are compressed into a tablet with potassium bromide as a diluent. The liquid dispersion is placed between plates of NaCl for support in the light path.

5. *Detector*. The human eye is an extremely sensitive detector, but it is not suited to quantitative measurement. Early in the development of spectroscopic techniques photographic plates were used as detecting elements, but they are slow and inconvenient to use. Visible and ultraviolet spectrophotometers now utilize electronic sensing devices, called phototubes and photomultiplier tubes, to detect the intensity of light transmitted by the sample. Phototubes contain a treated surface that, when struck by photons, emits electrons. These electrons are collected on a positive plate, producing a plate current that is proportional to the intensity of the incident radiation. If instead of being collected the electrons are accelerated through a large electric potential and made to strike a second photoactive surface, a multiple emission of electrons will occur. This results in an amplification of the plate current and an increased accuracy in its measurement. This is the principle of the photomultiplier tube.

Infrared spectrophotometers utilize a different detection system. The radiation is absorbed by the sensor and the radiation energy is converted to thermal energy, which is detected as a change in a property such as electrical resistance or potential.

6. *Meter or Recorder*. The signal from the detector is fed into a potentiometer circuit (see Chapter 6), which is balanced to give a reading of transmittance or absorbance, the instrument being suitably calibrated in these units rather than in the primary electrical signal. On manual spectrophotometers the potentiometer null point is found by hand. Some instruments provide a direct indicator dial of absorbance. Recording spectrophotometers trace a record of absorbance or transmittance on chart paper; with these instruments the entire absorption spectrum is recorded automatically, the instrument "scanning" the wavelength range and tracing the absorbance-wavelength curve.

Recall that transmittance is the ratio of the intensities of the transmitted and incident light: $T = I/I_0$. The minor diminution of light intensity caused by reflection from the cell surfaces and absorption by the solvent is compensated for by measuring I_0 as the intensity of light transmitted by a cell filled with pure solvent. I is then measured as the intensity of light transmitted by the sample solution contained in an identical cell. The instrument meter is calibrated to give directly the transmittance or, more usually, the absorbance, which is log $(1/T)$. Each value of A or T is therefore the result of two measurements, of I_0 and I.

In a single-beam spectrophotometer these two measurements are made sequentially by the operator. Figure 8.16 shows a schematic diagram of a typical single-beam manual spectrophotometer, the Beckman DU. Radiation from the light source A is directed by the mirrors B and C through slit D to the collimating mirror E. From E the light beam passes to the prism F, where it is dispersed. The reflecting back side of F sends the light back through the prism, further dispersing it. The light passes via E through the slit D and into the sample cell G. After passing through the sample, the light strikes the phototube H. The signal is brought manually to a null balance in a potentiometer circuit, and the absorbance or transmittance is read from a dial. The wavelength is selected by rotating a dial that changes the orientation of the prism. The analyst must, with a single-beam instrument, place the solvent (reference) cell in the light path and adjust the meter to read 100% transmittance; this effectively sets the value of I_0. The sample cell is next placed in the beam, and the meter gives T or A directly.

The necessity for making two separate measurements has been eliminated with double-beam spectrophotometers. With these instruments the monochromatic ray is split into two identical beams: one beam is passed through the reference cell and the other is simultaneously passed through the sample. The instrument in effect measures the ratio of the intensities of radiation transmitted by the cells. Recording spectrophotometers are, in most designs, double-beam instruments.

Sample Preparation. The concentration ranges suitable for studies in the visible and ultraviolet ranges were discussed on p. 193. Because the path length (b in Beer's law) can be varied from 0.1 to 10 cm, some latitude is gained in the concentration variable. The absorbance should be in the range 0.2–1.0

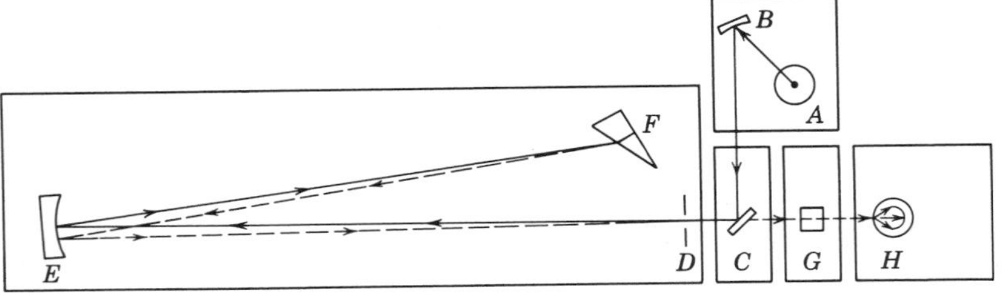

Fig. 8.16. Schematic diagram of the Beckman Model DU spectrophotometer, a single-beam, manually operated prism instrument. See text for details.

for most spectrophotometers, although some instruments permit accurate measurements to be made in the range 1–3.

The solvent should be transparent throughout the frequency range to be studied. Useful solvents for the entire visible and ultraviolet regions are water, methanol, ethanol, acetonitrile, *n*-hexane, and isooctane. Some solvents are used for studies at wavelengths longer than a "cut-off" point at which their own absorption begins; thus chloroform is transparent at wavelengths longer than about 250 nm. Chloroform is a very good solvent for quantitative measurements in the infrared.

The incorporation of buffers or the use of mixed solvents may alter the absorption characteristics of a solvent. The solvent placed in the reference cell should have the same composition as that used for the sample solution.

Infrared spectra for identification purposes may be obtained with the sample in the crystalline form. The powdered sample is dispersed in liquid petrolatum. (This preparation is called a Nujol mull, Nujol being a proprietary name for liquid petrolatum.) Alternatively the powdered sample is dispersed evenly in potassium bromide and the mixture is compressed into a tablet, which is placed in the light path. The KBr is transparent in the infrared.

Beer's Law Deviations of Instrumental Origin. Errors in measured absorbance values can result from malfunctions of the spectrophotometer (for example, nonlinear response of the phototube) or from operator error (for example, inaccurate setting of the wavelength selector). Other sources of imprecision in data and of curvature in Beer's law plots are possible.

The monochromator selects a beam of radiation of given wavelength by means of a dispersing element (prism or grating) and a slit. The band of radiation cannot be truly monochromatic, however, for its intensity would not then be measurable. A spectral interval of finite width must therefore be taken for passage through the sample. A plot of the intensity of radiation produced by the monochromator when the wavelength selector is set at λ_0 has the appearance of Fig. 8.17. λ_0 is the *nominal wavelength*, that is, the wavelength selected by the operator. $\Delta\lambda$ is the *effective band width*, or half-intensity band width; it is the width of the intensity band at one-half the maximum intensity.

Because the dispersion of a prism is not linear with wavelength (that is, the separation of adjacent wavelengths is more efficient at some wavelengths), the effective band width produced by the monochromator varies with wavelength. This variation is different for each instrument design. For example, the effective band widths for the Beckman DU, with a 1 mm slit width, are at 200 nm, 0.8 nm; at 300 nm, 3.7 nm; at 400 nm, 10.5 nm; at 500 nm, 20.1 nm; and at 600 nm, 35 nm. A monochromator using a diffraction grating for a dispersing element produces an effective band width that is constant at all wavelengths, because the dispersion of a grating does not vary with wavelength.

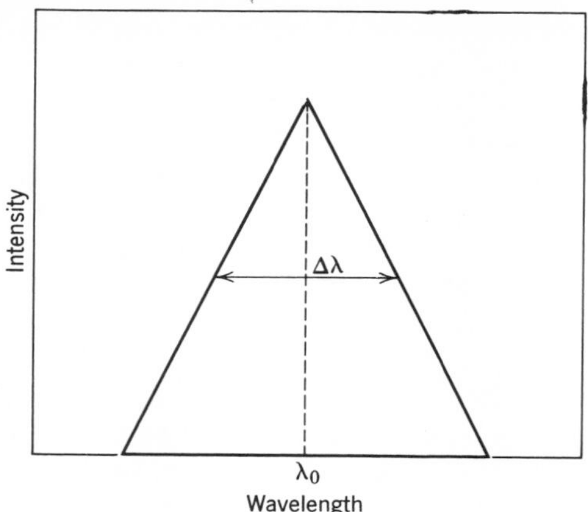

Fig. 8.17. Relation between the nominal wavelength λ_0 and the effective band width $\Delta\lambda$ for a monochromator.

Since the absorptivity of a compound varies with wavelength, the absorptivities at wavelengths different from λ_0, but included in the band width, may be several percent different from that at λ_0. The observed absorptivity is therefore different from the true absorptivity, and deviations are possible in the Beer's law plot. This effect is usually minimized by setting λ_0 at λ_{max}, the absorption maximum, for at this wavelength the absorptivity does not change rapidly with wavelength, unless the absorption band is extremely sharp.

Another cause of deviations is stray light, which is spurious radiation from uncontrolled sources, such as leaks in the cell compartment housing. At low absorbances a small amount of unabsorbed stray light causes little error, but at very high absorbances this same amount of unabsorbed stray light will produce a negative error in the observed absorbance. A negative deviation in the Beer's law plot will be observed.

The wavelength and absorbance scales of spectrophotometers should occasionally be checked to ensure that the wavelength scale calibration and the linearity of the absorbance scale are as accurate as specified by the manufacturer. Appendix B gives convenient procedures for making these checks.

Experiment 8.1. Colorimetric Analysis of Aromatic Amines by Diazotization and Coupling

PRINCIPLE

This experiment is a typical colorimetric analysis in which a colorless compound is converted to a derivative that absorbs in the visible region.

(This analysis could also be carried out on the original compound by measuring its uv absorption, but this would require an ultraviolet spectrophotometer.) In this analysis the structure of the colored derivative is known.

Diazotization of Aromatic Amines. Primary aromatic amines, which may be written $Ar—NH_2$, undergo reaction with an acidic nitrous acid solution to give diazonium salts, which are useful intermediates in the synthesis of many organics, especially dyestuffs. The overall diazotization reaction is

$$Ar—NH_2 + HNO_2 + HCl \rightarrow Ar—N_2{}^+Cl^- + 2H_2O \tag{8.25}$$

The reaction probably proceeds by means of an initial nitrosation of the amine (8.26), followed by tautomerization of the nitrosamine (8.27) and decomposition of the diazohydroxide (8.28) [13].

$$Ar—NH_2 + HNO_2 \rightarrow Ar—NH—N{=}O + H_2O \tag{8.26}$$

$$Ar—NH—N{=}O \rightleftharpoons Ar—N{=}N—OH \tag{8.27}$$

$$Ar—N{=}N—OH + HCl \rightarrow [Ar—N{\equiv}N]^+Cl^- + H_2O \tag{8.28}$$

Addition of these three reactions gives the net reaction (8.25). The nitrosamine is really not formed by reaction with nitrous acid; rather the actual reactant is the nitrous acidium ion H_2ONO^+, nitrous anhydride N_2O_3, or the nitrosonium ion NO^+, depending upon the reaction conditions. These species are formed from nitrous acid in acidic medium according to the following scheme:

$$H^+ + HNO_2 \rightleftharpoons H_2ONO^+ \begin{cases} \xrightarrow{X^-} NO^+X^- + H_2O \\ \xrightarrow{NO_2^-} N_2O_3 + H_2O \end{cases}$$

Reaction 8.25 forms the basis for a titrimetric analysis of sulfonamides (see Chapter 24).

Coupling of Diazonium Salts. The highly reactive diazonium salt $Ar—N_2{}^+Cl^-$ will react with a second organic compound containing a carbon atom of high electron density to yield a diazo compound, with the elimination of HCl. Phenol is a typical reactant. This reaction is called a coupling reaction. The

$$Ar—N_2{}^+Cl^- + C_6H_5—OH \longrightarrow Ar—N{=}N—C_6H_4—OH + HCl$$

product of a diazo coupling reaction is highly conjugated and therefore may be expected to absorb radiation of fairly long wavelengths. Most diazo compounds are, in fact, colored.

For many years an important method of analysis of sulfonamides has been a colorimetric procedure involving diazotization of the primary aromatic amine followed by coupling to a second component to give a strongly colored diazo compound, the concentration of which can be measured spectrophotometrically. The most satisfactory coupling agent was suggested in 1939 by Bratton et al. [14], and has since become known as the Bratton-Marshall reagent. This compound is *N*-(1-naphthyl)ethylenediamine, **7**. This reagent

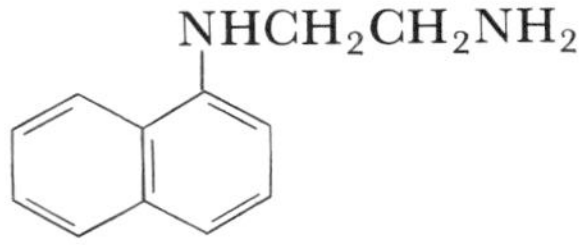

$NHCH_2CH_2NH_2$

7

is also applicable to coupling reactions with diazonium salts derived from substances other than the sulfonamides, and may be used to analyze local anesthetics containing the primary aromatic amine group, as in this experiment.

The technique involves diazotization of the amine in acid solution according to Eq. 8.25. The excess nitrous acid is then destroyed by reaction with sulfamic acid.

$$HNO_2 + H_2NSO_3H \rightarrow H_2SO_4 + N_2 + H_2O$$

Next the coupling agent **7** is added, producing a colored solution due to absorption of light by the coupled diazo product. The absorbance of the solution is measured at the band maximum; the unknown concentration is determined by reference to a standard Beer's law plot obtained by subjecting pure standard samples to the same procedure.

The probable reaction product of the coupling reaction between a diazonium salt and the Bratton-Marshall reagent is **8**, with coupling occurring in the 4 position [15].

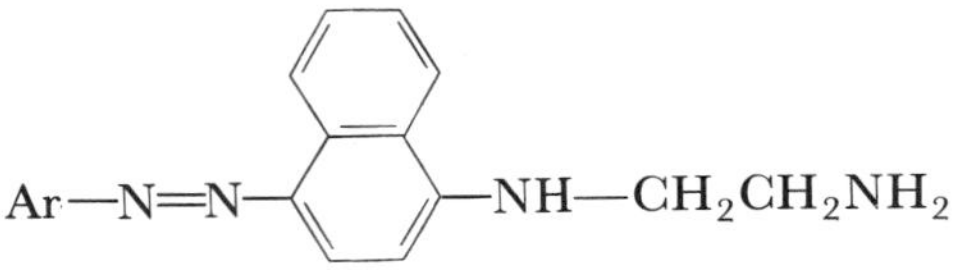

$Ar—N=N—$ $—NH—CH_2CH_2NH_2$

8

Procaine, **9**, was determined with this procedure by Bandelin and Kemp [16], who used ethanol to eliminate the excess nitrous acid. In the procedure described here sulfamic acid is used for this purpose.

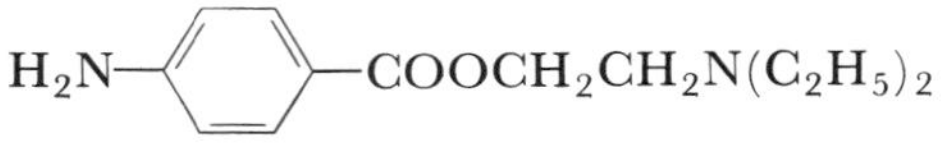

$H_2N—$ $—COOCH_2CH_2N(C_2H_5)_2$

9

APPARATUS AND REAGENTS

Spectrophotometer. Any ultraviolet or visible manual spectrophotometer is suitable. A filter colorimeter cannot be employed in the first part of the experiment (measurement of the absorption spectrum), but for the actual assay such an instrument is adequate.

Coupling Reagent. Dissolve 100 mg of good quality *N*-(1-naphthyl)ethylenediamine dihydrochloride in 100 ml of water. Store this solution in a dark bottle.

Standard Procaine Solution. Dissolve exactly 100.0 mg of procaine hydrochloride in enough water to make 100.0 ml. Dilute a 5.0 ml aliquot to 100.0 ml with water. Each milliliter of this diluted solution contains 50 μg of procaine hydrochloride.

Ammonium Sulfamate Solution. Dissolve 0.5 g of ammonium sulfamate in 100 ml of water.

Sodium Nitrite Solution. Dissolve 100 mg of sodium nitrite in 100 ml of water.

PROCEDURES

Measurement of the Absorption Spectrum. Pipet 0 and 2.0 ml of the diluted standard solution of procaine hydrochloride into two 50 ml volumetric flasks, each of which contains 1 ml of 4 *N* sulfuric acid. Add 5 ml of sodium nitrite solution to each flask, shake well, and allow to stand for 3 min. Add 5 ml of ammonium sulfamate solution to each flask, shake, and allow to stand for 2 min. Now add 5 ml of the coupling reagent to each flask, shake well, and dilute to volume with water. The color is stable for several hours. The solvent blank solution should be colorless.

Select two 1 cm cells, carefully clean them, and fill both with solvent blank (that is, the solution containing 0 ml of procaine solution). Designate one cell the solvent cell and the other the sample cell. Measure the absorbance of the sample cell relative to the solvent cell with a colorimeter or spectrophotometer, taking readings every 5 nm from 450 to 600 nm. (This step is necessary because the two cells may not be optically matched.) Now rinse the sample cell with the colored solution just prepared, and fill the cell with the solution. Measure the absorbance of the solution, relative to the solvent, over the same wavelength range, and apply any correction for mismatched cells. Make a plot of the corrected absorbance (vertical axis) against the wavelength.

Preparation of Standard Curve and Analysis of Unknown. Pipet 0, 1, 2, and 3 ml of diluted stock solution of procaine hydrochloride into four 50 ml volumetric flasks, each of which contains 1 ml of 4 *N* sulfuric acid. Into another 50 ml flask (containing 1 ml of 4 *N* sulfuric acid) pipet a suitable aliquot (1, 2, or 3 ml) of your unknown procaine hydrochloride solution. Carry all five solutions through the chemical procedure outlined above. Set the colorimeter wavelength selector at the wavelength of maximum absorption. Determine the corrected absorbance of each colored solution relative to the solvent blank.

Make a Beer's law plot of the absorbance of each known solution against the concentration of procaine hydrochloride in the final solution. From this graph read off the final concentration of your unknown solution, and calculate the concentration of the unknown solution that you obtained from the instructor, using the appropriate dilution factor.

From the slope of the Beer's law plot calculate the molar absorptivity of the coupled diazo product. (The molar concentration of the coupled product is identical to the molar concentration of procaine taken.)

Experiment 8.2. Analysis of Sulfonamides by Ultraviolet Spectrophotometry

PRINCIPLE

Sulfonamide drugs, which have the general structure $R_1R_2N—C_6H_4—SO_2—NHR_3$, absorb light in the ultraviolet region because they contain the phenyl chromophore. They do not all exhibit precisely the same absorption, however, because the R groups may cause additional absorption or may alter the basic aromatic spectral properties. The spectra differ sufficiently so that analysis of mixtures is often possible. In this experiment, which is based upon the work of Englis and Skoog [17], the ultraviolet absorption spectra of two sulfonamides are measured. Quantitative spectrophotometric analyses are made of a solution containing a single sulfonamide and of a solution containing both drugs. The calculations involved were given in detail in Section 8.2.

Any ultraviolet spectrophotometer is suitable for this analysis. The procedure is written for a manual instrument, but a recording spectrophotometer is more convenient.

PROCEDURES

Determination of Cell Correction. Because two absorption cells seldom have exactly the same optical characteristics, it is necessary to compare the "solvent" cell with the "sample" cell to determine the correction that must be applied. Carefully rinse a pair of 1 cm silica cells with 95% ethanol and fill them with this solvent. Dry and polish the cell faces with lens tissue and place the cells in the cell holder. Arbitrarily designate one cell the solvent cell, the other the sample cell. Put the instrument in operation in accordance with directions given by the instructor. Determine the absorbance of the sample cell relative to the solvent cell every 10 nm from 220 to 350 nm. This may be either a small positive or negative number. Plot these readings against the wavelength and draw a smooth curve through the points. The appropriate cell correction, which can be read from this graph, must be applied to all subsequent measurements to correct for the differences in these cells. The cells must not be interchanged during measurements.

Measurement of Absorption Spectra. Prepare a solution of sulfathiazole in 95% ethanol to contain about 5 mg/liter; the concentration must be accurately known. (Prepare this solution by successive dilutions of a stock solution; do not use large quantities of ethanol.)

Rinse the sample cell with the solution; then fill the cell. Fill the solvent cell with 95% ethanol. Determine the absorbance of the solution as a function of wavelength. Use increments of 10 nm for flat portions of the curve, 5 nm when on the side of an absorption band, and 2 nm in the region of a maximum or minimum. Scan from 220 to 350 nm. Make a graph of the spectrum on linear paper, plotting absorbance (corrected for cell differences) as the ordinate and wavelength as the abscissa.

Repeat this experiment with a solution of sulfanilamide.

Determination of Absorptivities. For each reading made in the preceding experiment calculate the corresponding molar absorptivity. Make a plot of molar absorptivity versus wavelength, superimposing the two spectra on the same graph. Examine this graph and choose two wavelengths that will be suitable for the analysis of a mixture of the two compounds.

Prepare five solutions of sulfathiazole in 95% ethanol to cover the concentration range 2–10 mg/liter. Determine the absorbance of each solution at the two chosen wavelengths. Repeat this with five solutions of sulfanilamide. Make Beer's law plots of absorbance (ordinate) against concentration. Four lines will be obtained. Calculate the four molar absorptivities.

Analysis of Unknown Samples. (1) A solution containing an unknown concentration of one of the compounds will be supplied you. Determine the identity of the compound and its concentration spectrophotometrically. (2) A solution containing unknown concentrations of both sulfathiazole and sulfanilamide will be furnished. Determine both concentrations.

Experiment 8.3. Spectrophotometric Determination of an Acid Dissociation Constant

PRINCIPLE

The pK_{a1} for pyridoxine hydrochloride (Vitamin B_6) will be measured.

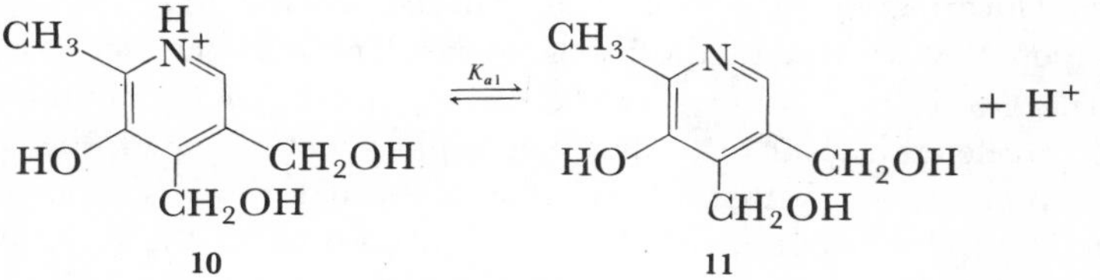

$$\mathbf{10} \overset{K_{a1}}{\rightleftharpoons} \mathbf{11} + H^+ \qquad (8.29)$$

Pyridoxine is stable in acid solution but is decomposed by light in neutral and alkaline solution, so it is good practice to protect the solutions from unnecessary light and to complete the spectral measurements shortly after preparing the solutions.

The spectrum of the conjugate acid, **10**, is elicited at pH 2, and that of the conjugate base, **11**, at pH 7. At higher pH's a further spectral change occurs because of dissociation of the phenolic proton.

This experiment is most conveniently carried out with a recording spectrophotometer.

REAGENTS

Pyridoxine Hydrochloride Stock Solution. Weigh about 25 mg of pyridoxine hydrochloride and dissolve it in water to make 100 ml.

0.05 M Sodium Acetate. Dissolve 4.1 g of anhydrous sodium acetate in water to make 1 liter.

pH 7.1 Phosphate Buffer. Dissolve 2.8 g of Na_2HPO_4 and 1.4 g of KH_2PO_4 in water to make 1 liter.

PROCEDURE

Preparation of Solutions. Prepare five solutions of different pH's, but each containing the same total pyridoxine concentration, according to these directions:

Solution	Vol of Pyridoxine Stock Soln (ml)	Vol of 0.1 *N* HCl (ml)	Vol of 0.05 *M* NaOAc (ml)	Vol of pH 7 phosphate (ml)	Total Vol. (ml)
A	10.0	10	0	0	100.0
B	10.0	6	25	0	100.0
C	10.0	4	25	0	100.0
D	10.0	2	25	0	100.0
E	10.0	0	0	50	100.0

Selection of Analytical Wavelength. Scan the uv spectra of solutions A (conjugate acid form) and E (base form) in a 1 cm cell over the range 230–375 nm. Superimpose the two spectra and choose a wavelength for the measurements.

Determination of pK'_{a1}. Measure the absorbance of each solution at the selected wavelength. (If a recording spectrophotometer is used, the spectra can be scanned to verify that all curves pass through the isosbestic points.) Measure the pH of solutions B, C, and D according to the procedure of Experiment 6.1. Record the solution temperature.

With Eq. 8.17 calculate the pK'_{a1} value of pyridoxine for solutions B, C, and D. Note that, since the total pyridoxine concentration is the same for all solutions, absorbances can be used instead of absorptivities. Compare your mean pK'_{a1} with values you find in the literature.

References

1. *Anal. Chem.*, **45,** 2449 (1973).
2. Bauman, R. P., *Absorption Spectroscopy*, John Wiley and Sons, New York, 1962, Chap. 9.
3. Rancke-Madsen, E. and J. A. Krogh, *Acta Chem. Scand.*, **10,** 495 (1956).
4. Snell, F. D. and C. T. Snell, *Colorimetric Methods of Analysis*, 4 vols., D. Van Nostrand, New York, 1948–1970.
5. Charlot, G., *Colorimetric Determination of Elements*, Elsevier Publishing Co., Amsterdam, 1964.
6. Sandell, E. B., *Colorimetric Determination of Traces of Metals*, 3rd ed., Interscience, New York, 1959.
7. Allport, N. L. and J. W. Keyser, *Colorimetric Analysis*, 2nd ed., Vol. 1, Chapman and Hall, London, 1957; Allport, N. L. and J. E. Brocksopp, Vol. 2, 1963.
8. *Organic Electronic Spectral Data*, a series published by Interscience, New York, 1960–1972.
9. Wiberg, K. B., *Physical Organic Chemistry*, John Wiley and Sons, New York, 1964, p. 7.
10. Gillam, A. E. and D. H. Hey, *J. Chem. Soc.*, **1939,** 1170.
11. Daglish, C., *Isolation and Identification of Drugs*, E. G. C. Clarke (ed.), The Pharmaceutical Press, London, 1969, pp. 84–102, 670–687.
12. Chapman, D. I. and M. S. Moss, *Isolation and Identification of Drugs*, E. G. C. Clarke (ed.), The Pharmaceutical Press, London, 1969, pp. 103–122, 688–793.
13. Ridd, J. H., *J. Soc. Dyers Colour.*, **75,** 285 (1959).
14. Bratton, A. C., E. K. Marshall, Jr., D. Babbitt, and A. R. Hendrickson, *J. Biol. Chem.*, **128,** 537 (1939).
15. Connors, K. A., *Am. J. Pharm. Educ.*, **29,** 29 (1965).
16. Bandelin, F. J. and C. R. Kemp, *Ind. Eng. Chem. Anal. Ed.*, **18,** 470 (1946).
17. Englis, D. T. and D. A. Skoog, *Ind. Eng. Chem. Anal. Ed.*, **15,** 748 (1943).

FOR FURTHER READING

Jaffe, H. H. and M. Orchin, *Theory and Applications of Ultraviolet Spectroscopy*, John Wiley and Sons, New York, 1962.

Dodd, R. E., *Chemical Spectroscopy*, Elsevier Publishing Co., Amsterdam, 1962.

Stearns, E. I., *The Practice of Absorption Spectrophotometry*, Wiley-Interscience, New York, 1969.

Edisbury, J. R., *Practical Hints on Absorption Spectrometry*, Plenum Press, New York, 1967.

Eriksen, S. P. and K. A. Connors, "Photometric Titrations," *J. Pharm. Sci.*, **53,** 465 (1964).

Bellamy, L. J., *The Infra-red Spectra of Complex Molecules*, 2nd ed., John Wiley and Sons, New York, 1958.

Szymanski, H. A., *Theory and Practice of Infrared Spectroscopy*, Plenum Press, New York, 1964.

Kramer, P. A. and K. A. Connors, "Determination of a Complex Stability Constant by the Spectral Technique," *Am. J. Pharm. Educ.*, **33,** 193 (1969).

Problems

1. Calculate, for radiation of wavelength 250 nm, these quantities: wavelength in cm and in angstroms; frequency; wave number; energy per photon in ergs; energy per einstein in kilocalories.

2. (*a*) A 6.40×10^{-5} *M* solution of a drug had an absorbance of 0.847 in a 1 cm cell at 255 nm. Calculate the molar absorptivity of the compound.

(*b*) Are the data of part (*a*) sufficient to tell if Beer's law is obeyed by this compound?

(*c*) Exactly 10.0 mg of a sample of this drug (MW 200.0) was dissolved in water to make 1 liter. At 255 nm the absorbance, in a 1 cm cell, was 0.556. Calculate the purity of the sample.

3. Poldine methylsulfate exhibits an absorption maximum at 257 nm (J. W. Poole and A. A. Monte, *J. Pharm. Sci.*, **53**, 158, 1964). Five solutions of this compound, in methanol, were prepared at the concentrations specified below, and the absorbance of each, in a 1 cm cell, was measured at 257 nm.

c (mg/ml)	A_{257}
0.1	0.105
0.2	0.207
0.3	0.318
0.4	0.420
0.5	0.529

(*a*) Is Beer's law obeyed by this system?

(*b*) Calculate the $A_{1\,\text{cm}}^{1\%}$.

(*c*) Calculate the molar absorptivity. The molecular weight of poldine sulfate is 451.

(*d*) A sample of poldine methylsulfate weighing 500.0 mg was dissolved in enough methanol to make 1 liter. The absorbance of this solution in a 2 cm cell at 257 nm was 0.946. Assume that any impurities present do not absorb light of this wavelength. Calculate the percent purity of the sample.

4. Estimate the pK_a' value of methyl orange from the spectra in Fig. 8.7. Compare your result with the literature value.

5. Calculate the molar absorptivities of tripelennamine hydrochloride at both maxima from the spectrum in Fig. 8.3.

6. Convert each of these transmittance values into the corresponding absorbance.

(*a*) $T = 0.001$

(*b*) $T = 0.25$

(*c*) $T = 0.75$

(*d*) $T = 0.99$

7. Convert each of these absorbance values into the corresponding transmittance.

(*a*) $A = 0.015$

(*b*) $A = 0.500$

(*c*) $A = 1.000$

(*d*) $A = 1.300$

(*e*) $A = 3.50$

8. Suggest analytical methods for the quantitative determination of each component in these mixtures. If you propose spectrophotometric analyses for any compounds, provide data from the literature to support your choice of wavelength and other experimental conditions.

(*a*) Phenol and mercuric chloride in water

(*b*) Aqueous solution of methyl red and phenolphthalein
(*c*) Fumaric acid and malic acid
(*d*) Aniline and *n*-butylamine

9. (*a*) Derive a formula for the interconversion of ϵ and $A_{1\,\text{cm}}^{1\%}$ values.
(*b*) Ethyl *trans*-cinnamate, $C_6H_5CH{=}CHCOOC_2H_5$, has $\epsilon_{max} = 2.21 \times 10^4$. Calculate $A_{1\,\text{cm}}^{1\%}$ for this compound.
(*c*) The $A_{1\,\text{cm}}^{1\%}$ of isoniazid at 266 nm in 378. Calculate its molar absorptivity at this wavelength.
(*d*) Under what circumstances would $A_{1\,\text{cm}}^{1\%}$ be preferable to ϵ as a means of expressing absorption intensity?

10. Derive a formula for the interconversion of wave number and wavelength in micrometers.

11. The absorbances of solutions of pure compound X and of pure compound Y, each in 5×10^{-5} *M* concentrations, are as follows:

Compound	A_{280}	A_{350}
X	0.510	0.192
Y	0.335	0.150

A solution of one of these pure compounds of unknown concentration yielded $A_{280} = 0.395$ and $A_{350} = 0.147$.
(*a*) Which compound (X or Y) is the unknown sample?
(*b*) What is the concentration of the unknown solution?

12. Metharbital, $C_9H_{14}N_2O_3$, has an absorption maximum at 245 nm in aqueous solution at pH 11. The following data were obtained in a 1 cm cell.

10^5c (*M*)	A_{245}
2.05	0.179
4.10	0.356
8.20	0.718
16.4	1.430

(*a*) Calculate the molar absorptivity.
(*b*) 1.200 g of pure metharbital was dissolved in pH 11 buffer to make 1 liter. 5.0 ml of this solution was diluted to 100.0 ml. 10.0 ml of the diluted solution was further diluted to 100.0 ml with buffer. What was the absorbance of the final solution at 245 nm in a 1 cm cell?

13. At 284 nm in ethanol solution, *p*-aminosalicylic acid has molar absorptivity 1.6×10^4 and phthalic acid has molar absorptivity 6.3×10^2.
(*a*) Calculate the absorbance of a 5×10^{-5} *M* solution of *p*-aminosalicylic acid in a 1 cm cell at 284 nm.
(*b*) What concentration of phthalic acid would be required to give a transmittance of 0.16 in a 1 cm cell at 284 nm?
(*c*) Calculate the absorbance of a solution containing 1×10^{-5} *M* *p*-aminosalicylic acid and 4×10^{-4} *M* phthalic acid in a 2 cm cell at 284 nm.

14. Tolbutamide, MW 270.4, has molar absorptivity 703 at 262 nm. If a single tablet of tolbutamide is dissolved in water and the solution is diluted to 2500 ml, its absorbance will be 0.520 at 262 nm in a 1 cm cell. What weight of tolbutamide is contained in the tablet?

15. Derive an equation giving the ratio of energies of photons of wavelengths λ_1 and λ_2.

16. Which compound in each pair would be expected to absorb light at the longer wavelength?

(*a*) C_6H_5COOH or $C_6H_5CH{=}COOH$

(*b*) $C_6H_5CH{=}CHC_6H_5$ (*cis*) or $C_6H_5CH{=}CHC_6H_5$ (*trans*)

(*c*) $C_6H_5NH_2$ or $C_6H_5NH_3^+$

17. The weak acid *p*-nitrophenol exhibits essentially no light absorption at 400 nm. The conjugate base, *p*-nitrophenolate, has molar absorptivity 2×10^4 liter/mole-cm at this wavelength. A spectrophotometric titration is carried out in this way: 100.0 ml of 10^{-3} *M* *p*-nitrophenol is titrated with 0.1 *N* NaOH. The absorbance of the solution is measured during the course of the titration.

(*a*) Calculate the end point volume.

(*b*) Calculate the absorbance of the solution at 400 nm in a 0.1 cm cell (assuming no volume change during titration) when the following volumes of titrant have been added: 0.0 ml, 0.3 ml, 0.7 ml, 1.0 ml, 1.5 ml.

(*c*) Sketch the titration plot of absorbance against titrant volume. Indicate the nature of the plot (i.e., straight lines or curves) and show where the end point is.

18. Amines form salts with picric acid (2,4,6-trinitrophenol). All amine picrates have the same absorption spectrum; $\lambda_{max} = 359$ nm, molar absorptivity 1.25×10^4 liter/mole-cm. 0.415 g of a pure amine was converted quantitatively to its picrate salt. This was dissolved in water to make 100.0 ml of solution. Exactly 1 ml of this solution was diluted to 1 liter. The absorbance of this final solution, at 359 nm in a 1 cm cell, was 0.875. Calculate the molecular weight of the amine.

19. A solution of chloramphenicol in water gave an absorbance of 0.610 at 278 nm in a 1 cm cell; the concentration was 20 μg/ml. The molecular weight of chloramphenicol is 323.1. Calculate its molar absorptivity.

20. Suppose this reaction takes place in solution

$$A \rightarrow B$$

and that at a given wavelength the molar absorptivities are 1.00×10^4 (for A) and 3.00×10^3 (for B). A solution of pure A had an absorbance of 0.750 in a 1 cm cell. After the reaction had proceeded for one half-life (that is, one-half of the original A has reacted), what was the absorbance?

9 FLUORESCENCE SPECTROSCOPY

9.1 Theory of Fluorescence

Fluorescence analysis is an analytical method closely related to spectrophotometry. As we learned in Chapter 8, a molecule can be excited from its ground electronic state to an excited electronic state by absorbing energy in the form of visible or ultraviolet light. Many molecules are capable of emitting this energy as radiation, thus returning to the ground state. The emitted radiation is called fluorescence. In order to appreciate this phenomenon more fully, it is necessary to consider the absorption process in greater detail than we did in Chapter 8.

Origin of Fluorescence. An electron in a molecule behaves as if it were spinning. There are two possible ways in which the electron can spin, and this characteristic of an electron is described by assigning to it a spin quantum number of $+\frac{1}{2}$ or $-\frac{1}{2}$. A molecule of the complexity encountered in pharmacy possesses many electrons. The spins of all electrons in closed shells are paired; that is, for every electron with a spin of $+\frac{1}{2}$ there is an electron with spin $-\frac{1}{2}$, so their spin components cancel. The resultant spin S of a molecule is calculated by adding the spins of all electrons outside the closed shells. If the total number of electrons is even, S will be zero or integral, whereas if the total number of electrons is odd, S will be an odd number of half-integers.

The *multiplicity* of a molecular energy state is equal to $2S + 1$, where the absolute value of S is taken. Most organic molecules contain an even number of electrons; moreover, the electronic transitions of spectroscopic interest are usually from the ground state to the lowest excited states, and only a pair of electrons is usually involved. These may be the electrons in a π orbital or an n orbital. The value of S for such molecules is therefore 0 (that is, $+\frac{1}{2} - \frac{1}{2}$) or 1 ($+\frac{1}{2} + \frac{1}{2}$ or $-\frac{1}{2} - \frac{1}{2}$), and the corresponding multiplicities are 1 and 3. The energy state of multiplicity 1 is called a singlet state, and the state of multiplicity 3 is called a triplet state.

The ground electronic state is usually a singlet. If an electron spin is represented as an arrow with its direction indicating the sign of the spin quantum

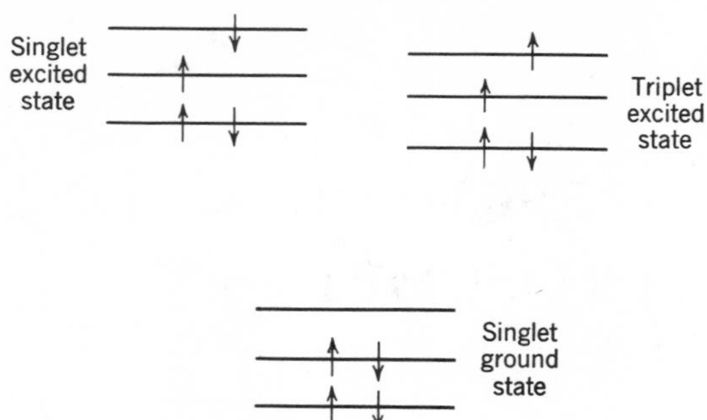

Fig. 9.1. Schematic representation of the lowest electronic states. Each line represents an orbital. Upon absorption of energy, one electron is excited into the unoccupied orbital. This can occur in two ways, as shown.

number, the ground singlet, first excited singlet, and first excited triplet states can be diagrammed as in Fig. 9.1. The excitation process shows the transition of an electron from the highest occupied orbital to the lowest unoccupied orbital. The lowest triplet state is usually of slightly lower energy than the lowest excited singlet state.

It is a result of quantum mechanics that transitions between states of different multiplicity have very low probability; such transitions are said to be "forbidden." Thus the absorption of uv or visible light does not cause excitation to the lowest excited state, which is the forbidden triplet, but to the next higher excited state, the singlet; this is an "allowed" transition. Once the molecule has been placed in the excited singlet state by absorption of energy, it can lose this energy by several mechanisms, thus returning to the ground state. Under many conditions this return is the result of loss of energy, via collisional processes, to surrounding molecules. In some molecules the return to the ground state is made stepwise, from the excited singlet to the excited triplet to the ground singlet. The transition from singlet to triplet required by this route is not forbidden if the transition is radiationless. The mechanism is as follows.

Each electronic state has associated with it many vibrational energy levels. Upon the absorption of radiant energy a transition occurs to the excited singlet, possibly to a high vibrational level of this singlet. The excess vibrational energy is soon lost to the surroundings until, for some molecules, the energy is equal to that of one of the higher vibrational levels of the triplet state. The molecule then makes an allowed radiationless transition to the triplet. The excitation from the ground state G to the excited singlet S, and the radiationless transfer to the triplet T are shown in Fig. 9.2.

A molecule in singlet state S can return to the ground singlet G by emitting light and making the allowed radiative transition. Light emitted by a singlet-singlet transition is *fluorescence*. Since this transition is allowed, the lifetime of the excited singlet is quite short, being of the order 10^{-8} sec. This means that fluorescence ceases as soon as the excitation source is removed.

If a molecule has passed over to the triplet state, the further transition to the ground state is forbidden. It can nevertheless occur, and the radiation emitted in this process is phosphorescence. Since the transition is forbidden, the lifetime of a triplet state may be quite long; usually this state exists for at least 10^{-4} sec, and it can last, for some substances, for days. Thus phosphorescence may persist after the excitation source is removed. The general term for fluorescence and phosphorescence is luminescence.

Excitation and Fluorescence Spectra. The electronic absorption spectrum (of a molecule capable of fluorescence) is also known as its excitation spectrum. In much the same way that an absorption spectrum is determined, it is possible to measure a fluorescence spectrum. From what has been said in the preceding paragraphs it would be predicted that the fluorescence spectrum of a compound should be identical with its excitation spectrum. This equivalence is not observed in practice, the fluorescence maxima nearly always appearing to the long wavelength side of the excitation maxima. This means that the difference in energy between the excited and ground states is greater in the absorption transition than in the emission process.

This result is explicable if we recall that associated with every electronic state is a large number of vibrational energy levels. The lowest vibrational level of the ground state is most highly populated. Upon absorption of light by molecules in the ground state a transition occurs to the excited singlet state, which also possesses many vibrational levels. Not all molecules will be excited to the same vibrational level; thus we observe a broad absorption band, whose width is controlled in part by the separation of vibrational levels within the excited state.

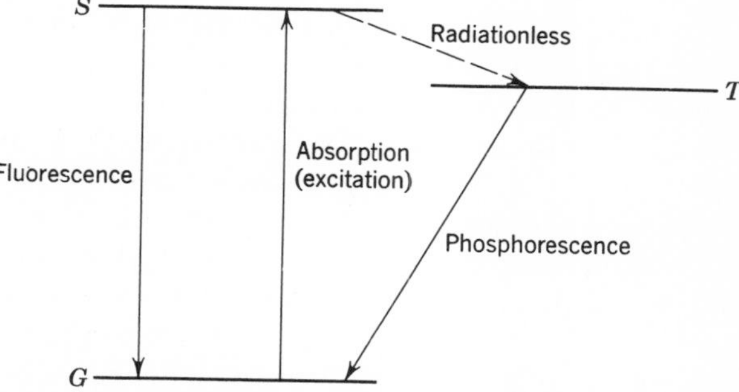

Fig. 9.2. Diagram showing the electronic transitions involved in excitation, fluorescence, and phosphorescence. (Vertical distances represent energy.)

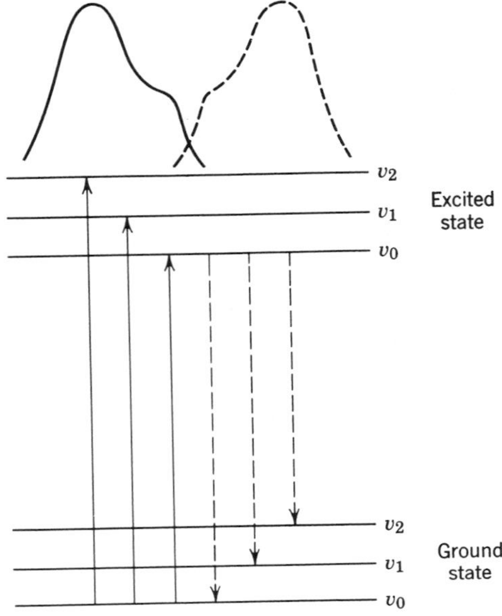

Fig. 9.3. Relationship between excitation spectrum (solid line) and fluorescence spectrum (dashed line). Each electronic state is shown with three vibrational energy levels.

Molecules in a higher vibrational level of the excited state quickly lose their excess vibrational energy by thermal dissipation, thus populating the lowest vibrational level of the excited state. Upon emission of radiation (fluorescence), these molecules can return to any of the vibrational levels of the ground state. The overall result has been that most molecules lose less energy by emission than they gained by absorption, so the fluorescence spectrum appears at longer wavelengths than the excitation spectrum. Figure 9.3 is an energy level diagram illustrating this process. Although this explanation predicts that the fluorescence and excitation spectra should be essentially mirror images, this close correspondence is not always observed.

Molecular Structure and Fluorescence. In order for a molecule to exhibit fluorescence it is necessary that the excited molecule return to the ground state via a radiative transition from the excited singlet. Other ways exist for the molecule to lose its energy, but these cannot result in fluorescence. One of these mechanisms leads to phosphorescence as described earlier. Most substances return to the ground state by radiationless transfer of heat energy to the surroundings; these compounds therefore do not fluoresce. If this thermal dissipation route is inhibited, the excited singlet state may persist long enough to yield fluorescence.

A necessary condition for fluorescence is, of course, strong light absorption by the molecule. Aromatic, heterocyclic, and highly conjugated structures, all of which cause intense absorption, are therefore apt to impart fluorescent properties to a molecule. Structural alterations that increase the absorption intensity may increase the intensity of fluorescence, but this correlation is not universal.

It has been found that the probability of a radiationless transfer from the singlet to the triplet state is much greater for an $n \rightarrow \pi^*$ singlet state than for a $\pi \rightarrow \pi^*$ state. Since fluorescence is emission by return from the lowest energy excited singlet to the ground singlet, this means that those compounds whose lowest excited singlet is a $\pi \rightarrow \pi^*$ state have a greater probability of fluorescing than do those whose lowest excited singlet is an $n \rightarrow \pi^*$ state [1]. Thus, for example, benzene fluoresces whereas pyridine does not. Most aromatics fluoresce [2]. Fluorescence intensity is enhanced by molecular planarity, which in turn is often established by molecular rigidity. For example, phenanthrene (**1**) fluoresces but *cis*-stilbene (**2**) does not.

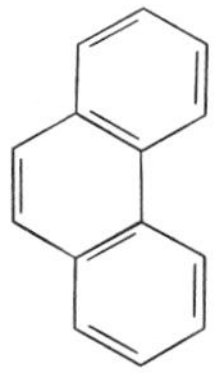

1 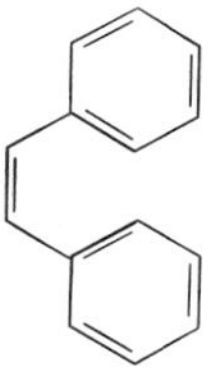 **2**

Many ionizable substances exhibit fluorescence by one ionic form but not by the other; therefore the fluorescence of such compounds is pH-dependent. These compounds are, in fact, fluorescent acid-base indicators.

Phenolic compounds fluoresce under many conditions. Since phenols are weak acids, it is not surprising that their fluorescence is sensitive to pH. Phenol itself fluoresces, but its anion does not. α-Napthol, on the other hand, does not fluoresce, although its anion does.

Udenfriend [3, 4] has given many examples of fluorescent molecules, including drugs and other substances of biological interest.

Quantitative Fluorescence Analysis. In order for a molecule to fluoresce it must first absorb radiation. If the concentration of the absorbing substance is very high, all the incident light may be absorbed by the first layers of solution, with very little light even reaching more distant portions of the sample. The fluorescence of such a sample will therefore be nonuniform and will not be proportional to the concentration of the substance. Because this is undesirable from the analytical point of view, solution concentrations of fluorescing substances are always held to very low levels to avoid the absorption of an appreciable fraction of the incident beam.

Although it is possible that all the light absorbed by a molecule may be emitted as fluorescence, it is more likely that part of the absorbed energy will be lost in other ways, as we have seen earlier. If F is the fluorescence intensity (the intensity of the emitted radiation) and I_{ab} is the intensity of the absorbed radiation, we may define a quantity Φ by Eq. 9.1,

$$\Phi = \frac{F}{I_{ab}} \tag{9.1}$$

where Φ is the *quantum yield of fluorescence*. Evidently Φ can have any value from 0 to 1.

The intensity of the absorbed radiation is equal to the intensity of the incident radiation I_0 minus the intensity of the transmitted radiation I. An expression for I was given in Chapter 8 (p. 177).

$$I_{ab} = I_0 - I_0 e^{-2.3abc} \tag{9.2}$$

In this equation a is the molar absorptivity, b is the path length, and c the molar concentration. If c is very small, Eq. 9.2 can be put in the approximate form

$$I_{ab} \cong \frac{2.3abcI_0}{1 + 2.3abc} \cong 2.3abcI_0 \tag{9.3}$$

where we have used the approximation $e^x \cong 1 + x$. Combining Eqs. 9.1 and 9.3, we obtain

$$F = 2.3I_0\Phi abc \tag{9.4}$$

showing that, at very low concentrations, the fluorescence intensity is directly proportional to concentration. Equation 9.4 also shows that F is proportional to I_0, so increased sensitivity can be achieved for a given concentration simply by increasing the intensity of the incident excitation radiation. This is a fundamental difference between fluorometry and spectrophotometry, for in the latter technique we saw that the absorbance was independent of the incident intensity.

According to Eq. 9.4, the fluorescence intensity is proportional to molar absorptivity. For this reason it is desirable to employ, as the excitation radiation, light corresponding to the absorption band maximum. A beam of radiation many wavelengths in width is usually used for excitation, with the wavelength range being selected to include the maximum in the excitation spectrum.

The analytical procedure is essentially that described in Chapter 8 for single-component spectrophotometric analysis. A standard curve, of fluorescence intensity versus concentration of fluorescing substance, is prepared with known solutions of a pure sample. The unknown sample then is carried through the same procedure, and its concentration is read from the graph. It is necessary to maintain the same experimental conditions (excitation source, solvent, pH, temperature) for the known and unknown measurements. Many foreign substances are capable of reducing the effective value of Φ, and therefore the sensitivity, of a fluorescent compound. This repression of fluorescence is called "quenching."

9.2 Practice of Fluorescence Analysis

Measurement of Fluorescence Intensity. Figure 9.4 indicates the essential components and their arrangement in a *fluorometer* (or fluorimeter), which is the instrument used to measure fluorescence intensity F.

The light source must be very intense* and very stable because F depends directly on I_0. Mercury arc lamps and xenon arc lamps are in common use. These lamps emit in the visible and ultraviolet regions. The xenon lamp emission is evenly distributed over a wide wavelength range, while the emission of a mercury lamp is concentrated in several very intense bands, of which those at 254 and 365 nm are of great value as excitation radiation.

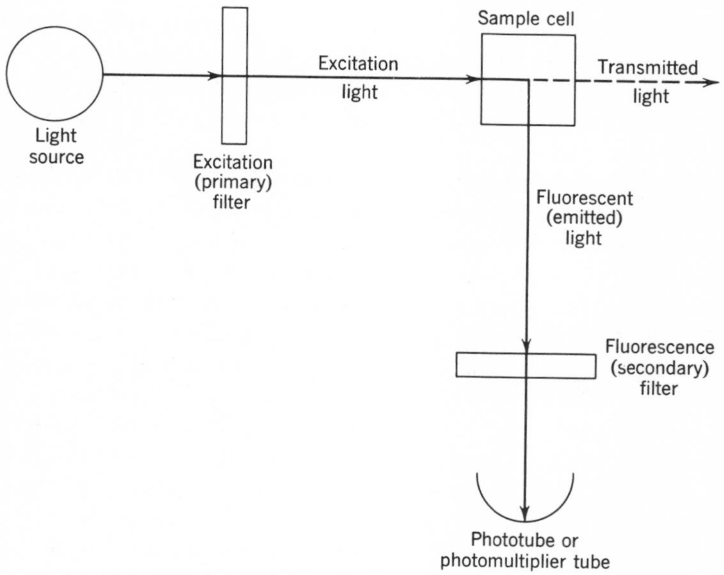

Fig. 9.4. Components of a filter photofluorometer.

* Radiation from the source can permanently injure the eyes. Never look at a fluorometer light source with unprotected eyes.

To achieve specificity of excitation, and to reduce stray light, a more or less narrow band of radiation is selected from the radiation emitted by the light source. This selection is performed by the excitation filter, which in most fluorometers is a glass filter that transmits light of the desired wavelength and absorbs all other radiation. Such filters may transmit a band of radiation 50–100 nm in width. The filters are exchangeable, and a selection is available to permit a filter to be chosen that transmits a band of radiation corresponding to the absorption maximum of the compound, but that cuts out light of shorter and longer wavelengths. The excitation filter is also known as the primary filter.

The excitation light now passes into the sample cell. Cells and solvents are capable of fluorescence and must be chosen carefully. Glass cells are adequate for most fluorescence analysis; quartz must be used below 320 nm.

The fluorescent light, of course, is emitted in all directions by the sample. Measurement of fluorescence intensity in the direction of propagation of the excitation radiation is extremely difficult because it involves measuring the emitted light against a high-intensity background of transmitted light. This problem is overcome by observing the fluorescence at a right angle to the beam of excitation light (see Fig. 9.4). Some of the transmitted light is apt to be scattered in this direction, and this undesirable light is removed with the fluorescence filter (secondary filter), which is selected so that it transmits maximally at the fluorescence maximum.

The fluorescence then contacts a phototube or photomultiplier, producing an electrical signal that is amplified and measured with a meter to indicate the fluorescence intensity.

The instrument described and shown in Fig. 9.4 is a filter fluorometer. Because it incorporates photoelectric detection of the fluorescence intensity, this instrument may be called a photofluorometer. Instruments are now available in which the excitation and fluorescence filters have been replaced with monochromators, permitting selection of very narrow bands of radiation. These instruments, which are termed spectrophotofluorometers, are capable of measuring excitation and fluorescence spectra in the same way that a spectrophotometer can be used to determine absorption spectra.

Applications. The outstanding advantage of fluorescence analysis is its sensitivity. Although the quantum yield Φ is nearly always less than one, the fluorescence intensity F can be forced to a very high level simply by increasing the intensity of the excitation radiation. Another contributor to high sensitivity is the excellent performance capabilities of modern photomultiplier tubes, so that very low intensities of emitted light can be accurately measured. Concentrations of fluorescent compounds in the range 10^{-4}–10^{-9} M can be measured quantitatively, and the plot of F versus c is usually linear.

Although the amounts of drugs present in dosage forms are seldom so small as to require sensitivity of this order, the concentrations of drugs and drug metabolites in blood, urine, and other biological samples may be extremely low, and fluorescence analysis finds wide application in quantitative studies of rates and mechanisms of drug absorption, metabolism, and excretion. Most compounds of biological origin also fluoresce, and therefore are potential interferences in these assays. Preliminary separation of these complex mixtures may be necessary before the fluorescence assay of the desired component can be carried out.

Perhaps the best-known fluorescent drug is quinine. The excitation maximum is at 350 nm and the fluorescence maximum at about 450 nm. Thus this compound absorbs ultraviolet light and emits visible light, the fluorescing solution appearing to be blue. In 0.1 N H_2SO_4 the quantum yield of fluorescence is about 0.3 for quinine; this value, together with the high molar absorptivity of quinine, means that this alkaloid produces a very intense fluorescence in sulfuric acid. In hydrochloric acid, however, the fluoresence is markedly quenched, although the absorption spectrum is not affected. This example illustrates the profound effect that solvent conditions may exert on fluorescence efficiency.

Vitamins are often assayed fluorometrically. The analysis of thiamine (Vitamin B_1) is an important example of the fluorescence method. Thiamine (**3**) is not itself fluorescent, but its oxidation product thiochrome (**4**) fluoresces strongly. Thiamine is oxidized with alkaline ferricyanide. The resulting

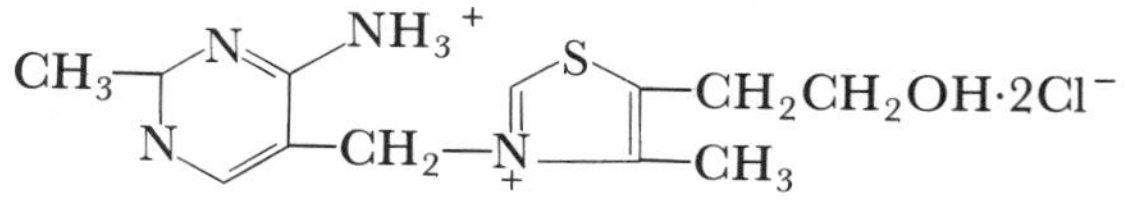

3

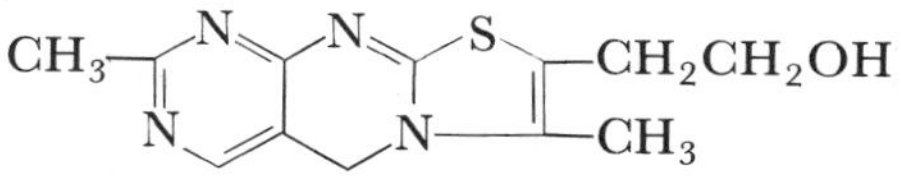

4

thiochrome is extracted into isobutyl alcohol and measured fluorometrically; the excitation maximum is at 365 nm and the fluorescence maximum at about 440 nm. If the thiamine is contained in tablets or capsules, it is necessary to separate it from interfering substances. Even when this separation is made, other fluorescent materials may be present in the oxidized sample, and these are corrected for by measuring the fluorescence of an aliquot of the thiamine solution that has not been subjected to oxidation.

It is common practice, in the thiamine assay and in many fluorescence analyses, to check the stability of the light source periodically by measuring the fluorescence of a standard quinine solution. The meter reading of the instrument can be arbitrarily adjusted to give the same response to the quinine reference even though the excitation source varies in intensity. Quinine is particularly convenient as a calibrating substance in the thiamine assay because the excitation and fluorescence maxima of quinine and thiochrome are nearly identical, so the same filters can be used for both measurements.

Many pharmaceuticals can be assayed fluorometrically. Vitamins [5], steroids, sedatives [6], tranquilizers, analgesics [7], antihistamines, and many other drugs can be determined [3, 4]. Qualitative applications of fluorescence are also important. Thus the tetracyclines yield different fluorescent colors (when examined visually) upon treatment with strong acids and pases, and their identification may be facilitated with these qualitative tests. Fluorescence is an extremely valuable property of molecules being subjected to a separation by paper or thin-layer chromatography. The location of zones on a paper chromatogram is accomplished readily by illuminating the chromatogram with suitable excitation radiation (a mercury lamp may be used) and observing the fluorescence of the compounds concentrated in zones on the paper. These zones can be outlined with pencil to give a permanent record. If the molecules being separated do not themselves fluoresce, they may be converted to fluorescent derivatives either before or after separation. For example, amino acids can be reacted with dansyl chloride [5-(dimethylamino)napthalene-1-sulfonyl chloride, **5**] to give dansyl amino acids, **6**, which are highly fluorescent and readily detected after chromatographic separation. Another way to

$$\underset{\mathbf{5}}{C_{10}H_6(SO_3Cl)N(CH_3)_2} + RCH(NH_2)COOH \longrightarrow \underset{\mathbf{6}}{C_{10}H_6(SO_3NHCHRCOOH)N(CH_3)_2} + HCl$$

detect nonfluorescent compounds is to incorporate a fluorescent substance in the chromatographic system; then wherever such compounds appear on the chromatographic plate they can be seen as dark spots against a fluorescent background.

Experiment 9.1. Fluorescence Analysis of Quinine

REAGENTS AND APPARATUS

Photofluorometer. Any filter photofluorometer should be satisfactory. Specific directions will not be given because these will be different for each model of instrument. Relative fluorescence intensities are measured in this experiment, as in most practical work.

The excitation filter should transmit maximally near 365 nm; the Coleman B_1 (Corning filter 5847) is suitable. The Coleman PC_1 (Corning filters 3389 and 4308) is a satisfactory fluorescence filter.

Quinine Sulfate Stock Solution. Accurately weigh about 10 mg of pure quinine sulfate, transfer it to a 1000 ml volumetric flask, and dissolve in enough 0.1 *N* sulfuric acid to make 1000 ml. Protect the solution from light.

PROCEDURE

On the day used prepare five quinine sulfate solutions by pipetting 1.0, 2.0, 3.0, 4.0, and 5.0 ml of quinine sulfate stock solution into 100 ml volumetric flasks. Dilute each to volume with 0.1 *N* sulfuric acid.

Fill the sample cell with the most concentrated of the five quinine solutions. Place the photofluorometer in operation as directed by the instructor. With the filled sample cell in position, adjust the instrument controls to yield a reading of maximum fluorescence intensity. Replace the solution with 0.1 *N* sulfuric acid and adjust the meter to read zero intensity. Then measure the intensity of the other four quinine solutions. Make a plot of fluorescence intensity against concentration of quinine sulfate.

Obtain an unknown solution of quinine sulfate from your instructor. Prepare a dilution, in 0.1 *N* sulfuric acid, such that its fluorescence intensity lies within the extremes produced by the standard solutions. Measure the intensity of your diluted unknown and read its concentration from the standard curve. Calculate the concentration of the original solution.

For the most accurate results the unknown solution should be measured at the same time the standards are examined. The stability of the instrument can be checked occasionally by remeasuring the most concentrated of the five standard solutions and resetting the controls to indicate the same intensity as in the initial adjustment.

References

1. Hercules, D. M., *Fluorescence and Phosphorescence Analysis*, Wiley-Interscience, New York, 1966, p. 23.
2. Berlman, I. B., *Handbook of Fluorescence Spectra of Aromatic Molecules*, 2nd ed., Academic Press, New York, 1971.
3. Udenfriend, S., *Fluorescence Assay in Biology and Medicine*, Academic Press, New York, 1962.
4. Udenfriend, S., *Fluorescence Assay in Biology and Medicine*, Vol. II, Academic Press, New York, 1969.
5. Hashmi, M.-U.-H., *Assay of Vitamins in Pharmaceutical Preparations*, John Wiley and Sons, New York, 1973.
6. Miles, C. I. and G. H. Schenk, *Anal. Lett.*, **4,** 61 (1971).
7. Schenk, G. H., F. H. Boyer, C. I. Miles, and D. R. Wirz, *Anal. Chem.*, **44,** 1593 (1972).

Problems

1. Derive Eq. 9.4.

2. The fluorescence of ethanolic solutions of griseofulvin were measured with the following results.

Concentration (μg/ml)	Fluorescence (arbitrary units)
0.02	13.0
0.04	23.0
0.06	36.6
0.08	49.4
0.10	61.5

(*a*) Is Eq. 9.4 followed?

(*b*) A solution of a griseofulvin sample of unknown purity contained 0.085 μg/ml. of sample. The fluorescence of the solution, on the same scale as the above data, was 46.4 units. Calculate the percent purity of the sample.

3. Speculate on the reason that thiochrome is fluorescent whereas thiamine is not.

10 REFRACTOMETRY

10.1 Principles of Refractometry

The Refractive Index. The velocity of light depends upon the medium through which it travels. The ratio of velocities of light in vacuum and in any substance is called the absolute refractive index of that substance. For all solids and liquids this definition is replaced by the more practical (and nearly equivalent) one

$$n_\lambda^t = \frac{v_{air}}{v_M}$$

where n_λ^t is the refractive index of the medium through which light travels with velocity v_M; the superscript indicates the temperature and the subscript the wavelength of the light. v_{air} is the velocity of the light in air.

It is possible to show that the refractive index is also given by

$$n = \frac{\sin i_{air}}{\sin r_M} \tag{10.1}$$

where i_{air} is the angle of incidence of the light, measured from the perpendicular to the boundary between air and medium M, and r_M is the angle of refraction in medium M, also measured from the normal. These relationships are shown in Fig. 10.1. Equation 10.1 is Snell's law of refraction.

The bending of a light ray on passing from one medium to another is called refraction. It will occur if the refractive indexes of the two media are different and if the angle of incidence is not zero. Liquids, gases, and solids whose properties are identical in all directions (cubic crystals) can be characterized with a single refractive index; such substances are *isotropic*. Other media are known, in particular crystals whose properties depend upon the relative orientation of the light beam and the crystal axis, that possess more than one refractive index. Such *anisotropic* crystals may have two or three refractive indexes, one for each optically different crystal axis. The refractive indexes of liquids fall in the range 1.3–1.7.

The refractive index of an organic liquid is quite sensitive to temperature; an increase of temperature of 1°C results in a decrease in n of 0.0004–0.0005.

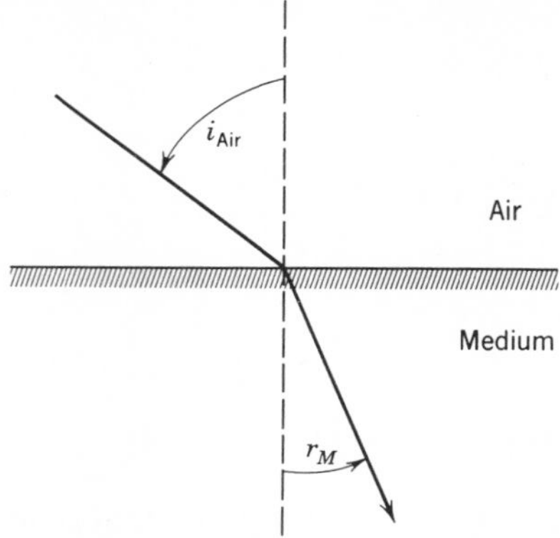

Fig. 10.1. Refraction of a light ray on passing from air into medium M.

Since even the most routine measurements of refractive index provide a reproducibility of about 0.0002, evidently temperature control is essential for accurate measurements.

The wavelength of the light used in measuring the refractive index is another important variable. The variation of n with wavelength is called optical dispersion. Nearly all tabulated refractive indexes for liquids refer to light of wavelength 589.3 nm; this is the radiation produced by a strong line in the emission spectrum of sodium, and it is referred to as the sodium D line. The refractive index may be written n_D to indicate this wavelength. If no subscript appears, the sodium D line may be assumed.

Besides the analytical uses of the refractive index, which will be considered shortly, it has been found useful in studies of molecular structure. The molar refraction R of a compound is calculated with

$$R = \frac{(n^2 - 1)M}{(n^2 + 2)d} \tag{10.2}$$

where M is the molecular weight of the compound and d is its density. R is, within limits, characteristic of molecular structure. In fact, it is possible to break down the molar refraction into component group refractions, which are roughly additive. The molar refraction of a compound can be calculated by adding together the appropriate group refractions, which have been tabulated [1]. Comparison of calculated and experimental refractions may enable helpful inferences to be made concerning the nature of bonding in the molecule.

Another important application of the molar refraction is in the determination of dipole moments of compounds; the measured quantities for this determination are the dielectric constant, refractive index, and density of dilute solutions of the substance [2].

TABLE 10.1
Refractive Indexes of Some Liquids[a]

Liquid	t (°C)	n_D	Liquid	t (°C)	n_D
Methanol	25	1.3276	Carbon tetrachloride	15	1.4631
Water	25	1.3325	Rosemary oil	20	1.4640–1.4760
Acetone	20	1.3589	Bergamot oil	20	1.4650–1.4675
Ethanol	18	1.3624	Turpentine oil	20	1.4680–1.4780
Acetic acid	20	1.3718	Orange oil	20	1.4723–1.4737
Ethyl acetate	19	1.3722	Bitter orange oil	20	1.4725–1.4755
Isopropyl alcohol	20	1.3776	Glycerin	20	1.4729
Paraldehyde	20	1.4049	Lemon oil	20	1.4738–1.4755
Dioxane	20	1.4232	Chenopodium oil	20	1.4740–1.4790
Cyclohexane	20	1.4264	Poppy seed oil	20	1.4766–1.4774
Ethylene glycol	20	1.4311	Pine oil	20	1.4780–1.4820
Cyclohexene	22	1.4451	Caraway oil	20	1.4840–1.4880
Chloroform	20	1.4476	Spearmint oil	20	1.4840–1.4910
Ethylenediamine	26	1.4540	Triethanolamine	20	1.4852
Rose oil	30	1.4570–1.4630	Thyme oil	20	1.4950–1.5050
Eucalyptus oil	20	1.4580–1.4700	Benzene	20	1.5014
Lavender oil	20	1.4590–1.4700	Bay oil	20	1.5070–1.5160
Peppermint oil	20	1.4590–1.4650	Sassafras oil	20	1.5250–1.5350
Coriander oil	20	1.4620–1.4720	Clove oil	20	1.5270–1.5350
Peanut oil	40	1.4625–1.4645	Pimenta oil	20	1.5270–1.5400
Cardamom oil	20	1.4630–1.4660	Methyl salicylate	20	1.5369

[a] From *The Merck Index*, 7th ed., Merck & Co., Rahway, N.J., 1960.

Table 10.1 gives refractive indexes of some liquids, including volatile oils and other substances of pharmaceutical importance. A refractive index range is specified for volatile oils because these substances are of variable composition.

Analytical Uses of the Refractive Index. An obvious application of the refractive index is in the identification of liquids. The refractive index is an important quantity in establishing the identity of pure organic compounds. Although identical values of n for an unknown substance and a known compound are not sufficient evidence to establish the identity of the two, it is at least a necessary condition if the two substances are the same.* The best way to make such a comparison is to measure the index of refraction of both samples on the same instrument at the same time, thus eliminating differences caused by variations in temperature and wavelength. If an authentic specimen is not available, it is necessary to make the comparison with a literature value, for example, the indexes in Table 10.1.

A similar use of refractive index measurements is their application as criteria

* Since, as noted earlier, the uncertainty in a refractive index measurement is about 0.0002, two values can be considered identical if they do not differ by more than about 0.0004.

of purity. Monographs for many liquids in the USP and NF specify ranges within which the refractive index of a sample must lie in order for it to meet the official requirements. These specifications help in the detection of adulteration of complex mixtures like volatile oils.

Quantitative analysis of solutions can sometimes be accomplished refractometrically. The refractive index of a solution will in general differ from that of the pure solvent. If a working curve of n against concentration is first prepared with solutions of known composition, then an unknown solution can be analyzed by measuring its refractive index and reading its concentration from the curve. This method is particularly valuable for the analysis of mixtures of two miscible liquids.

A recent application of refractometry is in monitoring effluents in high-speed liquid chromatography (see Chapter 17). In this separation technique a sensitive and general method for continuously detecting solutes in a flowing stream is necessary to take advantage of the capability of chromatography for resolving mixtures into their components. The column effluent is, at any given time, a binary solution whose refractive index reflects the presence of a solute. Actually a differential measurement is made, that is, the refractive index of the solution relative to that of the pure solvent. A difference in refractive index as small as 10^{-7} unit can be detected.

10.2 Measurement of Refractive Index

Refractive index is measured with a refractometer. The principle of this measurement is illustrated in Fig. 10.2. Consider the medium, whose refractive index $n(\mathrm{M})$ is to be measured, in contact with the prism P.* Figures 10.2*a*, *b*, and *c* show a light beam incident upon the surface of the prism, with successively greater angles of incidence i indicated. Combination of Eq. 10.1 as written for both the medium and the prism shows that the refractive index of the medium is given by

$$n(\mathrm{M}) = n(\mathrm{P}) \frac{\sin r}{\sin i} \qquad (10.3)$$

where $n(\mathrm{P})$ is the refractive index of the prism.

If the angle of incidence is made so large that it becomes essentially equal to 90°, as shown in Fig. 10.2*d* (this is called "grazing incidence"), the angle of refraction achieves its maximum possible value. This value is called the *critical angle of refraction*,† r_c. If $n(\mathrm{P})$ is known, measurement of r_c permits estimation of $n(\mathrm{M})$ according to Eq. 10.3, since $\sin 90° = 1$.

* The refractive index of the prism must be greater than that of the sample.

† Also known as the critical angle of reflection, because if a ray is sent in the reverse direction (that is, from inside the prism) at an angle greater than r_c, it will be totally reflected back into the prism. This phenomenon will be found useful in Chapter 11.

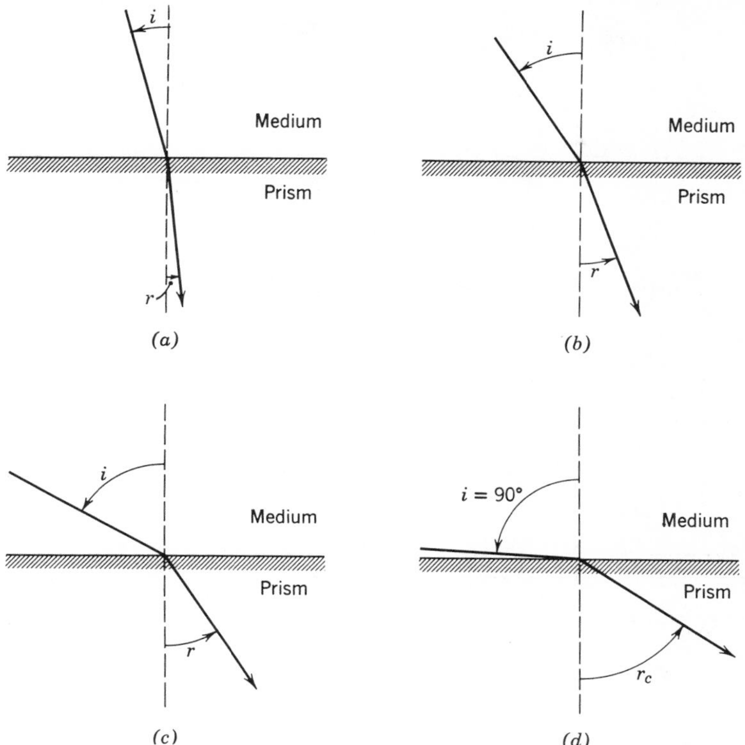

Fig. 10.2. Refraction of a light ray on passing from medium M into prism P. (*d*) shows the relationship between a grazing incident ray and the critical angle.

In practice, the light passing through the medium is not a single ray but a relatively broad beam. Part of this beam contacts the prism at grazing incidence, the rest of it at smaller values of the incident angle. Within the prism, then, all of that area swept out by angle r_c in Fig. 10.2*d* will be lighted, whereas that portion of the prism beyond the critical ray will be dark. A sharp boundary between the light and dark areas indicates the position of the critical ray.

A telescope is trained on the prism in the region of the critical boundary. Figure 10.3 shows the principle, although not the actual mechanism, of the measurement. The critical ray is represented, and the areas of light and darkness are shown. The circular area is the field of view of the telescope, with its superimposed cross hairs. The field of view is swept across the critical boundary, as in the four positions shown in Fig. 10.3, until the cross hairs center on the boundary. In the Abbe refractometer, which is the most widely used

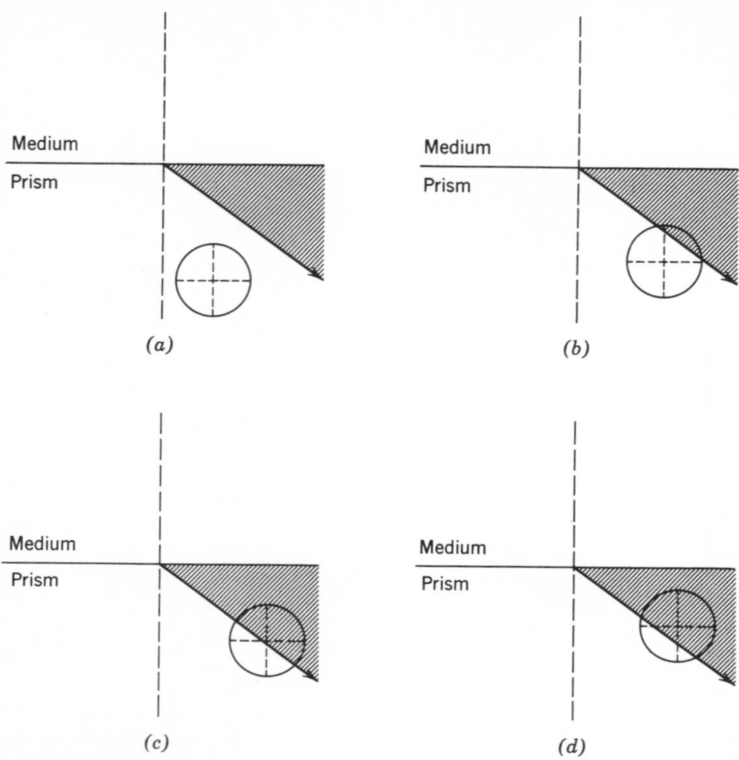

Fig. 10.3. Location of the critical boundary in the refractometer telescope. The boundary is properly positioned in (*c*).

instrument, the telescope is stationary and the prism is moved, but the effect is identical with that described. The angle through which the prism must be moved to center the critical boundary in the field of view corresponds to the critical angle of refraction. The scale of the Abbe refractometer is calibrated directly in refractive index, so no calculations are necessary.

The Abbe refractometer uses white light, which produces a critical boundary with a rainbow-like appearance, because the different wavelengths of the light are refracted to slightly different extents (this is the dispersion effect). To eliminate the color band and sharpen the boundary, an auxiliary optical system is incorporated that is capable of refracting the dispersed critical rays by exactly the same amount that they originally diverged from the D line critical ray. This optical "compensator" thus sharpens the boundary and yields a critical ray with white light that is equivalent to the ray that would be obtained with the sodium D line. The refractive index measured with the Abbe refractometer therefore is n_D.

The Abbe refractometer has facilities for thermostating the prism with flowing water of constant temperature. This refractometer is suitable for all general analytical work. For very demanding refractometric studies more elaborate instruments are available.

Experiment 10.1. Refractive Index Measurements in Identification and Quantitative Analysis

APPARATUS

Abbe Refractometer. For best results this refractometer should be thermostated to either 20 or 25°C. A constant temperature water bath with a circulating pump is connected with rubber tubing to the inlets and outlets provided for this purpose on the refractometer. Measurements adequate for many purposes can be obtained without careful temperature control; place the refractometer in a place free of drafts. It should be recognized that poor temperature control limits the reliability of the data.

PROCEDURES

Calibration with Water. In order to ensure that the refractometer yields correct values of the refractive index it is advisable to measure the refractive index of a substance whose index is accurately known. Water is suitable.

Set up the refractometer with the mirror facing away from you. Position an ordinary tungsten light above the mirror. Connect the constant temperature water bath, if available, to the refractometer. Adjust the angle of the telescope until you can look into it with comfort.

Unclamp the lower prism and swing it down. With a soft tissue moistened with alcohol, cleanse the faces of the upper and lower prisms. (The upper prism is the refracting prism; the lower one serves to hold the sample in place and to transmit light to the sample.) Allow the prisms to air-dry.

Support the lower prism in an approximately horizontal position, and place 2 or 3 drops of distilled water on it. Swing the prism to its closed position and clamp it firmly in place. Permit the sample to stand for several minutes so it may reach temperature equilibrium. Read the temperature of the circulating water (if used) or of the air in the vicinity of the refractometer.

Move the arm along the curved scale until the critical boundary comes into view within the telescope eyepiece. If the light source is either too intense or too weak, the boundary may not be readily discernible. When the boundary has been located, adjust the compensator knob on the barrel of the telescope until the boundary becomes colorless and sharp. Then with the fine adjustment control on the long arm bring the critical boundary into exact coincidence with the cross hairs.

Read the refractive index on the curved scale, sighting through the eyepiece on the arm. The refractive index is read to four decimal places, the final place being estimated. The refractive index of water has these values: $n_D^{15} = 1.3334$; $n_D^{20} = 1.3330$; $n_D^{25} = 1.3325$; $n_D^{30} = 1.3319$. If your experimental value differs from the accepted value by more than about 0.0004, a suitable correction may be applied to all subsequent measurements.

Immediately after a measurement has been made, clean the prism faces with ethanol and allow them to dry.

Measurement of Refractive Indexes. Using the same procedure as in the calibration with water, measure the refractive indexes of four pure liquids. Compare your values with literature values.

Measurements on volatile liquids should be made fairly quickly, before the sample can evaporate from between the faces of the prisms.

Obtain four samples from your instructor. Measure and report their refractive indexes.

Quantitative Analysis of Glycerin-Water Mixtures. Number and weigh, to the closest 0.01 g, seven 25 ml volumetric flasks. Add pure glycerin (glycerol) to the flasks in amounts such that successive flasks contain, very roughly 4, 8, 12, 16, 20, 24, 28 g of glycerin. Reweigh the flasks to the closest 0.01 g. Add water to the flasks, mix well, and dilute to the mark with water. Calculate the molar concentrations of glycerin in these solutions.

Measure the refractive indexes of pure water, pure glycerin, and the seven glycerin-water mixtures. Make a plot of refractive index (on the vertical axis) against molar concentration of glycerin.* Draw a smooth curve through all the points.

Obtain two samples of glycerin-water solutions from your laboratory instructor. Measure their refractive indexes and read their compositions from your graph. It is best to measure the indexes of the unknown samples at the same time you measure the indexes of the known solutions.

References

1. Lewin, S. Z. and N. Bauer, *Treatise on Analytical Chemistry*, I. M. Kolthoff and P. J. Elving (eds.), Wiley-Interscience, New York, Part I, Vol. 6, Chap. 70, 1965.
2. Smyth, C. P., *Physical Methods of Chemistry*, A. Weissberger and B. W. Rossiter (eds.), Wiley-Interscience, New York, Part IV, Vol. I, Chap. VI, 1972.

Problems

1. The angle of incidence of a ray of light on a liquid surface was 48°30′, and the angle of refraction was 31°45′. Calculate the refractive index of the liquid and the velocity of light within the liquid.

* Calculation of the molar concentration of pure glycerin requires its density, which (at 25°C) is 1.262 g/ml.

2. Calculate the molar refraction of chloroform.

3. Could you distinguish between samples of orange oil and bitter orange oil on the basis of refractive index measurements?

4. (*a*) Explain, by means of the concepts in this chapter, why it is that we can see a transparent solid (such as a glass rod) immersed in a transparent liquid.

(*b*) On the basis of the explanation given in (*a*), suggest a simple means for the determination of approximate values of refractive indexes of liquids.

11 POLARIMETRY

11.1 Theory

Polarization of Light. In Chapter 8 we saw that light can be described in terms of a wave motion. We must now examine this description more closely. Many of the properties of light are explicable if it is considered to be composed of an electric component and a magnetic component. Each of these components is a vector quantity; that is, each component has both magnitude and direction. The electric and magnetic components are normal to each other. Because of this simple relationship we need consider the behavior of only one of these vectors, and we select the electric component. The wave character of light is then a manifestation of the oscillatory motion of the electric vector. Figure 11.1 illustrates this concept. A head-on view of this wave, from the direction of propagation, would show the vector vibrating in a plane, varying in amplitude and direction with time.

Even this concept of light is oversimplified, and it is necessary to introduce the idea that this vector is the resultant of two vectors. Suppose a ray of light is viewed head-on, and suppose that it consists of two vectors of equal length, each rotating circularly but in opposite directions, as in Fig. 11.2. Then the vector addition of these components, when superimposed, will result in a vector varying in amplitude in a plane, as described above. Thus *linearly polarized light* (plane polarized light) is the resultant of two rays of circularly polarized light rotating in opposite directions.* A beam of natural light consists of a vast number of rays of linearly polarized light, the planes of the electric field vectors being randomly oriented, as indicated by Fig. 11.3*a*. Light with a random orientation of the field vector is said to be unpolarized. It is possible to isolate (by means described in Section 11.2) rays whose vectors all vibrate in a single plane, that is, linearly polarized light, Fig. 11.3*b*.

Interaction of Light and Matter. In Chapter 8 the absorption of light by molecules was described, and we noted that the intensity of absorption could be expressed in terms of the molar absorptivity ϵ. Chapter 10 showed that

* If the two vectors of circularly polarized light are of unequal length, their resultant vector will describe an ellipse. Linearly polarized light is a special case of this more general phenomenon.

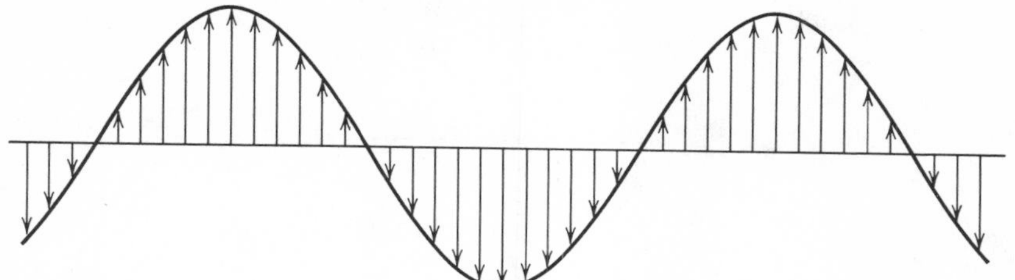

Fig. 11.1. Oscillation of the electric force vector of light. The arrows represent the magnitude and direction of the net vector and the horizontal axis represents time (or distance).

the refraction of light by matter can be represented by the refractive index n. Both ϵ and n are functions of the wavelength of light.

In view of our description of light as a resultant of two oppositely rotating vectors (circularly polarized light), we now must extend the concepts of absorption and refraction to consider the possibilities that left and right circularly polarized light may be absorbed or refracted to different extents. We therefore require, for the complete characterization of the interaction of light with matter, the four constants ϵ_L, ϵ_R, n_L, n_R.

First consider the refraction effect. According to Section 10.1 the refractive indexes for left and right circularly polarized light can be written $n_L = c/v_L$ and $n_R = c/v_R$, where v_L and v_R are the velocities of the corresponding rays. Now if for a given substance $n_L > n_R$, it follows that $v_R > v_L$; the right vector (rotating clockwise as the ray approaches the viewer) will travel faster than the left vector. Their vector addition will continue to yield a linearly polarized ray, but because of the velocity difference the direction of this ray will have changed from its direction before entering the matter. Figure 11.4 shows the construction leading to this conclusion. The angle through which the plane of the linearly polarized light is rotated is denoted α; if the rotation is clockwise as in Fig. 11.4, α is given a plus sign and the substance is said to be *dextrorotatory*. A substance rotating the plane counterclockwise ($n_L < n_R$, α negative) is *levorotatory*. The sign of rotation as well as its magnitude can depend upon the wavelength. Any substance capable of rotating the plane of polarized light is

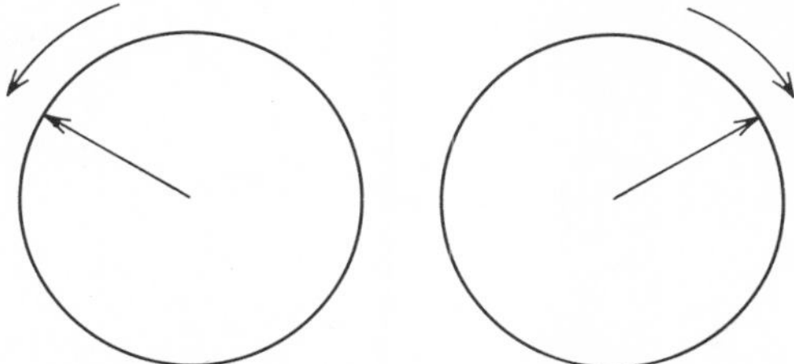

Fig. 11.2. Left and right circularly polarized light. Vectorial addition results in linearly polarized light.

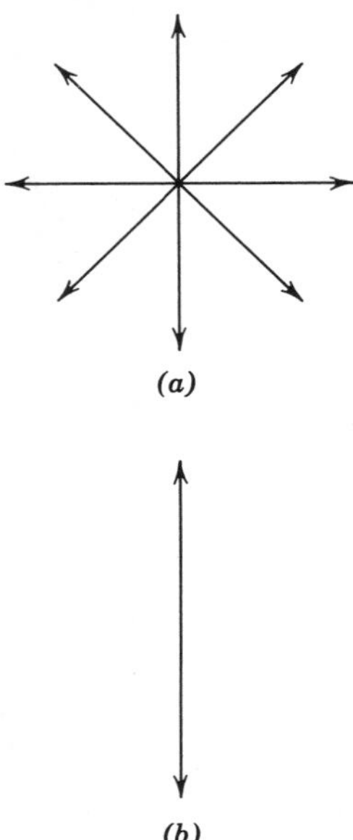

Fig. 11.3. (*a*) Schematic representation of the net electric force vectors of a ray of unpolarized light; (*b*) electric vector of linearly polarized light.

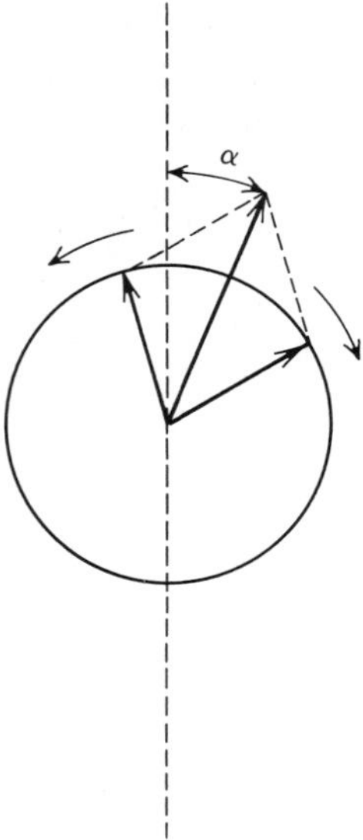

Fig. 11.4. Rotation of the plane of linearly polarized light through the angle α by a substance for which $n_L > n_R$.

said to be optically active. The phenomenon of the difference in velocity of left and right circularly polarized light is called circular birefringence.

The intensity of optical rotation is expressed as the *specific rotation* $[\alpha]$, given by

$$[\alpha]_\lambda^t = \frac{100\alpha}{lc} \tag{11.1}$$

where α is the observed rotation in degrees, c is the solute concentration in g/100 ml, and l is the path length in *decimeters*. The superscript indicates the temperature, the subscript the wavelength. If the rotation of a pure liquid is measured (the sample then being referred to as "neat"), the specific rotation is calculated with the formula $[\alpha] = \alpha/ld$, where d is the density. Comparisons of the rotatory power of compounds are facilitated by calculating the molecular rotation $[\Phi]$ by Eq. 11.2, where M is molecular weight.

$$[\Phi] = \frac{\alpha M}{lc} \tag{11.2}$$

The dependence of rotation on wavelength is called *optical rotatory dispersion* (ORD).

Turning now to the absorption effect, if the quantities ϵ_L and ϵ_R are different (for a given substance interacting with left and right circularly polarized light), then the lengths of the clockwise and counterclockwise vectors will differ as one is absorbed more intensely than the other. Their resultant will therefore no longer be linearly polarized, but will be elliptically polarized. The substance is said to exhibit *circular dichroism* (CD). The extent of this phenomenon is expressed as the molecular ellipticity $[\Theta]$,

$$[\Theta] = 3300(\epsilon_L - \epsilon_R) \tag{11.3}$$

The quantity $(\epsilon_L - \epsilon_R)$, the differential dichroic absorption, is accessible experimentally. Since the ellipticity is proportional to a difference of molar absorptivities, evidently the curve of $[\Theta]$ as a function of wavelength will have the same shape as the absorption spectrum; it may, however, be either positive or negative.

Clearly CD can be observed only if the molecule contains a chromophore, and a further condition is required, namely, that this be an optically active chromophore. The meaning and structural implications of this term will be considered in Section 11.3. At this point, however, it can be noted that if a chromophore exhibits circular dichroism ($\epsilon_L \neq \epsilon_R$) then it will also exhibit circular birefringence ($n_L \neq n_R$). The CD and ORD curves for a substance are related, and they contain essentially the same structural information. In a given instance, however, it may be easier to extract the information from one rather than the other, so both techniques are valuable.

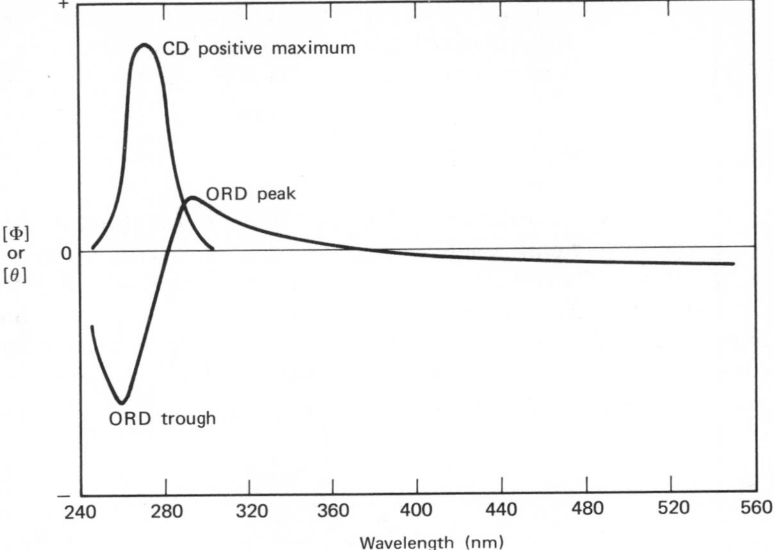

Fig. 11.5. ORD and CD curves and nomenclature. A positive Cotton effect is shown.

Figure 11.5 illustrates some features of ORD and CD curves, including nomenclature. The wavelength of maximal CD effect is called the CD maximum (positive or negative). In the region of the CD effect the corresponding ORD curve exhibits the complex behavior shown in Fig. 11.5; the highest point is called the peak, the lowest the trough (to distinguish clearly between these effects and absorption maxima and minima). When the peak occurs at longer wavelength than the trough, the curve is said to show a positive Cotton effect; the alternative is a negative Cotton effect. Far from the region of CD effects no Cotton effects are seen. Notice that it is possible for a substance to be dextrorotatory at some wavelengths and levorotatory at others. The CD maximum usually occurs very close to the uv absorption maximum for the same transition. CD is often more sensitive than uv absorption in resolving adjacent transitions.

11.2 Measurement of Optical Rotation

This section describes means for measuring optical rotation in the visible range of the spectrum, which traditionally has been the most important measurement. As pointed out in Section 11.1, ORD is most powerful in the uv region, since this is where most electronic transitions take place. The principles of polarimetry in the uv are similar to those discussed here, though obviously the components may be different.

Production of Linearly Polarized Light. Natural light cannot be employed directly for polarimetric measurements, for it includes electric force vectors in all planes. Optical rotation of these planes would merely result in another equivalent orientation that could not be differentiated from the initial one. It is therefore necessary to isolate light whose net electric vector is vibrating in a single plane, that is, linearly polarized light. This is accomplished with a polarizer.

The randomly oriented planes of oscillation of natural light can be reduced, in effect, to two planes perpendicular to each other; that is, unpolarized light can be represented by the symbol ✥. The process of polarization is then the process of separating natural light into its mutually perpendicular components ↕ and ↔. Either of these linearly polarized components can be used for polarimetric measurements.

Certain crystals have the property that through them the velocity of light polarized in one plane is different from the velocity of light polarized in the perpendicular plane. This means that the crystal has two refractive indexes, one for each linearly polarized ray, ↕ and ↔. Such a substance is said to be "double refracting." Calcite is a particularly important double refracting crystal; its refractive indexes are 1.4865 and 1.6584. When a ray of natural light is incident on a prism of calcite (with the angle of incidence different from 0°), the ray is separated into two linearly polarized rays with mutually perpendicular planes, each ray being refracted in accordance with its corresponding refractive index, with the result that natural light has been resolved into two rays of linearly polarized light. Figure 11.6*a* shows this behavior.

The simple polarizer of Fig. 11.6*a* is not particularly convenient, because it is not easy to select one of the rays with the complete exclusion of the other. The separation of rays can be accomplished with a small but important modification of the prism. The incident radiation enters the prism at an angle of incidence equal to 0°. The two polarized rays therefore do not separate (are not refracted), although their velocities differ. The angle at which they are incident upon the back face of the prism is selected such that the critical angle of reflection is exceeded for one ray but not for the other. The first ray will thus be totally reflected back into the crystal, whereas the second ray will pass on through for use in the polarimeter. Figure 11.6*b* illustrates this separation.

The emerging beam in Fig. 11.6*b* is not parallel to the incident beam, which is a practical disadvantage of this polarizer. In Fig. 11.6*c* a modification is shown that eliminates this disadvantage. A second prism is combined as shown to re-refract the polarized ray to be parallel with the incident ray. In order to reduce loss of intensity in the polarized ray by reflection at the prism interface, the two prisms are cemented together with Canada balsam, the refractive index of which is 1.55 (and therefore closer to that of the calcite than is n of air).

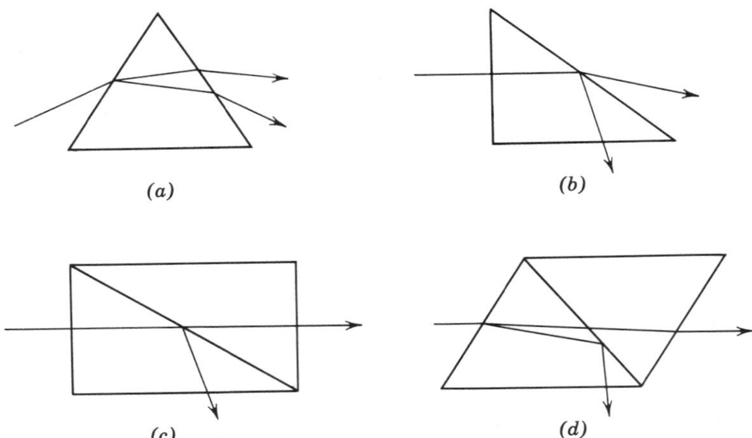

Fig. 11.6. Production of polarized light by double refraction. Both (*c*) and (*d*) are commonly called Nicol prisms, though (*c*) is more properly called the Glan-Thompson prism.

A polarizer design very similar to that of Fig. 11.6*c* is shown in Fig. 11.6*d*. Both of the polarizer designs pictured in *c* and *d* of the figure are referred to as Nicol prisms. They are used to obtain linearly polarized light from natural light in polarimeters.

Other means are available for the production of polarized light. A reflecting surface will polarize light, but this is an inefficient method. Crystals of iodoquinine, or certain other substances, all oriented in the same direction and embedded in sheets of plastic, have the property of absorbing one of the polarized rays more than the other. These sheets of oriented crystals are called Polaroid filters. They are not capable of producing pure linearly polarized light, the ray being contaminated with a small amount of the second component; hence they are not used as polarizers in precision polarimeters.

Determination of the Angle of Rotation. Linearly polarized light is produced with a polarizer, as described in the preceding paragraphs, and it is passed through the sample solution, which may alter the direction of the plane of the polarized light. It is next necessary to measure the angle α through which the plane has been rotated. This is accomplished with the analyzer. An analyzer is simply a second Nicol prism aligned to intercept the linearly polarized ray as it emerges from the sample solution. Since the polarizer Nicol has the ability to resolve natural light (✥) into its two components, rejecting one (say, ↔) and transmitting the other (↕), it is evident that the analyzer Nicol will transmit the ↕ ray if the prism is oriented identically with the polarizer Nicol. Maximum transmission of a linearly polarized ray by the analyzer is achieved with "parallel" Nicols. The arrangement is shown in Fig. 11.7*a*.

If the analyzer Nicol is turned by 90° from the parallel position, the plane of the linearly polarized ray will now strike the analyzer with exactly the same orientation as the ray (↔) that was rejected by total reflection in the polarizer. This ray will therefore be totally reflected in the analyzer. No light will be passed by this orientation of the polarizer-analyzer combination. This condition of maximum extinction is achieved by "crossed" Nicols (Fig. 11.7*b*).

At any intermediate position of the analyzer between the parallel and crossed positions, some light will be transmitted. Now suppose that a pair of Nicols is crossed so that maximum extinction is achieved. Next a solution of an optically active compound is placed in the light path between the polarizer and analyzer. The plane of the polarized light will be rotated by, say, α degrees upon passage through the sample solution. The new direction of the plane of light leads to transmission of light through the analyzer, because the plane is no longer oriented for total reflection. If the analyzer is rotated through α degrees, total extinction will be restored. The angle through which the analyzer must be turned to restore the condition of total extinction is therefore equal to the angle through which the sample rotated the plane of the light. This is the principle of the polarimeter.

The sensitivity of the measurement of α, the angle of optical rotation, by reproducing the condition of maximum extinction, is dependent upon the ability of the human eye and mind to *remember* degrees of darkness and light. This ability is not as great as the ability to *match* the intensities of adjacent illuminated fields. The measurement of α is therefore accomplished by a slight modification of the optical system already described. One such modification is shown in Fig. 11.8. The polarizer Nicol prism (seen end-on in the figure) is

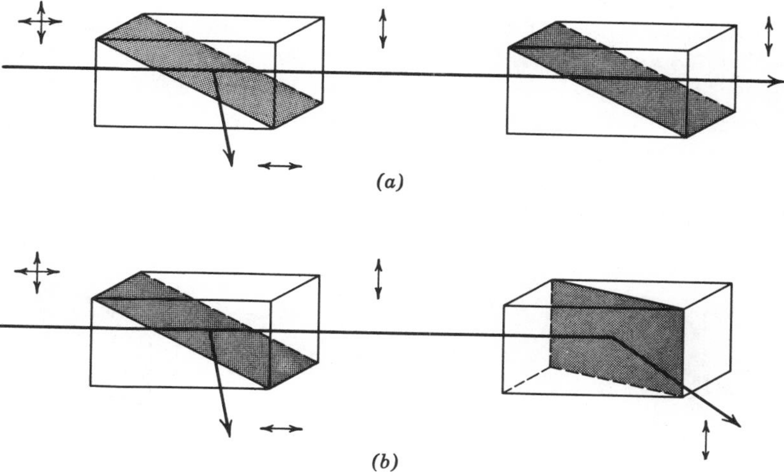

Fig. 11.7. (*a*) Parallel Nicols, giving maximum transmission; (*b*) crossed Nicols, giving maximum extinction.

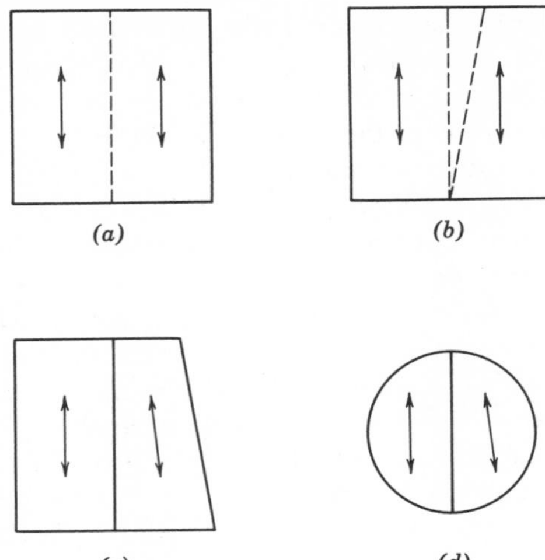

Fig. 11.8. Construction of the Jellett-Cornu half-shade modification of the Nicol polarizer (from Ref. 1).

sawed in half lengthwise along the dashed line. A wedge-shaped piece is cut out of one-half of the prism (*b*), and the two parts are cemented together as shown (*c*). A diaphragm gives a circular field of view (*d*). Light rays polarized by the two halves of the prism are oriented at a small angle, as indicated by the arrows.

An analyzer Nicol crossed with the left half of the polarizer will show maximum extinction for half the field of view, but since it cannot be simultaneously crossed with both halves of the polarizer, the other half of the field will be light. Similarly, if the analyzer is crossed with the right half of the polarizer, the right half of the field will be darker than the left half. The views in the analyzer corresponding to these settings are shown in Fig. 11.9*a* and *c*. When the analyzer is uncrossed to exactly the same degree with each half of the polarizer, both halves of the field will appear to be of equal intensity as in (*b*). This condition is highly reproducible. Instead of maximum extinction as the

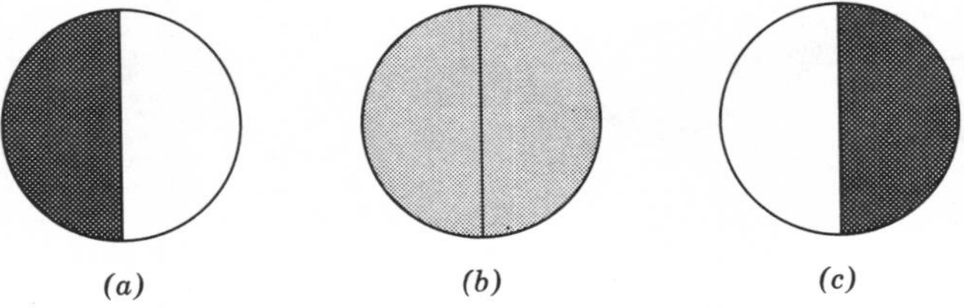

Fig. 11.9. Appearance of the half-shade field.

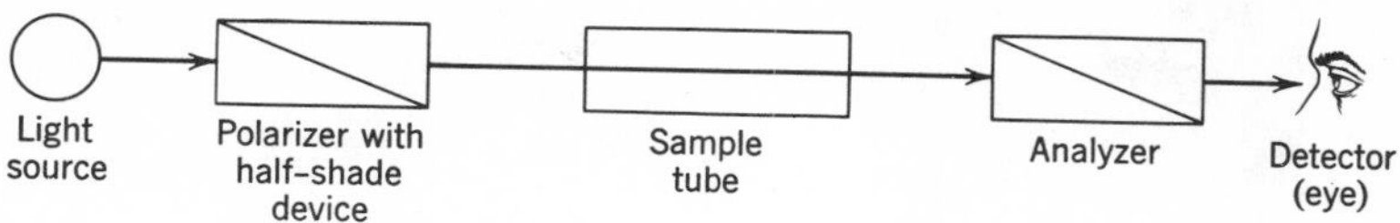

Fig. 11.10. Components of a polarimeter.

"end point" condition, the condition of equal intensity of the two half-fields is used. This is called the half-shade effect.

Maximum precision in locating the equal-intensity condition is achieved with a very small half-shade angle (the angle between the planes of polarized light produced by the two halves of the polarizer), but the angle must be sufficiently large to allow enough light to pass for ready visibility. The Jellet-Cornu half-shade device shown in Fig. 11.8 does not permit variation of the half-shade angle. Most polarimeters use another half-shade device, the Lippich modification, which provides a variable half-shade angle. Such polarimeters have a lever near the polarizer mounting with which the half-shade angle can be varied from 0 to 20°. On some instruments the circular field is split into three areas.

All the necessary components of a polarimeter are shown diagrammatically in Fig. 11.10. The light source is usually a sodium emission lamp, and the D line (589.3 nm) is isolated with a filter. A telescope is interposed between the analyzer and the eye (but is not shown in Fig. 11.10). The analyzer is mechanically connected to a large circle marked in degrees. By means of a vernier, measurements can be made to 0.01°; some high-precision polarimeters provide angle measurements to 0.001°.

11.3 The Optical Activity of Molecules

Steroisomers. Although many compounds can rotate the plane of linearly polarized light, many others cannot. Pasteur proposed that optical activity is associated with a lack of molecular symmetry. Le Bel and van't Hoff suggested that a frequent source of molecular asymmetry, and therefore of optical activity, is the presence of a carbon atom bonded to four different atoms or groups. The simplest molecule with this structural element may be represented *Cabcd.* The important contribution of Le Bel and van't Hoff was the concept of the tetrahedral arrangement of the four bonds to a saturated carbon atom; for the system C*abcd* this hypothesis predicts that two different *stereoisomers*, shown in Fig. 11.11, can exist. In these diagrams the carbon atom is not pictured, but it is understood to occupy a central position within the tetrahedron; the four single bonds extend from the C atom to the points of the tetrahedron. The two molecular representations in Fig. 11.11 are mirror

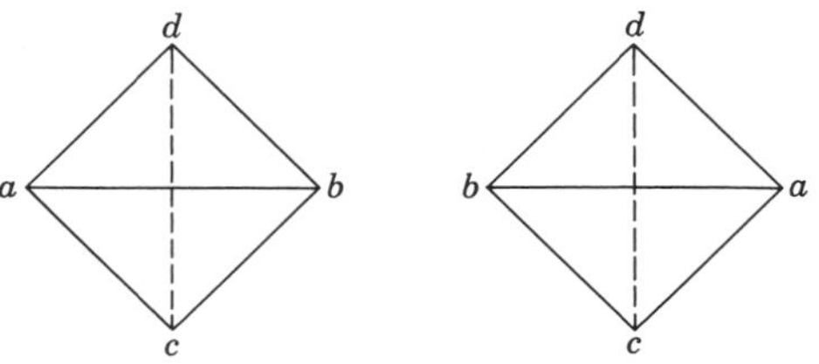

Fig. 11.11. Tetrahedral representations of the enantiomers of *Cabcd*.

images that are nonsuperimposable. They represent two different molecules, each of which is optically active and rotates light to the same extent but in opposite directions. The condition for optical activity is the existence of mirror images that are nonsuperimposable. Such isomers are called *enantiomers*. All the usual physical and chemical properties of the two enantiomers of a compound are identical except for their optical activity.

The three-dimensional representation of Fig. 11.11 is not convenient, and it is often replaced with a two-dimensional projection formula. The carbon atom is considered to be in the plane of the paper, the groups *a* and *b* to be above (in front of) the paper, and *c* and *d* to be behind the paper. Considering the compound α-aminopropionic acid (alanine), the projection formulas may be written

$$\begin{array}{c} \mathrm{COOH} \\ | \\ \mathrm{H{-}C{-}NH_2} \\ | \\ \mathrm{CH_3} \\ \mathbf{1} \end{array} \qquad \begin{array}{c} \mathrm{COOH} \\ | \\ \mathrm{H_2N{-}C{-}H} \\ | \\ \mathrm{CH_3} \\ \mathbf{2} \end{array}$$

Sometimes the relative orientations of the groups are more explicitly indicated as in formulas **3** and **4**.

$$\begin{array}{c} \mathrm{COOH} \\ \vdots \\ \mathrm{H{\blacktriangleright}C{\blacktriangleleft}NH_2} \\ \vdots \\ \mathrm{CH_3} \\ \mathbf{3} \end{array} \qquad \begin{array}{c} \mathrm{COOH} \\ \vdots \\ \mathrm{H_2N{\blacktriangleright}C{\blacktriangleleft}H} \\ \vdots \\ \mathrm{CH_3} \\ \mathbf{4} \end{array}$$

The carbon atom containing four different groups is called an asymmetric carbon. Of the enantiomers **1** and **2**, one will be dextrorotatory and the other other will be levorotatory; these conditions are indicated with a plus or minus sign. Thus the dextrorotatory enantiomer of alanine is (+)-alanine and the levorotatory enantiomer is (−)-alanine. The sign of rotation bears no relation to the configuration of the enantiomer; in fact, a simple change of solvent may alter the sign of rotation without any change in configuration about the asymmetric carbon.

```
            COOH                         COOH
                                          |
   H  (tetrahedron)  NH2      ≡     H  —  C  — NH2
                                          |
            CH3                          CH3

                                          |||

            CH3                          COOH
             |                            |
  HOOC  —   C  —  NH2       ≡    H2N  —  C  — CH3
             |                            |
             H                            H
```

Fig. 11.12. Equivalent representations of an enantiomer of alanine.

In comparing projection formulas to determine whether or not they represent nonsuperimposable mirror images (and therefore enantiomers) several limitations of these formulas must be recognized. Since the horizontal bonds are above the plane containing the carbon atom while the vertical bonds are below this plane, this relative orientation must be maintained. Thus the formula can be rotated 180° but not 90 or 270°. Moreover, the formula cannot be taken out of the plane of the paper. Although substituents cannot be switched in pairs, any three of them can be altered without changing the configuration of the enantiomer. Figure 11.12 shows equivalent formulas for an enantiomer of alanine. Ball-and-stick molecular models are useful aids in visualizing these comparisons.

A molecule containing a single asymmetric carbon can exist as one of only two possible enantiomers, as we have seen. The situation is more complex when there are two or more asymmetric carbons in the molecule. For most such compounds the number of stereoisomers is 2^n, where n is the number of asymmetric carbon atoms. Important examples in which $n = 2$ are the four-carbon sugars shown in Fig. 11.13. The two-dimensional projection formulas are interpreted as before; that is, the aldehyde and primary alcohol groups lie behind the paper, and the hydrogens and hydroxy groups lie above the paper.

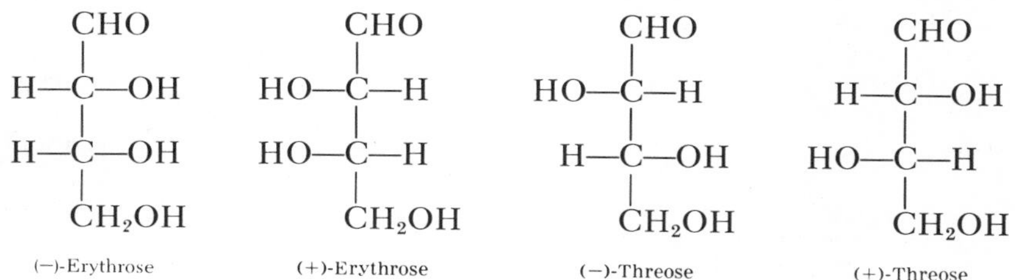

Fig. 11.13. Projection formulas of the four stereoisomers of the four-carbon sugars.

(For convenience in referring to these isomers, they have been identified with the correct configurational assignment.)

According to the criterion that nonsuperimposable mirror images are enantiomers, we can conclude that (−)-erythrose and (+)-erythrose are enantiomers. They have identical properties except that one is levorotatory and the other is dextrorotatory. Similarly, (−)-threose and (+)-threose are enantiomers. However, comparison of either erythrose enantiomer with either threose shows that, though stereoisomers, these are not mirror images, and they are therefore not enantiomers. Such stereoisomers are called *diastereoisomers.* Diastereoisomers may possess greatly different chemical and physical properties (unlike enantiomers) because their interatomic distances and angles may differ widely.

The erythroses and threoses are examples of substances containing two unlike asymmetric atoms, that is, the asymmetric carbons are not bonded to the same three groups. Tartaric acid is a compound containing two like asymmetric carbons. The four projection formulas of tartaric acid are shown in Fig. 11.14. The formulas labeled (−)-tartaric acid and (+)-tartaric acid are obviously nonsuperimposable mirror images and therefore represent enantiomers. The two other formulas, though mirror images, are superimposable by a 180° rotation in the plane of the paper. These cannot be enantiomers, therefore, and in fact these two formulas represent the same stereoisomer, which is called *meso*-tartaric acid. Only three distinct stereoisomers of tartaric acid exist, in contrast to the four stereoisomers possible for a compound containing two unlike asymmetric carbon atoms.

Since enantiomers rotate light to the same extent but in opposite directions, an equimolar mixture of a dextrorotatory enantiomer and its levorotatory enantiomer will appear to be optically inactive. Such a mixture is called a *racemic mixture*, *racemic modification*, or *racemate*. A racemic mixture may be labeled (±), *dl*, DL, or (*R*, *S*). The lack of observable optical rotation therefore does not necessarily mean that the sample contains no optically active molecules. Both *meso*-tartaric acid and *dl*-tartaric acid are optically inactive, but the first consists of a single optically inactive isomer, whereas the second is a

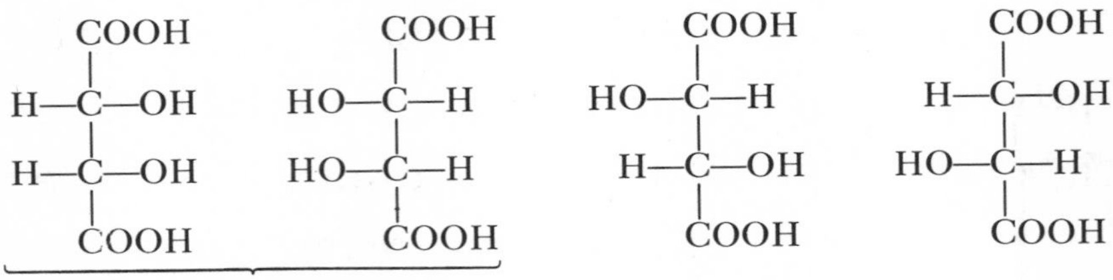

COOH	COOH	COOH	COOH
H—C—OH	HO—C—H	HO—C—H	H—C—OH
H—C—OH	HO—C—H	H—C—OH	HO—C—H
COOH	COOH	COOH	COOH
Meso-tartaric acid		(−) Tartaric acid	(+)-Tartaric acid

Fig. 11.14. Projection formulas of the three tartaric acids.

one-to-one mixture of the dextrorotatory and levorotatory enantiomers. It is possible to resolve the racemic modification into the optically active forms.

Atoms other than carbon can confer optical activity on a molecule, although carbon is undoubtedly the most important atom in this connection. Since the nonsuperimposability of mirror images (rather than the presence of an asymmetric atom) is the condition for the existence of enantiomers, it is possible to observe optical activity in certain molecules lacking asymmetric carbon but possessing the essential molecular dissymmetry as a result of other structural features. The general term *chiral* has come into use to denote molecules that lack certain symmetry elements and are therefore capable of being optically active [2, 3].

Configuration. The structure of a molecule is specified when the types and numbers of atoms, and the nature of the bonds between them, are known. Thus both enantiomers of alanine (**1** and **2**) have the same structure. They differ, however, in the arrangement of the groups about the asymmetric carbon; they are said to have different configurations. The study of optical isomerism is largely the study of molecular configuration.

The two possible configurations of a molecule with a single asymmetric carbon atom are easily represented by the two-dimensional projection formulas introduced earlier. The molecule may be written RCHXR′, where R—C—R′ is the main chain of the molecule. The No. 1 carbon of the chain (in the conventional numbering system) is placed at the top in the projection formula. Then if X is on the right the enantiomer has the D configuration, whereas if X is on the left it has the L configuration. Structure **1** is therefore D-alanine and **2** is L-alanine.

Configuration and sign of rotation bear no direct relationship to each other; thus **2** is L-(+)-alanine. Until relatively recently the true configuration of any substance was unknown. In order to make stereochemical studies possible, the convention (Fischer-Rosanoff) was adopted that (+)-glyceraldehyde, **5**,

```
     CHO
      |
  H—C—OH
      |
     CH₂OH
```

5

would be arbitrarily assigned the D configuration, and all other configurations would be related to this one. That is, an enantiomer with the same configuration as (+)-glyceraldehyde is to be assigned the D configuration. It is possible by chemical transformations to establish whether a given enantiomer possesses the same configuration as, or the opposite one to, (+)-glyceraldehyde, and thus to establish the *relative configuration* of the enantiomer. Since 1951 the absolute configurations of many compounds have been determined by physical methods. Fortunately, it was found that the arbitrary designation of the D configuration to (+)-glyceraldehyde is in fact the correct one (there was a 50% chance that it was incorrect), so all relative configurations may now be considered absolute configurations.

Molecules containing more than one chiral center are not easily described by the D,L system, and a newer method, proposed by Cahn, Ingold, and Prelog, has been adopted to permit the unambiguous specification of the configuration at every chiral center in a molecule. The procedure for assigning the configuration to a particular model uses these steps (simplified somewhat for our purposes). We consider the assignment of configuration to an asymmetric carbon atom, *Cabcd*.

1. List the four groups in a sequence of decreasing "priority," where the priority is determined by the atomic number of the atom bonded to the carbon. Atoms of higher atomic number have higher priority, giving the sequence

$$\mathrm{I > Br > Cl > F > O > N > C > H}$$

If two or more groups are bonded to the carbon by the same kind of atom, proceed to the second atom to establish priorities, and so on until all priorities are assigned.

2. View the model from the side of the tetrahedron opposite from the group having lowest priority.

3. Count around the exposed face of the tetrahedron containing the remaining three groups, proceeding in the direction of decreasing priority. If the order of this count is clockwise (right, *rectus*), the configuration is labeled *R*; if it is counterclockwise (left, *sinister*), it is *S*.

Consider the application of these rules to **1**, D-alanine. The priority sequence (in order of decreasing priority) is NH_2 (1), COOH (2), CH_3 (3), H (4). Figure 11.15 shows the tetrahedron oriented with the lowest-priority group,

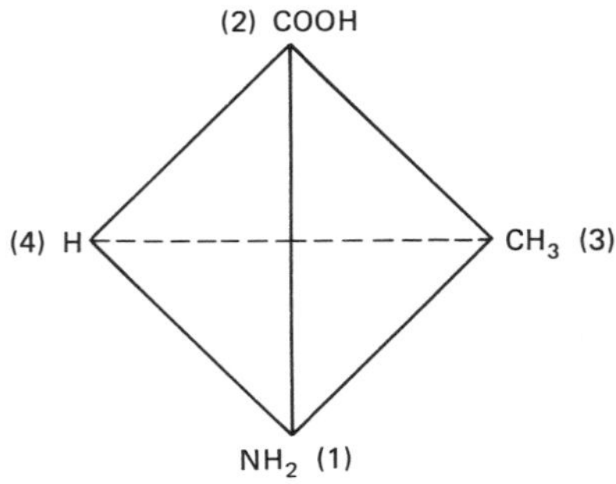

Fig. 11.15. Assignment of configuration to (*R*)-alanine. The numbers in parentheses represent group priorities, and the direction of view is from the right.

H, away from the viewer (compare with structure **1** and **3**). Proceeding around the forward face in the order NH_2, COOH, CH_3 requires a clockwise circuit, so this is (*R*)-alanine.

This is a very simple example. The rules for establishing priority have been refined to provide an unambiguous sequence for all groups, and the system can be applied to compounds whose chirality derives from dissymmetry other than that provided by an asymmetric carbon atom. Two points should be noted: the *R* assignment is not synonymous with the D configuration in the older method; and an assignment in the *R,S* system can change by changing the identity of the groups, even though no change in configuration has occurred.

Determination of Configuration. In order to produce ORD and CD phenomena, a molecule must possess an optically active chromophore. There are two types of such chromophores: (1) those that are inherently dissymmetric; and (2) those that are inherently symmetric but are perturbed by an asymmetric environment. In the first class are compounds like hexahelicene, **6**, and the twisted biphenyl **7**. These molecules do not possess asymmetric carbon atoms,

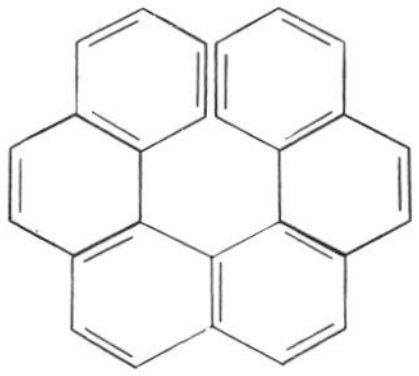

Y X

X Y

6 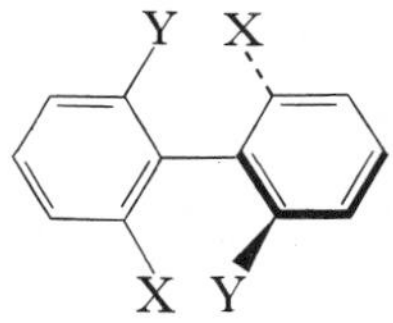 **7**

but they are chiral because of steric restrictions that produce a conformation with a nonsuperimposable mirror image.

The second class of optically active chromophore is much more common. The best studied of these chromophores is the carbonyl group, which itself has symmetry properties preventing it from being optically active. When the carbonyl group is located near a chiral center, however, its electronic transitions are perturbed and optical activity becomes possible; Cotton effects are observed in the region corresponding to the perturbed transition. Steroids have provided excellent molecular features for studying these effects [4–6]. The saturated steroid skeleton contains seven asymmetric carbons (**8**). No

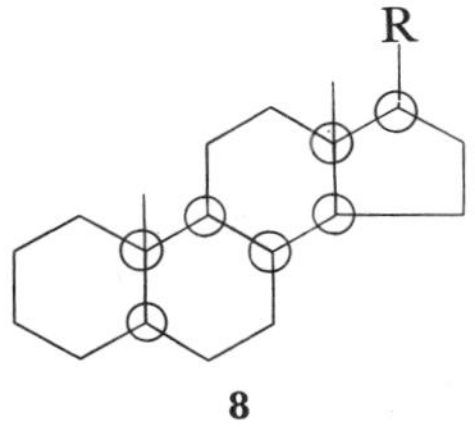

R

8

matter where a carbonyl group is located on the steroid nucleus, it will be close to a chiral center, and will therefore become an optically active chromophore. By means of observing the Cotton effects of many such molecules of known configuration and conformation, it has been found possible to make reliable correlations between the sign of the Cotton effect and the configuration of the chiral center. ORD and CD provide the single most useful technique for studying configuration. These studies have been extended to many other kinds of chromophores and molecules [4–6].

11.4 Analytical Applications

The main uses of ORD and CD have been for the study of configuration and conformation, beginning (in 1953) with the availability of instruments capable of measuring rotation into the uv region. Historically measurements of specific rotation at the sodium D line have been important; these quantities are symbolized $[\alpha]_D$. The concentration at which the measurement was made is usually specified. The specific rotation has some value as a criterion of identity and purity, and the USP and NF specify limits within which the specific rotation must fall for many substances. Often the biological activity of a compound can be correlated with its optical rotation. This is a result of the great specificity of many enzymes (and perhaps other components in biological phenomena) for certain structural and configurational features of their substrates, or substances with which they react. For example, some enzymes can hydrolyze esters of L-amino acids, but are ineffective in hydrolyzing D-amino acid esters. In fact, the L configuration appears to be greatly preponderant in naturally occurring substances. Nearly all biological processes (including drug action) are therefore dissymetric in some degree; that is, they proceed more readily with one enantiomer than with the other. This is why the rotation of an optically active drug is a good indication of its effective purity. Drugs of natural origin are often isolated as relatively pure enantiomers, though sometimes the isolation process causes partial or complete racemization (that is, formation of the optically inactive racemic mixture). Synthetic drugs, even if capable of optical activity, seldom rotate the plane of polarized light; the synthetic process, being symmetrical in nature, produces the racemate.

Table 11.1 gives the specific rotations of some substances important in pharmacy. The magnitudes of these rotations are typical. Notice the striking effect of the solvent on the sign of the rotation of chloramphenicol.

Since the observed rotation α is a function of concentration, quantitative analyses of optically active solutes may be carried out polarimetrically. Over a small concentration range, particularly at relatively low concentrations, the

TABLE 11.1
Specific Rotations of Some Compounds of Pharmaceutical Interest

Compound	$[\alpha]_D$	t	c	Solvent
L-Ascorbic acid	+ 48	23	1	Methanol
Benzyl penicillin	+269	20	0.6	Methanol
Camphor	+ 43.8	20	7.5	Ethanol
Chloramphenicol	+ 18.6	27	4.9	Ethanol
Chloramphenicol	− 25.5	25		Ethyl acetate
Cinchonidine	−109.2	20		Ethanol
Cinchonine	+229			Ethanol
Cocaine	− 16	20	4	Chloroform
Codeine	−112	15	2	Chloroform
Cortisone	+209	25	1.2	Ethanol
Diacetylmorphine	−166	25	1.5	Methanol
Digitoxin	+ 4.8	20	1.2	Dioxane
Ephedrine hydrochloride	− 34	25	5	Water
Epinephrine	− 52	25	5	0.5 *N* HCl
Erythromycin	− 78	25	2	Ethanol
Folic acid	+ 23	25	0.5	0.1 *N* NaOH
Hydrocortisone	+167	22	1	Ethanol
Kanamycin	+121	23	1	Water
Morphine	+132	25	1	Methanol
Prednisolone	+102	25		Dioxane
Quinidine	+258	17	1	Ethanol
Quinine	−169	15	2	Ethanol
Reserpine	−118	23	1	Chloroform
Strychnine	−139	18	1	Chloroform
Tetracycline	−239	25	1	Methanol

observed rotation is essentially linear with concentration. At higher concentrations the linear relationship fails. Then the quantitative analysis may be conducted by reading the unknown concentration from a standard curve of α versus c prepared from measurements on solutions of known concentrations. Quantitative polarimetric analysis is of particular value in the sugar industry; in fact, the polarimetric determination of sucrose has been given the name saccharimetry. Polarimetry is applied occasionally in quantitative pharmaceutical analysis, but its relative insensitivity is a disadvantage. It can be expected that ORD measurements in the uv region will find increasing use for quantitative analysis because of the higher rotations observed at shorter wavelengths.

Experiment 11.1. Polarimetric Measurements in Identification and Quantitative Analysis

PRINCIPLE

The quantitative analysis of sugars is an important application of polarimetry, and in this experiment a dextrose solution will be analyzed.

Sugars have more than one asymmetric carbon atom, so each structure may exist in several stereoisomeric forms. Diastereoisomers are usually specified with trivial names (for example, glucose, mannose, etc.). The configuration of a sugar is conventionally specified as the configuration of the carbon atom next to the primary alcohol group. Thus the naturally occurring (+)-glucose (also called dextrose), which has the configuration shown in **9**, is D-(+)-glucose.

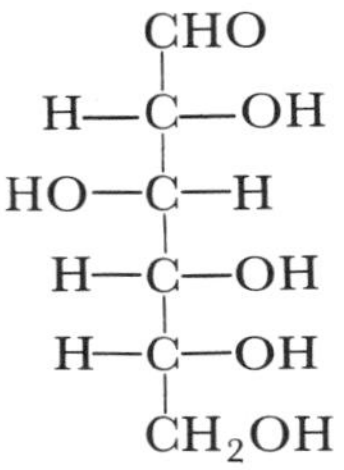

```
      CHO
       |
   H—C—OH
       |
  HO—C—H
       |
   H—C—OH
       |
   H—C—OH
       |
      CH2OH
```

9

In solution, D-glucose exists principally in a cyclic hemiacetal form in which the aldehydic carbon becomes asymmetric. This carbon therefore gives rise to two possible forms of D-glucose. These forms, which exist in equilibrium, are called α-D-glucose and β-D-glucose (Fig. 11.16). The specific rotation of a freshly prepared dextrose solution changes with time until a constant equilibrium value of $[\alpha]_D^{20} = +52.7°$ is attained; the same equilibrium value is

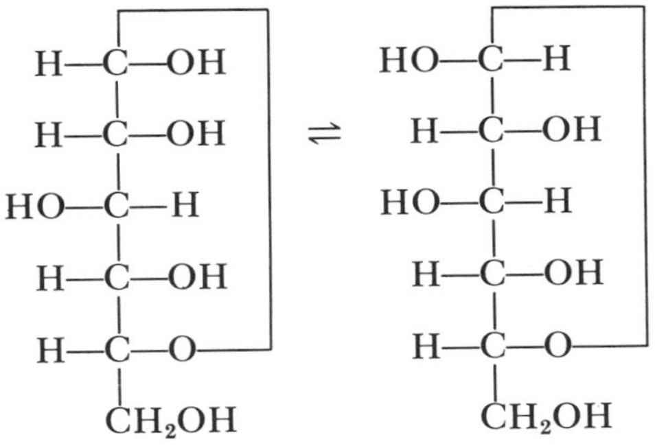

```
     ┌──────────┐                 ┌──────────┐
   H—C—OH       │              HO—C—H       │
     |          │                 |         │
   H—C—OH       │      ⇌        H—C—OH      │
     |          │                 |         │
  HO—C—H        │              HO—C—H       │
     |          │                 |         │
   H—C—OH       │               H—C—OH      │
     |          │                 |         │
   H—C—O────────┘               H—C—O───────┘
     |                            |
    CH2OH                        CH2OH
```

α-D-(+)-glucose $[\alpha]_D^{20} = +112.2°$

β-D-(+)-glucose $[\alpha]_D^{20} = +18.7°$

Fig. 11.16. Configurations of the alpha and beta forms of D-(+)-glucose.

reached whether the solution is prepared with pure alpha or pure beta form. The change of optical rotation with time is called *mutarotation.* It is usually caused by a configurational change, as with D-glucose. An equilibrium solution of D-glucose contains about 37% of the alpha form and 63% of the beta. The rate of mutarotation is increased by acids and bases.*

Another type of rotational change is undergone by solutions of sucrose, which is a disaccharide. Under the catalytic influence of acids, bases, or the enzyme invertase, sucrose is hydrolyzed into dextrose and levulose (this mixture of products is called "invert sugar"), with a change in optical rotation. This inversion process is negligibly slow in pure aqueous solution.

APPARATUS

Polarimeter. Any commercial polarimeter is suitable. Although all these operate according to the principles described in Section 11.2, the details of construction vary somewhat among instruments. Your instructor will explain the operation of your polarimeter.

Polarimeter Tubes. One decimeter and 2 dm tubes, with cover glasses and washers.

Sodium Lamp. The General Electric sodium vapor lamp or its equivalent.

PROCEDURES

Measurement of Specific Rotations. Accurately weigh 2–10 g of sucrose into a 100 ml volumetric flask and dissolve it in enough water to make 100 ml. Fill a 1 dm polarimeter tube with the solution. Measure the optical rotation of the solution. It is advisable to make several observations of the rotation, taking the mean value as the best estimate. Record the solution temperature.

Verify the direct proportionality between path length and optical rotation by measuring the rotation of the solution in a 2 dm cell.

Calculate the specific rotation of sucrose and compare your result with the literature value.

Obtain two samples of optically active compounds from your instructor. Accurately prepare solutions (in solvents suggested by the instructor) in the range 1–10%, and determine the specific rotations of the substances.

Quantitative Analysis of Dextrose Solutions. Accurately weigh samples of about 1, 2, 3, 4, 5, and 6 g of dextrose into six 100 ml volumetric flasks. Dissolve each sample in water, add 0.2 ml of 10% ammonia solution, dilute to 100.0 ml with water, and allow to stand at room temperature for 30 min. Measure the optical rotation α of each solution in a 2 dm tube and record the solution temperature. Make a graph of optical rotation against dextrose concentration.

Obtain a sample of dextrose injection from the instructor. Pipet an aliquot of injection containing 2–5 g of dextrose into a 100 ml volumetric flask. Add

* The interconversion of the alpha and beta forms proceeds through the open-chain form **9**.

0.2 ml of 10% ammonia, dilute to volume, and allow to stand for 30 min. Measure the optical rotation of the solution and read the concentration of dextrose from the standard curve.

References

1. Heller, W. and H. G. Curmè, *Physical Methods of Chemistry*, A. Weissberger and B. W. Rossiter (eds.), Vol. I, Part IIIC, Wiley-Interscience, New York, 1972, Chap. II.
2. Bentley, R., *Molecular Asymmetry in Biology*, Vol. I, Academic Press, New York, 1969.
3. Alworth, W. L., *Stereochemistry and Its Application in Biochemistry*, Wiley-Interscience, New York, 1972.
4. Djerassi, C., *Optical Rotatory Dispersion*, McGraw-Hill Book Co., New York, 1960.
5. Snatzke, G. (ed.), *Optical Rotatory Dispersion and Circular Dichroism in Organic Chemistry*, Heyden and Son, Ltd., London, 1967.
6. Crabbé, P., *Optical Rotatory Dispersion and Circular Dichroism in Organic Chemistry*, Holden-Day, San Francisco, 1965.

FOR FURTHER READING

Cahn, R. S., "An Introduction to the Sequence Rule. A System for the Specification of Absolute Configuration," *J. Chem. Educ.*, **41,** 116 (1964).

Mowery, D. F., Jr., "Criteria for Optical Activity in Organic Molecules," *J. Chem. Educ.*, **46,** 269 (1969).

Crabbé, P., *ORD and CD in Chemistry and Biochemistry*, Academic Press, New York, 1972.

Problems

1. 5.0 g of hyoscamine was dissolved in chloroform to make 50.0 ml. The observed optical rotation of this solution in a 2 dm tube at 20°C with the sodium D line was −5.04°. Calculate the specific rotation of hyoscyamine.

2. What will be the optical rotation of a 4.0% solution of chloramphenicol in ethyl acetate in a 1 dm tube? (Use Table 11.1.)

3. Consider the equilibrium $A \rightleftharpoons B$ with equilibrium constant $K = C_B/C_A$. If the specific rotations for pure A and pure B are $[\alpha]_A$ and $[\alpha]_B$, respectively, and if the equilibrium mixture has the apparent specific rotation $[\alpha]_{eq}$, show that

$$K = \frac{[\alpha]_{ep} - [\alpha]_A}{[\alpha]_B - [\alpha]_{eq}}$$

(Use an approach similar to that employed for spectrophotometric determinations of equilibrium constants.)

4. What is the equilibrium constant for the mutarotation of D-glucose?

5. Which of these compounds are capable of existing in stereoisomeric forms: lactic acid, glycine, benzaldehyde, phenylalanine, aspirin, urea, epinephrine?

6. (*a*) Derive an equation relating the specific rotation to the molecular rotation of a compound.

(*b*) Calculate the molecular rotation of hydrocortisone.

7. Devise an analytical procedure for the quantitative determination of each substance in these samples.

(*a*) Nicotinic acid and niacinamide in simple syrup.

(*b*) Reserpine and phenobarbital.

(*c*) Injection of dextrose and sodium chloride.

8. A compound was believed to have one of the isomeric structures A, B, or C. The compound had $pK_a = 10.2$ and $[\alpha]_D = -55°$. Which of the structures is consistent with the experimental data?

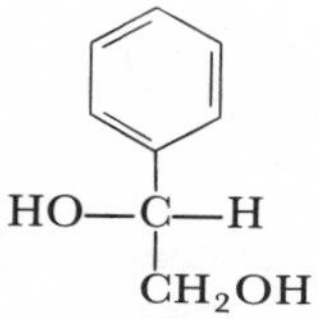

A: phenyl ring attached to HO—C—H, bottom CH_2OH

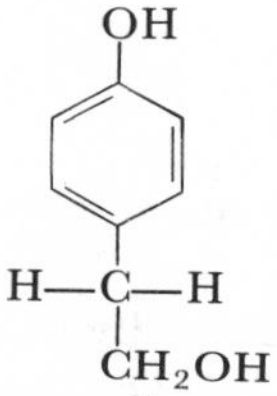

B: ring bearing OH (para) attached to H—C—H, bottom CH_2OH

C: ring bearing OH (para) attached to HO—C—H, bottom CH_3

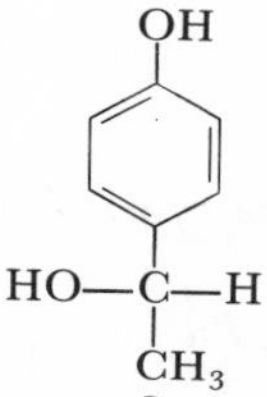

12 MAGNETIC RESONANCE SPECTROSCOPY

12.1 Theory of Nuclear Magnetic Resonance

Magnetic Properties of Nuclei. Usually the chemist is not concerned with the atomic nucleus except as it influences the electronic configuration of molecules, that is, except for its atomic number A and atomic weight Z. Our present subject, however, requires us to consider the magnetic properties of the nucleus. The nuclei of many isotopes possess an angular momentum, called spin, whose magnitude is described by the spin quantum number I. This quantity, which is characteristic of the nucleus, may have integral or half-integral values, that is, $I = 0, \frac{1}{2}, 1, \frac{3}{2}, \ldots$. If A is odd, I is half-integral; if A and Z are both even, $I = 0$; if A is even and Z is odd, I is integral. We are concerned only with nuclei having nonzero values of I. Table 12.1 lists the most important of these with their spin quantum numbers. Notice that $I = 0$ for the widely distributed ^{12}C and ^{16}O isotopes.

A nucleus having spin generates a magnetic moment μ, which is proportional to the angular momentum. Instead of the magnetic moment, sometimes the magnetogyric ratio γ (gyromagnetic ratio) is used to describe the magnetic properties of the nucleus; these quantities are related by Eq. 12.1, where h is Planck's constant.

$$\gamma = \frac{2\pi\mu}{Ih} \tag{12.1}$$

A nucleus can assume only $2I + 1$ energy states. Associated with each of these states is a magnetic quantum number m, where m takes the values I, $I - 1, I - 2, \ldots, -I + 1, -I$. In the absence of an external magnetic field, the allowed states are of identical energy, and are therefore equally populated in any assemblage of nuclei. In the presence of an applied steady magnetic field of strength H_0, these $2I + 1$ states will assume different energy levels. This separation of energy levels in a magnetic field is called nuclear Zeeman splitting. An intuitive model of the process can be given. Consider the proton, ^1H, with $I = \frac{1}{2}$. Then there are only two possible states, characterized by magnetic quantum numbers $m = +\frac{1}{2}$ and $m = -\frac{1}{2}$. In the absence

TABLE 12.1
Magnetic Properties of Some Important Nuclei

Nucleus	I	Resonance Frequency at 10 kG Field (MHz)	Natural Abundance (%)	Relative Sensitivity for Equal Numbers of Nuclei
^{1}H	$\frac{1}{2}$	42.58	99.985	(1.00)
^{2}H	1	6.54	0.015	0.00965
^{11}B	$\frac{3}{2}$	13.66	80.42	0.165
^{13}C	$\frac{1}{2}$	10.71	1.108	0.0159
^{14}N	1	3.08	99.63	0.0101
^{19}F	$\frac{1}{2}$	40.05	100	0.833
^{23}Na	$\frac{3}{2}$	11.26	100	0.0925
^{27}Al	$\frac{5}{2}$	11.09	100	0.206
^{31}P	$\frac{1}{2}$	17.24	100	0.0663
^{35}Cl	$\frac{3}{2}$	4.17	75.53	0.0047

of a magnetic field these states are equally populated. The states may be pictured as corresponding to opposite orientations of a tiny bar magnet, which is a crude way of visualizing the magnetic moment vector. Clearly in the absence of an applied field the orientation of the moment should not affect the energy of the nucleus.

Now let a steady field be applied. The two nuclear states now correspond to an orientation of the bar magnet parallel to the field (that is, N pole to S pole) or antiparallel to the field (N pole to N pole). There will be an energy difference between these states, the orientation with the field (N to S) being of lower energy than the orientation against the field.

The energy separation between these levels will be $\mu H_0/I$. Figure 12.1

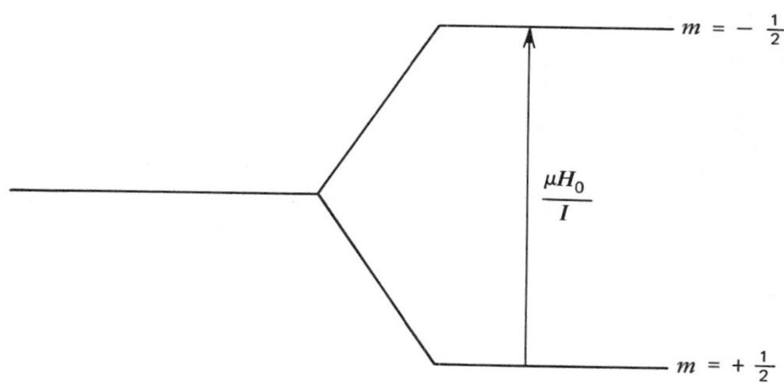

Fig. 12.1. Energy level splitting for a nucleus with $I = \frac{1}{2}$. Left side of diagram: no applied field. Right side of diagram: applied field H_0.

represents the situation that has been described for the proton. The analogy with optical phenomena, as described in Chapters 8 and 9, may now be obvious. It is possible to induce transitions from one energy level to another. (If splitting produces more than two levels, only transitions between adjacent levels are permitted.) The energy separation depends upon the kind of nucleus (through μ and I) and upon the strength of the applied field, H_0.

The frequency of the radiation that can be absorbed is given by the condition that the energy separation must exactly equal the energy absorbed. For electromagnetic radiation of frequency ν, therefore,

$$h\nu = \frac{\mu H_0}{I} \tag{12.2}$$

or, as it is sometimes encountered,

$$\nu = \frac{\gamma H_0}{2\pi} \tag{12.3}$$

where Eq. 12.3 is obtained from Eqs. 12.1 and 12.2. We can calculate the nuclear magnetic absorption frequency for the proton by using Eq. 12.2 and the experimental value $\mu = 1.42 \times 10^{-23}$ erg/G. Suppose $H_0 = 10{,}000$ G, a reasonable field strength. Then the frequency ν is 42.6 MHz, which is attainable as radio-frequency (rf) radiation. Table 12.1 gives absorption frequencies at 10,000 G for nuclei most apt to be encountered. The table also includes the natural abundances of these isotopes and, in the last column, the sensitivity of the response for equal numbers of nuclei, relative to ^{1}H. The actual relative responses can be obtained by correcting the sensitivity for the abundance; for example, the sensitivity of the ^{13}C absorption relative to ^{1}H is $(1.59 \times 10^{-2})(1.108 \times 10^{-2}) = 1.76 \times 10^{-4}$.

At this point we can summarize by observing that nuclei with nonzero spin numbers I can assume $2I + 1$ energy states. In an applied magnetic field H_0 these states are separated by an energy gap of $\mu H_0/I$. Transitions between adjacent states can be excited by the absorption of radio-frequency radiation. A significant difference between this phenomenon and optical spectroscopy is that the frequency of the radiation absorbed depends upon the strength of the applied magnetic field, according to Eq. 12.3.

The Resonance Condition. A nucleus that possesses a magnetic moment may be considered to be a spinning charged particle. If $I = \frac{1}{2}$ the nucleus behaves as if it were a spinning charged sphere. If I is greater than $\frac{1}{2}$, the nucleus is equivalent to a nonspherical spinning charge.* A nucleus with a magnetic moment, when placed in a steady applied magnetic field H_0, will tend to

* Such nuclei also possess an electric quadrupole moment, Q, which can have observable effects on the nmr spectrum.

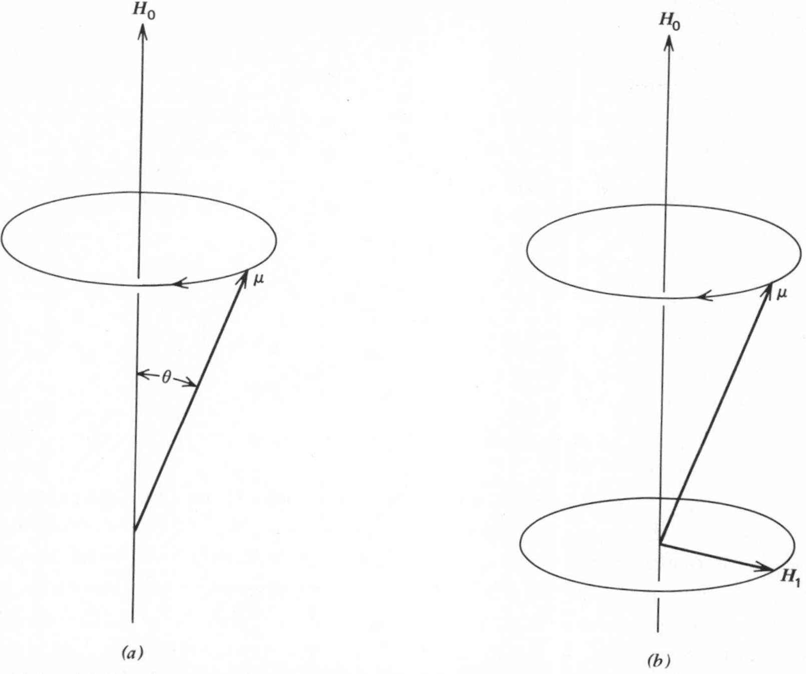

Fig. 12.2. (*a*) Magnetic moment vector μ precessing about applied field vector H_0. (*b*) Addition of rotating magnetic field H_1 normal to H_0.

adopt the orientation of the field, but because of its spin will instead assume an angle with the direction of the applied field; that is, the applied field vector and the magnetic moment vector will not be parallel. This situation is shown in Fig. 12.2*a*. The field H_0 tends to decrease the angle θ between the vectors, but because the nucleus is spinning the result is that the moment vector will precess about the field vector (Fig. 12.2*a*). This action is similar to that of a gyroscope. The angular velocity ω_0 (in rad/sec) of this precession is given by Eq. 12.4.

$$\omega_0 = \gamma H_0 \tag{12.4}$$

This velocity is called the Larmor precessional frequency.

Now suppose that an additional small magnetic field is applied perpendicular to H_0 in the plane formed by μ and H_0; call this field H_1 (see Fig. 12.2*b*). Field H_1 will act upon μ to increase the angle θ. If field H_1 is caused to rotate around H_0 at the Larmor precessional frequency of ω_0, the torque produced will steadily act to change the angle θ. On the other hand, if the frequency of rotation of H_1 is not the same as the precessional frequency, the torque will vary depending upon the relative phases of the two motions, and no sustained effect will be produced.

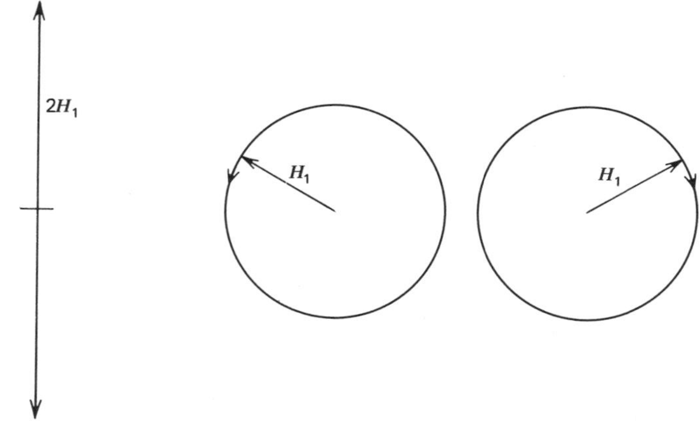

Fig. 12.3. A linearly oscillating field of amplitude $2H_1$ is equivalent to two oppositely rotating circular fields of amplitude H_1.

When the frequency of the rotating magnetic field H_1 equals the precessional frequency of the nucleus, energy is absorbed by the nuclear system and a transition occurs from a lower energy level to a higher one; in a sense the magnetic moment vector "flips" from one orientation to the other one. The nuclear absorption of energy from a rotating magnetic field in the presence of a constant magnetic field is called *nuclear magnetic resonance* (nmr). The resonance phenomenon occurs only when the angular velocity of the rotating field is equal to the Larmor precessional frequency of the magnetic moment. Comparing Eqs. 12.3 and 12.4 shows that this is the frequency ν that was calculated earlier.*

If a nucleus (actually a great many nuclei of the same substance, of course) is set precessing in field H_0, and the rotating field H_1 is altered in frequency, sweeping from a frequency lower than the Larmor frequency, through it, to a higher frequency, and if the energy absorbed from the rotating field H_1 is measured, the graph of energy absorbed against frequency of the rotating field is the nmr spectrum. It will consist of a sharp peak in the energy absorbed at the frequency corresponding to the Larmor resonance frequency of the nucleus at the given value of H_0.

It is not easy to apply a rotating magnetic field to the system of precessing nuclei. It is very easy, however, to generate a linearly oscillating field with an rf oscillator. This is perfectly satisfactory, since a linearly oscillating field of total amplitude $2H_1$ can be resolved into two rotating fields, each of amplitude H_1 but rotating in opposite directions (Fig. 12.3). Only the component rotating in the same direction as the precessing nuclei will interact; the other component has no effect.

* Angular velocity ω in radians per second is related to frequency ν in cycles per second (Hz) by $\omega = 2\pi\nu$.

It was suggested above that the field H_0 is held constant while the H_1 frequency is swept; this mode is called frequency sweep. An equivalent result is obtained by holding the rf field at a constant frequency and sweeping the field H_0. Nmr spectra obtained by field-sweep measurements are displayed with the field increasing from left to right; spectra obtained by frequency sweep are displayed with the frequency increasing from right to left, so that the two presentations are comparable.*

Nuclear Relaxation. Let us consider a set of nuclei (a spin system) with $I = \frac{1}{2}$ at thermal equilibrium in a steady magnetic field H_0. The two nuclear energy levels are separated by $2\mu H_0$, and the state for which $m = +\frac{1}{2}$ is the lower energy state, as in Fig. 12.1. Evidently the tendency is for all of the nuclei to pass to the lower energy level. This tendency, however, is opposed by thermal motion of the nuclei, which tends to produce an equilibrium distribution with identical numbers of nuclei in the two states. The net result is that a small but finite excess of nuclei will, at equilibrium, populate the lower energy level. The ratio of number of nuclei per unit volume in the lower energy level, N_+ (for $m = +\frac{1}{2}$) to the number N_- in the upper level is given by the Boltzmann distribution, Eq. 12.5, where k, the Boltzmann constant, is 1.38×10^{-16} erg/deg (k is the molar gas constant R divided by Avogadro's number).

$$\frac{N_+}{N_-} = e^{2\mu H_0/kT} \tag{12.5}$$

Since the energy separation $2\mu H_0$ is very small, the approximation $e^x \approx 1 + x$ is valid and we have

$$\frac{N_+}{N_-} \approx 1 + \frac{2\mu H_0}{kT} \tag{12.6}$$

showing the excess population of the lower energy state.

The nuclei constituting the spin system may be regarded as embedded in a medium, called the lattice, composed of the rest of the sample, that is, of atoms and molecules. Interaction between the spin system and the lattice (that is, transfer of energy) is possible but difficult. Now suppose this spin system is irradiated by an rf field at its resonance frequency, so that absorption of energy occurs. Some nuclei undergo transition from the lower to the higher energy state; thus the absorption of energy has reduced the excess of nuclei in the lower energy state. Equilibrium requires a return to the excess number present before the application of the rf field. Therefore transitions from the upper energy level to the lower one occur, with transfer of energy from the spin system to the lattice. The return of the spin system to its equilibrium

* This can be seen by writing Eq. 12.4 for two nuclei of different magnetogyric ratios and sketching the locations of the corresponding peaks in the nmr spectra plotted according to these two modes.

configuration is called relaxation, so this mechanism is called *spin-lattice relaxation*. We wish to find the rate of this process.

First consider the case in which the spin system and the lattice are in equilibrium at temperature T in field H_0. This means that the number of transitions upward must equal the number downward. If W_u is the probability of an upward transition per unit time and W_d is the probability of a downward transition, then $W_u N_+ = W_d N_-$, or $W_d/W_u = 1 + 2\mu H_0/kT$. Combining this with the mean transition probability $W = (W_u + W_d)/2$ gives

$$W_d = W\left(1 + \frac{\mu H_0}{kT}\right) \tag{12.7}$$

$$W_u = W\left(1 - \frac{\mu H_0}{kT}\right) \tag{12.8}$$

Therefore the probability of a downward transition in a magnetic field is slightly greater than the probability of an upward transition.

Now let energy absorption from an rf field take place. The excess number of nuclei in the lower energy state is denoted n, so $n = N_+ - N_-$. The rate of change of n is

$$\frac{dn}{dt} = 2N_- W_d - 2N_+ W_u \tag{12.9}$$

since for each nucleus that makes a transition n changes by 2. Combining Eqs. 12.7–12.9,

$$\frac{dn}{dt} = 2W(n_0 - n) \tag{12.10}$$

where $n_0 = N\mu H_0/kT$ and $N = N_+ + N_-$; n_0 is the value of n when the spin system is in equilibrium with the lattice. Integration of Eq. 12.10 gives

$$n_0 - n = (n_0 - n_i)e^{-2Wt} \tag{12.11}$$

where n_i is the initial value of n. A quantity T_1 is defined by $T_1 = 1/2W$, so that Eq. 12.11 expresses the result that the approach to spin-lattice equilibrium is a first-order process characterized by the first-order rate constant $1/T_1$. T_1 is called the spin-lattice relaxation time.* In liquids, T_1 values for nuclei of spin $\frac{1}{2}$ are often in the range 0.5–50 sec.

We have now to consider the interactions between vicinal nuclei in the spin system. This interaction is of a magnetic dipole-dipole nature. Each nucleus is within the steady field H_0, but is also subjected to a small local magnetic field H_{local}, produced by other nuclei, which are themselves small magnets.

* T_1 is also called the longitudinal relaxation time because it describes the relaxation of the component of the total magnetization vector that is parallel to the field vector H_0.

Since in general the disposition of neighboring nuclei is different for each nucleus, the magnitude of H_{local} will differ at each nucleus. The total magnetic field acting on a nucleus is the vector sum of H_0 and H_{local}. Since this is different at each nucleus, the Larmor precession frequency of each nucleus will be different by a small amount. The range of resonance frequencies for identical nuclei will be of the order $\delta\omega_0 = \gamma H_{local}$. This means that the absorption peak in the nmr spectrum will be not a sharp spike, but a band broadened by the amount $\delta\omega_0$.

There is another type of spin-spin interaction. Two adjacent nuclei can interact to cause a transition. For example, the precessing moment of nucleus A sets up an oscillating magnetic field at nucleus B. The oscillating field thus produced will, at some time, be in phase with the precession of B; nucleus B can absorb energy from this field and undergo transition to the upper level. Simultaneously nucleus A must pass to the lower level. Since the precessional frequencies of the two nuclei will differ by about $\delta\omega_0$, the length of time required for the two nuclei to come into phase will be about $1/\delta\omega_0$. This is the approximate lifetime of a nuclear spin state; it is symbolized T_2 and is called the *spin-spin relaxation* time.* T_2 incorporates both of the spin-spin relaxation mechanisms described.

We have seen that in a steady field H_0 a small excess, n_0, of nuclei are in the lower energy level. The absorption of rf energy reduces this excess by causing transitions to the upper spin state. This does not result in total depletion of the lower level, however, because this effect is opposed by spin-lattice relaxation. A steady state is reached in which a new steady value, n_s, of excess nuclei in the lower state is achieved. Evidently n_s can have a maximum value of n_0 and a minimum value of zero. If n_s is zero, absorption of rf energy will cease, whereas if $n_s = n_0$ a steady-state absorption is observed. It is obviously desirable that the absorption be time-independent, or in other words that n_s/n_0 be close to unity. Quantitative theory gives an expression for this ratio, which is called Z_0, the *saturation factor:*

$$Z_0 = (1 + \gamma^2 H_1{}^2 T_1 T_2)^{-1}$$

It is therefore desirable that the quantity $\gamma^2 H_1{}^2 T_1 T_2$ be as small as possible. The rf field H_1 should be of low power to prevent saturation.

12.2 Chemical Effects in nmr Spectra

The Chemical Shift. All that has been said so far implies that the nmr absorption by a particular isotope should occur at a single frequency for a

* Also called the transverse relaxation time because the magnetization component in the H_1 plane, that is, transverse to H_0, is responsible for exciting the spin-spin transfer of energy.

given field strength. Fortunately for the chemist, this is not the case. Each nucleus has associated with it an electronic environment consisting of electrons in motion. These moving electrons are equivalent to a current, which in the presence of the applied field H_0 will induce a small opposing magnetic field. Since the electronic environment of a nucleus depends upon the molecular structure of the molecule containing it, the magnitude of this secondary field can be different for the same kind of nucleus located in different molecular environments. The effective field may therefore be different at different nuclei because of this "screening" or "shielding" effect; consequently their resonance frequencies will differ slightly. This displacement in resonance frequencies because of differences in shielding is called the *chemical shift*.

According to Eq. 12.3 the resonance frequency is directly proportional to the field strength, so the chemical shift is directly proportional to a difference in frequencies (at constant field) or to a difference in field strengths (at constant frequency). In order to remove this dependency, the shift is expressed on a relative basis by

$$\text{chemical shift} = \frac{H_s - H_r}{H_r} = \frac{\nu_s - \nu_r}{\nu_r} \tag{12.12}$$

where subscript s refers to the sample nucleus and subscript r to a reference nucleus. Since spectra are calibrated in frequency (Hz or cps) rather than field, the definition in terms of frequencies is used. Moreover, since the absolute chemical shift $\nu_s - \nu_r$ is very small,* it is acceptable to replace ν_r in the denominator by the operating rf frequency of the spectrometer. The reference substance nearly universally used is tetramethylsilane, $(CH_3)_4Si$ (TMS), which has 12 equivalent protons. Incorporating these features gives Eq. 12.13 for the chemical shift on the *delta scale:*

$$\delta = \frac{\nu_s - \nu_{\text{TMS}}}{\text{spectrometer frequency}} \times 10^6 \tag{12.13}$$

The factor 10^6 converts δ values to a parts per million (ppm) basis, which gives convenient magnitudes. Nearly all organic protons are less screened than are those in TMS, so the δ scale of chemical shifts is a positive scale with $\delta_{\text{TMS}} = 0$.

Another scale, the *tau scale*, is used by some workers; in this scale the TMS absorption is assigned the value $\tau = 10$ ppm. The two scales are related by $\tau = 10 - \delta$. These definitions apply only to protons. Figure 12.4 is a graphic representation of the δ and τ scales, and corresponding features of nmr spectra as they are ordinarily presented. Figure 12.5 shows the proton nmr

* For the proton, the range of chemical shifts encompasses about 600 Hz at a field of 14.1 kG. Since the proton resonance frequency is 60 MHz at this field, this corresponds to a range of about $600/60 \times 10^6 = 10$ ppm within which most proton chemical shifts will be observed.

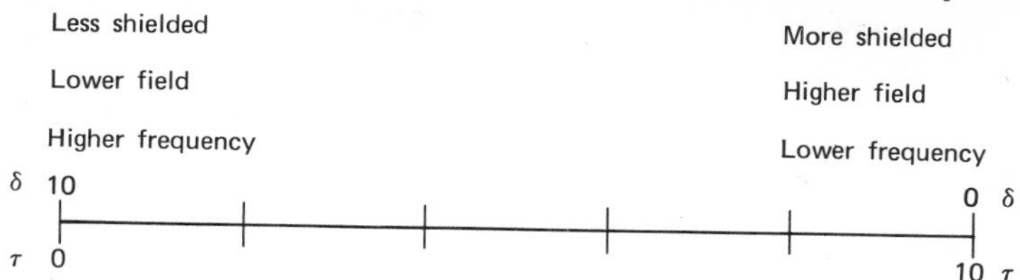

Fig. 12.4. Proton chemical shift scales. The term "less shielded" is synonymous with "more deshielded." "Downfield" and "upfield" refer to lower and higher fields, respectively. TMS has $\delta = 0$.

spectrum of 1,4-dimethoxybenzene, **1**. Because of the symmetry of this molecule the spectrum is very simple, the absorption at $\delta 3.68$ corresponding to the methyl protons and that at $\delta 6.67$ to the aromatic protons.

CH_3O—C_6H_4—OCH_3

1

Spin-Spin Coupling. Many nmr spectra reveal more absorption peaks than there are nonequivalent nuclei in the sample molecule. These peaks tend to appear in groups arranged in easily recognizable patterns, each group being located at a frequency characteristic of the chemical shift for a particular nuclear environment. Figure 12.6 shows an example of this behavior in the proton magnetic resonance (pmr) spectrum of ethyl acetate, $CH_3COOCH_2CH_3$. This division of an absorption peak into multiplets is called *spin-spin splitting;* it arises from a spin-spin coupling interaction between vicinal nuclei. This coupling takes place via the electrons associated with the nuclei, these electrons acting as a medium by which the magnetic spin states of one nucleus can affect the spin states of another nucleus. We therefore observe spin-spin coupling between nonequivalent nuclei that are fairly closely located in the molecule.

An analysis of spin-spin splitting is relatively simple for "first-order" effects, which occur when the chemical shift between two nuclei (or two groups of equivalent nuclei) is large compared with the splitting. The chemical shift, in hertz, between nuclei A and B is $\nu_A - \nu_B = \Delta\nu_{AB}$. The distance between the peaks within the multiplets produced by the splitting is measured in hertz and is called the spin-spin coupling constant J_{AB}. Then first-order spin-spin splitting is observed if Δ_{AB}/J_{AB} is large (at least 10). Spin systems are often described by assigning letters to the nuclei, letters close to each other in the alphabet denoting nuclei with similar chemical shifts. Thus the ethyl group $—CH_2CH_3$ is an A_2X_3 spin system, and a *p*-disubstituted benzene is an A_2B_2 system. An analysis of first-order spin-spin

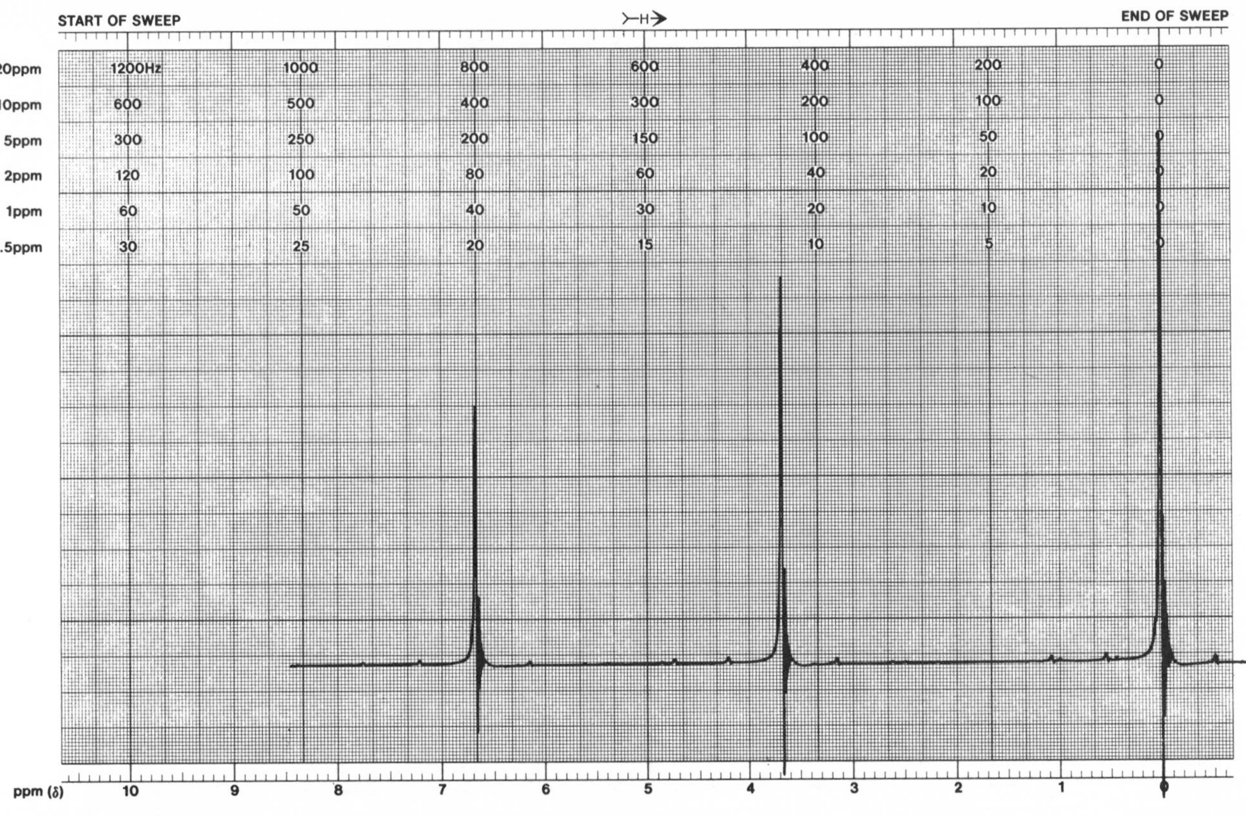

Fig. 12.5. Proton nmr spectrum of 1,4-dimethoxybenzene at 60 MHz; sweep width 600 Hz (10 ppm); solvent carbon tetrachloride; TMS absorption at $\delta = 0.00$.

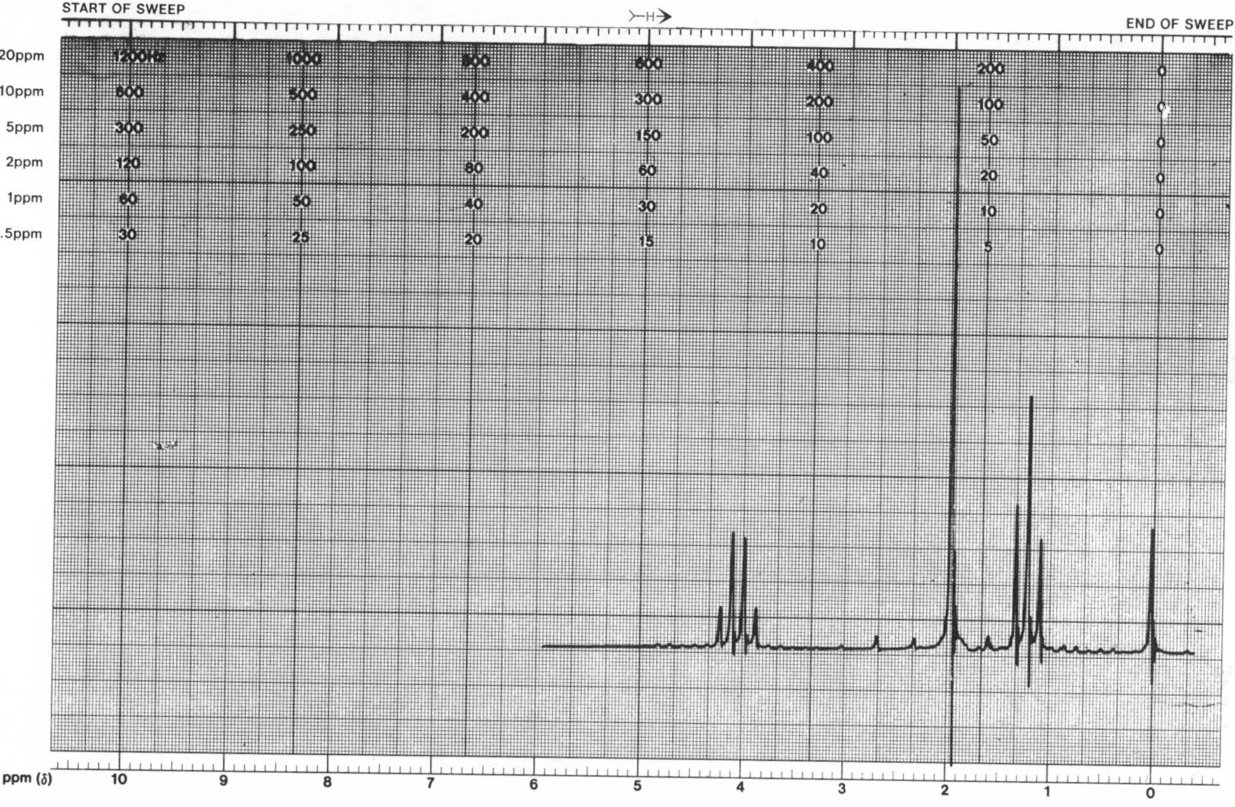

Fig. 12.6. Proton nmr spectrum of ethyl acetate (neat) at 60 MHz; sweep width 600 Hz (10 ppm); TMS reference.

splitting follows these rules:

1. $\Delta\nu/J$ must be large for all spin-spin couplings in the system.
2. A set of n_A equivalent nuclei of type A coupled with n_X equivalent nuclei of type X will produce a resonance signal for A having $2n_XI_X + 1$ peaks; likewise the X signal will be split into $2n_AI_A + 1$ components.
3. The coupling constant J_{AX} is obtained from the spacing of any two submultiplet lines. The coupling constant is the same for the A and X multiplets.
4. The multiplet is symmetrical about its center, which corresponds to the chemical shift for the set of nuclei. The relative intensities of the multiplet peaks are given by the coefficients of the binomial expansion (see the later discussion).

Since the chemical shift is field-dependent whereas J is not, a diagnostic test for whether two peaks represent spin-spin splitting or chemical shift differences is to change the field (or the spectrometer frequency). It is sometimes possible in this way to transform a spectrum into a first-order spin system.

Restricting our consideration to nuclei with $I = \frac{1}{2}$, we will amplify points 2 and 4 above. Splitting is caused by one or more equivalent nuclei in a sense imposing their spin states on one or more nearby nuclei. Therefore by counting the number of different spin states it is possible to predict the number of peaks in the resulting multiplet. Moreover, since each spin state has about the same probability, the intensities of the multiplet lines are determined by the numbers of states contributing to each distinguishable energy state. Figure 12.7 should clarify this. Here the splitting patterns produced by methenyl, methylene, and methyl protons are diagrammed. The single proton in the methenyl group has two states that can influence an adjacent nucleus, so this proton will split the signal of the nearby nucleus into a doublet of relative intensities 1:1. The methylene group has four spin states, but two of these are equivalent, so this group produces a triplet with intensities 1:2:1. This description is oversimplified, but it is adequate to illustrate some of the features and uses of spin-spin splitting. Thus the pmr spectrum of the ethyl group $—CH_2CH_3$ (Fig. 12.6) will contain a triplet and a quartet. This suffices to assign the peaks, since the triplet must be due to the methyl group (being split by coupling with $—CH_2—$), whereas the quartet is assigned to the methylene group (which is split by coupling to the $—CH_3$). Coupling constants, which are often in the range 2–8 Hz, are obtained from the spacings within multiplets. The coupling constant for the ethyl group, obtained from Fig. 12.6, is 7.0 Hz. The chemical shift is measured to the center of the multiplet.

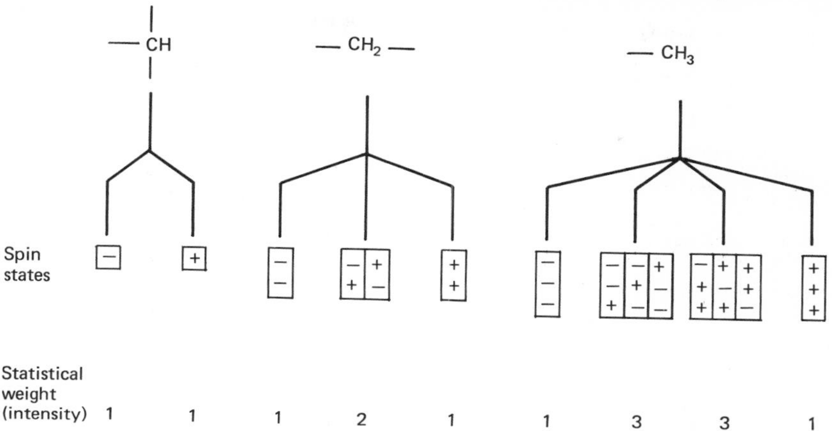

Fig. 12.7. Simplified representation of first-order spin-spin splitting patterns produced by methenyl, methylene, and methyl protons. A minus sign represents spin state $m = -\frac{1}{2}$ and a plus sign represents $m = +\frac{1}{2}$.

Chemical Exchange. If a nucleus can experience two different magnetic environments as a consequence of a chemical equilibrium, it might be expected that distinct resonance peaks will be observed for the two environments. Whether or not two peaks are seen is found to depend upon the rate of the exchange between the two environments. Consider a solution of the weak acid HA and the weak base B. This proton-transfer equilibrium is established:

$$\mathrm{HA + B \rightleftharpoons BH^+ + A^-}$$

At any moment some of the protons will be associated with "site" A and some with "site" B. Let ν_A and ν_B be the proton resonance frequencies of these environments. This system is a dynamic equilibrium, with protons undergoing exchange between A and B very rapidly. If τ_A and τ_B are the lifetimes of HA and BH^+, respectively, then the lifetime of the system is defined as $\tau = \tau_A\tau_B/(\tau_A + \tau_B)$. Then it is found that, if $\tau \gg 1/(\nu_A - \nu_B)$, two absorption lines are observed, at ν_A and ν_B; if $\tau \ll 1/(\nu_A - \nu_B)$, only a single line is observed at a frequency that is between ν_A and ν_B, its precise position being an average of ν_A and ν_B weighted by the proportion of sites occupied.

The intuitive view of this situation is that if the exchange process is much faster than the nmr time scale (which is given roughly by the reciprocal of the frequency), the nmr observation sees only the average environment of the rapidly exchanging nucleus. If the exchange process is slower than the nmr time scale, the nmr experiment detects the separate environments. Figure 12.8 is the nmr spectrum of ethanol containing a trace of strong acid, which catalyzes the exchange of the hydroxyl proton between different molecules. Only one line is seen for the hydroxyl proton, although it is adjacent to a

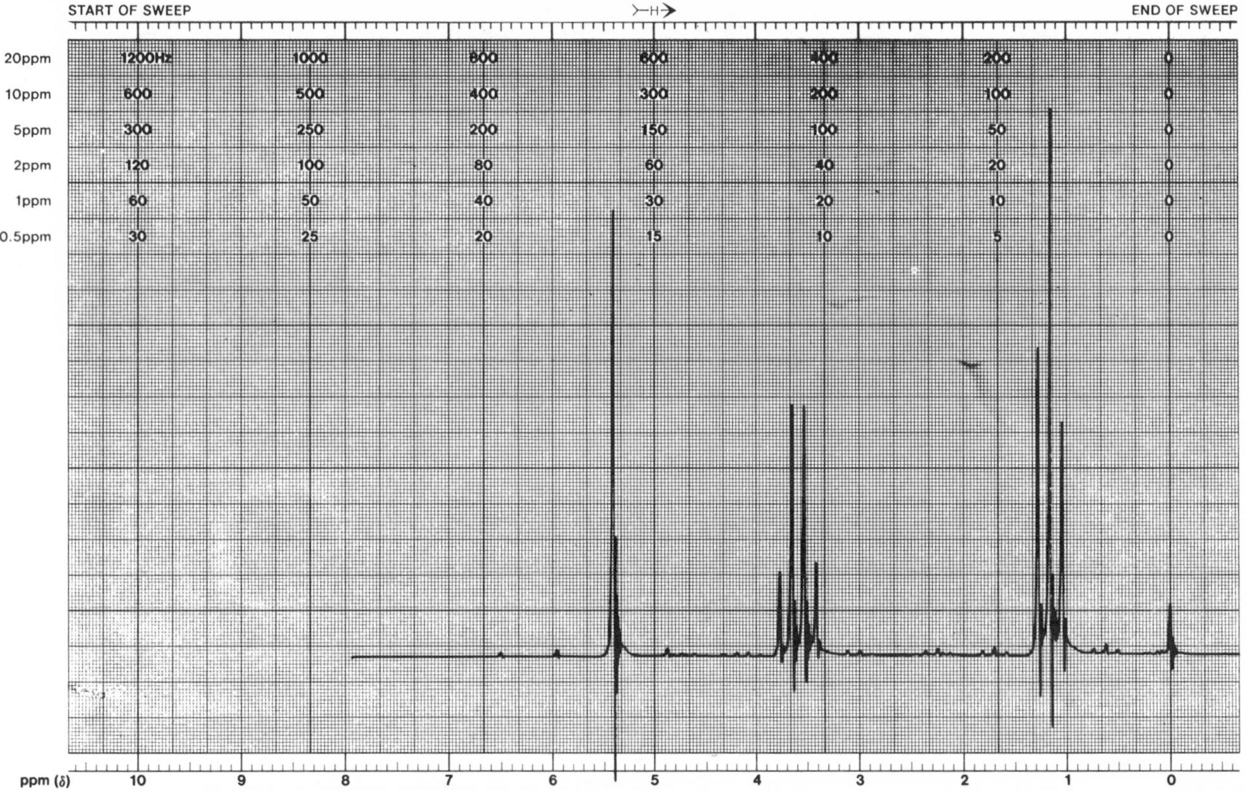

Fig. 12.8. 60 MHz nmr spectrum of ethanol containing a trace of hydrochloric acid; sweep width 600 Hz; TMS reference.

methylene group and might have been expected to be split into a triplet; moveover the methylene absorption, though split by spin-spin coupling with the methyl, is unaffected by the adjacent hydroxyl. This is a consequence of the time-averaging effects of rapid chemical exchange.

Proton transfer is one type of chemical exchange process. Rotation about single bonds (conformational change) is also usually very rapid, but steric or electronic effects may decrease these exchange rates. For example, in *N,N*-dimethylformamide, **2**, the acyl carbon-nitrogen bond has partial double-bond character because of electron delocalization. This results in restricted

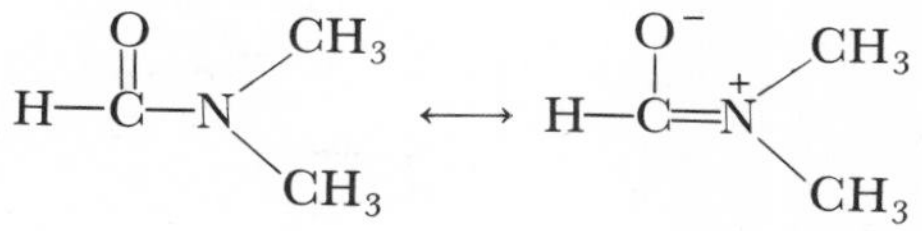

$$H{-}C({=}O){-}N(CH_3)_2 \longleftrightarrow H{-}C(O^-){=}N^+(CH_3)_2$$

2

rotation about this bond, so that the two methyl groups are nonequivalent. At room temperature separate resonances are observed for the protons on these two groups. At high temperature the rate of rotation increases and the two lines coalesce to a single averaged band.

12.3 Analytical Applications

Proton magnetic resonance has found the widest use. Studies of structure and conformation of organic molecules rely heavily on pmr. Chemical shifts can be correlated with structure as shown in Fig. 12.9 for a few kinds of proton environments. The chemical shift of a particular nucleus is sensitive to the nearby environment, so that relationships can be established between, for example, the electronegativity of aromatic substituents and the chemical shifts of aromatic protons. As another example, δ for the $—CH_3$ group depends on the kind of atom (C, O, N, etc.) to which it is bonded.

The assignment of spectral lines to particular protons uses several pieces of information. One of these is chemical shift correlations, as in Fig. 12.9. Another is spin-spin splitting patterns and coupling constants, as described in Section 12.2. A further piece of information is provided by the intensity of absorption, of which the area under the peak is the best measure. As long as the saturation factor is near unity, the area under the peak is proportional to the number of protons responsible for the resonance. Therefore the relative numbers of magnetically different protons in a sample can be obtained from the ratio of integrated areas. Figure 12.10 is the proton spectrum of *tert*-butyl acetate, $CH_3COOC(CH_3)_3$, with an integration trace superimposed on the absorption spectrum. The vertical distance under this trace is proportional to area.

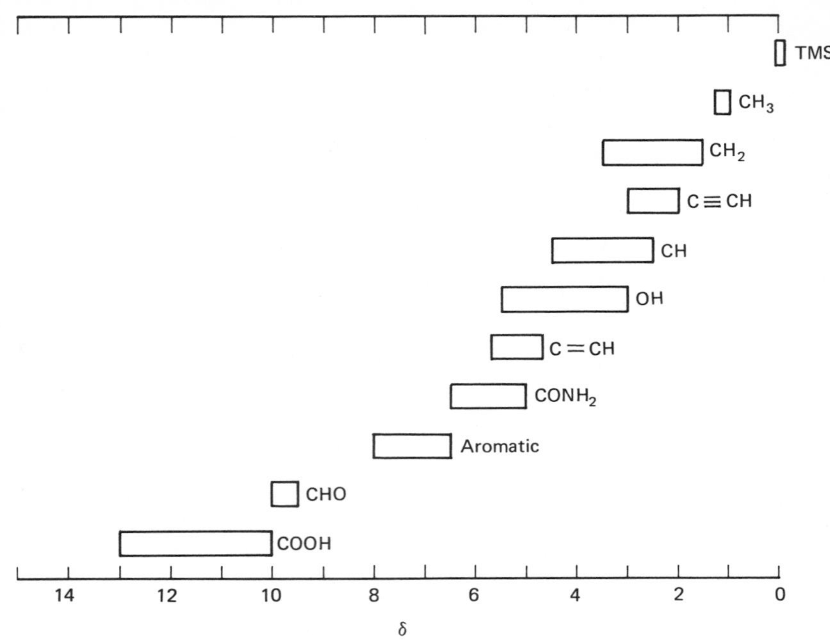

Fig. 12.9. A correlation chart of some proton nmr frequency ranges on the delta chemical shift scale.

Thus the peaks at $\delta 1.38$ and 1.87 have relative areas 3:1, respectively, which unambiguously assigns the former to the butyl group and the latter to the acetate.

The direct proportionality between integrated intensity and number of protons in a sample means that nmr can be used as a quantitative analytical tool. Since all protons absorb with equal intensity, it is not necessary to establish a calibration with the same compound that is being determined; any conveniently absorbing proton-containing compound can be used for calibration. Because of the high resolution of modern nmr spectrometers good selectivity is achieved in analyzing mixtures. An example of this application is the analysis of aspirin, phenacetin, and caffeine (APC) mixtures by pmr [1]. Nmr is not a very sensitive technique compared with other spectroscopic methods.

Table 12.1 shows that many other nuclei should provide information by nmr. ^{19}F nmr has been well studied. Much interesting work is now being done with naturally abundant ^{13}C nmr, which requires very sophisticated experimentation because of the low sensitivity and low abundance of this isotope. ^{13}C nuclei are spin coupled to nearby protons, resulting in very complex spectra. This problem has been overcome by subjecting the protons to rf

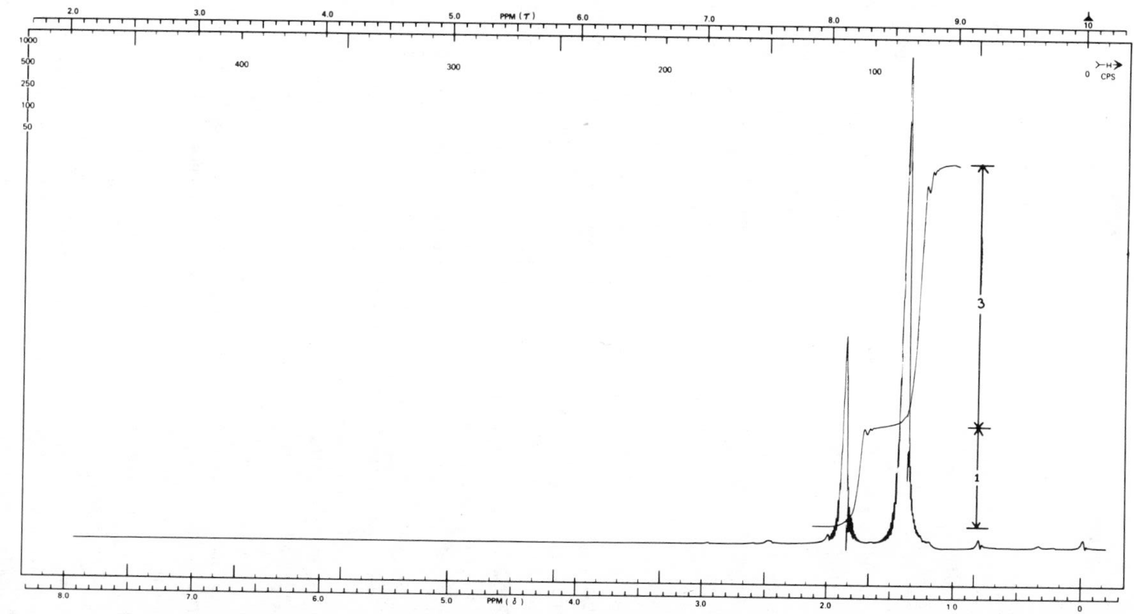

Fig. 12.10. 60 MHz nmr spectrum of *tert*-butyl acetate (neat); sweep width 500 Hz; TMS reference.

radiation corresponding to their own resonance frequencies, which eliminates $^{13}C—^{1}H$ coupling. This technique, called wide-band ^{1}H-decoupling, yields ^{13}C nmr spectra with a single absorption peak for each carbon atom [2]. ^{13}C chemical shifts cover a range of about 200 ppm.

12.4 Determination of nmr Spectra

These four components are basic to any nmr spectrometer [3]:

1. A magnet capable of producing the homogeneous field H_0; both permanent magnets and electromagnets are used.
2. A radio-frequency oscillator to generate the rf field H_1 as shown in Fig. 12.3.
3. A capability of sweeping either the magnetic field or the rf frequency over the range encompassing the chemical shift range of the nuclei of interest.
4. A radio-frequency receiver.

The magnet establishes field H_0, which causes splitting of the nuclear energy levels, making nuclear transitions possible. The other components are analogous to those required for optical absorption spectroscopy (Section 8.5): the rf oscillator is the source of energy, the sweep capability is analogous to a frequency selector, and the rf receiver is the detector. It is desirable to work at as high a value of H_0 as possible, because the absolute value of chemical shift, $\Delta\nu$, is directly proportional to H_0; however, the field must be highly homogeneous. Technological advances have allowed more powerful magnets to be used in modern instruments. According to Eq. 12.3 the rf oscillator frequency and the magnetic field strength are related by the magnetogyric ratio of the nucleus. Therefore if a more powerful magnet is incorporated into the spectrometer, its rf oscillator must generate a higher frequency field H_1. At this time the most commonly encountered nmr spectrometers have rf frequencies of 60, 90, or 100 MHz; some instruments operate at 220 MHz and above. Nmr spectrometers are described by specifying their rf frequency, which is also the quantity used in the denominator of Eq. 12.13 to calculate the chemical shift δ.

The sample, usually in solution at 5–15% concentration with TMS incorporated as an internal reference, is contained in a glass tube, which is placed between the poles of the magnet and within the coils of the rf oscillator. Magnetic field inhomogeneities within the sample are averaged out by spinning the sample tube on its axis. Solvents for proton nmr should preferably contain no protons themselves; carbon tetrachloride and deuterated chloroform are particularly useful.

12.5 Electron Spin Resonance

The electron has a spin number I of $\frac{1}{2}$; hence it has magnetic properties analogous to those of a proton. In a magnetic field electronic Zeeman splitting gives two energy levels, and transitions can be induced just as described for nmr. The resonance frequency is described by Eq. 12.14, which is comparable with Eq. 12.3 for nuclei.

$$\nu = \frac{g\beta H_0}{h} \tag{12.14}$$

In this equation β is the Bohr magneton; $\beta = 0.92732 \times 10^{-20}$ erg/G. The quantity g is called the g factor of the electron; for a free electron $g = 2.0023$.

If H_0 has the typical value 3400 G, then the resonance frequency of the electron is calculated to be 9.5×10^9 Hz (9.5 GHz). Radiation of this frequency is called microwave radiation (because its wavelength is much smaller than the more common radio-frequency radiation).

In most organic molecules all electrons are paired, the electrons within a pair differing in that one is in the $+\frac{1}{2}$ spin state and the other in the $-\frac{1}{2}$ state. A transition by one of these electrons would result in both electrons in the pair (orbital) having the same spin state, which is forbidden by the Pauli exclusion principle. Therefore paired electrons do not absorb energy from the microwave field as described above for the free electron. There are many substances, however, that contain unpaired electrons. These substances, which are said to be paramagnetic, include free radicals, transition metal ions, and the oxygen molecule. Such materials therefore can be studied by this form of spectroscopy, which is called electron spin resonance (esr) or electron paramagnetic resonance (epr).

For instrumental reasons the derivative of the absorption peak, rather than the absorption peak itself, is recorded in esr. The position of absorption is described by calculating the g factor of the electron using Eq. 12.14 and the experimental values of ν and H_0. More information can be obtained from the hyperfine structure of the esr spectrum, which is produced by spin-spin interaction between the unpaired electron and nearby magnetic nuclei. Esr has yielded some valuable information about biological systems such as proteins and membranes by chemically incorporating a paramagnetic substance (a "spin label") in the system and observing the perturbation of its esr signal. Inferences can then be made about the molecular environment in the vicinity of the spin label.

It is interesting to compare some important features of the several forms of absorption spectroscopy that we have studied [4, 5]; see Table 12.2. Notice the relationship between the energy gap separating different energy levels and the percentage population of the upper level.

TABLE 12.2
Comparison of Several Types of Absorption Spectroscopy[a]

Property[b]	nmr	esr	ir	uv-vis
ΔE between energy levels (cal/mole)	10^{-3}	1	300	10^5
λ of absorbed radiation (cm)	3×10^3	3	10^{-2}	3×10^{-5}
Population in excited state (%)	49.9999	49.9	20	Negligible
Lifetime of excited state (sec)	10	10^{-3}		10^{-8}

[a] From Ref. 5.
[b] Typical values are listed.

References

1. Hollis, D. P., *Anal. Chem.*, **35,** 1682 (1963).
2. Levy, G. C. and G. L. Nelson, *Carbon*-13 *Nuclear Magnetic Resonance for Organic Chemists*, Wiley-Interscience, New York, 1972.
3. Jackman, L. M. and S. Sternhell, *Applications of Nuclear Magnetic Resonance Spectroscopy in Organic Chemistry*, 2nd ed., Pergamon Press, Oxford, 1969, Chap. 1–2.
4. Bersohn, M. and J. C. Baird, *An Introduction to Electron Paramagnetic Resonance*, W. A. Benjamin, New York, 1966, p. 8.
5. Poole, C. P., Jr., in *Guide to Modern Methods of Instrumental Analysis*, T. H. Gouw (ed.), Wiley-Interscience, New York, 1972, p. 285.

FOR FURTHER READING

Bible, R. H., Jr., *Guide to the NMR Empirical Method*, Plenum Press, New York, 1967.

Dyer, J. R., *Applications of Absorption Spectroscopy of Organic Compounds*, Prentice-Hall, Englewood Cliffs, N.J., 1965.

Akitt, J. W., *NMR and Chemistry*, Chapman and Hall, London, 1973.

Assenheim, H. M., *Introduction to Electron Spin Resonance*, Plenum Press, New York, 1967.

Silverstein, R. M. and R. G. Silberman, "Troublesome Concepts in NMR Spectrometry," *J. Chem. Educ.*, **50,** 484 (1973).

Problems

1. Predict the number of lines and their relative intensities in a first-order multiplet produced by spin-spin coupling to four equivalent nuclei ($I = \frac{1}{2}$).

2. Why in uv spectroscopy can separate absorption bands be seen for a conjugate acid-base pair, whereas in nmr spectroscopy a single averaged band is seen?

3. The screening effect in nmr is represented by the equation

$$\nu = \frac{\gamma H_0(1 - \sigma)}{2\pi}$$

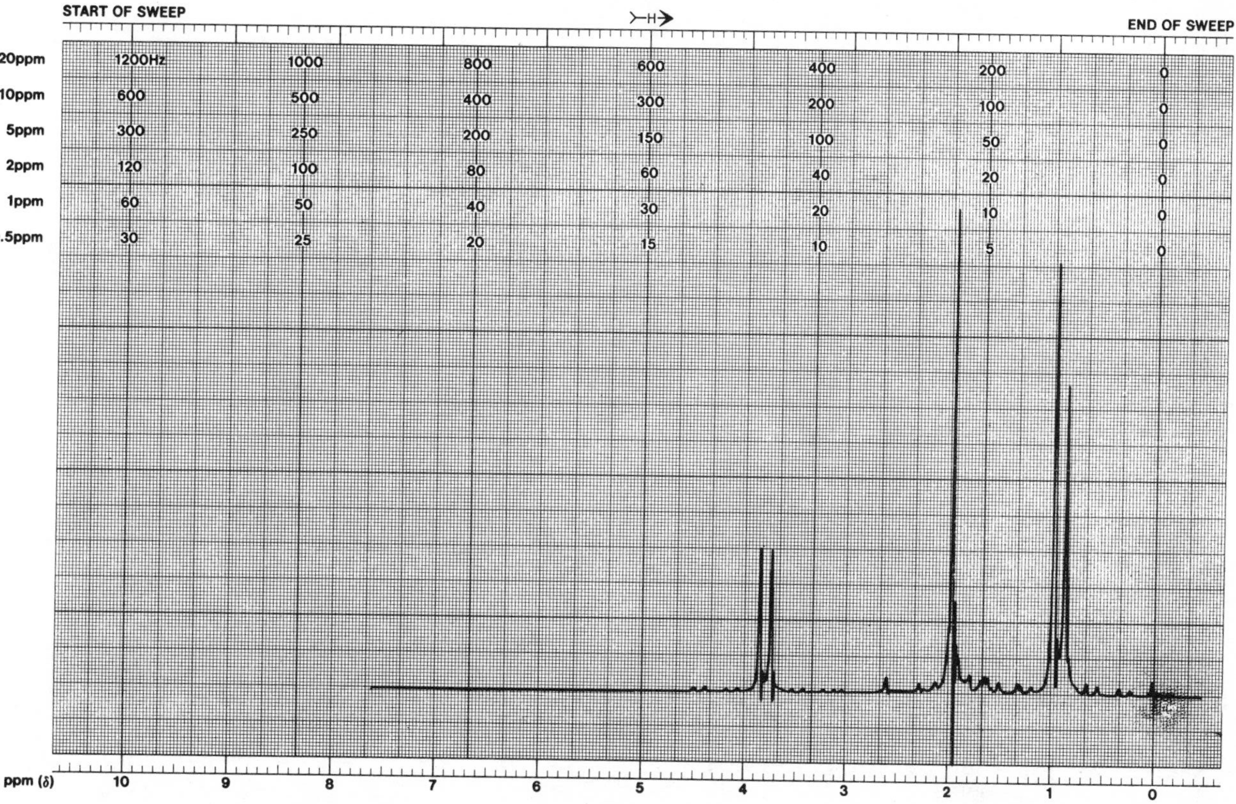

Fig. 12.11. 60 MHz nmr spectrum of isobutyl acetate (neat); sweep width 600 Hz; TMS reference.

where σ is the screening constant. Most organic protons are more deshielded (less screened) than are those of TMS. Show that most chemical shifts on the delta scale will be positive numbers.

4. Give the number of spin states and their magnetic quantum numbers (m) for nuclei of spin numbers $I = \frac{1}{2}$, 1, and $\frac{3}{2}$.

5. Sketch the proton nmr spectra you would expect to observe for these compounds on the basis of information in this chapter.

(*a*) Diethyl carbonate, $CH_3CH_2OCO_2CH_2CH_3$

(*b*) Cl—$CH_2CH_2COOCH(CH_3)_2$

(*c*) 2,4,6-Trimethylbromobenzene

6. Why does a 100 MHz spectrometer have greater sensitivity (i.e., greater response for a given number of nuclei) than a 60 MHz instrument? (Suggestion: see Eq. 12.6.)

7. Speculate on the reason for the relative analytical sensitivities of nmr and uv spectroscopy. (Suggestion: see Table 12.2.)

8. Figure 12.11 is the proton spectrum of isobutyl acetate,

$$CH_3COOCH_2CH(CH_3)_2.$$

Assign the peaks. (Note: the methenyl proton cannot be seen in the spectrum.)

9. Assign the peaks in the proton spectrum of ethyl acetate, Fig. 12.6. Estimate $\Delta\nu/J$ for the ethyl group.

13 MASS SPECTROMETRY

13.1 The Mass Spectrometer

Mass spectrometry (MS) is an old technique that has recently been exploited for organic analysis, particularly for identification and structure determination. In this section we consider the generation and collection of data by the *mass spectrometer*, which has three functions:

1. It produces a beam of ions from the sample substance.
2. It sorts these ions according to their mass-to-charge ratio.
3. It records the relative abundance of each species of ion.

Production of Ions. Many techniques are available to produce ions from neutral molecules, but at the present time the most widely used method is by bombardment of the neutral molecules (in the vapor state at very low pressure) with a beam of high-energy electrons. If an electron has sufficient energy, it can "shoot out" a valence electron from a neutral molecule, producing a positive molecule ion (a radical ion) having an odd number of electrons. Equation 13.1 shows this process, with an electron pair on the target molecule being explicitly shown.

$$\text{M:} + e\ (\text{fast}) \rightarrow \text{M}^{\dagger} + 2e\ (\text{slow}) \tag{13.1}$$

It is the ion $\text{M}^{\dagger}$, and other ions derived from it, that is detected in the mass spectrometer. This ion can be described by its mass-to-charge ratio, which, since it carries unit charge, can be denoted m/e, where m is its mass in atomic mass units (amu) and e represents unit electrical charge. It is conventional to describe ions in terms of m/e, and since most of them are singly charged this is equivalent to describing them in terms of mass.

Figure 13.1 is a schematic diagram of the ion source in a mass spectrometer. Point a represents a tungsten or rhenium filament, which upon heating emits electrons. These electrons are directed along the path of the dashed line by placing a positive potential on plate b. The energy of the electrons in this beam is determined by the potential drop from a to b; this is called the ionizing

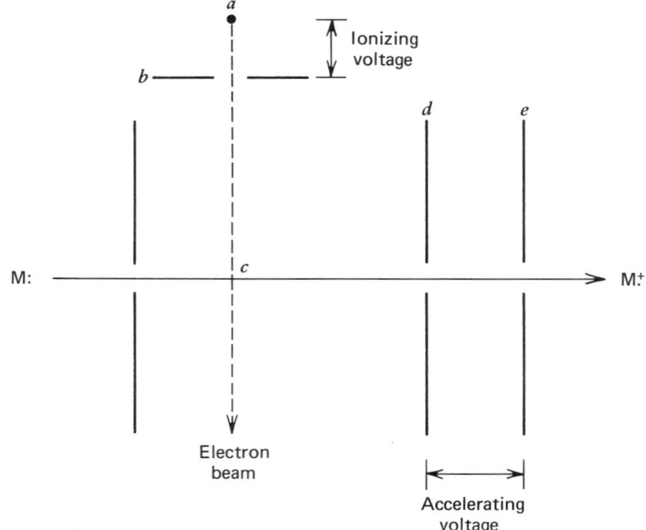

Fig. 13.1. Principle of the electron impact ion source.

voltage. The usual range of energies in the electron beam is 0–100 eV, with a 70 eV source being common.*

The ionizing voltage controls the energy of the electron beam, whereas the ionizing current controls the number of electrons emitted. An increase in ionizing current will therefore increase the probability of electron-molecule collisions at point *c*.

After production of positive ions at *c* by collision of high-energy electrons with neutral molecules, according to Eq. 13.1, the ions are directed and accelerated through slits by means of a potential drop between plates *d* and *e*. This potential drop, which is called the accelerating voltage, is variable within the approximate range 1000–4000 V.

Separation of Ions. Most commercial mass spectrometers use magnetic sorting to separate a beam of ions according to their m/e ratios. This sorting, or dispersion, is based on the principle that an ion injected into a magnetic field will describe a curved path whose radius depends upon m/e, or more exactly, upon mv/e, where v is the velocity of the ion.

A quantitative treatment is very simple. Figure 13.2 is a picture of a mass spectrometer using a so-called 180° magnetic sector. Ions leaving the source

* One electron-volt is the energy developed by unit electric charge falling through a potential of 1 V. The electronic charge is 1.602×10^{-19} C, so 1 eV = 1.602×10^{-19} J. Converting units and placing this on a molar basis shows that 1 eV corresponds to 23.04 kcal/mole. The energy of the MS ion source should be compared with the energies of the several types of absorption spectroscopy (Table 12.2).

have been given energy eV by the accelerating voltage V. Their kinetic energy is $mv^2/2$; therefore

$$eV = \frac{mv^2}{2} \tag{13.2}$$

The centrifugal force (force normal to the tangent) of a particle moving in a circle of radius r is mv^2/r, and this is exactly balanced by the centripetal force Hev exerted by the magnetic field H:

$$Hev = \frac{mv^2}{r} \tag{13.3}$$

Rearranging Eq. 13.3 gives

$$r = \frac{mv}{eH} \tag{13.4}$$

showing how the radius depends on the momentum mv. Eliminating v between Eqs. 13.2 and 13.3,

$$\frac{m}{e} = \frac{H^2r^2}{2V} \tag{13.5}$$

Equation 13.5 shows how the radius r of the trajectory of ions of ratio m/e can be varied by changing either the magnetic field H or the accelerating voltage V. Since the geometry of the instrument is fixed, variation of either H or V will bring ions of differing m/e into coincidence with the exit slit.

It is not necessary to use a 180° magnetic field sector, and Fig. 13.3 shows a 60° sector. The key feature is that the point of origin of the ion beam, the apex of the magnetic field sector, and the point of focus lie on a line. This type of magnetic analyzer produces "direction focusing" of ions having the same velocity but slightly different directions. This is the situation, to a first approximation, produced by the electron impact ion source, which imparts the same energy to all ions; therefore ions of identical mass have the same velocity, but

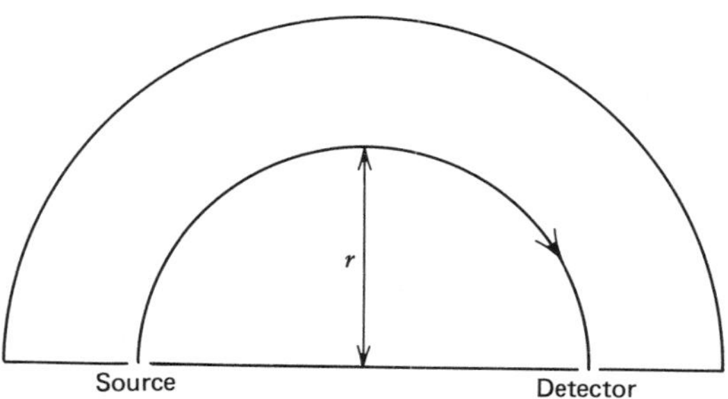

Fig. 13.2. Arrangement of a 180° magnetic sector, showing a trajectory of radius r. The magnetic field is perpendicular to the plane of the paper.

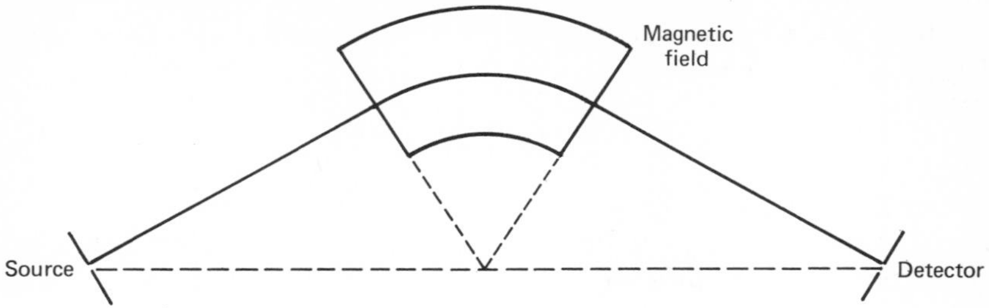

Fig. 13.3. Arrangement of a 60° magnetic sector.

they may have different directions because of the finite width of the slit at the ion source. These ions are brought to focus after traversing 180° [1].

As suggested above, the ion separation process really must accomplish two things: it must separate ions of different m/e values, and it must sharply focus all ions of the same m/e value. The magnetic analyzer carries out both functions, but a complicating factor in direction focusing is that not all ions of the same m/e have exactly the same velocity. One contributor to a variation in velocity is the variable kinetic energy possessed by the ions before acceleration. To achieve higher resolution, double-focusing mass spectrometers have been designed in which "velocity focusing" of ions with different velocities but the same direction is accomplished in an electrostatic field, followed by direction focusing in a magnetic field.

Detection of Ions. If a photographic plate is placed at the plane of focus of the ion beam, all the ions will be collected, each m/e ratio producing an image of the ion source entrance slit. The density of the image will be related to the intensity of the particular beam of ions. A mass spectrometer with photographic detection is called a mass spectrograph. Its advantage is high sensitivity, achieved since the ion beam can be collected over long periods of time to build up a photographic image from a very weak signal. A disadvantage is the long time required to develop and analyze the plate.

Most mass spectrometers now use electron multiplier detectors. The ion beam from the magnetic analyzer impinges on a sensitized electrode surface, which thereupon emits secondary electrons. These electrons are accelerated to another electrode, with a consequent multiplication of electron emission. This process is repeated for several stages until the electrons are collected at a final electrode and the resulting current is measured. Amplification factors of 10^7 can be realized, so this is a very sensitive form of detection. Its response is rapid.

Display and recording can be accomplished by pen-and-ink recorder, oscilloscope, a galvanometer with light-sensitive paper, and, more recently, by direct computer hookup permitting the computer to acquire and process the data from the detector.

13.2 The Mass Spectrum

Data Presentation. A mass spectrum is a plot of ion current intensity (in arbitrary units, plotted on the vertical axis) against *m/e* ratio. The data can also be presented in tabular form. The raw data are usually normalized by converting all intensities to relative intensities on a percentage basis; that is, the most intense peak in the spectrum (the *base peak*) is given the value 100, and the intensities of other peaks are expressed relative to this. Figure 13.4 is a mass spectrum of *n*-valeramide, $CH_3(CH_2)_3CONH_2$, plotted according to these conventions; the base peak is at *m/e* 59. Note that the base peak need not correspond to the *molecular ion* $M^{\dot{+}}$ that is first formed in the electron beam; thus the molecular ion of valeramide has *m/e* 101. Most other ions in the spectrum are derived from the molecular ion.

The presentation of mass spectral data in tables has the advantage that peaks of low intensity are less apt to be overlooked. Table 13.1 gives the mass spectrum of *n*-valeramide in this form.

Resolution. The resolution, or resolving power, of a mass spectrometer is its capability for separating two ion beams of similar *m/e* values. To place this on a quantitative basis a definition of "separation" is needed. Each ion beam will have a finite width, which is determined by instrumental characteristics,

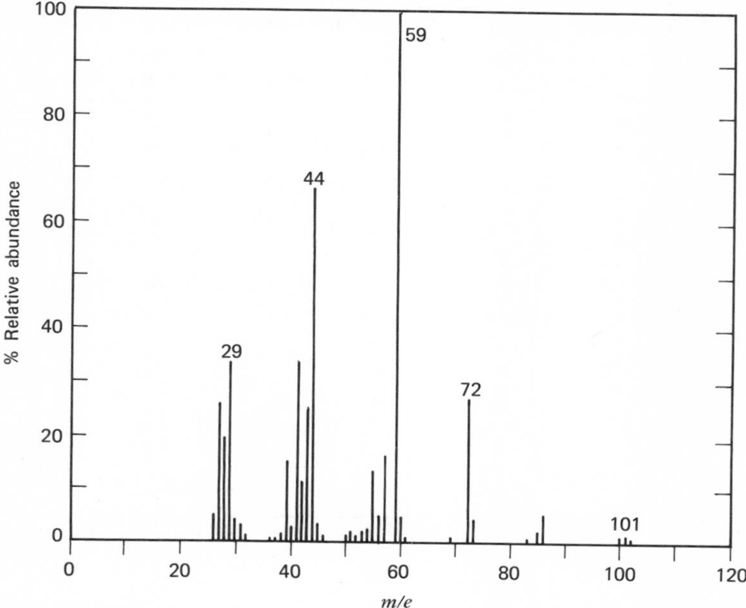

Fig. 13.4. Mass spectrum of *n*-valeramide with *m/e* values of some important peaks indicated (ionizing voltage 70 eV).

TABLE 13.1
Mass Spectrum of n-Valeramide[a]

m/e	% Abundance	m/e	% Abundance	m/e	% Abundance
26	5.3	42	11.7	59	100.0
27	26.7	43	25.0	60	4.7
28	20.0	44	66.7	61	0.4
29	33.3	45	3.7	69	0.5
30	4.3	46	1.3	72	26.7
31	3.2	50	1.2	73	4.7
32	1.2	51	1.3	83	0.7
36	0.4	52	0.8	85	2.7
37	0.7	53	2.3	86	5.3
38	1.8	54	2.7	100	0.8
39	15.0	55	13.3	101	1.1
40	2.7	56	4.7	102	0.4
41	33.3	57	16.7		

[a] See Fig. 13.4.

especially the slit width of the ion source. The detector slit width also is involved, since if two adjacent beams are incident on this slit simultaneously they will be recorded together. The resolution is therefore a function of the separation of adjacent beams (the distance d between centers of adjacent peaks, as in Fig. 13.5*a*) and the width of one of the peaks, w. Resolution is then calculated [2] by

$$R = \frac{d}{w} \cdot \frac{M}{\Delta M} \tag{13.6}$$

where M is the mass of the ion whose peak width is w, and ΔM is the mass difference between the two ions.

If the two peaks are completely but minimally separated, as in Fig. 13.5*b*, then $d = w$ and $R = M/\Delta M$; this condition is described as resolution with

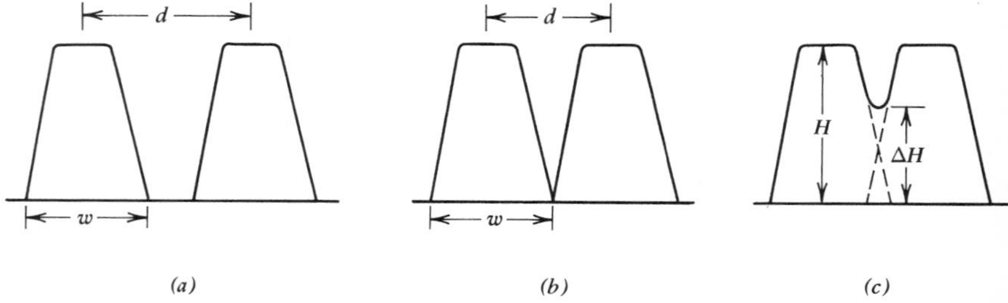

Fig. 13.5. Resolution of two idealized peaks of equal intensity: (*b*) shows resolution with 0% valley, and (*c*) shows resolution with 100 $\Delta H/H$% valley.

0% valley. Often it is unnecessarily conservative to insist on 0% valley resolution, and a more common criterion measures resolution with 10% valley. This means that $\Delta H/H = 0.1$, where these quantities are defined in Fig. 13.5*c*. The resolution of a pair of peaks at 10% valley is calculated with Eq. 13.6 by measuring w where $\Delta H/H = 0.05$; that is, one in effect draws a new base line at a height corresponding to one-half the selected valley definition; the peak width w is measured on this new base line.

Mass spectrometers are roughly categorized according to their resolution into these classes:

Low-resolution	$R < 200$
Medium-resolution	$R = 500\text{–}5000$
High-resolution	$R > 10{,}000$

For much organic analytical work medium resolution is acceptable, since it is required only to distinguish between ions whose nominal m/e values differ by 1 unit. High-resolution MS is required to resolve heavy ions with the same nominal mass but different exact masses. For example, a resolution of only 44 is needed to resolve the ions $C_3H_8{}^+$ (m/e 44) and $C_3H_7{}^+$ (m/e 43). To resolve the molecular ions of N_2 (m/e 28.006148) and CO (m/e 27.994915), both having nominal mass 28, requires a resolution of about 2500, and separation of $C_6H_5N_2{}^+$ from $C_6H_5CO^+$ requires a resolution of about 9300.

Types of Ions. Equation 13.1 is usually written without the electron pair explicitly indicated, that is,

$$M + e \rightarrow M^+ + 2e$$

The ion M^+ is the *molecular ion* or *parent ion*. Identification of the molecular ion in the mass spectrum immediately gives the molecular weight of the sample compound.

Organic compounds contain elements that occur naturally as mixtures of isotopes, for example, ^1H and ^2H; ^{12}C and ^{13}C; ^{16}O, ^{17}O, and ^{18}O; ^{32}S, ^{33}S and ^{34}S; ^{35}Cl and ^{37}Cl; and ^{79}Br and ^{81}Br. Molecules containing the less abundant isotopes give rise to *isotopic ions*, whose position and intensity in the mass spectrum depend upon the formula of the compound and the relative abundances of the isotopes. Thus the atom of chlorine in a monochloro compound could be either ^{35}C or ^{37}Cl. The relative abundance of these isotopes is about 3:1, therefore two molecular ion peaks will be seen in the mass spectrum, the peaks being separated by two mass units, with the lower mass peak having three times the intensity of the other.

The relative abundances of ^{12}C and ^{13}C are about 99% and 1%, respectively. Therefore the one-carbon compound CH_4 is expected to show a peak at m/e 17 due to $^{13}CH_4$ that is about 1% as intense as the molecular ion peak at m/e 16. The situation in ethane is more complicated, with each of the two carbons having an equal probability of being a ^{13}C. Besides the normal molecule $^{12}CH_3—^{12}CH_3$ with *m/e* 30, there will be a peak at *m/e* 31 with relative intensity 2% due to $^{13}CH_3—^{12}CH_3$, and a peak at *m/e* 32 with intensity 0.01% due to $^{13}CH_3—^{13}CH_3$. These ratios are a consequence of the natural abundance of ^{13}C and its random distribution.

The $M + 1$ peak (where M represents the *m/e* value of the molecular ion) can also gain intensity from other isotopic substitutions, including ^2H for ^1H and ^{15}N for ^{14}N. The $M + 2$ peak receives its greatest contribution from ^{18}O and ^{34}S. Halogen isotope ions are very distinctive because of their high abundances, as already noted for chlorine; ^{79}Br and ^{81}Br occur in about 1:1 ratio.

The molecular and isotopic ions account for a few of the peaks seen in a typical mass spectrum, but the majority of peaks are caused by *fragment ions*, which arise from bond cleavages within the molecular ion after it is formed but before it enters the magnetic analyzer. When the radical ion $M^{\ddagger}$ undergoes fragmentation by simple fission, a neutral radical is eliminated and an even-electron ion is produced and observed in the mass spectrum. The neutral fragment is not seen in the spectrum. A simple example is shown for the following hydrocarbon fragmentation:

$$[R_3C—CR_3]^{\ddagger} \rightarrow R_3C\cdot + R_3C^+$$

Isotopic ions fragment in the same way to yield isotopic fragment ions, whose identification can assist in establishing the pattern of fragmentation. The common fragmentation processes are described in Section 13.3.

Rearrangement ions are those arising from intramolecular processes. *Metastable ions* are those that undergo fragmentation while in transit in the magnetic analyzer. The apparent mass of a metastable ion therefore depends upon instrumental characteristics as well as the masses of the original and the product ions. Small amounts of *multiply charged ions* may be produced; the mass spectrometer actually sorts according to mass-to-charge ratio, which is equal to *m/e* if the ion is singly charged. Appearance of a peak at a half-integral value of *m/e* indicates a doubly charged ion of odd mass. Multiply charged ions are common in inorganic MS.

13.3 Fragmentation Processes

Conventions. As a result of much experimentation it has been learned that the mass spectrum of an organic compound often can be rationalized in terms of fragmentation processes that are closely similar to reactions that occur in solution. There is little evidence that fragmentation actually occurs in this way, but this "mechanistic" approach is nevertheless very successful in predicting and interpreting mass spectra [3].

It is very useful in this work to simplify the "electronic bookkeeping" with appropriate symbols. A curved arrow represents a two-electron shift, as in

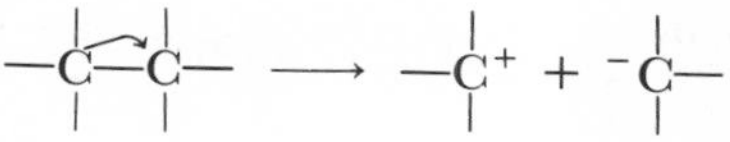

$$-\overset{|}{\underset{|}{C}}-\overset{|}{\underset{|}{C}}- \longrightarrow -\overset{|}{\underset{|}{C}}^{+} + {}^{-}\overset{|}{\underset{|}{C}}- \qquad (13.7)$$

A fishhook arrow signifies a one-electron shift:

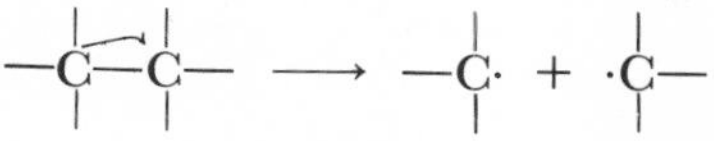

$$-\overset{|}{\underset{|}{C}}-\overset{|}{\underset{|}{C}}- \longrightarrow -\overset{|}{\underset{|}{C}}\cdot + \cdot\overset{|}{\underset{|}{C}}- \qquad (13.8)$$

As in normal usage, a dash represents a two-electron covalent bond.

Fission sites often are indicated on a molecular formula with the mass numbers of the ions generated, as shown in **1**, **2**, and **3**.

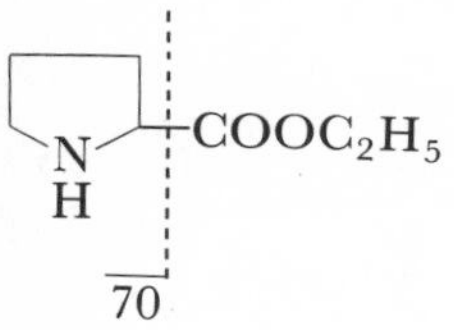

$COOC_2H_5$ N H 70

1

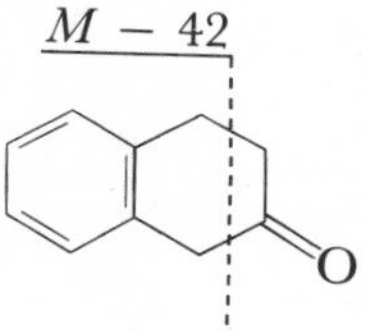

$M - 42$ O

2

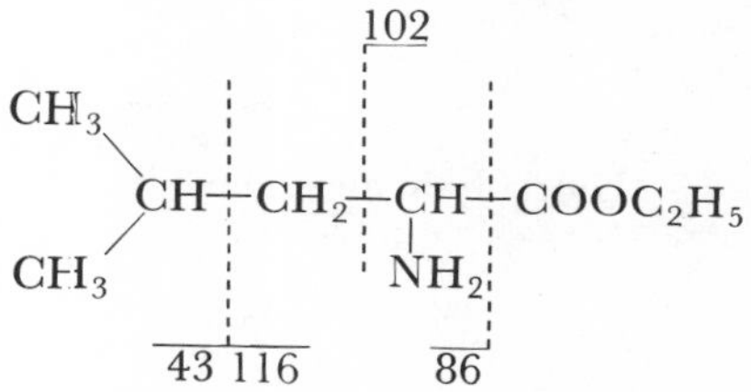

102 CH_3 $CH-CH_2-CH-COOC_2H_5$ CH_3 NH_2 43 116 86

3

The key premise of the mechanistic interpretation of fragmentations is that the positive charge on an ion is localized on one atom (or very few atoms), usually a heteroatom or π system, in accordance with familiar chemical principles. Thus the molecular ion produced from acetone is plausibly written as **4**.

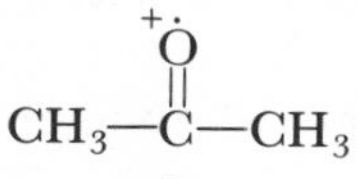

$$CH_3-\overset{\overset{+\cdot}{O}}{\overset{\|}{C}}-CH_3$$

4

This convention permits further reasonable electron shifts to be predicted, and these predictions are widely consistent with observed spectra.

Types of Fission. There is a very low probability that two molecular ions will collide, so it can be expected that most observed ions will be formed by unimolecular reactions of $M^{+\cdot}$. The most abundant ions in the spectrum will be formed as a consequence of these energetic features [4]:

1. The relative stabilities of the bonds in the ion undergoing reaction.
2. The relative stabilities of the ion and neutral fragments that can form via the several competing reaction paths.
3. The relative energetic advantage of possible intramolecular pathways.

Even-electron ions are usually more stable than odd-electron ions because of the stabilizing effect of electron pairing. Therefore the molecular ion $M^{+\cdot}$, unless stabilized by some structural feature, tends to fragment so as to produce an even-electron ion. This can happen in several ways [3]*:

1. Homolytic fragmentation alpha to the positive charge; this is called α fission.

$$-\overset{|}{\underset{|}{C}}-\overset{|}{\underset{|}{C}}-\overset{+\cdot}{X} \longrightarrow -\overset{|}{\underset{|}{C}}\cdot + \;>C{=}X^+$$

2. Intramolecular homolytic bond formation (rearrangement).

$$\begin{matrix} >C-\overset{+\cdot}{X} \\ C-Y \end{matrix} \qquad \begin{matrix} >C-X^+ \\ \qquad | \\ C\cdot \qquad Y \end{matrix}$$

3. Heterolytic cleavage of the bond.

$$-\overset{|}{\underset{|}{C}}-\overset{|}{\underset{|}{C}}-\overset{+\cdot}{X} \longrightarrow -\overset{|}{\underset{|}{C}}-\overset{|}{\underset{|}{C}}{}^+ + X\cdot$$

The ions thus produced from the molecular ion can themselves fragment by these processes. Some examples will now be given to illustrate these points. More systematic treatments can be found in many sources [2–6].

(*a*) Saturated hydrocarbons. Because the positive charge is not localized in these molecular ions, fragmentation patterns may not be easily predicted. A useful rule is that the relative abundances of fragment ions are determined by the stability sequence tertiary > secondary > primary.

(*b*) Fission of carbon-heteroatom bond. The two possibilities are heterolysis and homolysis.

$$R-\overset{+\cdot}{X} \longrightarrow R^+ + X\cdot$$

$$R-\overset{+\cdot}{X} \longrightarrow R\cdot + X^+$$

The second process if favored for X = I because of the stability of the iodonium ion; for X = F, Cl, Br, OR′, SR′, NR'_2 the first process is preferred.

(*c*) Fission of α carbon-carbon bond. The heteroatom may be singly or doubly bonded, and the resulting ion is often a relatively stable onium ion.

* If, however, an even-electron neutral fragment is very stable (such as H_2O, CO, N_2), its loss may be very favorable.

$$\overset{\text{H}}{\underset{}{\text{CH}_2}}\text{—}\overset{+\cdot}{\text{O}}\text{H} \xrightarrow{-\text{H}\cdot} \text{CH}_2\text{=}\overset{+}{\text{O}}\text{H}$$

m/e 31 (base peak for methanol)

$$\text{R—}\underset{\text{R}}{\overset{\overset{+\cdot}{\text{X}}}{\text{C}}}\text{—R} \longrightarrow \text{R—}\underset{\text{R}}{\overset{\overset{+}{\text{X}}}{\text{C}}} + \cdot\text{R}$$

When two substituents can be lost, usually loss of the larger one is preferred.

$$\underset{\substack{m/e\ 73 \\ (1.5\%)}}{\text{CH}_3\text{CH}_2\text{CH}_2\text{CH=}\overset{+}{\text{O}}\text{H}} \xleftarrow{-\text{H}\cdot} \text{CH}_3\text{CH}_2\text{CH}_2\text{—}\underset{\text{H}}{\text{CH}}\text{—}\overset{+\cdot}{\text{O}}\text{H} \xrightarrow{-\text{C}_3\text{H}_7\cdot} \underset{\substack{m/e\ 31 \\ (100\%)}}{\text{CH}_2\text{=}\overset{+}{\text{O}}\text{H}}$$

$$\text{CH}_3\text{—}\overset{\overset{+\cdot}{\text{O}}}{\text{C}}\text{—H} \longrightarrow \text{CH}_3\cdot + \underset{m/e\ 29}{\text{H—C}\equiv\text{O}^+} \qquad (13.9)$$

Because of this preference for loss of the larger radical, as in Eq. 13.9, aldehydes always show a peak at *m/e* 29. Methyl esters give two peaks corresponding to these fissions:

$$\text{R}\overset{a}{|}\overset{\overset{+\cdot}{\text{O}}}{\text{C}}\overset{b}{|}\text{OCH}_3 \begin{cases} \xrightarrow{a} \text{R}\cdot + {}^+\text{O}\equiv\text{C—OCH}_3 \quad m/e\ 59 \\ \xrightarrow{b} \cdot\text{OCH}_3 + \text{R—C}\equiv\text{O}^+ \quad m/e\ M-31 \end{cases}$$

(*d*) β Fission in unsaturated and aromatic systems. In these molecules the charge localization is not so clear-cut. β fission is favored when stabilization of the resulting ion by resonance is possible:

$$[\text{R—CH}_2\text{—CH=CH—R}']^{+\cdot} \longrightarrow \text{R}\cdot + \begin{cases} {}^+\text{CH}_2\text{—CH=CH—R}' \\ \updownarrow \\ \text{CH}_2\text{=CH—}\overset{+}{\text{C}}\text{H—R}' \\ \updownarrow \\ \overset{+}{\text{H}}\text{C—CH—R}' \text{ (bridged by CH}_2\text{)} \end{cases}$$

Substituted aromatics cleave β to the aromatic ring with the production of the benzyl ion, which rearranges to the more stable tropylium ion:

$$\left[C_6H_5\text{—}CH_2 \vdots X\right]^{+\cdot} \longrightarrow \left[C_6H_5\text{—}CH_2\right]^{+\cdot} \longrightarrow C_7H_7^+ \quad (m/e\ 91) \tag{13.10}$$

(*e*) The McLafferty rearrangement. This very general rearrangement illustrates the possibilities of intramolecular processes. The two requirements are a double bond at D—E and a γ hydrogen at A:

$$\text{H–}\gamma\text{A–}\beta\text{B–}\alpha\text{C–D(=E}^{+\cdot}\text{)–F} \longrightarrow \text{A=B} + \text{C=D(–F)–E}^{+\cdot}\text{–H} \tag{13.11}$$

Note that a neutral fragment and a radical ion result. Equations 13.12–13.14 show McLafferty rearrangements of ketones, esters, and aromatics, respectively.

$$\text{H–CH}_2\text{–CH}_2\text{–CH}_2\text{–C(=O}^{+\cdot}\text{)–CH}_3 \longrightarrow \text{CH}_2\text{=CH}_2 + \text{CH}_2\text{=C(–CH}_3\text{)–}\overset{+\cdot}{\text{O}}\text{H} \tag{13.12}$$

$$\text{R–CH(H)–CH}_2\text{–CH}_2\text{–C(=O}^{+\cdot}\text{)–OCH}_3 \longrightarrow \text{R–CH=CH}_2 + \text{CH}_2\text{=C(–OCH}_3\text{)–}\overset{+\cdot}{\text{O}}\text{H} \tag{13.13}$$

$$\left[\text{R–CH(H)–CH}_2\text{–CH}_2\text{–C}_6\text{H}_5\right]^{+\cdot} \longrightarrow \text{R–CH=CH}_2 + \left[\text{CH}_2\text{=C}_6\text{H}_6\right]^{+\cdot} \tag{13.14}$$

The base peak in Fig. 13.4 results from a McLafferty rearrangement.

(*f*) Four-membered cyclic rearrangements. A common rearrangement involves hydrogen radical transfer within a four-membered cyclic structure. Equation 13.15 shows the process for an alcohol, whose molecular ion (m/e 102) first undergoes α fission, the resulting m/e 59 ion then rearranging with hydrogen transfer.

$$\underset{m/e\ 102}{CH_3CH_2\overset{\overset{+\cdot}{O}H}{|}{CH}-CH_2CH_2CH_3} \xrightarrow{-C_3H_7\cdot} \underset{m/e\ 59}{CH_3CH_2\overset{\overset{+}{O}H}{\|}{CH}} \longleftrightarrow \begin{matrix} H & \overset{+}{C}H-OH \\ | & | \\ CH_2 - & CH_2 \end{matrix} \longrightarrow CH_2{=}CH_2 + \underset{m/e\ 31}{CH_2{=}\overset{+}{O}H \longleftrightarrow \overset{+}{C}H_2-OH} \quad (13.15)$$

Triethylamine undergoes two such rearrangements after an initial α fission:

$$\underset{m/e\ 101}{CH_3CH_2-\overset{CH_2CH_3}{\underset{+\cdot}{N}}-CH_2-CH_3} \xrightarrow{-CH_3\cdot} \underset{H}{CH_2}-CH_2-\overset{CH_2CH_3}{\underset{+}{N}}{=}CH_2 \quad m/e\ 86$$

$$\downarrow -CH_2{=}CH_2 \quad (13.16)$$

$$\underset{m/e\ 30}{H-\overset{H}{\underset{+}{N}}{=}CH_2} \xleftarrow{-CH_2=CH_2} \begin{matrix} H-CH_2 \\ CH_2 \\ H-\underset{+}{N}{=}CH_2 \end{matrix} \quad m/e\ 58$$

13.4 Interpretation of Mass Spectra

Usually the information sought is the structure of a compound, and the interpretation of the mass spectrum will provide part of the information required. Other data will usually be used in conjunction with MS, in particular uv, ir, and nmr spectra. Often the elemental composition will be known.

The mass spectrum should first be examined for the presence of an obvious molecular ion peak. This gives the molecular weight to the nearest mass unit. High-resolution MS may yield the empirical formula. The abundance of the molecular ion peak tells something about its stability. The isotope pattern may be significant (see Section 13.2).

If m/e is even for the molecular ion, it contains no, or an even number of, nitrogen atoms; if it is odd, it contains an odd number of nitrogen atoms.

The fragmentation ions should be examined for characteristic mass losses from the parent ion. Table 13.2 shows some of these and their possible

TABLE 13.2
Characteristic Neutral Fragment Losses

Ion m/e[a]	Neutral Fragment Lost	Tentative Inference
$M - 1$	H	Aldehyde
$M - 15$	CH_3	Methyl group
$M - 18$	H_2O	Alcohol
$M - 28$	C_2H_4, CO, N_2[b]	McLafferty rearrangement, CO present, etc.
$M - 29$	CHO, C_2H_5[b]	Aldehyde, ethyl group
$M - 31$	OCH_3	Methyl ester
$M - 34$	H_2S	Thiol
$M - 35$, $M - 36$	Cl, HCl	Chloride
$M - 43$	CH_3CO, C_3H_7[b]	Methyl ketone, propyl group
$M - 45$	COOH	Carboxylic acid
$M - 60$	CH_3COOH	Acetate

[a] M = mass of molecular ion.
[b] Alternatives can be distinguished by high-resolution MS.

structural meanings. Table 13.3 lists some characteristic fragment ions. Structural inferences drawn at this stage are very tentative. Upon preliminary identification of fragment ions and neutral losses, the responsible fragmentation processes are proposed. In this procedure it is helpful to know if two or more peaks are related by a fragmentation process. Table 13.4 gives the mass relationships between source and product ions. Whether two or more ions in the spectrum are related by a fragmentation process can sometimes be established by the mass of a metastable ion peak.

TABLE 13.3
Characteristic Fragment Ions

Ion m/e	Fragment
29	CHO
30	CH_2NH_2
31	CH_2OH, OCH_3
43	CH_3CO, C_3H_7
29, 43, 57, 71, . . .	C_2H_5, C_3H_7, . . .
39, 50, 51, 52, 65, 77	Aromatic fragmentations
60	CH_3COOH
91	$C_6H_5CH_2$
105	C_6H_5CO

TABLE 13.4
Mass Relationships in Fragmentation Processes

Process	m/e Source Ion	m/e Product Ion[a]
Simple fission	Even	Odd
	Odd	Even
Rearrangement	Even	Even
	Odd	Odd

[a] Unless a neutral fragment containing a nitrogen atom is lost.

The mass spectrum may also be used simply as confirmatory evidence of identity—the compound's "fingerprint"—by comparing the mass spectra of the sample compound and an authentic specimen. This comparison can be most efficiently carried out by computer, and one way to identify compounds is by computer matching of the mass spectrum of the unknown with a spectrum from a "library" of known spectra. The mass spectrum of a compound is unique; and is perhaps the single most powerful piece of evidence for establishing identity. A powerful use of MS is as the detector in gas chromatography (Chapter 18).

References

1. Beynon, J. H., *Mass Spectrometry and its Applications to Organic Chemistry*, Elsevier Publishing Co., Amsterdam, 1960.
2. Hamming, M. C. and N. G. Foster, *Interpretation of Mass Spectra of Organic Compounds*, Academic Press, New York, 1972.
3. Budzikiewicz, H., C. Djerassi, and D. H. Williams, *Mass Spectrometry of Organic Compounds*, Holden-Day, San Francisco, 1967.
4. McLafferty, F. W., *Mass Spectrometry of Organic Ions*, Academic Press, New York, 1963, Chapter 7.
5. Hill, H. C., *Introduction to Mass Spectrometry*, Heyden and Son, London, 1966.
6. McLafferty, F. W., *Interpretation of Mass Spectra*, W. A. Benjamin, New York, 1966.

FOR FURTHER READING

Kiser, R. W., *Introduction to Mass Spectrometry and Its Applications*, Prentice-Hall, Inc., Englewood Cliffs, N.J., 1965.

Biemann, K., "Applications of Mass Spectrometry," in *Elucidation of Organic Structures by Physical and Chemical Methods*, 2nd ed., K. W. Bentley and G. W. Kirby (eds.), Part I, Wiley-Interscience, New York, 1972, Chap. V.

Problems

1. What resolution (0% valley) is required to resolve the molecular ions of ^{35}Cl-chlortetracycline and ^{37}Cl-chlortetracycline?

2. Predict the two most probable fragment ions in the mass spectrum of ethanolamine, $H_2NCH_2CH_2OH$.

3. The mass spectrum of a compound showed significant peaks at *m/e* 27, 31, 41, 43, 56 (base peak), and 74 (molecular ion). Give a reasonable structure for the compound, and rationalize the *m/e* values.

4. Predict the *m/e* values of the major peaks in the mass spectrum of methyl isobutyl ketone.

$$CH_3\overset{\overset{\displaystyle O}{\|}}{C}CH_2CH(CH_3)_3$$

5. Figure 13.6 is the mass spectrum of *p*-hydroxybenzaldehyde. On the basis of information given in this chapter, identify the structural features or fragmentations responsible for the ions whose *m/e* values are given. Why is the *m/e* 29 peak much less abundant than the $M - 1$ peak?

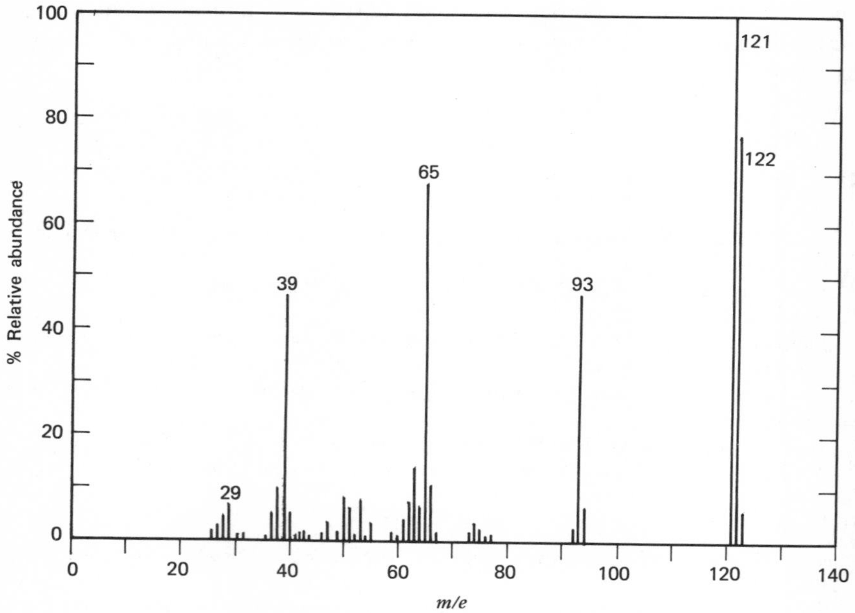

Fig. 13.6. Mass spectrum of *p*-hydroxybenzaldehyde.

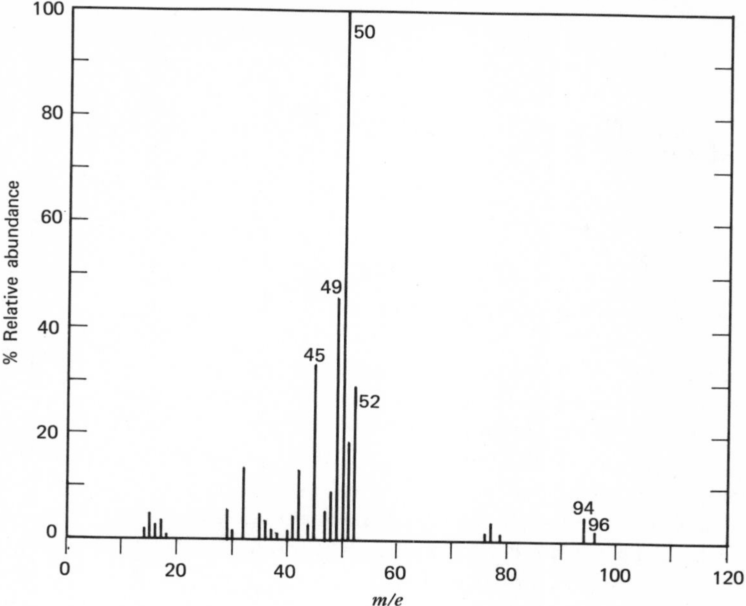

Fig. 13.7. Mass spectrum of a chlorine-containing compound; see Problem 7.

6. Identify the fragmentations responsible for the indicated ions in the mass spectrum of *n*-valeramide (Fig. 13.4).

7. A white solid compound known to contain chlorine gave the mass spectrum shown in Fig. 13.7. What is the structure of the compound?

14 DENSITY MEASUREMENT

14.1 Density and Specific Gravity

Measurements with the ordinary analytical balance are among the most accurate of determinations possible in a typical chemical laboratory. Suppose a 10 g sample is weighed on an analytical balance capable of 0.2 mg reproducibility; the precision of this measurement is about 2 parts per 100,000. With sufficient attention to possible sources of systematic error, accuracy of this order is also attainable. Gravimetric analysis makes use of this capability of the balance; the sample compound, or a suitable derivative of it, is quantitatively isolated and weighed to give a measure of the amount of compound in the portion of sample taken for analysis. The accuracy is limited by the derivatization and isolation steps, not by the final weighing.*

The amount of matter contained in unit volume of any substance is a quantity characteristic of that substance at constant temperature and pressure. This quantity is the density. In practical work the physical property usually encountered is the *specific gravity*, $d_{t'}^{\,t}$. The specific gravity of a substance is the weight of that substance at t°C relative to the weight of an equal volume of water at t'°C. Usually $t = t'$ in specific gravity measurements. The specific gravity of a liquid is easily measured to the third and fourth places, and measurements to six places are not uncommon. Specific gravities of solids are not so readily determined because of inhomogeneities of most solid samples.

The specific gravity of a liquid can be written as in Eq. 14.1, where m represents weight.

$$d_{t'}^{\,t} = \frac{(m/V)_{\text{liq}}^{t}}{(m'/V)_{\text{H}_2\text{O}}^{t'}} \tag{14.1}$$

This is evidently a dimensionless number. m and m' are expressed in grams and V in milliliters.

As a reference quantity in the denominator of equation 14.1, the weight per unit volume of water at 4°C (in g/ml) is very important. Water weighs

* The process of "weighing" on an analytical balance really involves a comparison of the forces exerted by two masses (the sample and the balance "weights") under the influence of gravity.

1.0000000 g/ml at 4°C. Therefore the specific gravity referred to 4°C becomes, from Eq. 14.1,

$$d_4{}^t = \left(\frac{m}{V}\right)^t_{\text{liq}} \tag{14.2}$$

The specific gravity relative to water at 4°C, $d_4{}^t$, is called the *density*. According to this description, it appears that the density is a dimensionless quantity, but it is conventional to ascribe the units of grams per milliliter to this property.

Density and specific gravity are related by Eq. 14.3, which results from suitable combination of 14.1 and 14.2,

$$d_4{}^t = d_{t'}{}^t \times d_4{}^{t'}\ (H_2O) \tag{14.3}$$

where $d_4{}^{t'}$ (H_2O) is the density of water at t'°C. For example, the specific gravity $d_{25}{}^{25}$ of methyl salicylate is 1.184. The density $d_4{}^{25}$ of methyl salicylate is therefore 1.184 × 0.99707, where $d_4{}^{25}$ (H_2O) = 0.99707 is available in reference tables. The density of water at a few temperatures is listed in Table 14.1.

TABLE 14.1
Density of Water[a,b]

t (°C)	$d_4{}^t$ (g/ml)
0	0.99987
4	1.00000
10	0.99973
15	0.99913
20	0.99823
25	0.99707
30	0.99567
35	0.99406

[a] At atmospheric pressure.
[b] This is ordinary distilled water free of air; it is not pure H_2O, but contains a normal ratio (1/4000) of D_2O.

14.2 Applications of Density Measurements*

The density is a fundamental property of a compound, because it reflects the type and arrangement of atoms in the molecule, and the arrangement of the molecules in the macroscopic sample. The molar volume, M/d, where M

* When speaking in general terms, we may employ the words *density* and *specific gravity* interchangeably to denote the property of mass per volume, as in the title of this chapter, but the distinction must be made when measuring or using this property.

TABLE 14.2
Specific Gravity of Some Liquids[a]

Liquid	$d_{t'}^{t}$	Liquid	$d_{t'}^{t}$
Diethyl ether	0.713	Peppermint oil	$0.896–0.908_{25}^{25}$
Cyclohexane	0.778	Ethyl acetate	0.902
Acetonitrile	0.783_{25}^{25}	Undecylenic acid	0.908_{4}^{25}
Isopropyl alcohol	0.785	Olive oil	$0.910–0.915_{25}^{25}$
Methanol	0.791	Cottonseed oil	$0.915–0.921_{25}^{25}$
Acetone	0.792	Spearmint oil	$0.917–0.9_{25}^{25}$
Ethanol	$0.798_{15.56}^{15.56}$	Paraldehyde	0.994
n-Butyl alcohol	0.810	Propylene glycol	1.036_{4}^{25}
95% Ethanol	$0.816_{15.56}^{15.56}$	Benzyl alcohol	1.045_{4}^{25}
Light liquid petrolatum	$0.828–0.880_{25}^{25}$	Acetic acid	1.049_{25}^{25}
Orange oil	$0.842–0.846_{25}^{25}$	Benzaldehyde	1.050_{4}^{15}
Lemon oil	$0.849–0.855_{25}^{25}$	Methyl salicylate	1.184_{25}^{25}
Liquid petrolatum	$0.860–0.905_{55}^{25}$	Glycerol	1.260
Toluene	0.866	Chloroform	1.498_{4}^{15}
Benzene	0.879_{4}^{15}	Mercury	13.546

[a] If no temperatures are specified, the value listed is d_4^{20} (that is, density at 20°C in g/ml.)

is molecular weight, is a useful quantity in structural studies. The molar refraction is a function of the molar volume. The density is also used in the calculation of the specific rotation of a pure liquid.

Density is a helpful criterion of identity and purity. The USP and NF specify narrow ranges within which the specific gravity (usually d_{25}^{25}) of liquids must lie. Table 14.2 gives some typical values of specific gravity.

The density of a mixture is a function of the composition of the solution, and in suitable instances may be utilized in a quantitative analysis of the mixture. The most important analytical application of density measurements is in the determination of alcohol content of aqueous solutions. A standard curve is prepared by measuring the specific gravity of numerous accurately prepared solutions of alcohol in water. The specific gravity of the unknown solution is then measured under identical conditions, and its concentration is read from the curve. Tables of specific gravity-alcohol concentration data have been published and may be utilized directly instead of preparing a standard curve. A preliminary distillation is required to separate the alcohol from other components when analyzing elixirs, tinctures, spirits, and fluid extracts (see Experiment 14.1).

14.3 Measurement of Density of Liquids

Density may be determined by weighing a known volume of the liquid. The accuracy of the volume measurement limits the accuracy of the density obtained in this way. It is easier and usually more accurate to determine the specific gravity by weighing a vessel filled with the liquid and then weighing the same vessel filled with water; the specific gravity is then calculated with Eq. 14.1.

A vessel designed for specific gravity determinations is called a *pycnometer*. Though many pycnometer designs are available, all are intended to provide a reproducible volume of liquid. Three common pycnometers are shown in Fig. 14.1.

The pycnometer is filled with the liquid and is placed in a constant temperature bath until equilibrium has been attained. The stopper is put into the neck of the Weld pycnometer, forcing excess liquid from the vessel. The overflow is carefully removed with tissue paper and the pycnometer may now

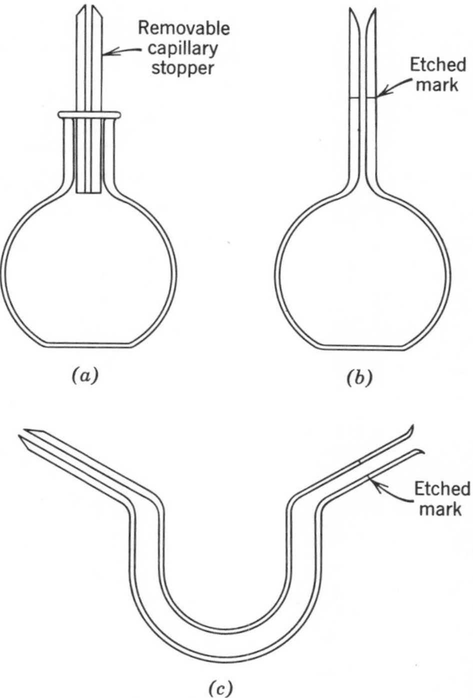

Fig. 14.1. (*a*) Weld pycnometer; (*b*) flask pycnometer; (*c*) Sprengel pycnometer.

be removed from the temperature bath. It is important that the room temperature be lower than the bath temperature when the design shown in Fig. 14.1*a* is used, in order that no liquid be lost from the vessel by expansion. Some Weld pycnometers have a cup around the neck to hold any expelled liquid.

The procedure with the flask and Sprengel pycnometers is slightly different. After the liquid has been brought to temperature equilibrium the meniscus is brought to the etched mark by removing excess liquid with a piece of paper. The fine capillary tip of the Sprengel design is used for this purpose. When the liquid has been brought to the mark the pycnometer can be removed from the water bath.

The outside of the pycnometer is wiped carefully with a slightly moist, lintless cloth, and the vessel is allowed to stand in the balance case for 15–20 min in order to reach equilibrium with the atmosphere. It is then weighed. This entire operation is repeated with water as the liquid contained in the pycnometer. Finally the empty pycnometer is weighed. These three weighings give all the information required to calculate the specific gravity with Eq. 14.1. The density, if desired, can be found with Eq. 14.3.

The technique described permits specific gravity determinations to be made accurate to the third place. Greater accuracy requires corrections for the buoyancy effect of the air on the weights and pycnometer [1]. For pharmaceutical applications such corrections are seldom necessary.

Another method of density determination is based on Archimedes' principle: a body immersed in a fluid is buoyed up with a force equal to the weight of the displaced fluid. A sinker suspended by a fine wire from the arm of a balance is weighed in air and when immersed in the liquid. The operation is repeated in water. The apparent loss of weight of the sinker on passing from air to the liquid divided by the loss of weight between air and water is the specific gravity of the liquid. The measurement in water may also be considered a determination of the volume of the sinker from the relation

$$d_4{}^t(\mathrm{H_2O}) = \frac{W_{\mathrm{air}} - W_{\mathrm{H_2O}}}{V}$$

where V is the volume of the sinker and $d_4{}^t(\mathrm{H_2O})$ is obtained from the literature. Then the density of the liquid is calculated with

$$d_4{}^t(\mathrm{liq}) = \frac{W_{\mathrm{air}} - W_{\mathrm{liq}}}{V}$$

The Westphal balance is an instrument designed to carry out specific gravity determinations according to this principle; the balance is calibrated directly in specific gravity.

Experiment 14.1. Specific Gravity Determinations in Identifications and Analysis

APPARATUS

Water Bath. A constant temperature water bath set at either 20 or 25°C is required.

Pycnometers. Any type of pycnometer is suitable. The 25 ml Weld pycnometer is particularly easy to use. Clean pycnometers with chromic acid-sulfuric acid cleaning solution and rinse them thoroughly with distilled water.

PROCEDURES

Specific Gravity of Pure Liquids. Select two pure liquids and determine their specific gravities with a pycnometer in the manner described in the preceding pages. Compare your results with literature values.

Obtain two samples from your instructor. Determine and report the specific gravity of each sample.

Analysis of Alcohol Solutions. Accurately prepare eight solutions of ethanol in water, using volumetric pipets and flasks, to cover the entire concentration range. Determine the specific gravity of pure water, pure ethanol, and the eight ethanol-water solutions, all at the same temperature. Make a plot of specific gravity against volume percent of ethanol.

Your instructor will give you two samples of aqueous alcohol. Measure their specific gravities and report the percent of alcohol in each sample.

Determination of Alcohol Content of Benzoin Tincture. Pipet 50.0 ml of benzoin tincture into a 500 ml round-bottom flask with 24/40 ₮ neck; measure the temperature at which the sample was taken. Add about 100 ml of water, and place some boiling chips in the flask. Connect a distilling head and water condenser, both with 24/40 joints, to the flask. Place a 100 ml volumetric flask in position as a receiver. Distill, and collect about 98 ml of distillate in the flask. Bring the distillate to the temperature at which the sample was taken. Dilute to 100.0 ml with water and mix thoroughly. This solution should have exactly one-half the alcohol content of the original tincture.

Bring the solution to 25°C and determine its specific gravity $d_{25}{}^{25}$. Using either your standard curve of alcohol concentration versus specific gravity, or the specific gravity tables in the USP or NF, determine the percent of alcohol in the final solution and from this the percent of alcohol in the tincture. (The official basis for the specification of alcohol content is percent by volume at 15.56°C. The specific gravity tables provide for the interconversion of $d_{25}{}^{25}$ and $d_{15.56}^{15.56}$.)

Reference

1. Bauer, N. and S. Z. Lewin, in *Techniques of Chemistry*, Part IV, Vol. I, A. Weissberger and B. W. Rossiter (eds.), Wiley-Interscience, New York, 1972, Chap. II.

Problems

1. Derive Eq. 14.3.

2. A dry pycnometer weighed 15.6527 g. When the pycnometer was filled with hamamelis water it weighed 39.6945 g, and when filled with ordinary water the weight was 40.1908 g; all measurements were made at 25°C.

(*a*) What is the specific gravity d_{25}^{25} of the sample of hamamelis water?

(*b*) Calculate the density d_4^{25} of hamamelis water.

(*c*) What is a synonym for hamamelis water?

15 PHASE SOLUBILITY ANALYSIS

15.1 Phase Solubility Diagrams and Their Interpretation

The equilibrium solubility of a pure substance in a given solvent, at constant temperature, is a quantity characteristic of the substance, and may therefore be utilized as a criterion of identity and purity. If a sample exhibits a solubility in excess of that expected for the pure compound, then the additional quantity of solute may be ascribed to the presence of a second component (that is, impurity). The refinement of this basic idea for the determination of purity is known as phase solubility analysis.

To introduce the principle of phase solubility analysis, let us first consider its application to a pure compound. The experimental operation consists of adding successively larger portions of the sample to constant volumes of a solvent in which it is slightly soluble. The systems are brought to equilibrium by prolonged agitation at constant temperature. The supernatant solution phases are then analyzed for total solute content. A phase solubility diagram is constructed by plotting the weight of solute found per unit of solution on the vertical axis against weight of sample added per unit of solvent on the horizontal axis. Figure 15.1 shows the hypothetical phase diagram for the pure compound being considered. This diagram is readily interpreted. Along the segment *AB* all of the solid added to the system dissolves and is found in solution; the slope of *AB* is therefore unity. Since at point *B* the solution becomes saturated with the compound, further addition of sample cannot lead to an increase in solution concentration; the slope of *BC* is zero. Extrapolation of *BC* to the vertical axis yields the solubility *S* of the compound.

Now consider the same experiment carried out on a two-component mixture. The phase diagram will take the form of Fig. 15.2. As in Fig. 15.1, the slope of *AB* is unity, for all solid added goes into solution. At point *B* the solution has become saturated with respect to one of the components. Along *BC*, therefore, only the second component passes into solution. At *C* the solution becomes saturated with the second component, so the slope beyond *C* is zero.

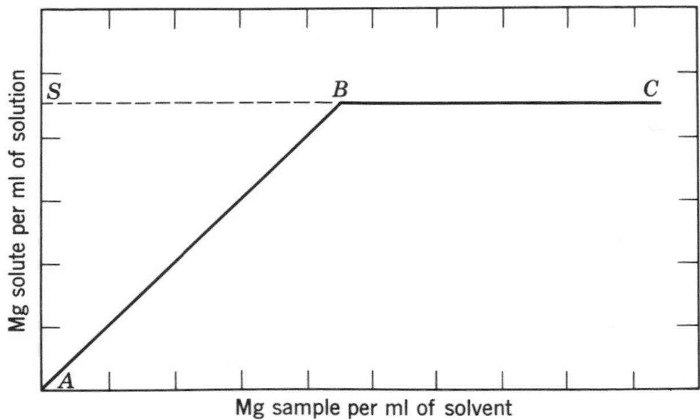

Fig. 15.1. Phase solubility analysis of a pure compound.

From B to C only the fraction of original sample consisting of the second component (usually the minor component) is going into solution; therefore the slope of BC is equal to the fraction of minor component in the sample. Subtraction of this fraction from unity gives the fraction of the major components. Suppose, for example, that a sample contains 25% by weight of an impurity. A phase diagram is obtained similar to that of Fig. 15.2. Along the second segment (BC), for each gram of sample added only 0.25 g passes into solution (because the solution is saturated with the major component). The slope of BC is therefore 0.25, which is the fraction of impurity in the sample.

Extrapolation of CD to the vertical axis gives the sum of the solubilities of the two components. Extrapolation of BC gives the solubility of the first component to reach saturation. Thus, in addition to a quantitative analysis

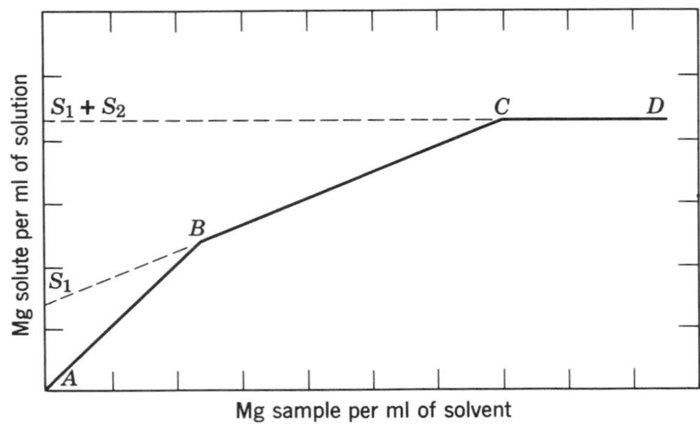

Fig. 15.2. Phase solubility analysis of a two component mixture.

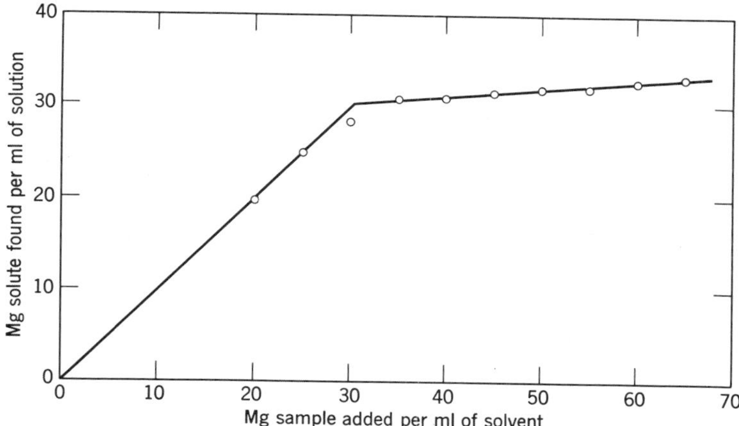

Fig. 15.3. Phase solubility analysis of a mixture of glycine and alanine; the solvent was 50% ethanol-water and the temperature was 30.0°C.

of the mixture, this method yields the equilibrium solubilities. A further use of this type of analysis is in the isolation of small quantities of very pure substances. Along *BC* in Fig. 15.2 the system contains two phases: one of these is a solution of both components, and the second is a solid phase consisting of a pure compound—that component whose solubility limit was reached at point *B*. This pure sample can be isolated readily and its purity checked by subjecting it to phase solubility analysis; if it is pure, the resulting phase diagram should look like Fig. 15.1.

A peculiarity of phase solubility analysis is that it is inapplicable to a mixture whose components are present in the ratio of their solubilities. In this unique instance both components will reach saturation at the same point in the diagram, and the sample will give the same phase diagram as a pure substance.

Figure 15.3 shows a phase solubility analysis of a glycine sample containing some alanine. (The procedure is described in Experiment 15.1.) Note that for the determination of the purity of the major component it is unnecessary to establish the entire phase diagram; only the slope of the second segment is needed. In the analysis shown this slope is 0.083, so the sample contains 91.7% glycine.

15.2 Practical Aspects and Applications

The selection of a solvent for a phase solubility analysis is governed partly by the solubility of the major component and partly by the method of analysis to be employed in determining the concentration of the solution phase. It is essential to analyze the total solute in the solution, so the analytical method must respond to all possible components of the mixture. The most general method is gravimetric. An aliquot of the supernatant is evaporated to dryness and the residue is weighed. This method requires that the solvent be readily vaporized at temperatures too low to decompose the solutes, and that sufficient solute be contained in the aliquot to permit accurate weighing. Low solubilities minimize anomalies from solute-solute interactions. A solvent is usually selected so that the solubility will be in the range 1–30 mg/ml.

It is essential that equilibrium be attained before the solution phases are analyzed. A constant-temperature water bath, capable of holding the temperature constant to within 0.1°, is necessary, and means must be provided to agitate the sample. For most samples equilibrium is reached in 1–3 days. Decomposition of the sample during the equilibration period is a possible complication.

Phase solubility analysis is employed routinely for purity determination, particularly in the pharmaceutical industry. It is an absolute method of analysis. Since the slope of the second segment is equal to the fraction of impurity in the sample and the accuracy of the slope determination is approximately 0.5%, evidently a sample that contains about 0.5% impurity is indistinguishable from a pure compound. Despite this insensitivity the method is extremely valuable. The examples of steroid analysis given by Tarpley and Yudis [1] are typical.

Experiment 15.1. Phase Solubility Analysis of Glycine-Alanine Mixtures

REAGENTS AND APPARATUS

Water Bath. A water bath capable of maintaining the temperature constant to within 0.1° is necessary. The bath should be set at either 25 or 30°C. A device is required to agitate the samples continuously; a motor-driven rotor that will tumble the attached sample containers end-over-end is satisfactory.

Aluminum Weighing Pans. These are numbered and tared.

Solvent. Prepare a 50% ethanol-water mixture.

Known Mixture. Accurately prepare a mixture of glycine and DL-alanine. Make the mixture to contain 10–30% by weight of alanine. Mix the solids thoroughly to ensure homogeneity of the sample.

PROCEDURE

Known Mixture Analysis. Ten 15 ml screw-cap vials will be used. Accurately weigh into the numbered vials the following approximate amounts of the known mixture.

Vial	Mg of known mixture
1	200
2	250
3	300
4	350
5	400
6	450
7	500
8	550
9	600
10	650

Pipet 10.0 ml of solvent into each vial, cover the vials tightly, and place them in the constant temperature water bath. Subject them to continuous agitation.

Equilibration should be complete in 2–3 days. Withdraw a 5.0 ml aliquot form each vial, wrapping a bit of cotton about the pipet tip to filter out any particles of solid; use a clean pipet for each sample. Transfer each aliquot to a separate numbered and tared aluminum pan. Evaporate the solutions to complete dryness in an oven at 70–80°C. The residue should not be permitted to char. Weigh the pans, redry them, and reweigh to constant weight.

Make a plot of milligrams of sample added per milliliter of solvent (x axis) versus milligrams of solute found per milliliter of solution (y axis). Find the percent of alanine in the sample and compare it with the known value. Determine the solubility of glycine.

Unknown Mixture. Obtain a sample of glycine contaminated with alanine. Carry out a phase solubility analysis and report the purity of the glycine.

Reference

1. Tarpley, W. and M. Yudis, *Anal. Chem.*, **25,** 121 (1953).

FOR FURTHER READING

Mader, W. J., "Phase Solubility Analysis," *Org. Anal.*, **2,** 253 (1954).

Higuchi, T. and K. A. Connors, "Phase-Solubility Techniques", *Advan. Anal. Chem. Instrum.*, **4,** 117 (1965).

Cohen, J. L. and K. A. Connors, "Determination of a Complex Stability Constant by the Solubility Technique," *Am. J. Pharm. Educ.*, **31,** 476 (1967).

Problems

1. Explain the difference between the solubility of a nonelectrolyte and the solubility product of a slightly soluble salt.

2. A phase solubility analysis was carried out on a sample of cortisone acetate by adding the weights of sample per milliliter of methanol as given in the left-hand column and analyzing the solution phase after equilibration; the weights found per milliliter are given in the right-hand column.

Mg Added/ml	*Mg Found/ml*
4.0	4.0
8.0	8.0
12.0	12.0
16.0	14.2
20.0	14.8
24.0	15.4
28.0	16.0
32.0	16.5
36.0	16.5
40.0	16.5

(*a*) What is the percent purity of the cortisone acetate?
(*b*) What is the solubility of cortisone acetate?
(*c*) What is the solubility of the impurity?

3. The equation of the second segment of a phase solubility diagram was found to be $y = 0.164x + 4.35$, where y = mg of solute found per milliliter and x = mg of solute taken per milliliter.

(*a*) What is the purity of the sample and the solubility of the major component?
(*b*) Reconstruct the phase diagram.

Summary: Part Two

Subsequently in this book the material of Part Two will be utilized as a matter of routine, as for example in a statement ". . . the analysis is completed by determining the concentration spectrophotometrically," or ". . . the end point is located potentiometrically." The analytical literature in general assumes knowledge of these fundamental techniques, and familiarity with them is essential. Many more physical methods are used routinely, and some of these will be briefly described here. This listing does not exhaust the topics that could be considered, but it includes some important ones.

Conductometric Titration. The electric current through a chemical cell is carried by the ionic species in the solution. The ease with which current is conducted through a solution (under the influence of a potential difference applied across two electrodes) depends upon the concentrations and kinds of ions in the solutions. The *conductance*, which is the reciprocal of the electrical resistance, is a measure of the ease of current flow through the solution.

That the conductance will depend upon the concentration of ionic species is not surprising, since the greater the number of ions in unit volume, the greater the current flow. But the conductance also depends upon the identity of the ions carrying the current. In short, some ions move faster than others in an electric field. Hydrogen and hydroxyl ions are particularly powerful contributors to the conductance. Now suppose that a solution of hydrochloric acid is titrated with sodium hydroxide, and that the conductance is measured at several points in the titration. The titration reaction is

$$H^+ + Cl^- + OH^- + Na^+ \rightarrow H_2O + Cl^- + Na^+$$

The important result has been the replacement of the highly mobile hydrogen ions by the less mobile sodium ions. Therefore the conductance of the solution steadily decreases during the titration. After the end point, however, further addition of titrant increases the concentration of Na^+ and OH^-, both species (but especially the hydroxide ion) causing an increase in the conductance of the solution. A plot of conductance versus volume of titrant will be a V-shaped graph, with the intersection of the straight lines marking the end point. This is an example of a *conductometric titration.* These titrations can be extremely helpful in analyzing weak acids and bases, especially in mixtures, and in locating the end point in precipitation titrations. They are obviously useless if the solution contains large concentrations of ionic species other than those involved in the titration reaction. An advantage of conductometric titration is that the important data are obtained well before and after the end point, rather than in the immediate region of the end point.

Coulometric Titration. In coulometry a chemical reaction is made to occur in a chemical cell by the passage of electricity. The process is called electrolysis, and it differs from the electrochemical techniques described in Chapters 6 and 7 in that the reaction is carried to completion, all of the electroactive substance being reacted; in voltammetric methods only a minute amount of the solute undergoes reaction. In coulometry the quantity measured is the amount of electricity, which is related to the amount of chemical reaction by $Q = \mathbf{F} \times$ no. of equivalents, or $Q = n\mathbf{F}w/M$, where Q is the number of coulombs, $\mathbf{F}$ is the faraday, n is the number of electrons transferred per molecule, w is the weight of reactant, and M is its molecular weight. Thus by carrying the electrolysis (oxidation or reduction) to completion and measuring Q, the amount of reactant can be calculated. If the current i is maintained constant throughout the electrolysis, then $Q = it$, where t is the time of electrolysis.

In effect coulometry is a titrimetric method in which electrons serve as the titrant. If a direct electrode reaction of the sample substance is not feasible, an indirect coulometric titration may be carried out by generating a titrant coulometrically *in situ;* the titrant species then reacts with the sample, and the end point is detected by any of the conventional means. Again the measured quantity is the amount of charge Q. For example, acids can be titrated by coulometric generation of hydroxide according to the reaction

$$2H_2O + 2e \rightarrow H_2 + 2OH^-$$

Coulometric titration can be very sensitive because small quantities of electricity can be accurately measured. Another advantage is that titrants can be generated that are impossible or difficult to prepare as standard solutions because of their instability.

Emission Spectroscopy. In Chapters 8 and 9 the absorption and emission of energy by molecules were shown to be phenomena upon which fruitful analytical techniques could be based. The same general considerations apply to atoms. One of the oldest branches of analytical chemistry utilizes the emission of radiation from excited atoms to identify and determine quantitatively many elements. This is emission spectroscopy.

The sample to be analyzed is placed between two electrodes across which a high-temperature electric arc is produced. The atoms in the sample are raised to higher energy levels. Upon their return to the ground state, they emit radiation in very sharply defined lines. This emitted radiation is dispersed with a prism or grating, and the resulting line spectrum is photographed. By comparing the frequencies of the observed lines with spectra of known samples, the element present in the sample can be identified. A great advantage of this method is that a sample containing a mixture of elements can be analyzed, because the sharply defined line spectra of many elements can be distinguished in a mixture. The method is sensitive, 0.001% of an element being detectable, with this limit being lower for some substances. Quantitative analysis is accomplished by measuring the intensities of the spectra and comparing them with standard samples. Emission spectroscopy is used primarily for the identification and determination of metals in trace amounts.

Flame Photometry. This technique is a type of emission spectroscopy, differing from the analytical method discussed previously in its experimental procedures. The sample is a solution of the metal in the form of one of its salts. This solution is dispersed with an atomizer into a hot flame, where some of the atoms (0.01–1%) are excited to higher energy levels. Upon their return to the ground state, the characteristic line spectra are emitted. The emitted radiation is dispersed with a monochromator and the spectrum is detected with a phototube, exactly as in a spectrophotometer. In fact, many conventional spectrophotometers may be utilized as flame photometers with commercially supplied modifying apparatus.

The fundamental difference between emission spectroscopy and flame photometry is a result of the different means of excitation. Since the flame is not nearly as hot as an electric arc, fewer high-energy orbitals are occupied in the flame. The resulting spectra are less complex.

The flame photometer is widely used for the quantitative analysis of sodium, potassium, and lithium. These elements are very difficult to determine, especially in mixtures, by chemical methods. In the flame photometer they give intense emission lines. Concentrations down to 1 ppm are readily determined. This method has been applied to biological fluids. Other alkali metals also can be analyzed by flame photometry.

Atomic Absorption Spectroscopy. It will be clear from the theoretical considerations in Chapter 8 that an atom is capable of absorbing light of exactly the same frequency as that that it emits, since the frequency depends solely upon the energy difference between energy levels. In flame photometry a small fraction of the atoms in a dispersed solution of the metal is excited into higher energy levels. The emission of radiation by these excited atoms as they return to their ground states is measured; the frequency of the emitted light permits identification of the element and its intensity provides a quantitative measure.

A newer spectroscopic method utilizes the same sampling system, but instead of measuring the light emitted by the very small proportion of atoms in the excited state, this method measures the light absorbed by the very large proportion of atoms in the ground state. This technique is atomic absorption spectroscopy.

The light source for atomic absorption spectroscopy can in principle be any source that includes the frequency that is to be absorbed and monitored by the detector. In practice, great specificity is achieved by using as the source a discharge tube constructed of, or containing, the same element that is to be analyzed. Then any light absorbed by the sample must have been absorbed by atoms of the element in the source. The diminution of source intensity, at a frequency selected with a monochromator, is a measure of the amount of element in the flame, and therefore of the concentration of the element in the original sample solution.

Atomic absorption spectroscopy is very sensitive because it takes advantage of nearly all the atoms in the flame, unlike flame photometry. Its use is rapidly being extended to the trace analysis of metals in many products. A few parts per million of a metal can be measured. Among the elements that have been determined in pharmaceutical preparations are Na, K, Cu, Au, Mg, Ca, Zn, Hg, As, Fe, and Co.

Radiochemical Analysis. The chemical behavior of atoms and molecules depends upon their electronic configurations outside of the nucleus, and the chemist has until recently been able to ignore the properties of the nucleus. Many substances are now known with electronic configurations identical with those of well-known elements but with different nuclear compositions. Elements with identical atomic numbers (that is, identical numbers of protons in their nuclei and therefore identical numbers of orbital electrons) and different atomic weights (that is, different numbers of neutrons in their nuclei) are called isotopes. Many isotopes are radioactive, which means that they are unstable and will change, with the emanation of some form of radioactivity, into another isotope.

The energy emitted by a radioactive isotope appears as doubly charged helium atoms (alpha particles), as electrons (beta particles), as positively charged electrons (positrons), or as high-energy electromagnetic radiation (gamma rays). The rate at which radioactive "decay" occurs is expressed as the half-life of the isotope, which is the time taken for the radioactivity to decay to one-half its initial value. Radioactivity can be detected and measured by measuring the ionization of matter caused by the passage of the radiation. The Geiger counter and scintillation counter are instruments capable of registering radioactivity (in events per unit time).

The most valuable chemical application of radioactive isotopes takes advantage of the chemical indistinguishability of a stable element and one of its radioisotopes. The compound of interest is synthesized with the incorporation of some of the radioactive isotope as a tracer. In subsequent reactions the progress of the tracer can be followed by measuring its radioactivity. This method is much used by organic chemists and biochemists to elucidate reaction mechanisms. A tracer is used in an important analytical technique called the isotope-dilution method. This method is often applied when it is necessary to analyze a component of a mixture from which it is relatively easy to isolate a pure sample of the component but impossible to effect a quantitative separation. A known quantity (say, W_a grams) of the pure component labeled with a radioactive tracer is added to the mixture to be analyzed, which is thoroughly mixed. Next a pure sample of the component is isolated; it makes no difference whether all of the component is isolated as long as the portion isolated is pure. The specific activity A_m (radioactivity in counts per minute per gram) is measured. Since the total activity in the mixture must be equal to the total activity of the added labeled compound,

$$A_a W_a = A_m W_m$$

where A_a and A_m are the specific activities of the added compound and of the recovered compound, respectively, W_a is the weight of added compound, and W_m is the weight of compound in the mixture; evidently $W_m = W_a + W_i$, with W_i being the weight of compound in the mixture before addition of the labeled compound. All these quantities are known except W_i, which may be readily calculated. The success of the isotope-dilution method is based upon the chemical identity of the labeled and unlabeled samples, so that any information (in particular, the radioactivity) about the isolated portion applies equally to the unisolated fraction.

Neutron Activation Analysis. This is another technique based on radioactivity; it is used for the sensitive determination of elements. The sample is bombarded with neutrons, resulting in the production of one or more radioisotopes of the element. The radioisotope decays and the resulting radioactivity is measured.

A neutron is a neutral particle having unit mass. When ordinary sodium, as an example, is subjected to a flux of neutrons, this nuclear reaction occurs:

$$^{23}_{11}\text{Na} + ^{1}_{0}\text{n} \rightarrow ^{24}_{11}\text{Na} + \gamma$$

The sodium nucleus captures the neutron, increasing its mass, and gamma radiation is emitted. This reaction is abbreviated $^{23}\text{Na}(\text{n}, \gamma)^{24}\text{Na}$. Another example is the conversion of $^{75}_{33}\text{As}$, the natural isotope of arsenic, to $^{76}_{33}\text{As}$ upon neutron capture.

Suppose a sample containing N nuclei of the isotope of interest is bombarded in a nuclear reactor with a neutron flux ϕ, where ϕ has the units neutrons/cm^2-sec. Each type of nucleus has an effective nuclear cross section σ, which is a measure of the probability that the nucleus will capture a neutron; σ is measured in barns, where one barn is 10^{-24} cm^2/nucleus. The number of neutrons captured per second is then $N\phi\sigma$. Nuclear reactors produce fluxes of 10^{11}–10^{13} neutrons/cm^2-sec.

The radioisotope produced at once begins to decay with its characteristic half-life. Thus the radioactivity measured is a function of the rate at which neutrons are captured (which depends on time in the reactor) and the decay half-life. A compromise is made, with the time of irradiation being selected corresponding to 1–2 half-lives, since longer irradiation times do not increase the radioactivity proportionately. Often the radioactivity is not measured immediately upon removal from the reactor, and then the permissible time lapse between removal and measurement depends upon the half-life.

Neutron activation analysis is extremely sensitive and is finding increasing use for trace element analysis in environmental samples.

Chemical Microscopy. Qualitative analysis (identification) of compounds is an important aspect of pharmaceutical analysis. Observations through the microscope can provide valuable evidence for identification purposes, and many properties can be determined rapidly and simply with inexpensive apparatus. The microscope must be fitted with an electrically heated stage and with means for measuring its temperature. With such a microscope the melting point can be determined with a minute amount of sample. Much more information can be obtained during the melting of the compound and its subsequent cooling. The occurrence of sublimation, decomposition, loss of water of crystallization, the refractive index of the melt, polymorphic transformations (change of crystal form), and rate of crystallization all may be helpful in identifying the sample. Mixed fusion tests, in which a second substance is mixed with the sample and the mixture is melted, yield characteristic eutectic behavior. If the added substance is identical with the sample, the melting point of the mixture should not be lower than that of the sample; such mixed melting points can be very critically observed under the microscope.

Thermal Analysis. Thermal methods of analysis are based on changes in physical properties of samples that are subjected to temperature changes. Several techniques are used. In differential thermal analysis (DTA) the solid sample and a reference substance are both subjected to an increase of temperature with time. The difference in temperature, ΔT, between the sample and the reference is recorded as a function of the time. If the sample undergoes phase transitions (e.g., melting) or chemical reactions within the temperature range studied, it will absorb or evolve more heat than the reference, with a resulting peak in the ΔT signal corresponding to the period during which the process is taking place. The DTA curve (thermogram) can be analyzed to obtain the enthalpy change for the process. If the sample is a mixture it can sometimes be analyzed quantitatively by DTA. The method is useful for the empirical differentiation of materials by comparison of their thermograms.

Differential scanning calorimetry (DSC) is carried out much like DTA, but, instead of measuring the temperature difference ΔT between the sample and reference, the electrical power necessary to keep $\Delta T = 0$ is measured. DTA and DSC give much the same information. In thermogravimetric analysis (TGA) the weight of a sample is recorded continuously as it is heated or cooled. Since the sample may undergo reactions (dehydration, etc.) resulting in weight changes, the thermogram of weight change against temperature is characteristic of the sample.

Thermometric titrimetry measures the temperature of a titration solution as a function of the titrant volume added. The temperature change during a titration is determined in part by the enthalpy change for the reaction. From the titration plot of temperature against volume the end point can be determined and thermodynamic properties can be obtained. A key feature of thermometric titrations is that they are controlled by ΔH^0 for the titration reaction, whereas all other kinds of titrations are controlled by ΔG^0, the free energy change (or, equivalently, the equilibrium constant). This means that it may be possible to carry out a titration for which the equilibrium constant is unfavorable, provided the enthalpy change is finite. For example, boric acid is too weak an acid (pK_a 9.1) to titrate directly with alkali potentiometrically; however, it can be titrated thermometrically with the same ease as can a strong acid.

Radioimmunoassay. Radioimmunoassay (RIA) and some related techniques are based upon highly specific antigen-antibody interactions. An antibody (Ab) is a serum protein whose production is induced by injection of a large protein (the antigen, Ag) foreign to the species; this is the immunogenic response. An Ag-Ab complex is formed in an equilibrium process. RIA is used to determine the antigen on the basis of competitive binding by radioactively labeled antigen and unlabeled antigen. This competition can be represented as

$$\begin{array}{ccc} \underset{\text{(free)}}{Ag^*} + & Ab \rightleftharpoons & \underset{\text{(bound)}}{Ag^* - Ab} \\ & + & \\ & Ag & \\ & \Updownarrow & \\ & Ag\text{—}Ab & \end{array}$$

where Ag* is the labeled antigen. A standard curve is prepared with a series of solutions each containing the same total amounts of Ag* and Ab, but with increasing amounts of unlabeled antigen. After equilibration, the solutions are analyzed for free labeled antigen (Ag*) and bound labeled antigen (Ag*-Ab). Since the equilibrium is competitive, introduction of unlabeled antigen into the system will displace some labeled antigen from the bound form, thus decreasing the percentage of bound labeled antigen. The standard curve is a plot of percent labeled antigen bound against total antigen present. A sample solution is analyzed by adding labeled antigen, determining the percent bound, and reading the total antigen from the curve.

This method achieves selectivity from the specificity of the immunogenic response, and sensitivity from the radioactivity measurement. It has been applied widely to the determination of protein hormones. Small molecules, such as most drugs, do not function as antigens, but if they are covalently linked to proteins they become antigenic and can be assayed by RIA. Steroids, barbiturates, and narcotics are among the drugs that can be determined.

Part Three: Separation Techniques

Nearly all the samples presented to the pharmaceutical analyst are mixtures, sometimes very complex ones. The determination of the amount of each isolated component is usually a simple matter with the techniques already described in Parts One and Two, and methods to be treated in later chapters. The analysis of these same components in each other's presence may, however, be difficult or even impossible because of interference by one substance in the assay of another. Interference can take several forms. The interfering substance can respond quantitatively to the analytical method for the desired component. An example is the interference caused by acetic acid in the assay of hydrochloric acid by titration with alkali. This is not an entirely hopeless situation, for the analysis will at least yield the sum of the amounts of the desired component and the interfering component. Another common example is the interference observed in absorption spectroscopy when two solutes have overlapping absorption bands. Sometimes the interference is a partial, nonquantitative response to the assay. For example, the nonaqueous titration of weakly acidic drugs in tablets containing stearic acid may be unsuccessful because of consumption of titrant by the stearic acid; this is not a reproducible effect, probably because of incomplete dissolution of stearic acid in the titration medium. It is very difficult to compensate for interferences of this type. Another commonly encountered form of interference is an impairment of the analytical method for the desired component, leading to nonquantitative results even for this component. A trace of copper in a sample of magnesium can vitiate a visual complexometric titration of the magnesium by poisoning the indicator. Another instance is the quenching of quinine fluorescence by hydrochloric acid.

When an analytical method cannot be applied directly to a mixture because of possible interference, a separation of the mixture into its components may be necessary. Part Three describes many of the ways in which mixtures can be separated.

16 SOLVENT EXTRACTION

16.1 Liquid-Liquid Extraction

Extraction is the process of removing a constituent from one phase by bringing this phase into contact with a second, immiscible, liquid phase. This section treats liquid-liquid extraction, which is the transfer of a solute from one liquid phase to another liquid by contact. This process is also called *partitioning* or *distribution.*

The Partition Coefficient. Consider a single solute species distributed between two immiscible liquids (as in a separatory funnel). Equilibrium 16.1 is established in this system.

$$\text{Solute in lower phase} \rightleftharpoons \text{Solute in upper phase} \qquad (16.1)$$

According to thermodynamics, at equilibrium the ratio of activities of the solute species in the two phases is a constant; this is called the Nernst distribution law. Usually concentrations are substituted for activities; then the distribution law is written

$$K = \frac{c_\mu}{c_l} \qquad (16.2)$$

where c_μ is the concentration in the upper phase, c_l is the concentration in the lower phase, and K is the *partition coefficient* or distribution coefficient. Notice that K is the equilibrium constant for reaction 16.1. The partition coefficient is dependent upon the temperature, but it is not a function of the absolute concentrations or the volumes of the phases.

The symbol P is often used to represent the partition coefficient. Usually one of the phases is aqueous, and some authors define the partition coefficient as the ratio $c_{\text{organic}}/c_{\text{aqueous}}$, or $c_{\text{oil}}/c_{\text{water}}$, etc.; all of these definitions are acceptable as long as the one being used is clearly specified.

The determination of a partition coefficient can be accomplished very simply. The solute, present in an amount small enough so that its solubility is not exceeded in either solvent, is distributed between the two immiscible phases; this distribution can be carried out in a separatory funnel. After equilibration, the phases are separated and analyzed for the solute. The partition coefficient is calculated with Eq. 16.2. It is good practice to determine K at several absolute concentrations of solute; a constant K value should be obtained if the solute does not undergo dissociation or association in one of the solvents. Another way to examine such data is to plot c_μ against c_l; this is called a distribution, or partition, isotherm. The slope of this plot is equal to K, and a linear partition isotherm over the concentration range examined indicates constancy of K over this range. More refined experimental techniques have been described [1]. A valuable collection of partition coefficient data has been published [2].

A nonlinear partition isotherm usually indicates that the solute is not present solely as the undissociated monomer in both solvents. Thus a neutral carboxylic acid, which can dissociate into the carboxylate anion in aqueous solution, may yield a curved partition isotherm for a distribution between water and benzene, for only the undissociated portion of the solute is benzene-soluble, and as the absolute concentration of the solute changes, the fraction present as the undissociated acid varies. Another equilibrium that can produce a curved isotherm is formation of a dimer (or higher aggregate) in one of the solvents. Because of these possible complications, the partition coefficient usually determined must be labeled an apparent partition coefficient that reflects the overall distribution behavior of all species present. The true partition coefficient, as defined earlier, applies only to a single species.

Single Extraction. If the partition coefficient for a solute between two solvents is known, it is possible to calculate the fraction of that solute present in each of the phases at equilibrium. Let p be the fraction of solute in the upper phase and q the fraction in the lower phase at equilibrium. The quantity p is defined by

$$p = \frac{\text{Amount of solute in upper phase}}{\text{Total amount of solute}} \tag{16.3}$$

The amounts specified in Eq. 16.3 can be expressed in terms of concentrations c and volumes v, where the subscripts indicate the phase:

$$\text{Amount of solute in upper phase} = c_\mu v_\mu \tag{16.4}$$

$$\text{Total amount of solute} = c_\mu v_\mu + c_l v_l \tag{16.5}$$

For convenience the ratio of phase volumes is denoted as in

$$U = \frac{v_\mu}{v_l} \tag{16.6}$$

Equations 16.2–16.6 can be combined to give

$$p = \frac{KU}{KU + 1} \tag{16.7}$$

which relates the fraction of solute extracted into the upper phase to the partition coefficient and the ratio of phase volumes. Since p is the fraction extracted into the upper phase, $100p$ is the percent extracted into the upper phase.

By definition, $p + q = 1$, so q is given by

$$q = \frac{1}{KU + 1} \tag{16.8}$$

The larger the partition coefficient, the larger the percent of solute that will be found in the upper phase after equilibration; of course the ratio of the phase volumes is an equally important factor, and the product KU is called the capacity factor.

EXAMPLE 16.1. A solute is known to have a partition coefficient of 4.0 between water and ether. If 15 ml of an aqueous solution of the compound is extracted with one 20 ml portion of ether, what percentage of the original solute will be found in the ether?

Equation 16.7 can be applied directly, with $K = 4.0$ and $U = 1.33$. The fraction p is found to be 0.842, so 84.2% of the solute is in the ether layer and 15.8% in the aqueous layer after equilibration.

Multiple Extractions. Unless K is extremely large, a significant portion of the solute will be present in both phases after a single extraction, as illustrated by Example 16.1. It is common practice, therefore, to reextract with additional portions of fresh solvent (the *extractant*) until essentially all of the solute has been removed from the phase being extracted (the *raffinate**). It is possible to calculate the fraction extracted after any number of extractions, or to calculate the number of extractions necessary to achieve any desired extent of extraction.

As before, let p represent the fraction of the solute present that is partitioned into the upper phase in a single equilibration. Then q is the fraction of solute in the lower phase. Suppose that the lower phase is the raffinate and the upper phase the extractant; then the state of the extraction after one equilibration is specified in the first row of Table 16.1, where n is the number of extractions.

If the partition isotherm is linear, then the same fraction p of the solute remaining in the raffinate is extracted into the upper phase each time (assuming identical volumes of extractant are used in each extraction). Then the fraction of the *total* solute removed in the nth extraction (with fresh upper phase) is equal to the product of the fraction of the total remaining in the raffinate and the fraction extracted in a single extraction.

$$\begin{matrix}\text{Fraction of total extracted} \\ \text{in } n\text{th extraction}\end{matrix} = \begin{matrix}\text{Fraction of total left after} \\ (n-1)\text{th extraction} \times p\end{matrix}$$

* From the French *raffiner*, to refine.

TABLE 16.1
Calculation of the Progress of Extraction

n	Fraction of Total Extracted in nth Extraction	Total Fraction Extracted	Fraction Remaining
1	p	p	$1 - p = q$
2	pq	$p + pq$	$1 - (p + pq) = q^2$
3	pq^2	$p + pq + pq^2$	$1 - (p + pq + pq^2) = q^3$
.	.	.	.
.	.	.	.
.	.	.	.
n	$pq^{(n-1)}$	$\sum_{n=1}^{n} pq^{(n-1)}$	q^n

When we apply this formula to the second extraction,

$$\text{Fraction of total extracted in 2nd extraction} = pq$$

This quantity is entered in the second column of Table 16.1. The total fraction extracted after two extractions is the sum of the fractions extracted in the first and second extractions, or $p + pq$, and the fraction remaining in the raffinate is one minus the total fraction extracted, or q^2, as shown in column 4 of Table 16.1.

This calculation can be carried out for any number of extractions, and the final row of Table 16.1 shows the result for n extractions. The third column gives an expression for calculating the total fraction extracted after n extractions. An equivalent, and more convenient, expression is obtained with the relation

$$\text{Total fraction extracted} = 1 - \text{fraction remaining}$$

giving, from Table 16.1,

$$\text{Total fraction extracted} = 1 - q^n \tag{16.9}$$

This can also be expressed in terms of p by using the relation $q = 1 - p$. The fraction extracted may, if desired, be expressed as percent extracted simply by multiplying by 100.

Consider the extraction of a solute with $K = 4.0$ in the ether/water system; for simplicity let $U = 1.0$. The results of the calculation are given in Table 16.2. For most analytical purposes the extraction would be considered quantitative after the fourth extraction.

This type of calculation can be carried out without the general formula

TABLE 16.2
Extraction of a Solute with K = 4.0 and U = 1.0

Number of Extractions, n	Total Extracted (%)
1	80.00
2	96.00
3	99.20
4	99.84
5	99.97

given above. Thus, in this example, 0.80 of the solute is extracted in the first step. (This figure is of course obtained by applying Eq. 16.7.) In the second extraction 0.80 of the remaining 0.20, or 0.16 of the total, is extracted; the total extracted is therefore 96%. This calculation can be continued indefinitely.

EXAMPLE 16.2. With our familiar example of the solute whose partition coefficient is 4.0 in the ether/water system, compare the efficiency of extraction of a 10 ml aqueous solution of the compound with (*a*) one 40 ml portion of ether or (*b*) four 10 ml portions of ether.

(*a*) Applying Eq. 16.7 we find that 94.12% of the solute is extracted into the 40 ml of ether when the extraction is carried out in a single step.

(*b*) Applying Eq. 16.9, we find (in Table 16.2) that 99.84% of the solute is extracted into the 40 ml of ether when the extraction is carried out in four steps.

This calculation illustrates a very important practical result of extraction theory. A more efficient extraction is achieved with several extractions than with a single extraction utilizing the same total volume of extractant. In Example 16.2 the multiple extractions gave an essentially quantitative removal of the solute from the raffinate, while the single extraction was far from complete. In fact, comparison of the figure 94.12% with the results of Table 16.2 shows that just 20 ml of ether, used in two 10 ml portions, removes more solute (96.00%) than does 40 ml used in a single portion.

If the extracting solvent is heavier than the raffinate, the previous equations are applicable merely by interchanging p and q.

The Analytical Problem. The preceding discussion has been concerned with the distribution of a single solute. In practice, however, we most frequently wish to separate a pair of substances by taking advantage of their distribution behavior. The feasibility of resolving two substances is sometimes discussed in terms of the separability factor α:

$$\alpha = \frac{K_1}{K_2}$$

where the K's are the partition coefficients of the two substances in the liquid-liquid system. Evidently a separation factor of unity means that the two substances cannot be separated by extraction. The greater the deviation of α from unity, the more feasible is the separation.

A complete separation of two solutes by simple liquid-liquid extraction (as carried out with separatory funnels, for example) requires that one of the partition coefficients be so small (or large) that this substance is essentially not extractable from the raffinate. Then, if α is at least moderately different from unity, the second substance can be removed quantitatively by successive extractions with fresh portions of the extracting solvent. When presented with a separation problem, the analyst must, in using liquid-liquid extraction as his method of separation, influence the values of the apparent partition coefficients so they meet the requirements just outlined. He can accomplish this in several ways.

1. Choice of Solvents. Sometimes the analyst may select both solvents, but often the sample is an aqueous solution, which fixes the nature of the raffinate. The partition coefficients obviously will be influenced markedly by the chemical nature of the second solvent. Widely used extractants are diethyl ether, chloroform, and hydrocarbons. A simple example of a separation by liquid-liquid extraction would be the analysis of a mixture of caffeine and sodium benzoate. The mixture is dissolved in water, in which both solutes are appreciably soluble. It is then extracted completely with chloroform, in which caffeine is quite soluble but sodium benzoate is very insoluble. The final result is that the caffeine is contained totally in the combined chloroform extracts, whereas the sodium benzoate remains behind in the aqueous raffinate. It is a simple matter to assay the separated components (spectrophotometrically, for example).

Often, when more than one extracting solvent appears to be satisfactory, the choice is based on their densities, that is, whether they are heavier or lighter than water.

A rough idea of the size of a partition coefficient may sometimes be obtained from the equilibrium solubilities of the solute in the two solvents. This estimate will not be quantitative, however, because of the different forces involved in the two situations. The equilibrium solubility is a function of a comptetition between solute-solute and solute-solvent interactions, whereas the partition coefficient depends upon two types of solute-solvent interactions. The situation is complicated by the partial miscibility of all solvents, so that (for example) the two-phase ether/water system contains ether saturated with water in equilibrium with water saturated with ether. Nevertheless, useful indications of magnitudes of partition coefficients can be obtained by cautious use of solubilities. For example, the solubility of acetanilide in ether and water, respectively, is about 5.6 g/100 ml and 0.55 g/100 ml, giving an estimated value of $K = 10.2$ in the ether/water system. The experimental value is 3.0. This agreement, which is as good as can be expected, is sufficiently close to permit a decision to be made regarding the suitability of the solvent system.

2. Control of pH. Many, perhaps most, of the compounds encountered by the pharmaceutical analyst are weak acids or bases. The solubility characteristics of these substances depend upon their ionic form, with the neutral species usually being soluble in nonpolar, organic solvents, and the ionic species being more soluble in polar (especially aqueous) solvents. These forms can be interconverted at will merely by altering the pH of the medium, and so pH control is the most powerful means for influencing the value of the partition coefficient. A mixture of a base and an acid is readily separated by solvent extraction. For example, acetylsalicylic acid and an antihistamine could be separated by dissolving in water, acidifying the solution with hydrochloric acid, and completely extracting the acid with ether; the antihistamine will be retained, as its hydrochloride salt, in the aqueous solution. Next the aqueous raffinate can be made basic and the antihistamine can be removed by extraction.

It is necessary to know, approximately, the pK_a of the solute in such a separation. Suppose it is desired to retain a weak neutral acid, with $pK_a = 5$, in the aqueous raffinate while extracting a second, basic substance. The acid must be quantitatively converted to its anion. How basic must the aqueous solution be to ensure that no significant portion of the neutral acid is present? According to the equation

$$pH = pK_a + \log \frac{[A^-]}{[HA]}$$

at pH = 5, equal amounts of the acid are present in the anion and neutral forms, at pH = 6 about 10% remains as the neutral form, at pH 7 about 1% exists as the neutral form, and at pH 8 only 0.1% is present as the acid. If the neutral form is soluble in the extracting solvent, it is therefore essential that the pH be at least 3 units more basic than the pK_a to ensure "complete" conversion to the anion form. A similar argument applies in the conversion of a neutral base to its protonated acid form; in this instance the pH must be at least 3 units more acidic than the pK_a. The simultaneous effect of pH on the partition coefficient of the solute being extracted must also be considered.

A quantitative relationship between the apparent partition coefficient and the pH is easily derived (see Problem 6). Practical applications of these principles are described in Chapter 26.

3. Control of Ionic Strength. If the salt concentration of an aqueous solution is made very high, the solubility of a nonelectrolyte will usually be decreased. This reduction of solubility by an increase in ionic strength is the

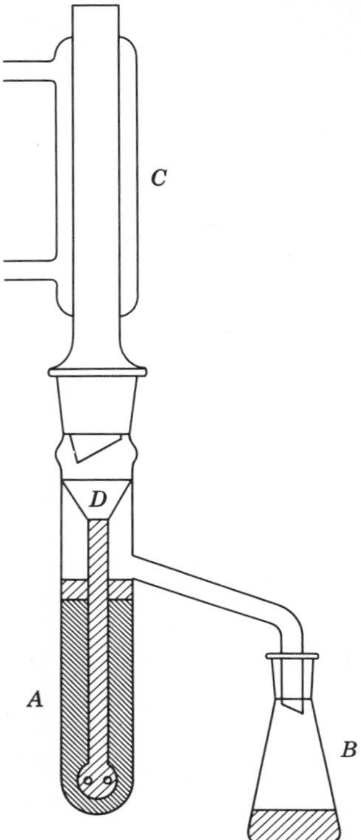

Fig. 16.1. Continuous extractor for extractants lighter than the raffinate.

"salting-out effect." In a crude way it may be associated with the reduced availability of water molecules to act as the solvent for the nonelectrolyte, the ions of the salt tying up much of the water (through strong ion-dipole forces) as a hydration shell around the ions. This phenomenon can be used to advantage in solvent extraction. By incorporating a large amount of sodium chloride in the aqueous phase, the solute is salted out into the organic extracting phase. (The salt also helps to break emulsions that may form when shaking the two phases together.) In the terms of this chapter, the salting-out effect alters the apparent partition coefficient of many substances.

Continuous Extractors. Most quantitative separations by solvent extraction are performed by multiple extraction with separatory funnels. Some assays have been rendered more efficient and less tedious by using continuous extraction devices. Figure 16.1 shows a continuous extractor designed for separations in which the extractant is less dense than the raffinate; this design is often utilized for extractions of aqueous solutions with ether. The raffinate is contained in the body A. Ether is placed in the flask B, which is immersed in a beaker of warm water to volatilize some of the ether. The ether vapors are condensed in the condenser C, and the ether drops into the inner tube. When the column of ether in this tube rises to a sufficient height to overcome the hydrostatic pressure of the raffinate solution, drops of ether are forced out of the holes in the bottom of the inner tube. These drops rise through the aqueous raffinate, collect on its surface, and return to the flask. This process may be continued until the extraction is complete. Figure 16.2 shows a continuous extractor for extractants more dense than the raffinate. The operation parallels the one just described. The condensed extractant drops through the raffinate, extracting the desired component, and it collects on the bottom of the extractor until the side tube is filled sufficiently to allow return to the flask.

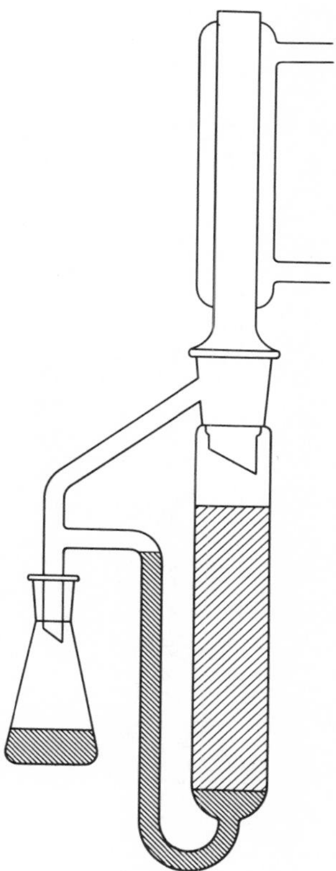

Fig. 16.2. Continuous extractor for extractants heavier than the raffinate.

16.2 Extraction of Solids

The extraction of solids is an important step in the preparation of many pharmaceuticals. Tinctures, for example, are prepared by percolation (process P) or maceration (process M) of the ground crude drug with a hydroalcoholic menstruum. Alkaloids and other compounds of plant and animal origin commonly are separated from the crude sources by solvent extraction ("leaching"). Crude drugs are assayed for their content of active ingredient in this way, and extraction of the active component from solid dosage forms is often the first step in their quantitative analysis.

In many instances it is necessary merely to agitate a weighed portion of the ground drug or finely powdered dosage form with the extracting solvent; after extraction is complete the exhausted solid is removed by filtering and an aliquot of the filtrate is taken for analysis. Sometimes it is advisable to heat the mixture to hasten the extraction; this is often done when extracting the active ingredients from ointments.

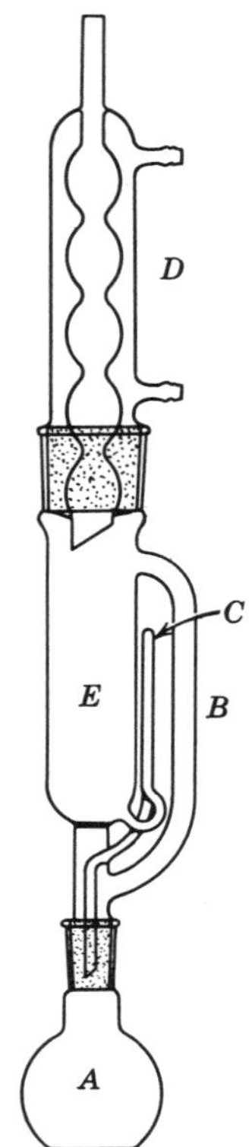

Fig. 16.3. A Soxhlet extractor.

When sustained extraction is necessary to leach all the active component from the crude material, as with plant drugs, an automatic extractor is used. The most popular of these is the Soxhlet extractor (Fig. 16.3). The finely ground crude drug, held in a porous bag or "thimble" made of strong filter paper, is placed in chamber E. The extracting solvent in flask A is heated. Its vapors rise through side arm B and are condensed in the condenser D. The condensed extractant drips into the thimble containing the crude drug, extracting it by contact. When the level of liquid in the chamber E rises to the top of the siphon tube C, the liquid contents of E are automatically filtered through the thimble and siphoned into A. This process is continued until extraction is complete.

16.3 Countercurrent Distribution

Countercurrent distribution (CCD) is a refinement of basic liquid-liquid extraction that permits separation of substances with very similar partitioning behavior. The term "countercurrent" indicates that the two phases move in opposite directions; actually in the CCD procedure as it is usually used, one phase is stable and the other moves; hence the two phases are in relative motion.

Principle of Countercurrent Distribution. Let us consider the distribution of a single solute between two immiscible liquids. It was shown in Section 16.1 that the fraction p distributed into the upper phase is a function of the partition coefficient K and the ratio U of upper- to lower-phase volumes:

$$p = \frac{KU}{KU + 1}$$

The fraction of solute in the lower phase at equilibrium, q, is given by

$$q = \frac{1}{KU + 1}$$

since $p + q = 1$. The greater the value of KU, the larger the fraction p of solute that passes into the upper phase.

The countercurrent distribution process utilizes a train of tubes within which the individual equilibrations occur. At the beginning of the experiment each tube is charged with an identical volume of the lower phase (for example, water or an aqueous buffer). These tubes are numbered 0, 1, 2, . . . , r. Into tube 0 a suitable volume of the upper phase solvent (for example, ether) is introduced. The solute is added to tube 0; it is immaterial whether the solute is added in the upper or the lower phase. Figure 16.4 is a schematic rendering of a countercurrent distribution of a single solute; it is assumed, in this case, that $p = q = 0.5$. Figure 16.4*a* represents the train of tubes as it has been

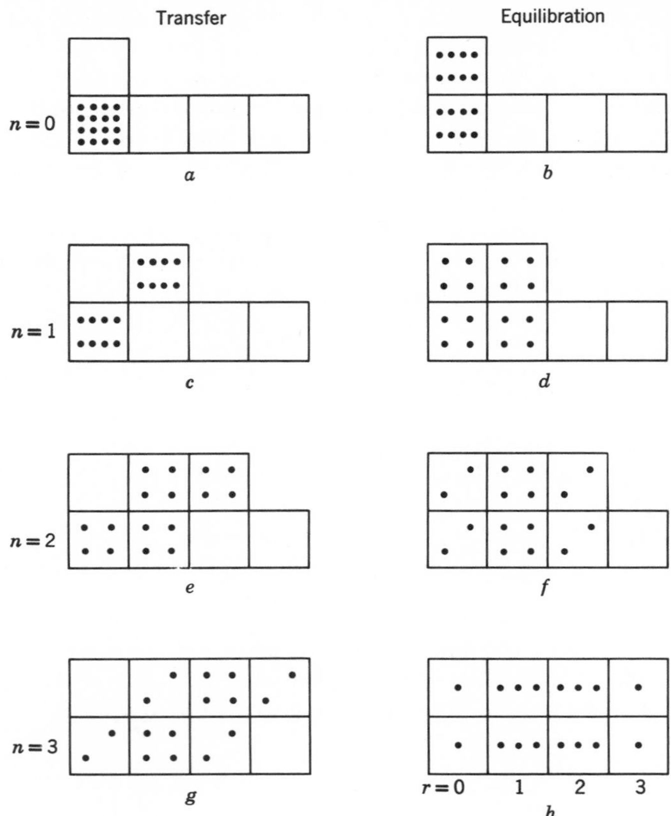

Fig. 16.4. Schematic representation of countercurrent distribution with three transfers of a solute with $p = 0.5$.

described above, with 16 parts of solute added to the lower phase of tube 0.

Now the tube is shaken to allow distribution to occur; in Fig. 16.4*b* the resulting partitioning of the solute is shown as eight parts in each phase, since $p = q$ for this particular solute.

Next the upper phase of tube 0 is transferred to tube 1 (this is called the first transfer) and fresh solvent is added to tube 0 (Fig. 16.4*c*). The tubes are equilibrated to give the distribution shown in Fig. 16.4*d*. This sequence is repeated until three transfers have been effected ($n = 3$), as shown in Fig. 16.4*h*.

The result of these operations has been to transfer the solute in the direction of motion of the upper phase. This process may be repeated many times. Since only the upper phase is transferred, clearly the solute can progress along the train of tubes only by being extracted into the upper phase. Therefore the greater the value of p, the farther along the tube train the solute will progress in a given number of transfers. Actually the solute is distributed over many tubes, as can be seen by the example shown in Fig. 16.4.

If the original sample contains two solutes with different partition coefficients, they will progress along the tubes at different rates, the substance with the larger partition coefficient traveling faster. In order to separate the solutes it is necessary only to perform enough transfers. An instrument has been designed that will carry out hundreds of transfers automatically [3]. Countercurrent distribution is a very efficient process for the separation of closely related compounds. It has been widely utilized in investigations of natural products, and has been especially valuable in the study of peptides. Several authors have reviewed the theory and practice of this separation method [3, 4]. A bibliography of separations by CCD has been given by Casinovi [5].

Calculation of the Distribution. It is possible to predict quantitatively the countercurrent distribution behavior of a solute if its partition coefficient is known for the liquid-liquid system. We assume that the partition isotherm is linear. Since K and U are known quantities, p and q may be calculated.

Suppose that one unit of a single solute is placed in the lower phase of tube 0; the situation may be represented as in the first row of Table 16.3, where, as in

TABLE 16.3
Calculation of the Distribution through Four Transfers

Transfer Number, n		Tube Number, r				
		0	1	2	3	4
0	B^a	$0/1$				
	A^a	p/q				
1	B	$0/q$	$p/0$			
	A	pq/q^2	p^2/pq			
2	B	$0/q^2$	pq/pq	$p^2/0$		
	A	pq^2/q^3	$2p^2q/2pq^2$	p^3/p^2q		
3	B	$0/q^3$	$pq^2/2pq^2$	$2p^2q/p^2q$	$p^3/0$	
	A	pq^3/q^4	$3p^2q^2/3pq^3$	$3p^3q/3p^2q^2$	p^4/p^3q	
4	B	$0/q^4$	$pq^3/3pq^3$	$3p^2q^2/3p^2q^2$	$3p^3q/p^3q$	$p^4/0$
Totals after four transfers		q^4	$4pq^3$	$6p^2q^2$	$4p^3q$	p^4

[a] B represents *Before equilibration*, and A, *After equilibration*.

the earlier discussion, the tubes are numbered 0, 1, 2, . . . , r, and transfers 0, 1, 2, . . . , n. Before equilibration all of the solute is in the lower phase, and after equilibration a fraction p of the solute is in the upper phase and q is in the lower phase.

Next the upper phase of tube 0 is transferred to tube 1 (which contains fresh lower phase) and fresh upper phase is placed in tube 0. The phases are equilibrated. The fraction of total solute extracted into the upper phase of tube 0 will be p times the fraction of solute in the tube, or pq. Similarly, the fraction of solute in the lower phase is q times the fraction of solute in the tube, or q^2. In this way the distribution has been calculated through four transfers (Table 16.3).

In the last row of the table the total fraction of original solute in each tube is listed. The distribution exhibits a marked symmetry in p and q. Obviously the calculation of such a distribution for many transfers would be extremely laborious, but it is fortunately not necessary to proceed as in the previous example. It has been observed that the total fraction of original solute in each tube is given by the corresponding term in the binomial expansion, $(q + p)^n$. Two implications of this result are: (1) for n transfers there are $n + 1$ terms, and therefore $n + 1$ tubes; (2) the sum of all the terms is 1, since $p + q = 1$, and 1 to any power is 1.

The expansion of the function $(q + p)^n$ is laborious for large n, and an easier calculation is available. The binomial expansion may be written

$$(q + p)^n = q^n + nq^{n-1}p + \frac{n(n-1)}{2} q^{n-2}p^2 + \cdots + p^n$$

which can be expressed

$$(q + p)^n = \sum_{r=0}^{n} \frac{n!}{r!(n-r)!} p^r q^{(n-r)}$$

where r is the number of the corresponding term in the expansion.* Interpreting this in the context of CCD, we write Eq. 16.10 for the rth term in

* The quantity $n!$ is called "n factorial" and is defined $n! = 1 \cdot 2 \cdot 3 \cdot 4 \cdots n$. The identity $0! = 1$ must be accepted. Note that the numerical factor $n!/r!(n-r)!$, which is called the binomial coefficient, is generated for any n by Pascal's triangle:

n									*Binomial Coefficients*
0					1				
1				1		1			
2			1		2		1		
3		1		3		3		1	
4	1		4		6		4		1
.									
.					etc.				
.									

the binomial expansion,

$$T_{nr} = \frac{n!}{r!(n-r)!} p^r q^{(n-r)} \tag{16.10}$$

where the quantity T_{nr} is read "the fraction of total solute contained in both layers of the rth tube after n transfers." A calculated countercurrent distribution is usually exhibited as a plot of T_{nr} versus r. Equation 16.10 is called the binomial distribution.

The calculation of the CCD curve may be further simplified. According to statistical theory, the mean of the binomial distribution is equal to np. The mean corresponds to the maximum; therefore the tube number of the maximum in the curve, $r_{\max}$, is given by

$$r_{\max} = np \tag{16.11}$$

This simple expression permits one to calculate the maximum in the CCD curve if p is known. Although n must be an integral number, $r_{\max}$ need not be. Notice that $r_{\max}$ is directly proportional to p. If Eq. 16.10 is written for T_{nr} and for $T_{n(r-1)}$, these expressions can be combined to give

$$\frac{T_{nr}}{T_{n(r-1)}} = \frac{p(n-r+1)}{qr} \tag{16.12}$$

with which the fraction of solute in any tube can be calculated if the fraction in an adjacent tube is known.

The easiest way to calculate an entire distribution curve with these equations (assuming p is known) is first to find $r_{\max}$ with Eq. 16.11. Next calculate T_{nr} with Eq. 16.10 for one tube in the vicinity of $r_{\max}$. Finally calculate the fractions of solute in all surrounding tubes by means of Eq. 16.12. Figure 16.5 shows the results of such a calculation for a typical separation of two solutes: it was assumed that $K_1 = 0.5$, $K_2 = 2.0$, and $U = 1.00$ for this system. In Fig. 16.5*a* the distribution of each solute is shown after four transfers. In an actual experiment the tube contents would be analyzed for total solutes present, and the experimental curve would therefore represent the sum of the fractions of the individual solutes; this curve is shown as the solid line in Fig. 16.5*a*. Separation is not yet apparent in this curve. The individual distribution curves, however, show that a partial resolution has occurred, with tubes 0 and 1 enriched in solute 1, tubes 3 and 4 enriched in solute 2, and tube 2 containing equal fractions of solutes 1 and 2.

Figure 16.5*b* shows the same system after 24 transfers. Separation of the solutes is now apparent. Tubes 0–9 contain essentially only solute 1, whereas tubes 15–24 contain only solute 2. Portions of both solutes will be found in tubes 10–14. If the experiment were extended to a larger number of transfers, a complete separation could eventually be achieved. Note, however, that the

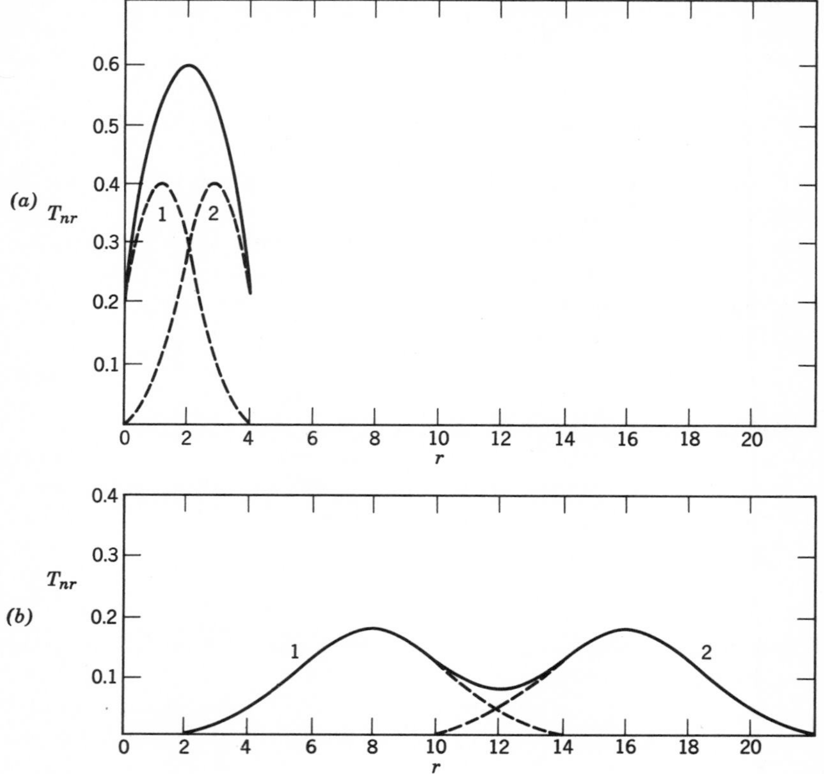

Fig. 16.5. Countercurrent distribution of two solutes in a system where $K_1 = 0.5$, $K_2 = 2.0$, $U = 1.0$: (*a*) distribution after 4 transfers; (*b*) distribution after 24 transfers. The calculated points are connected by smooth curves, though in fact the distribution is discontinuous.

width of the "zones," or distribution curves, increases as the number of transfers increases.

In a real experimental situation, the quantity plotted on the vertical axis would usually be an analytical quantity, such as weight of solute per tube, rather than the fraction T_{nr}. It may be noted that from such an experimental distribution curve the quantity $r_{\max}$ may be read and, by utilizing Eqs. 16.11 and 16.7, the partition coefficient may be estimated.

The countercurrent distribution curve is not symmetrical (unless $p = q$), but as n becomes larger, the curve approaches very closely a symmetrical distribution.

Normal Approximation to the Binomial Distribution. CCD is a discontinuous process; that is, it occurs in discrete, countable steps. Its exact mathematical description, the binomial distribution, is therefore a discontinuous function. As we have seen, the calculation of the CCD for large n is very laborious with the binomial distribution. As n becomes larger, however, the CCD plot becomes more symmetrical, and it is found that the binomial distribution can be closely approximated, at large n, by a continuous function that permits calculations to be more easily made.

The procedure in finding this function is to express $n!$ by Eq. 16.13, which is called Stirling's formula, and which gives a close approximation when n is large.

$$n! \approx \sqrt{2\pi}\, n^{(n+1/2)} e^{-n} \tag{16.13}$$

This is substituted into Eq. 16.10, and ultimately it can be shown that Eq. 16.14 can be obtained.

$$T_{nr} = \left[\frac{1}{2\pi npq}\right]^{1/2} e^{-(r-np)^2/2npq} \tag{16.14}$$

According to statistical theory, the mean (μ) in the binomial distribution is given by Eq. 16.15, and the standard deviation (σ) by Eq. 16.16.

$$\mu = np \tag{16.15}$$

$$\sigma = \sqrt{npq} \tag{16.16}$$

Substituting these into Eq. 16.14,

$$T_{nr} = \frac{1}{\sigma\sqrt{2\pi}} e^{-1/2[(r-\mu)/\sigma]^2} \tag{16.17}$$

Equation 16.17 is variously called the normal distribution, normal error curve, or Gaussian error curve. Although we derived it as an approximation to the binomial distribution, it is an important distribution function in many physical contexts.

The normal distribution can be displayed as a plot of T_{nr} against r. The appearance of a particular normal curve is completely determined by its mean μ and standard deviation σ; μ is the maximum in the curve and therefore determines its position on the r axis, and σ is a measure of the width of the curve. These relationships are illustrated in Fig. 27.1.

Experience has shown that the normal curve gives a good approximation to the binomial distribution as long as $np > 5$ when $p \leq 0.5$, or $nq > 5$ when $p > 0.5$. That is, n must be large and p must not be very small. Under these conditions the entire CCD curve is easily calculated. We first note that an expression for the fraction of solute in the tube corresponding to the maximum is obtained by letting $r = \mu$; thus $r - \mu = 0$ and we have

$$T_{max} = (2\pi npq)^{-1/2} \tag{16.18}$$

For the general problem of plotting the entire CCD curve, let

$$t = \frac{r - \mu}{\sigma} \tag{16.19}$$

Then Eq. 16.17 becomes

$$T_{nr} = \frac{1}{\sigma\sqrt{2\pi}} e^{-t^2/2} \tag{16.20}$$

If we define the function $f(t)$ by

$$f(t) = \frac{1}{\sqrt{2\pi}} e^{-t^2/2} \tag{16.21}$$

we have the standard normal curve, that is, the normal curve with mean 0 and standard deviation 1. Combining Eqs. 16.20 and 16.21,

$$T_{nr} = \frac{f(t)}{\sigma} \tag{16.22}$$

All collections of mathematical tables list values for the standard normal curve. These tables give $f(t)$ (the ordinate) as a function of t; they also give the area under the curve from 0 to t. Since the curve is symmetrical about $t = 0$, the other half is obtained by symmetry. To calculate the CCD curve we must know n and p; then μ and σ can be calculated. Next t is calculated for several tubes on one side of the maximum, the corresponding values of $f(t)$ are obtained from the tables, and finally T_{nr} is found with Eq. 16.22. If the curve is to be expressed as weight of solute per tube, each T_{nr} value is multiplied by the total weight of solute.

EXAMPLE 16.3. Calculate the theoretical CCD curve for a solute that gave $r_{max} = 150$ after 200 transfers.

From this information we obtain $p = \frac{3}{4}$, $q = \frac{1}{4}$, $\mu = 150$, $\sigma = 6.12$. Table 16.4 shows the calculation for several tubes. Tube 149 contains the same fraction as tube 151, and so on. The sum of T_{nr} over all tubes must equal unity.

From the mathematical tables of area as a function of t we find that the area from $t = 0$ to $t = 1$ is 0.34. Therefore the area under the normal curve within the limits $\mu \pm \sigma$ is 68% of the total area under the curve. Similarly the area in the range $\mu \pm 2\sigma$ is about 95% of the total, and in $\mu \pm 3\sigma$ it is more than 99%. We can therefore calculate the tubes within which any fraction of the solute is contained. Thus in Example 16.3 95% of the solute will be recovered if the contents of tubes 138–162 ($\mu \pm 2\sigma$) are pooled.

TABLE 16.4
Calculation of a CCD Curve Using the Normal Approximation[a]

r	$r - \mu$	t	$f(t)$	T_{nr}
150	0	0	0.399	0.0654
151	1	0.163	0.394	0.0643
152	2	0.327	0.378	0.0617
154	4	0.653	0.323	0.0528
156	6	0.98	0.247	0.0404
158	8	1.31	0.169	0.0276
160	10	1.63	0.106	0.0173
164	14	2.28	0.030	0.0049
168	18	2.94	0.005	0.0008
172	22	3.59	0.001	0.0000

[a] See Example 16.3.

Experiment 16.1. Development of a Liquid-Liquid Extraction Assay of Ephedrine-Phenobarbital Mixtures

PRINCIPLE

A mixture of ephedrine (as its hydrochloride or sulfate salt) and a barbituric acid derivative is a common combination of drugs. This mixture is perfectly suited to separation by liquid-liquid extraction. Briefly, the procedure involves bringing the mixture into an alkaline aqueous solution. The ephedrine is quantitatively extracted with several portions of ether, the alkali salt of the barbiturate being retained in the water phase. The aqueous solution is next acidified, and the free barbituric acid derivative is extracted. The ether extracts may be assayed in any convenient and reliable manner for the separated substances. The assay is developed from the principles outlined earlier in this chapter, with a preliminary determination of a partition coefficient being made [6]. An alternative extraction plan would be first to extract the barbiturate from an acid solution, then to make the aqueous raffinate basic and to extract the ephedrine.

REAGENTS

Standard 0.1 N Acetous Perchloric Acid, Mercuric Acetate Solution, p-Naphtholbenzein Indicator Solution. See Experiment 2.1 for the preparation of these solutions.

Ephedrine Hydrochloride. If desired, the purity of the sample can be checked. Accurately weigh about 500 mg into an Erlenmeyer flask and dissolve it in 25 ml of glacial acetic acid. Add 25 ml of mercuric acetate solution and several drops of indicator. Titrate to the green color with standard 0.1 *N* perchloric acid. Calculate the purity of the ephedrine hydrochloride.

PROCEDURES

Determination of Ephedrine Partition Coefficient. Prepare the aqueous phase by mixing 100 ml of water, 50 ml of 1 *N* sodium hydroxide, and 30 g of sodium chloride. Shake this in a large separatory funnel with 150 ml of diethyl ether to saturate each phase with the other. Separate the phases.

Accurately weigh about 400 mg of ephedrine hydrochloride and transfer it to a 250 ml separatory funnel. Add 50.0 ml of the aqueous phase just prepared and dissolve the sample. Now add 50.0 ml of the ether phase and shake vigorously to achieve equilibrium distribution. Record the temperature.

Run out the aqueous layer and accurately collect all of the ether phase in a flask. Evaporate the ether solution to dryness in a hood. Dissolve the residue in about 50 ml of glacial acetic acid, add *p*-naphtholbenzein indicator, and titrate with standard 0.1 *N* perchloric acid.

Calculate the amount of ephedrine in the ether phase. Obtain the amount of ephedrine in the aqueous phase by subtracting the amount in the ether from the total amount of ephedrine *base* taken, making any necessary adjustment for the purity of the ephedrine hydrochloride. Calculate the partition coefficient according to Eq. 16.2.

Repeat this experiment starting with 600 and 800 mg samples of ephedrine hydrochloride. Construct a partition isotherm by plotting concentration of ephedrine in the aqueous phase against concentration in the organic phase.

Quantitative Extraction of Ephedrine. Calculate, with Eq. 16.9, the number of extractions required to extract 99.9% of the ephedrine from an aqueous solution of the composition prepared previously; use $U = 1.0$ and the partition coefficient evaluated in the preceding experiment.

Accurately weigh about 2 g of ephedrine hydrochloride into a 100 ml volumetric flask and dissolve it in enough water to make 100.0 ml. Pipet a 30.0 ml aliquot into a 250 ml separatory funnel and add 15.0 ml of 1 *N* NaOH and 9 g of sodium chloride. (The final volume of this solution is about 50 ml.) Now add 50 ml of ether and shake to equilibrate. Run the aqueous layer into another separatory funnel and transfer the ether layer to a 250 ml erlenmeyer flask. Add a fresh 50 ml portion of ether to the aqueous raffinate and extract a second time, running the aqueous phase into a separatory funnel and adding the ether layer to the flask containing the first ether extract. Repeat this extraction as many times as the calculation showed was necessary to achieve 99.9% extraction.*

Evaporate the combined ether extracts to dryness on a steam bath in a hood, dissolve the residue in acetic acid, and titrate to the *p*-naphtholbenzein

* Two separatory funnels are sufficient for the entire operation; the funnels are used alternately.

end point with standard perchloric acid. Calculate the percent recovery of ephedrine.

Analysis of Ephedrine-Phenobarbital Mixtures. The complete separation scheme can be carried out by pipetting 30.0 ml of the aqueous ephedrine hydrochloride solution prepared previously into a separatory funnel, adding 15 ml of 1 *N* NaOH and 9 g of NaCl, as before, and then adding an accurately weighed sample of about 500 mg of phenobarbital to the solution. A more realistic experiment consists of adding a weighed 1 g sample of an accurately prepared mixture of ephedrine hydrochloride and phenobarbital to a separatory funnel containing 30 ml of water, 15 ml of 1 *N* NaOH, and 9 g of NaCl.

Carry out the quantitative extraction of the ephedrine exactly as described in the preceding paragraphs. Titrate the residue and calculate the percent recovery of ephedrine.

Find in the literature the solubility of phenobarbital in water and in ether. Use this information to estimate the partition coefficient of phenobarbital in the ether/water system. Calculate the number of extractions necessary for 99.9% extraction of the phenobarbital.

Acidify the aqueous raffinate with sufficient concentrated hydrochloric acid to make the solution distinctly acidic (at least pH 4). Completely extract the phenobarbital with 50 ml portions of ether. Evaporate the combined ether extracts in a tared flask, dry the residue at 100° for 1 hr, cool, and weigh the dry phenobarbital. Calculate the percent recovery of phenobarbital.

The ephedrine extraction, and subsequent acidification of the raffinate, should be carried out without delay, for the barbiturate is subject to decomposition in basic medium.

Analysis of Unknown Sample. From your instructor obtain capsules or a bulk sample of ephedrine-phenobarbital mixture. If your sample is capsules, completely empty a counted number of capsules and mix the contents. Accurately weigh the pooled example.

Weigh about 1 g of the powder into a separatory funnel and analyze it for ephedrine and phenobarbital by solvent extraction. Perform a duplicate analysis. Calculate the percentage composition of the mixture. If your sample was capsules, report the average weights of ephedrine and phenobarbital per capsule.

Experiment 16.2. Determination of Alkaloidal Content of Belladonna Leaf by Solvent Extraction

REAGENTS AND APPARATUS

0.02 N Sulfuric Acid, 0.02 N Sodium Hydroxide. These solutions are prepared and standardized as described in Experiment 1.1.

Soxhlet Extraction Apparatus (medium size), with thimbles.

PROCEDURE*

Weigh about 10 g of belladonna leaf, in moderately coarse powder, into a Soxhlet extraction thimble. Place the thimble in the extractor. Moisten the crude drug with a mixture of 8 ml of concentrated ammonium hydroxide, 10 ml of 95% ethanol, and 20 ml of ether; thoroughly mix the drug and solvent. Allow it to macerate overnight. Extract the drug in the Soxhlet extractor with ether for at least 3 hr.

Transfer the ether extract, containing the alkaloids, to a separatory funnel; rinse the flask with a small quantity of ether and add the rinsings to the funnel. Extract the alkaloids with five 20 ml portions of approximately 0.5 *N* sulfuric acid, filtering the aqueous solutions into a second separatory funnel. Add 10% ammonia to the combined aqueous solution until it is distinctly alkaline. Extract the alkaloids with five 20 ml portions of chloroform. Evaporate the combined chloroform extracts to dryness on a steam bath. Dissolve the residue in a few ml of chloroform, add 15.0 ml of standard 0.02 *N* sulfuric acid, heat to drive off the chloroform, cool, add methyl red indicator solution, and titrate the excess acid with standard 0.02 *N* sodium hydroxide.

Calculate the alkaloidal content of the belladonna leaf as atropine. Compare your result with the official requirement.

References

1. Reese, D. R., G. M. Irwin, L. W. Dittert, C. W. Chong, and J. V. Swintosky, *J. Pharm. Sci.*, **53,** 591 (1964).
2. Leo, A., C. Hansch, and D. Elkins, *Chem. Revs.*, **71,** 525 (1971).
3. Craig, L. C. and D. Craig, *Technique of Organic Chemistry*, Vol. III, Part I, 2nd ed., A. Weissberger (ed.), Interscience, New York, 1956, Chap. II.
4. Weisiger, J. R., *Org. Anal.*, **2,** 277 (1954).
5. Casinovi, C. G., *Chromatographic Reviews*, Vol. 5, M. Lederer (ed.), Elsevier Publishing Co., Amsterdam, 1963.
6. Kelsey, J. E. and K. A. Connors, *Am. J. Pharm. Educ.*, **29,** 500 (1965).

FOR FURTHER READING

Hansch, C. and W. J. Dunn, III, "Linear Relationships Between Lipophilic Character and Biological Activity of Drugs," *J. Pharm. Sci.*, **61,** 1 (1972).

Flynn, G. L., "Structural Approach to Partitioning: Estimation of Steroid Partition Coefficients Based upon Molecular Constitution," *J. Pharm. Sci.*, **60,** 345 (1971).

Jackson, J. V., "Extraction Methods in Toxicology," *Isolation and Identification of Drugs*, E. G. C. Clarke (ed.), The Pharmaceutical Press, London, 1969, pp. 16–30.

Connors, K. A. and S. P. Eriksen, "A Simple Apparatus for the Demonstration of Countercurrent Distribution," *Am. J. Pharm. Educ.*, **29,** 509 (1965).

* This follows the official procedure.

Problems

1. A 25.0 ml aliquot of a 0.4% (*w/v*) aqueous solution of acetanilide was extracted with three 10.0 ml portions of ether. The combined ether extracts were evaporated to dryness and the residue was weighed. The ether/water partition coefficient for acetanilide is 3.0. What was the weight of the residue?

2. The following spectrophotometric data are available for acetanilide.

Solvent	λ_{max} (nm)	Molar Absorptivity
Water	240	10,000
Benzene	239	13,000

One milligram of acetanilide was dissolved in 100 ml of water. This solution was extracted once with 50 ml of benzene. The phases were separated and their absorbances measured at the appropriate wavelengths in a 1 cm cell. The absorbance of the aqueous solution was 0.245, whereas the absorbance of the benzene solution was 1.290. What is the partition coefficient of acetanilide in the benzene/water system?

3. Outline a method of analysis for the caffeine content of a sample of tea. Does your method sound practical enough for you to be willing to try it in the laboratory?

4. The partition coefficient of an alkaloidal drug between chloroform and water is 8 (it is more soluble in the organic solvent). Fifty milliliters of a 0.01 *M* aqueous solution of the alkaloid is extracted with one 10.0 ml portion of chloroform, and the chloroform solution is evaporated to dryness. What is the weight of the residue? The MW of the alkaloid is 210.

5. Outline a practical method for the quantitative analysis of the active ingredients in a tablet containing codeine phosphate, aspirin, and lactose.

6. (*a*) Consider the distribution of a weak acid HA between an organic phase and an aqueous phase. If the true partition coefficient is $K = [HA]_{org}/[HA]_{aq}$, and if the anion is not detectably soluble in the organic phase, show that the apparent partition coefficient K_{app} is related to K as follows:

$$K_{app} = \frac{K[H^+]}{[H^+] + K_a}$$

where K_a is the acid dissociation constant of HA and K_{app} is the ratio of total concentrations of solute in the organic and aqueous layers.

(*b*) How is K_{app} related to K in the limits of very high and very low hydrogen ion concentration? What is their relationship when pH = pK_a?

(*c*) Calculate K_{app} as a function of pH for a solute whose pK_a = 5.0 and whose K = 8.0. Plot K_{app} versus pH.

7. How many extractions are necessary to remove 99.9% of a drug from 50 ml of an aqueous solution if it is extracted with 25 ml portions of ether and its partition coefficient is 1.0?

8. The partition coefficient of a compound (benzene/water system) was known to be 0.6. One millimole of the compound was dissolved in 50 ml of water and was shaken

with 100 ml of benzene. A sample of the benzene layer was examined spectrophotometrically in a 1 cm cell at a wavelength where the molar absorptivity of the compound in benzene is 3.2×10^2. What was the absorbance?

9. 100 ml of an aqueous solution containing 1 mg/ml of acetanilide and 3 mg/ml of aspirin is extracted with one 50 ml portion of ether under conditions such that the partition coefficients (ether/water) are 3.0 for acetanilide and 0.5 for aspirin. The ether layer was separated and evaporated to dryness. What was the total weight of the dried residue?

10. Suppose the aqueous solution described in Problem 9 is subjected to countercurrent distribution, with 10 ml of the solution being placed in Tube 0, and 10 ml portions of ether being used in the CCD. Let 12 transfers be carried out.

(*a*) Calculate the positions of the maxima in the CCD curve for acetanilide and aspirin.

(*b*) Calculate the total weight of solute in Tube 8. (Note that both acetanilide and aspirin will be found in each tube.)

11. 50.0 ml of a 1% (w/v) aqueous solution of a drug is extracted with three 25 ml portions of ether, the partition coefficient (ether/water) being 0.8. The ether extracts are combined and evaporated to dryness. What is the weight of the residue?

12. 0.750 g of acetic acid was dissolved in 20 ml of ether. This was shaken with 10 ml of water, the phases were separated, and the aqueous phase was titrated with 0.250 *N* NaOH, 32.50 ml being required to reach the phenolphthalein end point. Calculate the partition coefficient of acetic acid between ether/water.

13. Recall that for any equilibrium process we have $\Delta G^\circ = -RT \ln K$, where ΔG° is the standard molar free energy change and K is the equilibrium constant. If the process is

$$\text{Caffeine in } CHCl_3 \rightleftharpoons \text{Caffeine in } H_2O$$

define the appropriate K to be used in the equation, and explain the meaning of the resulting ΔG°.

14. Imagine the system consisting of a single solute distributed among three mutually immiscible phases (A, B, C), the system being at equilibrium.

(*a*) Define the three partition coefficients.

(*b*) Derive an equation relating one of the partition coefficients to the other two.

(*c*) Derive an equation relating the fraction of solute in phase A to the partition coefficients and the volumes of the phases.

15. 100.0 ml of a 1% drug solution was extracted with two 20 ml portions of ether. The combined ether extracts were evaporated and the dry residue was found to weigh 865.5 mg. Calculate the partition coefficient.

16. The pK_a of ephedrine is 9.5, its partition coefficient is 8.4 (ether/water), and its molecular weight is 165.2.

(*a*) 100.0 ml of 0.10 *M* ephedrine solution in water was made strongly alkaline with NaOH. It was extracted with two 50 ml portions of ether; the ether extracts were combined and evaporated to dryness. Calculate the weight of the dried residue.

(*b*) Suppose the extraction in part (*a*) was carried out with the aqueous phase being buffered at pH 9.5. Now estimate the weight of dried residue obtained by following the same extraction procedure.

17. What is the fundamental difference between the multiple extraction technique (Section 16.1) and countercurrent distribution?

18. The partition coefficients of two compounds are 0.8 between benzene and water. A CCD separation of a mixture of these substances is conducted, with 5 ml of water and 4 ml of benzene contained in each tube. Calculate the positions of the distribution maxima after 60 transfers.

19. A mixture of three compounds was subjected to countercurrent distribution. After 150 transfers in an apparatus containing 5 ml of water and 5 ml of ether per tube, the maxima in the distribution curves for these compounds appeared at tubes 30, 75, and 120. Calculate the partition coefficients of these three compounds.

20. Calculate the fraction of total solute in the upper phase of the fourth tube after 10 transfers in a countercurrent distribution if the partition coefficient is 2.0 and the ratio of phase volumes is 1.0.

21. After 150 transfers in a countercurrent separation of two compounds, the maxima in their distribution curves appeared at tubes 27.5 and 83.0. The distribution was carried out with 10 ml of aqueous buffer as the lower phase and 10 ml of ether as the upper phase in each tube. Calculate the partition coefficients of the two compounds.

22. (*a*) Calculate the entire CCD curves for the separation of two solutes having partition coefficients 0.5 and 2.0 if $U = 1.0$ and $n = 20$. Use the binomial distribution. Plot the results.

(*b*) Repeat the calculation using the normal approximation. Superimpose the results on the calculations of part (*a*) to see how good the approximation is.

23. Calculate and plot a graph of percent extracted in a single extraction ($100p$) against $\log K$ (for $U = 1$) over the range $K = 0.001$ to 1000. (Let K vary by factors of 10).

24. (*a*) Calculate, with the normal approximation to the binomial distribution, the theoretical CCD curve for a solute with $K = 2.0$ in the ether/water system if each tube contains 10 ml of each solvent and 300 transfers are carried out.

(*b*) If 1.50 of solute was taken initially, how many milligrams will be present in the upper phase of the maximum tube after the distribution?

(*c*) The contents of which tubes should be pooled to yield 95% of the original solute?

25. Show that the absolute width of the CCD curve increases as n increases, whereas its relative width decreases. (The standard deviation, or some multiple of it, is a convenient measure of width.)

17 LIQUID CHROMATOGRAPHY

17.1 Introduction to Chromatography

The Chromatographic Process. In 1903 the Russian biochemist Tswett developed a new separation technique that involved passage of the mixture to be separated through a column of a finely powdered adsorbent. A portion of the mixture was applied to the top of such a column, and it was washed through with an organic solvent. As the washing step proceeded, the several components in the mixture were washed down the column at different rates; finally they separated completely, and could be recovered by washing them out of the column and collecting them in separate fractions, or by extruding the column from the tube in which it was contained and cutting the column apart between the zones of separated compounds. Most of Tswett's samples were plant pigments, so the colored bands formed by the compounds on the column were readily visible; in fact, these colored zones gave rise to the name chromatography for this method of separation. Tswett accounted for the separation by proposing that the molecules of solute were adsorbed to the surface of the powdered column material. Those substances that were very strongly adsorbed to the solid were not readily desorbed by the solvent, and these compounds moved very slowly down the column. Less strongly adsorbed solutes were transported down the column at greater rates; thus a separation was achieved because of the varying affinities of the solutes for the solvent and the solid adsorbent. The American geologist Day, at about the same time, effected partial separations of crude petroleum by passage through columns of adsorbents.

Many forms of chromatography have now been developed, but they are all based on this simple principle: the separation results from different rates of zone migration caused by differences in relative affinities for two phases. This, of course, is the same principle underlying the countercurrent distribution method of separation. Chromatography is a process for the separation of molecular mixtures by distribution of the solutes between two phases, the phases being contacted in a continuous countercurrent manner.

Before considering the theory and application of chromatography it will be helpful to have a conception of the physical system and the actual conduct of a chromatographic separation. Since all forms of chromatographic separations are based on the same principle, any one of them will serve as an example. We will consider liquid-liquid column chromatography; that is, both the phases are liquids, so the distribution process is liquid-liquid partitioning, and the process is carried out in a column.

In all types of chromatography one phase is held motionless and the other is moved past it in a continuous manner. The thin phase is always the stationary phase and the bulk phase is the mobile one; we shall often use the terms stationary and mobile to refer to these two phases. The stationary phase in column liquid-liquid chromatography is a very thin layer of solvent held as an adsorbed coating on fine particles of a supporting powder. The only function of the solid is to hold the stationary phase (sometimes called the internal phase). This combined system of solvent adsorbed on a solid support is packed more or less firmly into a glass tube, being supported at the lower end of the tube by a sintered glass disk or other device. The interparticle space on the column is filled with the mobile phase, which must be a solvent immiscible with the stationary phase. A cork or stopcock on the bottom of the tube controls the flow of mobile solvent.

Now the sample mixture is added to the top of the column in a fairly small portion to form a narrow band at the top of the packing. Suppose that the sample is a mixture of compounds A and B, and that the stationary and mobile phases have been selected so that the partition coefficients of A and B in the mobile phase (M)/stationary phase (S) system are different. Let $K_B(=c_S{}^B/c_M{}^B)$ be larger than K_A.* The chromatographic column at this point may be represented as in Fig. 17.1*a*, where the sample zone at the top of the column contains both A and B.

Now mobile phase is added to the top of the column and is allowed to percolate into the packing. As this fresh solvent enters the sample zone, the distribution equilibrium requires that a fraction of each A and B pass into the mobile phase in order to satisfy the expressions for K_A and K_B; and since K_A is smaller than K_B, a larger proportion of A than of B will enter the mobile phase. As more mobile phase (the *eluent*) enters the packing, the portion of eluent carrying A and B enters the lower region of the column below the initial sample zone. Now the distribution equilibrium requires that the solute pass from the mobile into the stationary phase, since in this region of the column the stationary phase contains no solute. Thus both A and B are caused to migrate down the column, with the solute being removed from the stationary phase at the trailing (upper) edge of the zone and being deposited at the leading

* The definition $K = c_S/c_M$ is universally used in chromatography, so it is adopted here. In discussing CCD in Chapter 16 we used the reciprocal, the moving phase concentration appearing in the numerator.

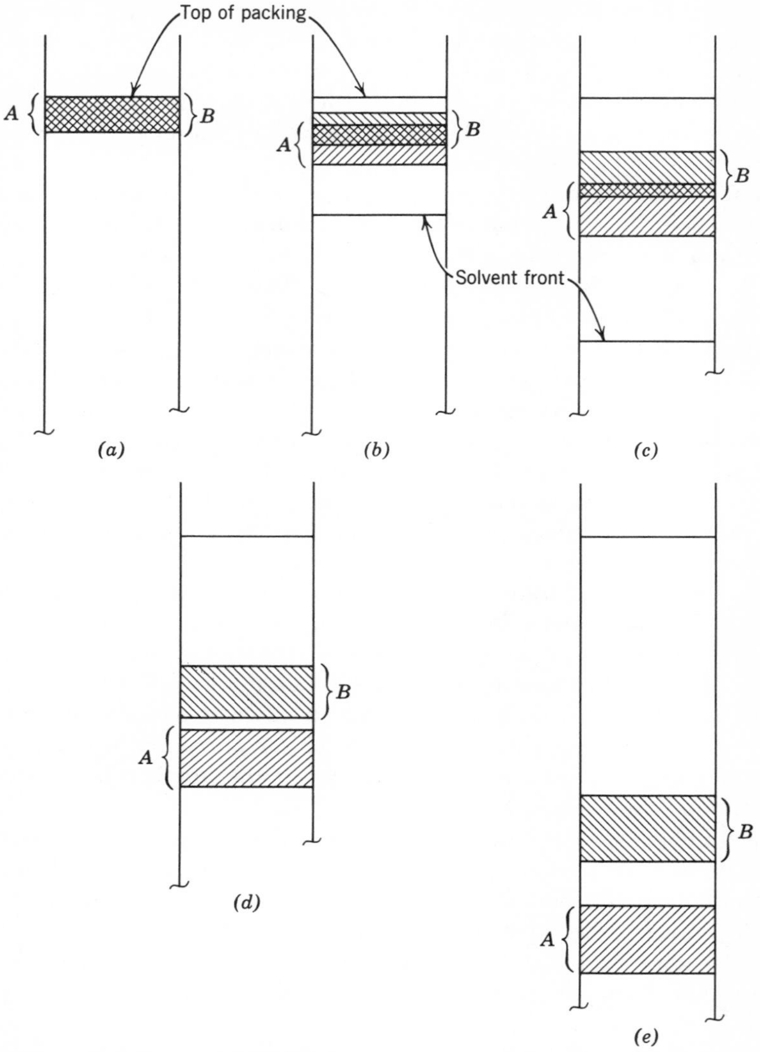

Fig. 17.1. Progress of a column chromatographic separation of solutes A and B.

edge of the zone; this process is due solely to the operation of the distribution equilibria.

Now since the solute can move downward only while it is in the mobile phase, the solute that spends more time in the mobile phase will migrate faster down the column. In the example being considered evidently compound A, which possesses the smaller partition coefficient, will be the faster migrating component. This effect is illustrated in Fig. 17.1*b*, which shows the zone of A pulling slightly ahead of B. Meanwhile the leading portions of solvent have been completely divested of solute by the partition process, and the solvent front, which obviously moves faster than solute A unless K_A is extremely small, is indicated in Fig. 17.1*b* slightly in advance of the solute zones.

The process of passing eluent through the column (this is called *elution*) is continued with the results seen in Fig. 17.1*c*–*e*. The zones, which are traveling at different rates, eventually draw completely apart if the column is sufficiently long. Simultaneously the zones become broader, and the success of the separation depends upon both the extent of separation of the centers of the zones and the extent of zone broadening.

If the development were stopped at the stage shown in Fig. 17.1*e*, the column packing could be removed from the tube, carefully cut between the two zones, and the individual components A and B recovered by extraction from the column material. This technique is seldom utilized. Usually the elution is continued until the zones are washed completely out of the column, the mobile solvent issuing from the column (the *eluate*) being collected in fractions. The fractions containing A can be pooled, and similarly for B. Thus the original sample has been resolved into its components, which are available for identification and quantitative determination.

It is instructive to compare this separation process with the countercurrent distribution method. The essential differences between the two are (1) that CCD is based upon a distribution between two bulk phases, whereas chromatography utilizes a distribution between a bulk and a thin phase; and (2) that the movement of the mobile phase is discontinuous (occurs in discrete, countable steps) in CCD but is continuous in chromatography. In some respects partition chromatography can be regarded as continuous countercurrent distribution. If the eluate from a chromatographic column is collected in small portions, which are analyzed for their solute content, a chromatogram can be constructed by plotting quantity of solute per portion against the eluate volume. Each zone on the column will give rise to a peak or band in the chromatogram. The chromatogram is therefore a concentration profile of the zones as they emerge from the column. Figure 17.2 is a hypothetical chromatogram of the separation carried out in Fig. 17.1. The chromatogram is very similar in appearance to the CCD curves in Fig. 16.5. This close correspondence is another reflection of the common basis of these two methods.

Types of Liquid Chromatography. The physical nature of the phases and the mechanics of bringing them into contact give rise to several types of chromatography. As long as the mobile (bulk) phase is a liquid, the technique is called liquid chromatography (LC). The kinds of LC can be classified in several ways.

1. By Mechanism. When the stationary phase is a liquid so that the

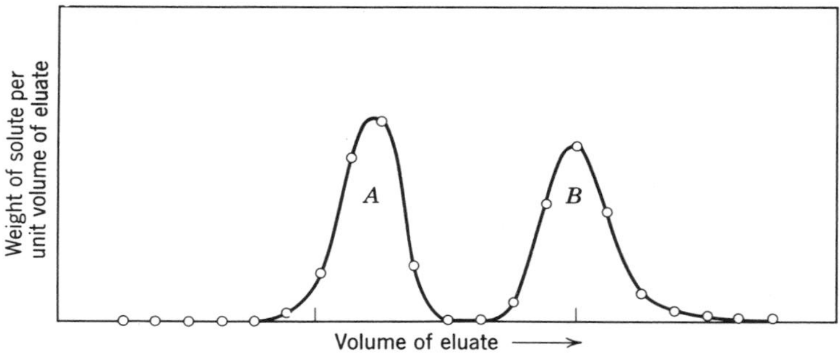

Fig. 17.2. Elution chromatogram of the separation of A and B shown in Fig. 17.1.

distribution mechanism is liquid-liquid partitioning, the technique is called *partition chromatography* or liquid-liquid chromatography (LLC). If the stationary phase is a solid (more properly, the interface between a solid and a liquid), the method is *adsorption chromatography* or liquid-solid chromatography (LSC). Other distribution mechanisms may operate, as in ion-exchange chromatography and molecular exclusion chromatography; these are discussed in Section 17.3.

2. By Experimental Form. In *column chromatography* the chromatographic system (the "bed") is enclosed in a cylindrical tube, usually of glass or metal. *Flat-bed chromatography* is carried out on a plane surface. The forms of flat-bed chromatography are paper chromatography (which usually operates by a partition mechanism) and thin-layer chromatography, TLC (which usually is a form of adsorption chromatography).

3. By Isotherm Linearity. In *linear chromatography* the partition or distribution coefficient is independent of concentration, that is, the partition isotherm is linear over the concentration range encountered in the zone. In *nonlinear chromatography* the isotherm is nonlinear. Partition chromatography is usually linear, and adsorption chromatography is often nonlinear. Linear chromatography is much easier to treat theoretically.

Extent of Zone Migration. The practical chromatographer wants to be able to specify the distance that a sample compound migrates (in flat-bed chromatography) or the volume of mobile phase required to elute it (in column chromatography). Several quantities have been defined to describe zone migration behavior. The most fundamental of these is the R value, defined by

$$R = \frac{\text{Velocity of movement of center of zone}}{\text{Velocity of movement of solvent}} = \frac{i}{v} \tag{17.1}$$

These are linear velocities, with units of distance/time. R can be expressed in several other ways. Since a molecule can move only when it is in the mobile

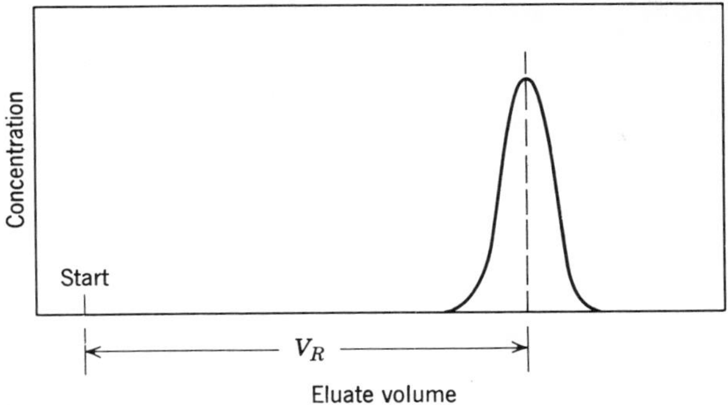

Fig. 17.3. The retention volume in elution chromatography.

phase, R is equal to the fraction of time that a molecule spends in the mobile phase. We can write the velocity of the zone as the product of the velocity of the solvent and the fraction of solute in the mobile phase, or $i = vp$. Therefore $R = p$, with the partition coefficient being defined $K = c_S/c_M$.*

R is not easily measured directly, so other quantities are used to describe migration behavior. With column operation the eluted zone can be characterized by the volume of mobile phase required to elute the zone maximum from the column. This quantity is the *retention volume*, V_R; it is indicated in Fig. 17.3. For a given set of column variables (kind and amount of mobile and stationary phases, column length, temperature, etc.) the retention volume of a compound is essentially constant. If the flow rate of the mobile phase is constant, the retention volume is related to the *retention time* t_R by $V_R = Ft_R$, where F is the flow rate (ml/min); the retention time is the time required to elute one-half of the zone, that is, to reach the zone maximum (Fig. 17.3).

In flat-bed chromatography the zone is not often eluted; instead the development is usually halted before the solvent front has reached the end of the bed. Zone migration is then given by the R_f value, defined by Eq. 17.2 and calculated as shown in Fig. 17.4; evidently $R_f = x/y$.

$$R_f = \frac{\text{Distance from initial point to center of zone}}{\text{Distance from initial point to solvent front}} \tag{17.2}$$

Since the distances are equal to velocities multiplied by the time of development, $x = it$ and $y = vt$, and we find, by the argument given for R, that $R_f = p$.

R and R_f have the character of a fraction, as pointed out above. These

* This definition of K results in the relationship $p = 1/(KU + 1)$.

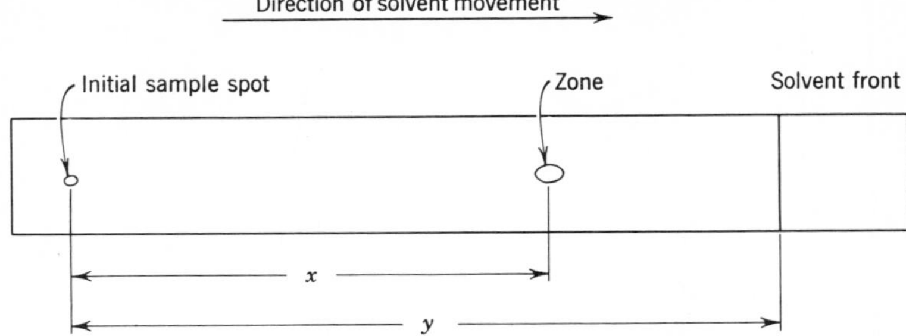

Fig. 17.4. Calculation of R_f value in paper chromatography and thin-layer chromatography.

quantities must lie between 0 and 1.* If R (or R_f) is 0 for a solute, clearly its partition coefficient is extremely large and the solute remains in the stationary phase and therefore immobile. If $R = 1$ the solute has no affinity for the stationary phase and travels with the solvent front. Chromatographic phases are chosen to achieve intermediate values of R or R_f.

17.2 Theory of Chromatography

The Plate Theory. Column partition chromatography was introduced by Martin and Synge in 1941 [1] in a paper that has had great impact on further developments in chromatography. These authors gave a theory for the chromatographic process that can be developed easily by drawing an analogy between liquid-liquid chromatography and countercurrent distribution (see Section 16.3). The point of view is adopted that although a partition chromatographic column is a continuous system, it is equivalent to a series of units within each of which equilibrium is achieved between the mobile and stationary phases. That is, the column is compared to a train of countercurrent distribution tubes. Since the external phase is always moving, equilibrium is really never established, but we can act as if it were by dividing the column into layers or slices (transverse to the direction of flow) of thickness such that the solution leaving each layer is in equilibrium with the average concentration of solute in the stationary phase throughout the layer. Each of these layers is called a plate, and the thickness of a plate is called the height equivalent to a theoretical plate (HETP or simply H). Therefore the plate in a column is analogous to the tube in a CCD system.

In order to obtain a description of the concentration profile of the zone as it

* Some authors tabulate $100R_f$ instead of R_f, simply for typographical convenience.

moves through the column, it is now only necessary to reinterpret the quantities applied in Section 16.3 to CCD.

r = plate number (numbered 0, 1, 2, 3, . . . , r)
n = number of mobile phase volumes passed into the column
V_m = volume of mobile phase per plate
V_s = volume of stationary phase per plate
$U = V_s/V_m$
c_M = concentration of solute in mobile phase at equilibrium (at any point)
c_S = concentration of solute in stationary phase at equilibrium (at any point)
$K = c_S/c_M$ = partition coefficient (assumed constant)
$p = 1/(KU + 1)$ = fraction of solute per plate in mobile phase at equilibrium
$q = KU/(KU + 1)$ = fraction of solute per plate in stationary phase at equilibrium
T_{nr} = fraction of total solute in rth plate after n mobile phase volumes have passed into the column

Then T_{nr} is given by Eq. 17.3, the binomial distribution, by arguments given in Section 16.3.

$$T_{nr} = \frac{n!}{r!(n-r)!} p^r q^{(n-r)} \tag{17.3}$$

When n is large and p is not small (as in CCD), the binomial distribution closely approaches the normal (Gaussian) distribution, Eq. 16.17, with mean $\mu = np$ and standard deviation $\sigma = \sqrt{npq}$. When n is large and p is small (as in chromatography), the binomial distribution can be approximated by a function called the Poisson distribution. However, when n is very large, the Poisson distribution can itself be approximated by the normal distribution, whose mean will be np. Since p is small, q is close to unity, so the standard deviation of this distribution will be $\sqrt{np}$. We therefore conclude that the zone in a chromatographic column will have a Gaussian concentration profile (shape) with $\mu = np$ and $\sigma = \sqrt{np}$.

Now consider the zone while it is still in the column. Its concentration profile can be visualized as a plot of T_{nr} (or concentration) against position down the column as denoted by plate number r (exactly as for a CCD curve). Let us now specify position along the column in length units, that is, we write $L = kr$, where L is the distance along the column corresponding to plate r, and the proportionality constant k is chosen to give L the units of length. Then for the concentration maximum (mean) in the zone one can write $\mu = kr$, where r is the plate number corresponding to the mean, and for the standard deviation of the zone $\sigma = kr^{1/2}$.

The plate height can be found by dividing column length by number of plates in that length, or $H = L/r = k$. Therefore $\sigma^2 = k^2 r = HL$, or

$$\sigma = \sqrt{HL} \tag{17.4}$$

We have obtained the extremely important result that the standard deviation of a chromatographic zone (which is a measure of its width) is related to H. As we shall later see, the ability of a chromatographic system to separate compounds is a function of the width of the zones, so H is a measure of column efficiency. The smaller the value of H, the narrower the zone.

The preceding discussion has considered the zone while in the column, the concentration profile being, in effect, a plot of T_{nr} against r at constant n (as in CCD). In column elution chromatography, however, the zone is eluted from the column. Each portion of solute therefore passes through the same number of plates r (where r equals the total number of plates in the column), but different parts of the zone are subjected to different numbers of mobile phase volumes n before emerging from the column. An elution chromatogram is therefore in essence a plot of T_{nr} versus n at constant r. We wish to find the number of plates r on the column.

Figure 17.5 is a chromatogram showing the basis of the calculation. The horizontal axis is in units of n (number of mobile phase volumes passed through the column), but this information is not available. Instead the chromatogram will be plotted with eluate volume, time, or simply distance on the chart paper as the abscissa. According to our earlier results the mean in this chromatogram occurs at $r = np$, so we can write

$$d = cr \tag{17.5}$$

where d is the distance from the beginning of the chromatogram to the peak maximum, and c is a proportionality constant that includes p and a factor determined by the units (volume, time, or distance) of d. The width of the peak is defined in terms of standard deviation units, and it is conventional to define the width w as four standard deviations, that is, $\mu \pm 2\sigma$, which includes about 95% of the area under the curve. Accordingly we have

$$w = 4cr^{1/2} \tag{17.6}$$

where w has the same units as d. Combining Eqs. 17.5 and 17.6,

$$r = 16\left(\frac{d}{w}\right)^2 \tag{17.7}$$

where r is the total number of plates on the column. The height equivalent to a theoretical plate is then calculated by

$$H = \frac{\text{column length}}{r} \tag{17.8}$$

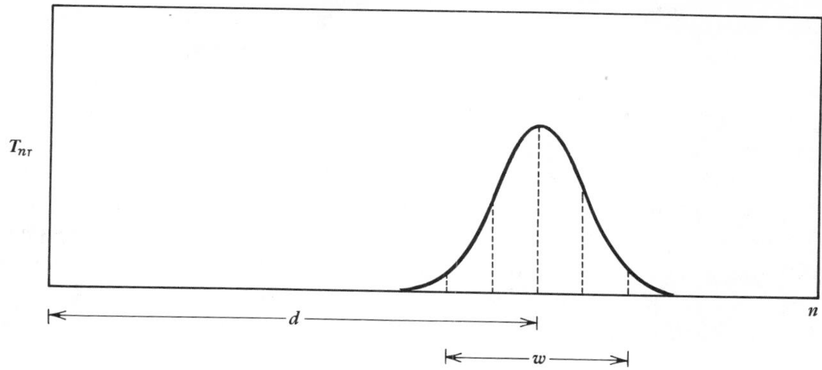

Fig. 17.5. Generalized chromatogram showing the measurements required to calculate the number of plates in the column. The vertical dashed lines are each separated by one standard deviation.

An important relationship can be found between the retention volume, column parameters, and partition coefficient. At the maximum in the elution curve we have $r = np$. Combining this with $p = 1/(KU + 1)$ and $U = V_s/V_m$ gives

$$nV_m = rV_m + rKV_s$$

where V_m and V_s are the mobile and stationary phase volumes per plate, respectively. Therefore rV_m is equal to the total mobile phase volume of the column, V_M, whereas $rV_s = V_S$ is the total stationary phase volume of the column. Moreover, since n is the number of mobile phase volumes required to elute the zone maximum, $nV_m = V_R$. Thus we obtain

$$V_R = V_M + KV_S \tag{17.9}$$

as the relationship between V_R, the partition coefficient, and the column parameters. A similar expansion of the equality $R = p$ shows that $R = V_M/V_R$. The column mobile phase volume can be experimentally determined by measuring the retention volume of a compound with a very small partition coefficient (little affinity for the stationary phase); then $V_R = V_M$ according to Eq. 17.9.

Three important assumptions were made at the beginning of this theoretical treatment: (1) equilibrium conditions apply in the continuous system; (2) all of the sample was in the first plate ($r = 0$) at the beginning of the development; (3) the partition isotherm is linear; that is, K is a constant, being independent of concentration. The first of these is not true, and because it is only an approximation, the quantitative theory developed here is not an exact representation of the chromatographic process. This is to be compared with the countercurrent distribution separation, where the same theory is exact because true equilibrium can be attained at each step in the procedure.

The second condition is seldom fulfilled because H is so small that all of the sample will not fit into the first plate, and several plates are occupied by the sample even before the elution is begun. The observed chromatographic peak can be thought of as resulting from the superposition of several successive chromatograms whose initiation positions have been successively advanced by one plate. The effect is to broaden the peak in the direction of the leading edge. It is therefore desirable to make the initial sample zone as narrow as possible.

The third requirement is necessary to make the mathematics manageable. If in fact the partition isotherm is not linear, that is, if the partition coefficient varies with concentration, then different regions of the zone will migrate at different rates. The effect is to produce a highly asymmetric ("skewed") peak, with accompanying broadening. By working at low concentrations (that is, with small samples), where the partition isotherm may be expected to be fairly linear, this problem is usually avoided in partition chromatography.

The essential results of the plate theory are embodied in Eqs. 17.4, 17.7, 17.8, and 17.9. The limitations of this theory are a consequence of its neglect of the dynamic, nonequilibrium, aspects of chromatography.

Zone Broadening Processes. According to Eq. 17.4 the width of a chromatographic zone, which can be taken equal to 4σ, increases as the zone progresses down the column, σ increasing with the square root of the distance migrated. The plate theory, which is an equilibrium theory, gives no insight into the molecular basis of this zone broadening effect. For this purpose it is necessary to consider the rates of molecular processes in the chromatographic system. This can be done in several ways; we will outline the *random walk* theory of Giddings [2].

Suppose a molecule is placed on the X axis at a position $X = Z$ at time $t = 0$. At successive times $t = 1, 2, 3, \ldots$, the molecule moves one unit step to the right or to the left depending upon the outcome of a random trial (such as the toss of a coin). Let the probability of a move to the right be p and of a move to the left be q. If $p = q$ the particle will tend to remain at its original position Z. If $p > q$ the particle will tend to drift to the right of Z. The motion described by the molecule is called a random walk. Molecular diffusion can be viewed as the consequence of random walks by a large number of molecules.

In chromatography each molecule in a zone can be pictured as undergoing a random walk, independently of all other molecules. If a great many molecules were placed, at time $= 0$, at a given point in a chromatographic column, and they were allowed to undergo random walks for a prolonged period, some of the molecules would be found to the left of the starting point and others to its right. Thus the initially sharp concentration spike will have been broadened due to random time-dependent processes. It is in this manner that zone spreading can be accounted for by a random walk model. Concurrently, of course, the center of the zone is migrating down the column in accordance with the requirements of equilibrium, as specified by the R value. Equilibrium controls the position of the zone center, whereas rate processes control zone width.

From plate theory we derived Eq. 17.10,

$$\sigma^2 = HL \tag{17.10}$$

from which we concluded that H is a measure of zone spreading and therefore of column efficiency. The quantity σ^2 is called the variance; it has the convenient attribute of additivity. Now although H, as a theoretical concept of the plate theory, has no real validity in a rate theory, *all* theories of chromatography predict a final Gaussian zone concentration profile, so the variance of the zone can always be related to H through Eq. 17.10. In other words, it has become conventional to express zone broadening, and hence column efficiency, in terms of contributions to plate height H. The goal of theory is to evaluate these contributions. There are three independent processes responsible for zone broadening.

1. *Longitudinal Molecular Diffusion.* All solute molecules tend to diffuse from a region of high concentration to a region of lower concentration. In a chromatographic system, solute molecules will therefore diffuse out of the zone both forward and backward, thus broadening the zone. The more time the zone spends in the column, the more extensive will be this longitudinal molecular diffusion, so we anticipate that this effect will be inversely proportional to the mobile phase flow velocity v. First consider the zone spreading caused by diffusion of the solute in the mobile phase. Let t_m be the time spent by the molecules in the mobile phase while migrating the distance L. Then

$$L = vt_m \tag{17.11}$$

According to diffusion theory, the variance of a concentration profile produced by molecular diffusion for a time t is given by Eq. 17.12, Einstein's equation,

$$\sigma^2 = 2Dt \tag{17.12}$$

where D is the diffusion coefficient (units of cm^2/sec). Combining these gives

$$\sigma^2_{\text{diff}-m} = \frac{2D_mL}{v} \tag{17.13}$$

The flow path is actually complicated by constrictions and tortuosities, so this equation is modified by introducing an empirical factor γ, which has the value of about 0.6, so $\sigma^2_{\text{diff}-m} = 2\gamma D_m L/v$. Combining this with Eq. 17.10 gives the plate height contribution of diffusion in the mobile phase.

$$H_{\text{diff}-m} = \frac{2\gamma D_m}{v} \tag{17.14}$$

Similar reasoning can be applied to the effect of diffusion in the stationary phase, but here the solute's R value enters, for the time it spends in the stationary phase depends on R. Summing the two effects gives for the total plate height contribution from diffusion

$$H_{\text{diff}} = \left[2\gamma D_m + \frac{2\gamma_s D_s(1 - R)}{R}\right]\frac{1}{v} \tag{17.15}$$

Note that this is of the form

$$H_{\text{diff}} = \frac{B}{v} \tag{17.16}$$

where parameter B is a function of molecular and chromatographic properties.

2. *Mass Transfer* (*Sorption-Desorption Kinetics*). True partition equilibrium cannot be attained in a flowing chromatographic system because mass transfer between the two phases is not instantaneous. The equilibrium condition is approached by making one of the phases very thin. Nevertheless, equilibrium is only approximated, and the greater the flow velocity, the less complete is the approach to equilibrium, because solute molecules in the mobile phase may fail to pass into the stationary phase and are swept ahead of the zone, whereas some of the molecules in the stationary phase may be slow in passing into the mobile phase and therefore lag behind.

The situation in LSC can be described easily by the random walk model. Passage from the stationary to the mobile phase (desorption from the surface) is a random step forward, since when the molecule becomes desorbed it is carried onward in the moving phase. Passage from the mobile to the stationary phase (adsorption) is in effect a step backward, since the zone continues to move forward. The total number of steps by a molecule is equal to the number of desorptions plus the number of adsorptions. Since each adsorption is followed by a desorption, the total number of steps is twice the number of adsorptions.

Let t_a be the average time a molecule remains in the mobile phase before it is adsorbed. The distance it covers in this time is therefore vt_a, where v is the flow velocity. In order to go a distance L, a total of L/vt_a steps must therefore be taken. The total number n of random steps is therefore

$$n = \frac{2L}{vt_a} \tag{17.17}$$

While the molecule in each desorbed stage is moving forward the distance vt_a, the zone center is also moving, though at a slower rate; the zone center moves distance Rvt_a in the same time. The net advance made by the molecules, which is the true step length l, is then $vt_a - Rvt_a$, or

$$l = (1 - R)vt_a \tag{17.18}$$

According to random walk theory, $\sigma^2 = l^2n$, so $\sigma^2 = 2(1 - R)^2 vt_a L$. Combining this with Eq. 17.10,

$$H_{s-d} = 2(1 - R)^2 vt_a$$

This can be combined with the relationship $t_a/t_d = R/(1 - R)$ to give

$$H_{s-d} = 2R(1 - R)vt_a \tag{17.19}$$

where t_d is the average time a molecule spends in the stationary phase. H_{s-d} is the plate height contribution produced by the finite time required for sorption-desorption between the mobile and stationary phases. For LLC a similar expression is found in which the diffusion coefficient in the stationary phase and the thickness of the stationary phase appear. Note that Eq. 17.19 has the form

$$H_{s-d} = Cv \tag{17.20}$$

3. *Eddy Diffusion.* Within a flow system like a chromatographic column the actual flow velocity of the mobile phase varies from point to point depending on proximity to particle surfaces, wall effects, and packing inhomogeneities. Even flow in a simple tube exhibits such an effect, with velocity of flow being essentially zero at the walls (because of viscous drag) and maximal in the center. In a packed chromatographic column the flow patterns are extremely complex.

The random walk model pictures a step as the distance a molecule travels at a given flow velocity. The step is terminated by a change in flow velocity. This can happen in two ways: (*a*) the molecule can be carried by *flow* from one flow stream to another with a different velocity; (*b*) the molecule can *diffuse* laterally from one flow stream to another. Together these are called eddy diffusion. They contribute to zone broadening by dispersing molecules through their residence in streams of different velocities.

The flow and diffusion mechanisms of eddy diffusion are coupled, which means that they are not independent; the step length of a molecule in a flow path may be shortened by lateral diffusion, and vice versa. Thus their plate height contributions H_F and H_D are not additive. Instead it is found [2] that

$$H_{\text{eddy}} = \frac{1}{1/H_F + 1/H_D} \tag{17.21}$$

It is found that H_F is independent of flow velocity and H_D is directly dependent upon average flow velocity, so Eq. 17.21 takes the form

$$H_{\text{eddy}} = \frac{1}{1/A + 1/Ev} \tag{17.22}$$

The quantities A and E include the particle diameter.

The total plate height can now be obtained by adding the three contributions, $H = H_{\text{eddy}} + H_{\text{diff}} + H_{s-d}$; from Eqs. 17.16, 17.20, and 17.22,

$$H = \frac{1}{1/A + 1/Ev} + \frac{B}{v} + Cv \tag{17.23}$$

This is Giddings' equation for plate height. If E vanishes an approximate version, the van Deemter equation, is obtained:

$$H = A + \frac{B}{v} + Cv \tag{17.24}$$

Figure 17.6 is a generalized plot of Eq. 17.24, showing the dependence of H on v. At very high flow velocities zone broadening is dominated by the mass transfer term, the deviation from equilibrium being greater at high velocities. The longitudinal diffusion term has its greatest effect at low velocities. In LC the mobile phase is a liquid, typical values of the diffusion coefficient D_m are of the order 10^{-5} cm^2/sec, and the B/v term seldom plays an important role. In gas chromatography, however, D_m is several orders of magnitude larger, and the rise in H at low v, as shown in Fig. 17.6, is commonly observed.

Resolution. Chromatography is used to separate compounds, so it is useful to be able to describe the extent of separation and to relate it to molecular and chromatographic properties. Figure 17.7 is an elution chromatogram for two solutes, with retention volumes and peak widths indicated. Define the separation of zone centers as $\Delta d = d_B - d_A$ and the zone width as $w = 4\sigma$, where σ is the average standard deviation of the two peaks; thus $w = (w_A + w_B)/2$. The extent of separation is a competition between the drawing apart of zone centers due to differential migration rates and the merging of zones due to zone broadening processes. We define the chromatographic *resolution*, R_s:

$$R_s = \frac{\Delta d}{w} \tag{17.25}$$

Since the distance migrated by a zone is proportional to n (or, equivalently, to L), the quantity Δd is also proportional to n. The standard deviation σ, however, is proportional to $\sqrt{n}$ (or $\sqrt{L}$). This means that R_s increases with increase in column length. Two zones are conventionally considered to be

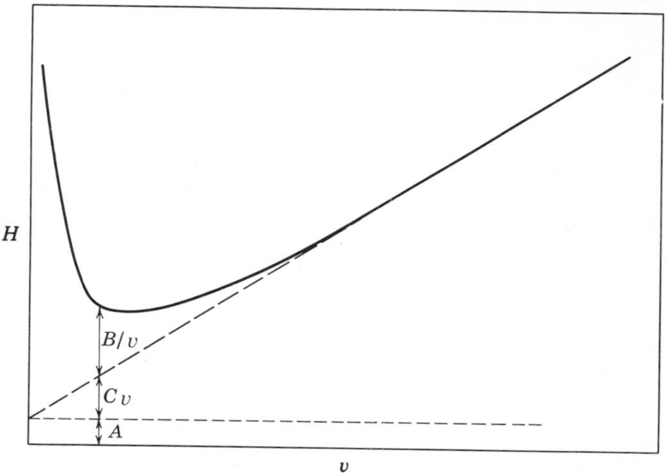

Fig. 17.6. Variation of H with mobile phase flow velocity according to Eq. 17.24.

resolved when $R_s = 1$. Thus in principle it should be possible to resolve any two compounds (unless they have identical R values) by chromatographing them on a long enough column. In practice this may not always be feasible because of experimental difficulties. The calculation of R_s from experimental data may be made in distance, time, or volume units as long as Δd and w are expressed in the same units.

R_s can be related to chromatographic parameters in a useful way. According to Eq. 17.1 zone velocity is equal to Rv, so in time t the zone migrates a distance $L = Rvt$. The distance between two zone centers is therefore $\Delta d = vt\,\Delta R$ or

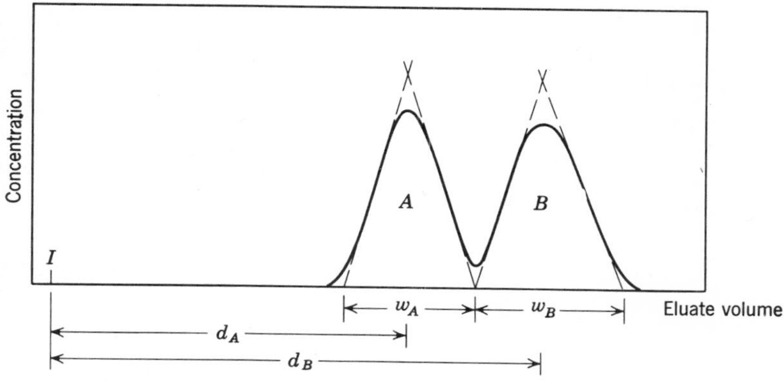

Fig. 17.7. Quantities used to define chromatographic resolution, R_s. The figure shows the condition in which $R_s = 1$.

$\Delta d = L\,\Delta R/R$. Combining this result with Eqs. 17.4 and 17.25,

$$R_s = \sqrt{\frac{L}{16H}} \cdot \frac{\Delta R}{R} \tag{17.26}$$

If the zones are eluted, then L is the column length and L/H is the total number of plates on the column. R in Eq. 17.26 refers to the mean R value of the two closely spaced zones. Further algebraic manipulation combining Eq. 17.26 with $R = p = 1/(KU + 1)$ leads finally to [2]

$$R_s = \frac{1}{4}\sqrt{r}\left(\frac{\alpha - 1}{\alpha}\right)\left(\frac{k'}{k' + 1}\right) \tag{17.27}$$

where r is the number of plates on the column, α is the ratio of partition coefficients ($\alpha \geq 1$), and $k' = KU$ (the average value for the two compounds). The first term in this equation describes column *efficiency*, the second term describes *selectivity*, and the last term is the *capacity* factor.

Equation 17.27 is useful in identifying the factors that can be influenced to modify resolution. Column efficiency can be increased by decreasing plate height (H) or by increasing column length (L). If a separation has very high resolution ($R_s \gg 1$) it may be desirable to sacrifice some resolution by decreasing L in order to shorten the time of analysis. The selectivity can be altered by changing the nature of the stationary and mobile phases. The capacity term can be placed in an equivalent form, as in

$$\frac{k'}{k' + 1} = 1 - R$$

Thus if R is close to unity (small k'), resolution is degraded. Moreover, this shows that as k' becomes large, $1 - R$ increases very slowly. This equation reveals that resolution is optimized (through the capacity factor) if k' is in the range 1–10.

The selectivity and capacity factors are easily evaluated from the elution chromatogram. From the definition $k' = KU$ we find

$$k' = \frac{V_R - V_M}{V_M} \tag{17.28}$$

and since $\alpha = K_2/K_1 = k'_2/k'_1$,

$$\alpha = \frac{V_{R,2} - V_M}{V_{R,1} - V_M}$$

17.3 Types of Liquid Chromatography

Partition Chromatography. In partition chromatography both phases are liquids, so this is also called liquid-liquid chromatography (LLC). The process responsible for retention (that is, for different zone migration rates) is liquid-liquid partitioning, just as described for solvent extraction and countercurrent distribution in Chapter 16.

As LLC is normally carried out, the stationary phase (internal phase) is the more polar of the two liquids. This phase is adsorbed, in a very thin film, to the surface of a finely divided solid (the support). Ideally, the only role of the support in LLC is to hold the stationary phase. The mobile phase is a less polar solvent immiscible with the stationary phase. Very often the stationary phase is water or an aqueous solution, and the mobile phase is an organic solvent. In paper chromatography the stationary phase consists of water adsorbed to the paper fibers.

When the stationary phase is a nonpolar solvent and the mobile phase is polar, the technique is referred to as *reversed-phase* LC.

A practical difficulty with the type of stationary phase described above is that with prolonged use the stationary phase solvent tends to be stripped from the column, thus changing the column characteristics. Recent developments in LC column design have led to stationary phases that are chemically bonded (rather than physically adsorbed) to the solid support. A typical chemically bonded phase is prepared with a solid support of very small controlled-porosity glass beads. To the free hydroxy groups on the glass surface this series of reactions attaches an "ether silicone" polymer phase [3].

$$\text{glass—OH} \xrightarrow{Me_2SiCl_2} \text{glass—O}\underset{\displaystyle Me}{\overset{\displaystyle Me}{Si}}\text{Cl} \xrightarrow{H_2O} \text{glass—O}\underset{\displaystyle Me}{\overset{\displaystyle Me}{Si}}\text{OH}$$

$$\big\downarrow \; (1)\ R_2SiCl_2 \quad (2)\ H_2O$$

$$\text{glass—O}\underset{\displaystyle Me}{\overset{\displaystyle Me}{Si}}\text{O}\left(\underset{\displaystyle R}{\overset{\displaystyle R}{Si}}\text{O}\right)_n\text{SiMe}_3 \xleftarrow{Me_3SiX} \text{glass—O}\underset{\displaystyle Me}{\overset{\displaystyle Me}{Si}}\text{O}\left(\underset{\displaystyle R}{\overset{\displaystyle R}{Si}}\text{O}\right)_n\text{H}$$

The polarity of the resulting bonded coating depends upon the nature of the R groups.

The selectivity in LLC is usually controlled by choice of solvents, for these control the partition coefficient. Further selectivity control has been achieved by incorporating into the stationary phase a solute that can undergo noncovalent complex formation with the compounds being chromatographed; then the selectivity is influenced by the extent of complex formation. A recent development in biochemical separations uses a modification of this technique, in which a small molecule is covalently bonded to the solid support, this molecule being chosen as a specific complex former with a biological macromolecule, which is thereupon selectively retarded when chromatographed. For example, an enzyme substrate can be attached to the stationary phase support, and then the enzyme for the substrate can be removed selectively from a mixture because of the specific enzyme-substrate complexation, which will increase the retention time. This technique is called affinity chromatography.

Adsorption Chromatography. The distribution process in adsorption chromatography (liquid-solid chromatography, LSC) is an equilibrium distribution of the solute between the mobile phase solvent and the solid surface, where it can be (noncovalently) bound by interactions between functional groups on the molecule and on the surface.

It is possible to develop distribution isotherms (adsorption isotherms) analogous to the partition isotherms for liquid-liquid systems. The common types of isotherm are shown in Fig. 17.8. In these plots C_M is the concentration (at equilibrium) of solute in the solvent (that is, mobile phase in the case of adsorption chromatography), and X is the weight of solute adsorbed per gram of solid adsorbent. Figure 17.8*a* is a linear isotherm, signifying that the distribution coefficient, which is defined $K = X/C_M$, is constant. Although this is the usual situation in partition chromatography, it is less often observed in adsorption chromatography.

Figure 17.8*b* shows the most commonly encountered adsorption isotherm, the Langmuir isotherm. The equation describing this curve can be derived from the assumptions that the solid surface is homogeneous, and that the surface forces can adsorb a film only one molecule thick. The equation is

$$X = \frac{k_1 k_2 C_M}{1 + k_1 C_M} \tag{17.29}$$

Thus at low concentrations the equation reduces to $X = k_1 k_2 C_M$, and the isotherm approaches linearity, while at very high concentration the equation becomes $X = k_2$, indicating that the amount of adsorbed solute reaches a maximum. In terms of the physical theory, this means that the entire surface is covered with a monomolecular layer of adsorbed solute, and a further increase in the solution concentration cannot produce an increase in the amount adsorbed.

Figure 17.8*c* shows a Freundlich isotherm, which has the equation

$$X = k{C_M}^n \tag{17.30}$$

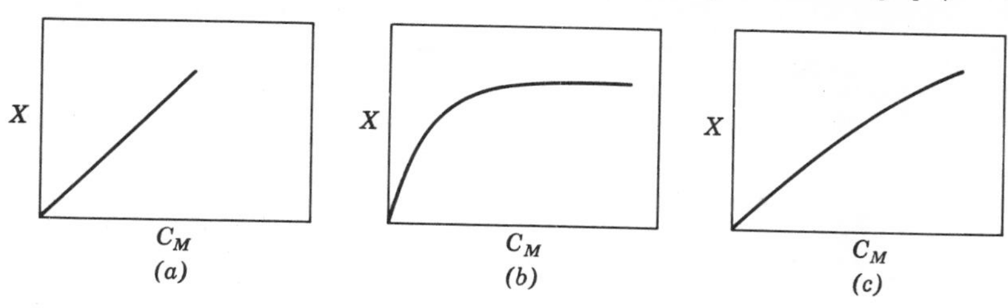

Fig. 17.8. Types of adsorption isotherms: (*a*) linear isotherm; (*b*) Langmuir isotherm; (*c*) Freundlich isotherm. C_M is the equilibrium solution concentration and X is the weight of solute adsorbed per gram of adsorbent.

where n is less than 1. The Freundlich isotherm does not achieve a constant limiting value.

An adsorption isotherm can be experimentally determined very simply. A known weight of the adsorbent is shaken with a solution of known concentration of the solute. After equilibrium is reached, an aliquot of the solution is analyzed to find C_M. The quantity X is then found by difference. This experiment is repeated for several values of the concentration. The curve obtained (and the constants in the isotherm equation) depend upon the solute, solvent, and solid.

We noted, in Section 17.2, that if the distribution isotherm is linear, the zone of solute as it migrates down the column or along the paper increases in width and assumes a symmetrical concentration profile. The concentration of solute is maximal in the center of the zone and falls off toward the leading and trailing edges in a manner quantitatively described as a Gaussian distribution. Figure 17.9*a* shows the linear isotherm and the corresponding shape of the peak in the chromatogram.

The isotherm in an adsorption system is seldom linear, however (except at extremely low concentrations). Usually the Langmuir isotherm describes the adsorption equilibrium. The distribution coefficient K is the slope of a line from the origin to a point on the adsorption isotherm at any given value of C_M. For the Langmuir isotherm, the slope decreases with increasing concentration, so K decreases with increasing concentration. The solute in a chromatographic zone migrates only when it is in the mobile phase, and we have seen that the smaller the distribution coefficient, the greater the fraction of solute in the mobile phase. We therefore concluded that the zone migrates faster, the lower the value of K.

In the present situation K varies within the zone. In the center section of the zone K is smallest because the concentration is highest. Toward both the leading and trailing edges the concentration decreases and therefore K increases. Therefore the center of the zone migrates faster down the column than does

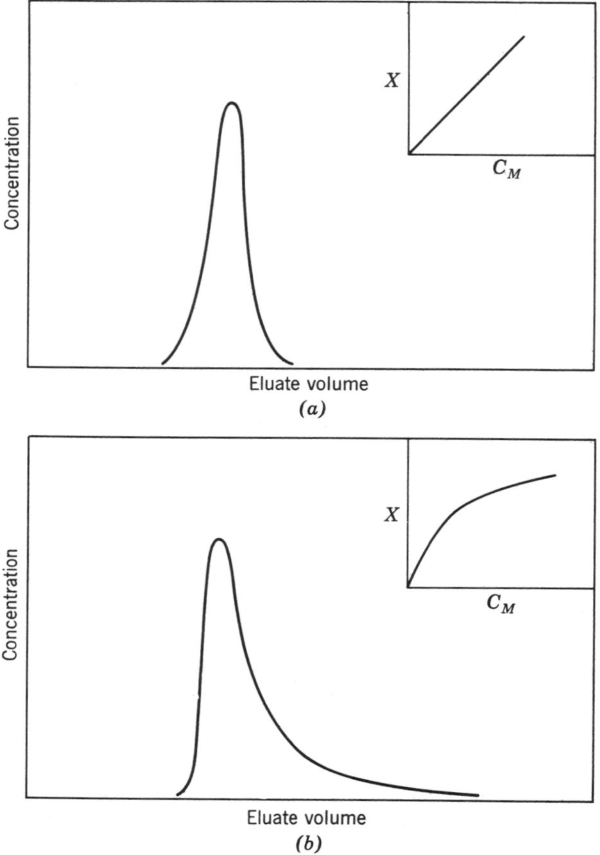

Fig. 17.9. Shape of the adsorption isotherm and its effect on the chromatographic peak. (*a*) Linear isotherm, peak is symmetrical; (*b*) curved isotherm, peak shows serious tailing.

either edge. This means that the center of the zone overtakes the slower-moving leading edge and leaves behind the trailing edge. The resulting chromatographic peak is shown in Fig. 17.9*b*. The leading edge has been sharpened, but the trailing edge exhibits serious tailing that could render a quantitative separation and recovery impossible.

The best way to overcome tailing is with the gradient elution technique, in which the eluting power of the mobile phase is gradually increased, so that the tail of the zone is subjected to a more potent desorbing action than is the leading edge. This counteracts the effect produced by a nonlinear isotherm; in fact, gradient elution is a "trick of the trade" that, in effect, straightens out the adsorption isotherm.

Table 17.1 lists some of the solids that are widely used in LSC. The most popular adsorbent is aluminum oxide (alumina, Al_2O_3). The surface of this solid is highly polar, its precise nature depending upon pretreatment conditions. Alumina is capable of adsorbing practically all polar molecules, including unsaturated hydrocarbons, and by judicious selection of the eluent most pairs of solutes can be separated on an alumina column. The more highly polar a compound is, the more strongly adsorbed it will be.

The alumina surface may be pictured as possessing active sites of adsorption. If an adsorption site is occupied by an adsorbed molecule it is unavailable for further adsorption (unless the adsorbed molecule is displaced by another solute that has a greater affinity for alumina). One of the strongest adsorptives (adsorbable solutes) is water, which is highly polar. The adsorbent power of alumina is therefore markedly affected by its water content, with the freshly dried alumina having the highest adsorbent activity. The activity of alumina is specified by its ability to retard the migration of certain dyestuffs through a column prepared with the alumina. This empirical method permits alumina to be classified into five activity grades, I–V, with Grade I alumina being the most active. Any grade of alumina can be transformed into a grade of lower activity by exposing it to water (this is called deactivation). Alumina is activated by heating it (not above 200°C).

Alumina is available in forms exhibiting either a basic, neutral, or acidic reaction depending upon its treatment prior to activation. The neutral alumina is fairly chemically inert; the other forms are capable of extensive ionic interactions with solutes, and may function as ion exchangers. Basic alumina may be contraindicated for samples of labile substances such as esters.

Silicic acid or silica gel, SiO_2, is a useful adsorbent. It can be activated by heating or by prewashing the column with an anhydrous solvent to remove adsorbed water. Charcoal is a powerful adsorbent. It has long been used to remove impurities from solutions during recrystallization purifications; it is particularly effective in removing colored impurities, because colored compounds always are large polar molecules. This common procedure is a batch process, and is therefore not chromatographic. However, charcoal is a good chromatographic adsorbent.

TABLE 17.1
Adsorbents Listed in Order of Decreasing Strength

(1) Fuller's earth	(6) Calcium carbonate
(2) Activated charcoal	(7) Potassium carbonate
(3) Activated alumina	(8) Talc
(4) Activated silicic acid	(9) Starch
(5) Magnesium oxide	

The relative adsorbent strength of a series of materials depends partly upon the solute and solvent selected for the comparison. A list of relative strengths, as in Table 17.1, is therefore somewhat arbitrary, but it can be useful in designing a chromatographic separation.

The function of the developer (mobile phase, eluent) is to cause the zones to migrate, selectively, down the column. It does this by competing for the solute materials with the adsorbent surface and, to some extent, by displacing the solute from the adsorbent active sites. It is therefore reasonable to expect that highly polar solvents will be more powerful eluting agents than will slightly polar solvents. This is in general true, although the exact relationship of pairs of similar solvents is arbitrary, depending as it does on the nature of the adsorbent and solute. Table 17.2 grades the common eluents in approximate order of increasing eluting power. In the gradient elution technique the developer eluting power is gradually increased by incorporating increasing concentrations of a polar solvent into a nonpolar solvent.

Ion-Exchange Chromatography. It has been known for many years that certain solids are capable of giving up ions to a solution in exchange for the ions of the solution. Clays have this property. Such solids are called ion exchangers. Although many inorganic ion exchangers are known, and some of them are utilized in industrial processes, few are of value in the analytical laboratory. For analytical purposes the inorganics have largely been replaced by synthetic organic ion exchangers called ion-exchange resins. These substances are very insoluble polymeric materials with functional groups capable of ionization. They are available in the form of beads or granules.

Two general types of ion-exchange resins can be distinguished: (1) *cation exchangers* possess exchangeable cations, the anionic portion of the molecule being part of the resin, and therefore immobile; (2) *anion exchangers* can exchange anions with the solution. The "backbone" of an ion-exchange resin is (for most resins) a copolymer of styrene and divinylbenzene (DVB). Figure 17.10 shows the partial structure of such a resin. This resin contains no ionizable groups. It can be transformed into an ion-exchange resin by the chemical introduction of suitable functional groups.

TABLE 17.2
Eluents Listed in Order of Increasing Eluent Power

(1) Petroleum ether	(6) Acetone
(2) Carbon tetrachloride	(7) Ethyl acetate
(3) Benzene	(8) Ethanol
(4) Ether	(9) Methanol
(5) Chloroform	(10) Water

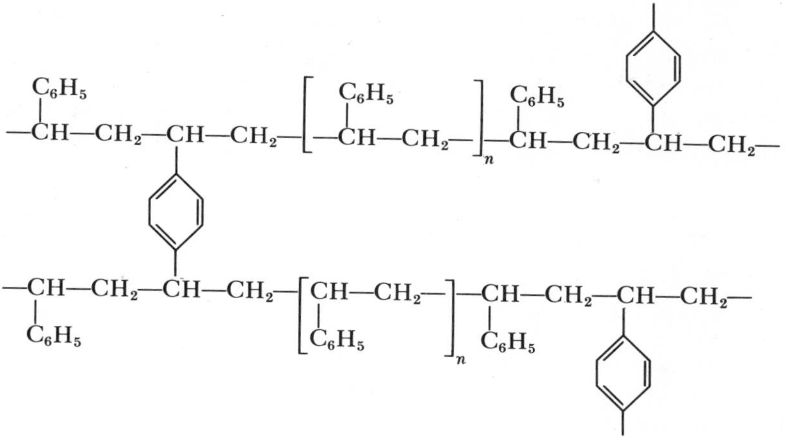

$$
\begin{array}{l}
-\underset{|}{\overset{C_6H_5}{CH}}-CH_2-\underset{|}{CH}-CH_2-\left[-\overset{C_6H_5}{CH}-CH_2-\right]_n-\overset{C_6H_5}{CH}-CH_2-\overset{C_6H_4}{CH}-CH_2- \\
\qquad\qquad\qquad\quad C_6H_4 \\
-\underset{C_6H_5}{CH}-CH_2-CH-CH_2-\left[CH-CH_2-\right]_n-\underset{C_6H_5}{CH}-CH_2-\underset{C_6H_4}{CH}-CH_2-
\end{array}
$$

Fig. 17.10. Partial structure of a styrene-divinylbenzene resin.

If the styrene-DVB resin is sulfonated, approximately one sulfonic acid group per phenyl group will be introduced, to give benzenesulfonic acid groups. A sulfonic acid resin is a strong acid cation exchanger. Weakly acidic

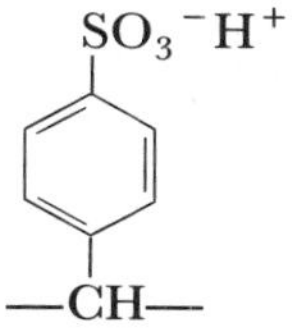

$$
\begin{array}{c}
SO_3{}^-H^+ \\
| \\
C_6H_4 \\
| \\
-CH-
\end{array}
$$

cation exchange resins are available in which the ionizable functions are carboxylic acid groups.

Strong base anion exchangers possess quaternary ammonium groups in a styrene-DVB resin:

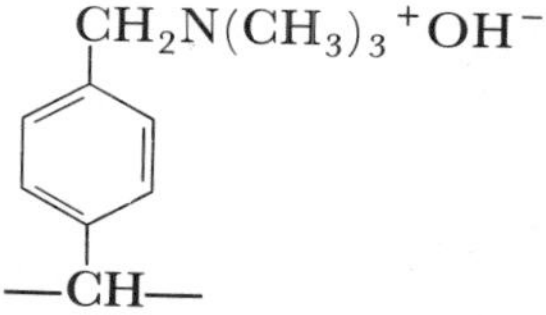

$$
\begin{array}{c}
CH_2N(CH_3)_3{}^+OH^- \\
| \\
C_6H_4 \\
| \\
-CH-
\end{array}
$$

Weakly basic anion exchangers are made with amine groups as the ionizable groups.

An ion-exchange resin may be considered an insoluble acid or base. It undergoes the usual acid-base reactions, but the species bound to the polymer structure cannot go into solution. Ions with the charge of the exchangeable ions (that is, cations for cation exchangers, anions for anion exchangers) are called counterions. Ions with the charge of the resin-bound groups are co-ions. The type of counterion on a resin is usually specified; for example, a sulfonic acid resin is said to be in the hydrogen form if all its ionizable groups exist as the acid —SO_3H, whereas it is in the sodium form when the counter-ion is Na^+.

If we represent a sulfonic acid resin in the hydrogen form as Resin—$SO_3^-H^+$, the exchange reaction between this resin and a solution containing sodium ions is

$$\text{Resin—}SO_3^-H^+ + Na^+ \rightleftharpoons \text{Resin—}SO_3^-Na^+ + H^+$$

Sodium ions are removed from solution, being replaced by an equivalent amount of H^+. Similarly, the anion exchange between a strongly basic resin in the hydroxide form and a solution of chloride ions is

$$\text{Resin—}N(CH_3)_3{}^+OH^- + Cl^- \rightleftharpoons \text{Resin—}N(CH_3)^+Cl^- + OH^-$$

It is not necessary that one of the exchangeable ions be either H^+ or OH^-.

The numerous uses of ion-exchange resins will be considered shortly, but it may be helpful at this point to give an example of one of these applications. Suppose the concentration of an aqueous solution of potassium nitrate is to be determined. A small aliquot of the solution is passed into a column packed with a sulfonic acid resin in the hydrogen form. As the first portion of sample contacts the resin, the exchange reaction Resin—$SO_3^-H^+ + K^+ \rightleftharpoons$ Resin—$SO_3^-K^+ + H^+$ occurs. Since this is an equilibrium, it may not necessarily go completely to the right, but as the solution, now partly depleted of K^+, passes further into the column it contacts fresh acid resin, which exchanges more of the counterions. The result is, finally, that all of the potassium nitrate is converted to nitric acid, which is washed from the column with water and is titrated with standard alkali to give a measure of the original solution concentration. Usually many such analyses can be carried out before the resin becomes exhausted (completely converted to the potassium form). The H^+ form of the resin can be regenerated simply by passing a large excess of mineral acid through the column, thus reversing the direction of the exchange reaction.

The same KNO_3 solution could have been analyzed by passing it through an anion exchanger in the OH^- form. The column effluent would then contain an equivalent amount of KOH, which can be titrated with standard acid.

A characteristic property of an ion-exchange resin is its exchange capacity, which is defined as the number of milliequivalents of exchangeable ions per gram of dry resin. This quantity is easily determined. The exchange capacity of a sulfonic acid resin, as an example, may be measured by passing a large volume of sodium chloride solution through a column prepared with a known weight of the resin, until no more acid emerges from the column; at this stage the resin has been completely converted to the sodium form. The acidic effluent is titrated with standard alkali to determine the total milliequivalents of exchangeable hydrogen ion on the resin.

Another important property of resins is the effective size of the "pores" within the polymer network structure. The greater the degree of "cross-linking" between the styrene chains by DVB units, the smaller the pore size. This factor controls the extent of swelling undergone when dry resin beads are immersed in water; a higher degree of cross-linking leads to less swelling. The swelling is caused by the penetration of water molecules and of ions into the resin network. The degree of cross-linking may be specified as the percent of DVB in the polymerization process. A number preceded by an X in the manufacturer's code indicates the cross-linkage; for example, Dowex 50W-X4 is a 4% DVB resin. Many ion-exchange resins are available. The principal types were described earlier: polystyrene-DVB sulfonic acid cation exchangers and quaternary ammonium anion exchangers, and the weakly acidic carboxylic cation exchangers and weakly basic amine anion exchangers. Each type is available in several sizes and with various degrees of cross-linking. The capacity may be expressed in meq/g (dry basis) or in meq/ml (wet basis). The particle size is given as a mesh size; some selected mesh sizes and their corresponding measurements in mm are 20 mesh, 0.84 mm; 50 mesh, 0.30 mm; 100 mesh, 0.15 mm; and 200 mesh, 0.074 mm. The mesh size refers to the dry resin, and for some companies' products it refers to the resin before conversion to the functional group form. A particle size range is specified because a distribution of sizes is present in all commercial resins. Table 17.3 lists a few of the common ion-exchange resins.

The exchange of two ions A and B between a suitable ion-exchange resin and a solution can be written

$$\mathrm{A}_r + \mathrm{B}_s \rightleftharpoons \mathrm{B}_r + \mathrm{A}_s \tag{17.31}$$

where the subscripts indicate the resin and solution phases. We shall consider the simple case in which the ions A and B possess equal charges; the more complicated situation can be treated similarly by taking into account the appropriate stoichiometric relation.

Reaction 17.31 is an equilibrium, and an equilibrium constant can be defined

$$k = \frac{[\mathrm{B}]_r[\mathrm{A}]_s}{[\mathrm{B}]_s[\mathrm{A}]_r} \tag{17.32}$$

where k is the selectivity coefficient for the exchange reaction between A and B. The selectivity coefficient is a measure of the relative affinity of the two ions for the resin.

TABLE 17.3
Properties of Some Ion Exchange Resins

Name and Number	Chemical Type	% Cross-linkage	Form Available	Capacity maq/g	Capacity maq/ml
Dowex 50 or 50 W	Sulfonic acid	1–16	H^+	5.0	1.7
Dowex 1	Quat. ammonium	1–10	Cl^-	3.5	1.3
Dowex 2	Quat. ammonium	1–10	Cl^-	3.5	1.3
Dowex 3	Amine	—	Cl^-	5.5	2.5
Amberlite IR-120	Sulfonic acid	—	Na^+	4.3	—
Amberlite IRC-50	Carboxylic acid	—	H^+	10.0	—
Amberlite IRA-400	Quat. ammonium	—	Cl^-	3.3	—
Amberlite IR-45	Amine	—	OH^-	5.0	—
Permutit Q	Sulfonic acid	—	Na^+, H^+	4.8	2.0
Permutit H-70	Carboxylic acid	—	H^+	7.9	3.6
Wolfatite KPS200	Sulfonic acid	8	Na^+	4.5	2.0

The thermodynamic selectivity coefficient must of course be defined in terms of activities rather than concentrations. Although the activities of the ions in the external solution are reasonably close to their concentrations, this is not true of these quantities in the resin phase. This is because the interior of the resin is analogous to a highly concentrated electrolyte solution, and we saw in Chapter 6 that activity coefficients can deviate markedly from unity in such solutions. The concentration selectivity coefficient defined in Eq. 17.32 is therefore not a true constant, but varies with concentration.

The selectivity coefficient is characteristic of a pair of ions and of the resin. As the degree of cross-linking decreases, the selectivity coefficient approaches unity; more extensive cross-linking produces a more selective resin. Selectivity coefficients can be useful in predicting order of emergence in chromatographic separations. The relative affinities of some univalent cations for an 8% DVB sulfonic acid resin (relative to lithium, which is arbitrarily set at 1.00) are Li^+, 1.00; H^+, 1.27; Na^+, 1.98; $NH_4{}^+$, 2.55; and K^+, 2.90.

It is helpful to recognize that ion-exchange procedures fall into two distinct classes. In one procedure, of which an example was given earlier, a quantitative exchange of ions is achieved, with the eluate containing the resin counterion. This exchange of counterions is the function of the resin in this type of operation. The second important procedure is ion-exchange chromatography. The purpose of this technique, as in all chromatography, is to separate components of a mixture. This is accomplished by the elution technique. A narrow band of sample is placed on the top of the column, where the sample counterions exchange with the resin counterions. The development is now carried out with an eluent consisting of an electrolyte solution; the operation of the exchange equilibrium (Eq. 17.31) between the eluent counterion and the ions of the sample displaces the sample ions down the column. The rate of migration of each type of ion is determined by its selectivity coefficient with respect to the eluent counterion. The sample ions are collected in the eluate in the usual manner.

The ion-exchange equilibrium in both types of operation can be described in terms of selectivity coefficients. In ion-exchange chromatography, however, which commonly involves the distribution and migration of traces of the sample ions in the presence of high concentrations of the eluent ion, attention is focused on the sample ions by defining a distribution coefficient D:

$$D = \frac{\text{Amount of sample ion in resin phase}}{\text{Amount of sample ion in solution phase}} \tag{17.33}$$

D will be a function of the nature and concentration of the eluent counterion, but for a specified eluent and resin, the distribution coefficient is a constant for a given ionic species. Ion-exchange chromatography is formally analogous to liquid-liquid partition chromatography. Usually aqueous solutions are employed, and the mobile phase is an aqueous electrolyte solution. The interior of the resin, which we have observed has the character of a concentrated electrolyte solution, represents the stationary phase. Although both phases are aqueous, they are essentially immiscible because of insolubility of the resin and the fineness of its network structure. The partition coefficient of partition chromatography is replaced by the ion-exchange distribution coefficient. The retention volume is related to D by Eq. 17.34, which differs from Eq. 17.9 because of the way in which D is defined.

$$V_R = V_M + DV_M \tag{17.34}$$

Ion exchangers provide simple solutions to many industrial and analytical problems. Although our present concern is with ion-exchange chromatography, some of the other important applications are described briefly.

1. *Water treatment.* The softening of "hard" water, which contains appreciable concentrations of calcium and magnesium ions, is accomplished by passing the water through a cation exchanger in the sodium form. The Ca^{2+} and Mg^{2+} are retained by the column, which releases sodium ions to the solution. When the column has been exhausted it may be regenerated by treatment with sodium chloride.

Water can be "deionized" by successively passing it through a cation exchanger in the H^+ form, which exchanges all cations for hydrogen ions, and an anion exchanger in the OH^- form, which exchanges anions for hydroxide ions. Thus all foreign ions are replaced by the elements of water. (This process is properly referred to as demineralization rather than deionization, because some ions —H^+ and OH^-— are always present in water.) This treatment does not remove nonelectrolytes from the water.

Removal of foreign cations from water may be essential for sharp visual end points in complexometric titrations (Chapter 4); this is accomplished by passing the water through a cation exchanger in the H^+ form.

2. *Determination of total salt concentration.* This is the simplest analytical application of ion exchangers, and one of the most widely used. The aqueous solution of one or more salts is passed through a strong acid cation exchanger in the H^+ form. All cations are exchanged for hydrogen ion. The column effluent is titrated with standard alkali. This method is applicable to salts of acids strong enough to titrate accurately. It evidently does not distinguish between different salts if their acids are of similar strength, and it therefore yields the total salt concentration of the solution. If the two acids are of different strengths it may be possible, by potentiometric titration, to distinguish between them. A sample containing an acid and a salt can be analyzed for each component by titrating aliquots before and after passage through the column.

Examples of some of these techniques are given in Experiment 17.5.

3. *Separation of oppositely charged ions.* In the identification and determination of many ions interference is encountered when certain oppositely charged ions are present. A particularly important example is the analysis of phosphate by precipitation as magnesium ammonium phosphate. Many cations, in particular calcium and iron, interfere by forming precipitates themselves. These cations may be eliminated by classical precipitation methods prior to the phosphate analysis, but these methods are time consuming and subject to error. Ion exchange provides a rapid, simple solution to this separation problem. The sample solution is passed through a cation exchanger in the H^+ form, and the liberated phosphoric acid is washed out of the column. It can then be determined by the gravimetric method, by titration with alkali, or colorimetrically. If it is desired to analyze the cations in the original sample, these can be eluted from the column and determined in the effluent. The principle illustrated here has been applied in many other separations [4].

4. *Concentration of dilute solutions.* Ion exchangers provide a very simple means of concentrating solutions of ions. The conventional method is by evaporation of the solvent, often a slow and cumbersome technique.

The method may be illustrated by the analysis of cations in water. A large volume of the water is passed into a cation exchanger in the H^+ form. The cations are retained in the column. Elution is performed with a powerful eluting agent (4 N HCl), so that the volume of eluent required to remove the cations from the column is much smaller than the volume of original sample. The result is an increase in concentration. Conventional methods of analysis may now be applied. Anions may also be concentrated by using an anion exchanger.

5. *Separation of ions from nonelectrolytes.* The applicability of ion exchangers to this separation problem is obvious. The type of resin to be used depends upon whether cations or anions are to be removed from the solution. All ions can be removed by successive passage through an anion exchanger and a cation exchanger, as described on p. 385.

Since ion-exchange resins may act as adsorbents for nonelectrolytes, their undesired retention by the column may occur; adsorption effects are often complicating factors in ion-exchange separations.

6. *Ion-exchange chromatography.* True chromatographic separation based on difference in selectivities is a powerful application of ion-exchange resins. There are two fields in which ion-exchange chromatography is the method of choice: metal separations and amino acid analyses. All elements can be separated on suitable ion-exchange resins. The nature of the eluent is the decisive factor in determining the chromatographic behavior of metal ions. Usually the differential migration is based upon differences in extent and type of complex formation between the metal ions and the anions of the eluent. An example is the separation of barium and lead. Lead forms a complex in an ammonium acetate solution, whereas barium does not. Lead is therefore eluted more rapidly than barium when ammonium acetate is the eluting agent.

Amino acid analysis has been revolutionized by the introduction of ion-exchange chromatography. Sulfonic acid resins are used. The procedure has been made automatic, including the analysis of the effluent, with a great saving in time. Automatic amino acid analysis is employed to determine the amino acid composition of proteins and of biological fluids.

Molecular Exclusion Chromatography. Inorganic and organic substances are known that possess a network structure of molecular dimensions. The effective "pore size" of the network depends upon the crystal or molecular structure of the substance. These materials have the property of permitting the entrance into the internal network of ions and molecules smaller than the network pore size and excluding from the interior those species larger than the pore size. The descriptive term *molecular sieve* has been given to these selective filters. Separation by molecular sieve is a form of chromatography in which the relative affinities of the migrating substances are based on differences in molecular size.

The first known molecular sieves were minerals known as zeolites. These naturally occurring substances are aluminosilicate crystalline materials built up, in various arrays, of AlO_4 and SiO_4 tetrahedrons. The crystalline structure encloses channels and cavities of fairly regular size, and it is these openings that permit the zeolites to function as molecular sieves. (Zeolites also are cation exchangers.)

Synthetic zeolites are now available with various pore sizes. These molecular sieves are widely employed industrially. Their action appears to be describable as surface adsorption, with access to the surface limited by the molecular size of the adsorptive. Because of the polar nature of the zeolite surface, polar molecules are strongly adsorbed. This accounts for the effectiveness of zeolites as drying agents; the small, highly polar water molecule is adsorbed strongly. Gases and liquids can be dried effectively by passage through a zeolite. Zeolites are also used as adsorbents in the gas-solid chromatography of permanent gases and hydrocarbon mixtures. Because of their high affinity for water, zeolites are not useful for analyses of aqueous solutions.

Nonionic organic molecular sieves are now available, and these permit chromatographic separations to be made on the basis of molecular size. These molecular sieves, which are polymeric materials, are called gels. Hydrophilic gels, prepared with cross-linked dextran or polyacrylamide, are used with aqueous solvents, the technique then being called *gel filtration chromatography*. Hydrophobic gels, used with organic solvents, are employed in *gel permeation chromatography* (GPC) [5]. Both techniques are used to separate macromolecules.

These methods are formally similar to partition chromatography. The retention volume is given by

$$V_R = V_M + K_D V_S$$

which is similar to the expression for the partition system. K_D, in this equation, is a distribution coefficient defined $K_D = c_S/c_M$. If the solute is completely excluded from the interior of the gel, $K_D = 0$ and the solute is not retarded as it passes down the column. If the solute is able to pass within the gel without hindrance, $K_D = 1$, indicating that the interior and exterior of the gel are equally accessible. Thus if a true molecular sieve effect is operative, K_D can vary between the limits 0 and 1. This is a markedly different situation from that in partition chromatography. If K_D should be greater than 1, evidently an additional mechanism is exerting an effect, increasing the affinity of the solute for the internal phase. This additional effect is usually ascribed to adsorption.

Gel filtration is widely used to desalt protein solutions. High concentrations of salts are employed in protein purification procedures, and it may be necessary to remove the salt. This is very simply accomplished on a gel column. $K_D = 0$ for the protein if the gel is properly selected, whereas $K_D = 1$ for the salt. Therefore the protein passes unretarded through the column, whereas the salt, which enters the gel particles and therefore effectively travels a longer path than the protein, is retarded. Complete separation can be achieved.

Sometimes it is desired to replace one salt with another in a protein solution. The exchange is carried out on a gel column that has previously been loaded with the replacement salt solution, which is also used as the eluent.

Finally, true chromatographic separations may be effected. A series of closely related molecules, such as homologous polymers, can be separated on a gel column if their K_D values are sufficiently different. Besides its use in separating mixtures, gel chromatography can give estimates of molecular weights of macromolecules. For this purpose a calibration curve is prepared of V_R against MW for a series of substances of known molecular weights. Then the molecular weight of an unknown substance can be determined by measuring its retention volume.

17.4 Practice of Liquid Column Chromatography

Although LC has been a standard separation technique for decades, fresh developments have greatly increased its potential. This section briefly surveys the uses of LC. Several books have dealt with these topics at greater length [6–8].

Selection of Mode. The choice of one of the four basic types of LC to solve a particular separation problem is largely based on prior experience rather than general principles, but some guidelines can be given [7]. For separations of molecules with molecular weights in the approximate range 200–2000, LLC, LSC, or ion exchange usually will be used; for larger molecules molecular exclusion chromatography may be better. The solubility characteristics of the substances to be separated are important. Water-soluble compounds are best handled by LLC or ion-exchange chromatography, water-insoluble substances by LSC or reversed-phase LLC. The molecular structures of the sample compounds may suggest the best mode. Thus the presence of ionic groups, including acidic or basic functional groups, on a molecule may make ion exchange the method of choice. Polymers can be approached with GPC. LSC is very good for separating mixtures into functional group classes, whereas LLC is superior for resolving homologous classes into their members. Of course, such generalizations may be inappropriate in any given instance, and experimentation is the best guide.

Selection of Column and Solvent. After the mode has been chosen the stationary and mobile phases must be selected. These obviously depend upon the mode. Section 17.3 discussed some of the factors that must be considered, such as adsorbent strength and solvent polarity. Practical matters such as the stability of the column packing toward multiple use and the means of monitoring the eluate may control the phases that can be used. The experimental technique (whether gravity flow or high-pressure LC, as discussed below) may limit the choices.

In general terms, the stationary and mobile phases are selected so as to achieve adequate chromatographic resolution. Equation 17.27 provides a theoretical basis for modifying column conditions in order to alter resolution. In developing a separation a mobile phase solvent is often selected that has moderate solvent polarity; then adjustments are made on the basis of trial experiments. Mixed solvents offer a means for adjusting eluent polarity over a wide range. The first step in optimizing a separation is to calculate k' (Eq. 17.28) and then to adjust solvent polarity so that k' is brought into the optimum range of 1–10. Next column efficiency may be improved by increasing column length. The selectivity α should finally be adjusted, by solvent selection, so that $\alpha > 1.1$ for the two most closely spaced compounds.

A multicomponent mixture may contain compounds possessing a wide range of retention volumes, thus requiring very long development times to elute the compounds with low R values (k' values greater than 10). This is called the "general elution problem." In LC the most satisfactory solution to this problem is the gradient elution technique, in which the polarity of the solvent is gradually increased so that the k' values of the most strongly retained compounds are decreased into the optimal range.

Apparatus and Techniques. In classical LC the mobile phase passes through the column under the influence of gravity. The equipment required is very simple and inexpensive. A chromatographic column need be little more than a glass tube. Figure 17.11 shows two designs. The dimensions are not critical, with diameters ranging from a few millimeters to a few centimeters and lengths from centimeters to meters. For a given weight of column packing greater efficiency (more plates) will be obtained with a long narrow column than with a short thick one, but if the column is too long the flow rate will be very low.

The method of packing the column depends on the LC mode. Ion-exchange columns are packed by pouring the wet ion-exchange resin into a column full of water and allowing the beads to settle. Since resins swell markedly upon absorbing water, columns must never be packed with dry resin beads. Addition of water to a dry resin bed would result in shattering of the glass column.

Columns for LSC can be packed dry or as a slurry formed with the mobile phase solvent. If a series of solvents is to be used in the elution, the slurry is made (or the dry column is wetted) with the least polar of the planned eluents.

In LLC the column material is prepared by causing the stationary phase to be adsorbed to the surface of the support particles and dispersing this in the mobile phase. Two procedures give good results. In one of these the stationary phase solvent is thoroughly stirred into the solid support until it is uniformly dispersed. With an aqueous stationary phase and silicic acid as the support a

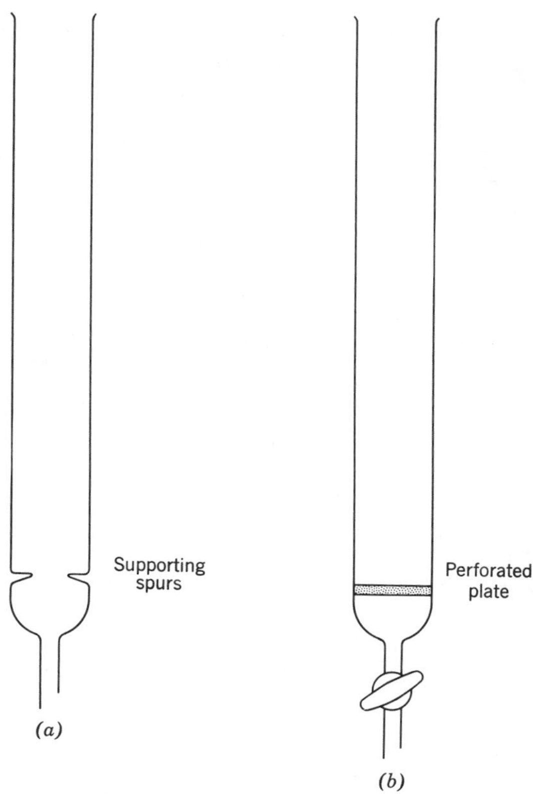

Fig. 17.11. Glass columns for gravity flow LC.

1:1 ratio (v/w) of solvent to support is usually satisfactory. The resulting mixture is stirred into enough mobile phase to make a smooth slurry. The other general procedure is to form a slurry of the solid support and the mobile phase, and then to add the stationary phase and stir until a smooth mixture is obtained.

The slurry is packed into a chromatographic column. It is supported at the bottom by a perforated disk or by a plug of glass wool. The packing technique is described in detail in Experiment 17.4. If the separation is a difficult one (because the partition coefficients are very similar), the column must be packed with care to minimize eddy diffusion. If the compounds are readily separable, an indifferent technique will still yield an acceptable column. The flow rate is controlled by the firmness with which the column is packed and by the height of liquid in the tube above the column. It is possible to increase the flow rate by applying air pressure to the top of the column or vacuum to its lower end.

The sample can be applied to the column in the mobile phase or in the stationary phase. The former method is the simpler one. A solution is prepared by dissolving the sample mixture in some of the mobile solvent. An aliquot of this solution is carefully pipetted onto the top of the column. The partitioning process begins as it passes into the column packing. The other method for adding the sample is especially useful if the sample is an aqueous solution. This cannot be pipetted directly onto the column, so an appropriate amount of solid support is mixed with the aqueous sample, and this mixture is packed on the top of the column in a narrow zone. This procedure is described in Experiment 17.4.

The packed column, containing the sample in a narrow zone at its top, is now ready for development. The mobile phase solvent is added to the tube and the lower end of the tube is opened. The eluent will percolate through the packing, and the column effluent (the eluate) can be collected in small fractions for analysis.

For an accurate picture of column performance the eluate concentration should be determined in a differential manner. This means that the concentration of solute in each infinitesimal portion of eluate should be measured, the plot of this value against the corresponding eluate volume constituting the chromatogram. This is actually done in instrumental chromatographic techniques, but when fractions are collected for analysis a true differential chromatogram is not obtained. If the fractions are small relative to the volume required to elute a peak, this procedure will yield a fairly satisfactory picture of the peak shape. If relatively large fractions are collected, it is not possible to deduce peak shapes from the data, although the results are fully valuable for quantitative analysis, because the total solute under the peak will be the same regardless of the number of fractions it is collected in. Figure 17.12 is a typical column chromatogram. The first two peaks, which are narrow, have not been well-defined because the fractions collected were too large. The third and fourth peaks, being quite wide, have been outlined reasonably well with the use of 10 ml fractions.

Modern LC differs from classical LC primarily in using high pressures to drive the mobile phase through the column, and the technique is referred to as high-pressure liquid chromatography (HPLC), or high-speed liquid chromatography. The essential components of a high-pressure liquid chromatograph are shown in Fig. 17.13.

Operating pressures in HPLC are in the range 500–7000 psi. Columns are 1–3 mm in diameter, made of glass or stainless steel. Mobile phase flow rates are up to 10 ml/min. An essential requirement is a constant flow rate with pulse-less flow of solvent. If gradient elution is required, a gradient mixing chamber must be incorporated in the design.

The detector in HPLC is critical in the performance of the system. For most

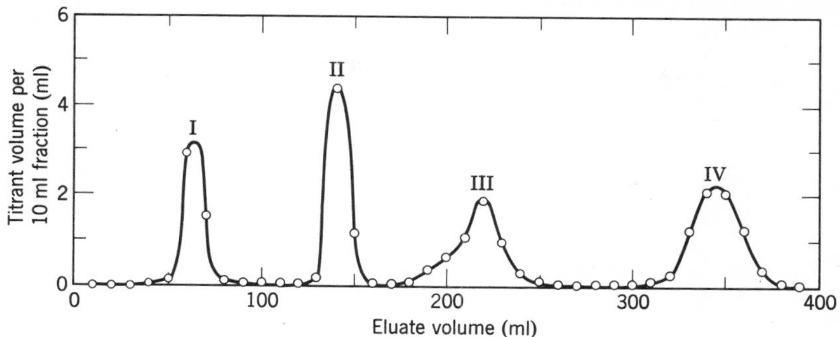

Fig. 17.12. Column LLC separation of aminopyrine (I), antipyrine (II), procaine (III), and nicotinamide (IV). Solid support, Celite 545; stationary phase, pH 6.5 phosphate buffer; mobile phase; 0–90 ml, 10% $CHCl_3$ in petroleum ether; 90–170 ml, 50% $CHCl_3$ in petroleum ether; 170–260 ml, $CHCl_3$; 260–390 ml, 20% *n*-butanol in $CHCl_3$. 10 ml eluate fractions were titrated with perchloric acid.

applications the ideal detector would have a universal response (that is, would detect all compounds except the solvent), it would be sensitive, and the response would be directly proportional to concentration. No single detector exists with these properties, but several widely applicable detectors are available. At this time the most used detector is the ultraviolet absorption detector. In essence, the column effluent is passed through a microcell that is continuously monitored for light absorption at a preselected wavelength. For compounds that absorb in the uv region (or that can be converted to absorbing derivatives), this is a very sensitive detector. The recorder plots absorbance against time to give a differential chromatogram. Figure 17.14 shows a HPLC separation with uv detection. A more general detector measures the refractive index (RI) of the eluate, or rather the difference between the refractive indices of the eluate and the pure solvent. Though its response is more general than is that of the uv detector, the RI detector is less sensitive, and it cannot easily be used with gradient elution.

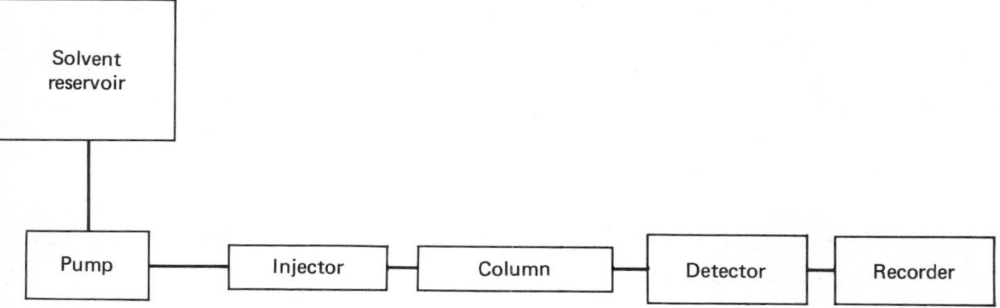

Fig. 17.13. Schematic diagram of a high-pressure liquid chromatograph.

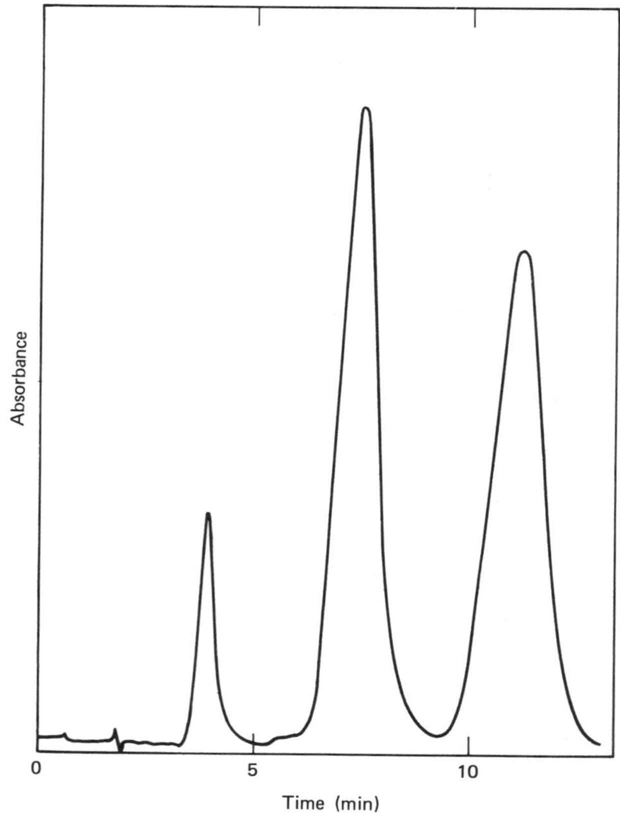

Fig. 17.14. High-pressure liquid chromatogram of a mixture of steroids. Column, β,β'-oxydipropionitrile on Zipax; mobile phase, 1% ethanol in hexane; flow rate, 0.8 ml/min; pressure, 500 psi. In order of elution: flumethasone pivalate, prednisolone, dexamethasone [J. A. Mollica and R. F. Strusz, *J. Pharm. Sci.*, **61,** 444 (1972)].

The immediate advantage of HPLC over classical LC is the sharp reduction in time of separation, which is accompanied by narrower zones and therefore improved resolution.

Applications. LC can be used for qualitative analysis (identification) and for quantitative analysis. The manipulations and calculations required for these purposes are described in Chapter 18.

Classical LC has long been a standard separation technique with certain well-accepted applications, including amino acid analysis by ion-exchange chromatography and the separation of complex mixtures of natural products by LSC. With the development of HPLC, however, liquid chromatography is becoming the preferred method for separating many mixtures on a routine

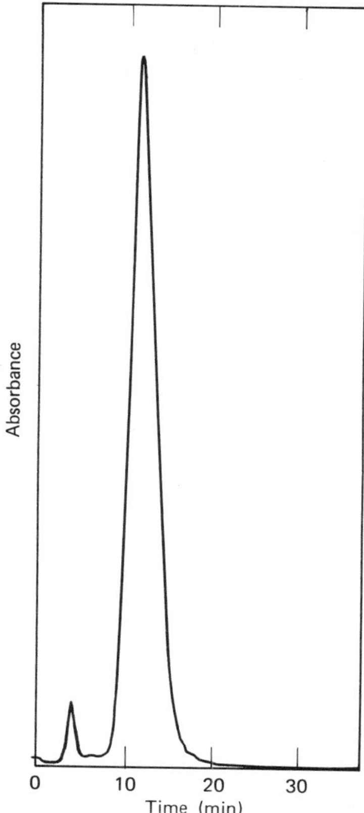

Fig. 17.15. High-pressure liquid chromatogram of a commercial preparation containing 0.5% antazoline phosphate and 0.05% naphazoline hydrochloride. Column, strong cation resin on Zipax; mobile phase, pH 12.45 phosphate buffer with ionic strength 0.95 adjusted with Na_2SO_4; flow rate, 0.8 ml/min; pressure, 1800 psi; detector, uv at 254 nm [J. A. Mollica, G. R. Padmanabhan, and R. Strusz, *Anal. Chem.*, **45,** 1859 (1973)].

basis. The analysis of pharmaceutical dosage forms, especially those containing mixtures of drugs, can often be done by HPLC. Figure 17.14 is an example of such a separation. Figure 17.15 shows another separation of a drug mixture by HPLC. Drug stability studies, in which the intact drug molecule must be distinguished from its degradation products, are also facilitated by LC.

17.5 Flat-Bed Chromatography

Paper Chromatography. Consden, Gordon, and Martin in 1944 [9] introduced a variation of Martin and Synge's column partition method that utilizes sheets of paper as the solid support. Thousands of articles have since been published dealing with this technique. Although the physical arrangement in paper chromatography is different from that in column chromatography, the fundamental separation process is the same. Zones on paper chromatograms are seldom eluted, the development being stopped while the zones and the solvent front are still within the bounds of the paper. The extent of zone migration is specified in terms of the R_f value.

Many variations in the apparatus and experimental details have been developed. Some of the basic equipment and methods are briefly described here. Fuller treatments are available [10–12].

Developing chambers may be as simple as a test tube, or may be more elaborate arrangements designed to hold many chromatograms simultaneously. The chamber holds the paper in place during the development and provides an atmosphere saturated with the eluent; this is necessary because in the paper chromatographic method the system is not surrounded by the walls of a column, and loss of mobile phase to the atmosphere would distort the zones. Paper strips may be supported from a cork or otherwise supported in a test tube; the lower end of the strip dips into the eluent, which rises through the paper by capillary action. Sheets of paper require larger developing tanks. The equipment is commercially available, but for occasional use it is easily improvised. Experiment 17.3 utilizes a simple experimental setup.

Filter paper is usually the support material. Whatman No. 1 filter paper is probably the most popular paper, but other types can be used. The type of paper controls the flow rate, with coarse-grained papers having relatively high flow rates. The internal (stationary) phase is probably a water-cellulose complex—even untreated paper in equilibrium with the atmosphere contains about 20% water—and it is possible that the distribution equilibrium is not simply a liquid-liquid partitioning alone. The paper (cellulose) probably exerts some direct adsorptive effect in addition to the liquid-liquid equilibrium. It nevertheless appears that paper chromatography is best described as a partition chromatographic method. The adsorbed atmospheric moisture may provide an adequate internal phase, but usually the paper is "conditioned" by exposing it for some time to the vapors of the mobile phase. The polar component of the developer (which is usually a mixed solvent) is adsorbed to the paper and acts as the stationary phase. The paper may also be impregnated by dipping it into the stationary phase solvent.

The mobile phase is usually a mixed solvent. It may be neutral, basic, or acidic. Typical mixtures are isopropanol-ammonia-water, *n*-butanol-acetic acid-water, and aqueous phenol. Some of these mixtures form two-phase systems when shaken together; the polar phase is used to condition the paper prior to development (the polar phase being preferentially adsorbed to the paper), and the less polar phase (the nonaqueous phase) is used to develop the chromatogram. The eluting power of a developer can be varied widely by alterations in the proportions of the solvent mixture.

A few microliters of the sample solution are applied by micropipet in a small spot near an end of a paper strip or an edge of a sheet; the position of the spot is marked with a pencil. The paper is then placed in the chromatography chamber, which contains the polar stationary solvent in a separate vessel. After conditioning is complete, the mobile phase is added to contact the paper, care being taken that the developer liquid does not touch the sample spot.

The physical orientation of the development may be arranged in three ways.

1. *Ascending* chromatography is easily carried out without special equipment. The strip of paper is lowered into the developer, which rises through the paper by capillary action. As the mobile phase passes across the sample spot the liquid-liquid distribution occurs that is the basis of all partition separations. The compounds with the greatest affinity for the mobile phase migrate fastest on the paper.
2. *Descending* chromatography utilizes a downward flow of the developer. The paper strip or sheet is suspended with its top edge dipping into a trough of the developer. As the solvent flows down the paper, it passes over the sample spot, which is placed near the upper end of the paper.
3. *Radial* chromatography is used with circular filter paper. The sample spot is applied at the center of the paper, which is supported in a horizontal position across a dish containing the developer. A wick conducts the developer to the center of the paper disk. The radial movement of the solvent on the disk produces concentric rings, rather than spots, as the sample is resolved into its components.

Some samples cannot be resolved completely by chromatography with a single solvent system. A successful variation utilizes development of the sample spot with a solvent capable of effecting separation of some of the components (starting with the spot applied at one corner of a square sheet of paper), followed by development with a second solvent in a direction at 90° to the first development. The second solvent is selected to effect resolution of the components unresolved in the first development. This technique is called two-dimensional paper chromatography. Figure 17.16 shows a paper chromatogram after the first (Fig. 17.16*a*) and second (*b*) stages of development.

After the development of a paper chromatogram has been completed (usually when the solvent front has advanced most of the distance on the paper), the solvent front is marked with a pencil and the chromatogram is dried. Since most compounds are colorless; it is necessary to locate the zones by the

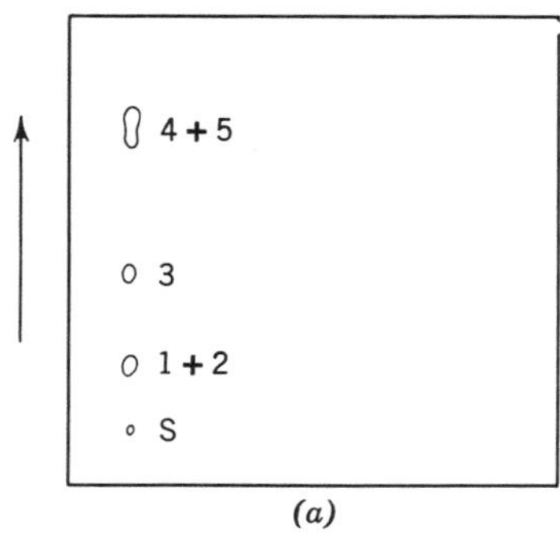

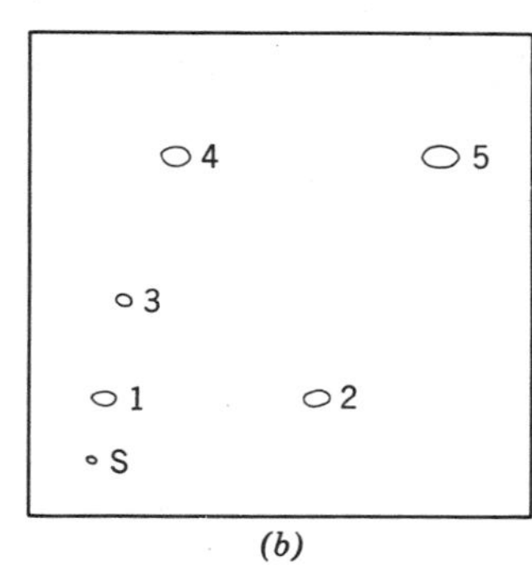

Fig. 17.16. Two-dimensional paper chromatogram of a five component mixture. (*a*) After development with the first solvent, showing partial resolution into three zones; (*b*) after second development, with complete separation.

application of a suitable chemical or physical test. If the compounds are fluorescent, illumination with a mercury lamp will probably cause fluorescence, and the spot can be outlined in pencil for permanent reference. Many substances can be induced to form colors upon reaction with properly selected reagents. Most amino acids, for example, produce purple spots when their chromatograms are sprayed with a ninhydrin solution. Nitrogen compounds give a yellow color with *p*-dimethylaminobenzaldehyde. Phenols react with ferric salts to produce colored spots. These are just a few of the color reactions available to locate the zones on a paper chromatogram.

After the zone is revealed, the R_f value for each substance is calculated with Eq. 17.2. This value should be characteristic of each compound on a given paper-solvent combination. Unfortunately, R_f values are found to be dependent upon many other variables, such as temperature, sample size, distance from solvent reservoir to initial sample spot, geometry of the paper, and type of development (ascending, descending, or radial). To increase the reliability of the R_f as a criterion of identity it is therefore necessary to chromatograph an authentic specimen side-by-side, on the same paper sheet, with the suspected sample. Both the standard and the unknown are thus subjected to the same conditions.

Paper chromatography can form the basis of quantitative analytical methods, although it is inferior to column chromatography for this purpose. After the zone has been located (usually one runs a pair of samples, using one as a locator and the other, undisturbed one for analysis), it is cut out of the paper and eluted with a solvent. The solution can then be analyzed, for example, by spectrophotometry or fluorometry. Quantitative analysis of the substance in the in situ zone may also be possible by direct spectrophotometry of the zone on the paper. A visual method may give semiquantitative results; the size and intensity of the sample spot are compared with several adjacent spots produced with known amounts of the pure substance, which is also subjected to chromatography.

A technique related to paper chromatography that has been of special value in the separation of biochemical mixtures is *paper electrophoresis*. If a mixture of substances carrying ionic charges is chromatographed on paper and simultaneously subjected to a strong electric potential difference imposed across the paper at 90° to the direction of flow, the substances will be deflected from the flow direction by angles depending upon their charges. A neutral substance will be unaffected by the applied field. Positively and negatively charged ions will be deflected in opposite directions. Since all proteins, and many other important compounds of biological origin, exist in forms whose charges depend upon pH, paper electrophoresis introduces an additional effect that can be manipulated to achieve separations. By altering the pH of the stationary phase, the electrophoretic behavior of the solutes can be influenced. Electrophoresis is also carried out on gels.

It is not an exaggeration to state that every type of compound has been subjected to paper chromatography. Not all separations are equally successful, but a vast number of difficult separation problems can be solved. Paper chromatography is very sensitive, requiring only micrograms of substance for many separations. Its principal value is probably for the detection and identification of components in complex mixtures. The literature of pharmaceutical analysis contains many reports of the fruitful use of paper chromatography [12].

Thin-Layer Chromatography. Thin-layer chromatography (TLC) is a form of adsorption chromatography in which the adsorbent is spread in a thin layer on a glass plate; usually it is held in place by a chemical binder. The sample addition and development steps are similar to the same procedures in paper chromatography. This technique has become extremely popular.

Although TLC as usually carried out is an adsorption chromatographic method, it is perfectly feasible to perform thin-layer partition chromatography. There probably are many solvent systems that give rise to a combination partition-adsorption effect during the separation. If, for example, the developer contains water, methanol, or another very polar solvent, this liquid may be adsorbed from the developer that is running ahead of the zone, thus converting the adsorption system into a partition chromatographic system.

Equipment is commercially available for the preparation of the thin layer of adsorbent slurry on the glass plate. This layer can be formed by spreading (the usual technique), spraying, sifting, or any other method that produces a layer of uniform thickness. Some very simple methods have been developed;

one of these is used in Experiment 17.2. The commercial applicator is essentially a reservoir under which the glass plates (usually 20 × 20 cm) are passed to receive a uniform coating of adsorbent slurry. A typical layer is 250 μ thick. Prepared plates of many types of adsorbent can be purchased.

Alumina and silica gel are the most versatile adsorbents. A binding agent (calcium sulfate) may be incorporated. The particle size of the adsorbent is smaller than that of column materials, and this fine-grain character of the adsorbent accounts for the great sensitivity of TLC. The mobile phase may be any of the solvents, or mixtures of them, already discussed as column developers, and the same principles govern the selection of the developer.

The adsorbent is mixed with water to form a smooth slurry, which is applied to the clean glass plate in a uniform layer. After the slurry has dried, the layer will be more or less firmly bound to the plate by the added binder. Since in the preparation of the slurry the adsorbent has been deactivated by contact with water, the prepared plate must be activated. This is accomplished by heating in an oven. Activated plates are stored in a desiccator.

The development in TLC is carried out by the ascending technique. After development is complete the plates are allowed to air-dry prior to examination of the migrated zones. The zones can be revealed by an adequate physical or chemical method. Illumination with ultraviolet light is particularly convenient for compounds that fluoresce. Nonfluorescent compounds can be located by incorporating a fluorescent substance in the adsorbent slurry. After development is complete the zones will appear as dark spots against a fluorescent background. As with paper chromatography, specific color-forming reactions are valuable indicators of zone position. The thin-layer chromatogram is superior to a paper chromatogram as a medium for color reactions, because many corrosive reagents, which might react with paper, can be applied directly to the TLC chromatogram to reveal the zones.

R_f values are calculated as usual. The thin-layer R_f value is reproducible if the chromatographic conditions are reproduced. The thickness and uniformity of the layer are important factors in determining reproducibility. It is always wise to chromatograph known specimens on the same plate as the unknown to compensate for variations in uncontrolled factors.

Quantitative analysis of the material in separated zones of the thin-layer chromatogram is accomplished by scraping the adsorbent layer containing the zone from the plate. The adsorbed solute is dissolved from the adsorbent, and is determined by a sensitive analytical method, usually spectrophotometry or fluorometry.

A major advantage of TLC over paper chromatography is its inherently greater sensitivity because of the finer grained character of the adsorbent particles compared with paper fibers. The sample remains concentrated in a smaller zone in TLC, and a smaller sample can therefore be detected. Another advantage of TLC is its rapidity of development, which requires only minutes compared with hours for most paper chromatographic separations. Undoubtedly many problems could be solved by either of these two methods, and then the choice is based upon the time and materials available or the analyst's familiarity with and preference for one or the other method.

The principal application of TLC is for the detection and identification of compounds in complex mixtures. The correspondence of R_f values of an authentic specimen and the unknown substance is a criterion of identity (though not a proof). If the R_f's again coincide when the solvent system is altered, the chromatographic evidence is usually considered to be strengthened, though caution is indicated in establishing identity on such evidence alone [13]. Usually some nonchromatographic evidence (such as sample history, uv, ir, MS, nmr, color reactions, etc.) is combined with the TLC or paper R_f data to establish proof of identity.

TLC (like all chromatographic methods) is a powerful tool for the detection of impurities. If chromatography of a substance gives but a single zone or peak in the chromatogram, certain inferences may be made about possible impurities in the sample. Although we can never prove that a chemical is pure, it is possible to demonstrate that specified impurities are not present (or if present, they occur in amounts below detectable levels). For example, acetylsalicylic acid and salicylic acid can be separated by thin-layer chromatography. If a sample of aspirin is chromatographed with the appearance of a single zone corresponding to the R_f value of aspirin, then it may be said that salicylic acid, if present in the sample at all, occurs at a concentration smaller than a level determined by the sensitivity of the detection method. Such semiquantitative information is often adequate.

Experiment 17.1. Separation of 2,4-Dinitrophenylhydrazones by Column Adsorption Chromatography

INTRODUCTION

In this experiment carbonyl compounds are separated as their 2,4-dinitrophenylhydrazones (see p. 481). Many separations of these derivatives by column adsorption chromatography have been reported; the procedure described here is a modification of the method of Schwartz et al. [14]. Because 2,4-dinitrophenylhydrazones produce colored bands on a chromatographic column, this experiment is suitable as a demonstration of the progress of a separation. On magnesium oxide, the adsorbent used here, the normally yellow compounds exhibit colors characteristic of their structures. The color of the band is therefore an indication of identity. The extent of zone migration is most conveniently specified in terms of a relative R value. The derivative of camphor has been selected as the reference compound because it moves faster than most other substances on this column. Calculation of the "R_C" value is made with the equation

$$R_C = \frac{\text{Distance from top of column to sample zone}}{\text{Distance from top of column to camphor zone}}$$

Combination of the R_C with the zone color may permit identification of the parent carbonyl. Separation of a four-component mixture is described here; undoubtedly other carbonyls could be substituted for the ones used. The zone color and R_C value may vary slightly with different lots of magnesium oxide.

Two methods for applying the sample mixture to the column are given. The purified 2,4-dinitrophenylhydrazones may be prepared, mixed, and placed on the column, or the derivatives may be extemporaneously prepared from the carbonyl compounds just before use without preliminary purification. If the carbonyl samples contain impurities, use of the second procedure may lead to more bands in the chromatogram than were anticipated.

REAGENTS

2,4-Dinitrophenylhydrazine Reagent. Dissolve 1 g of 2,4-dinitrophenylhydrazine in 7.5 ml of concentrated sulfuric acid. Add this solution to 75 ml of ethanol, dilute to 250 ml with water, and filter if necessary.

Magnesium Oxide. Use heavy magnesium oxide, USP grade.

Alumina. Use chromatographic grade neutral (pH 7.6) aluminum oxide.

Eluent. Dilute 40 ml of chloroform to 100 ml with Skellysolve B.

PROCEDURES

Packing the Column. Suspend 1.5 g of alumina and 13.5 g of heavy magnesium oxide in just enough Skellysolve B to make a free-flowing slurry. Mix this thoroughly and pour it into a 2.4 × 20 cm chromatographic column containing a pledget of glass wool at its lower end to support the packing. Do not tamp the column. Allow the liquid to flow from the column until it is level with the top of the packing. With a plunger force a circle of filter paper (slightly greater in diameter than the tube) down the column and seat it on top of the packing. This piece of paper will protect the column packing from disruption during addition of eluent.

Sample Preparation. To 3 ml of 2,4-dinitrophenylhydrazine reagent in a test tube add several drops of a liquid carbonyl compound or a methanolic solution of a solid carbonyl compound. If a precipitate does not appear, add a few drops of water. Filter with suction in a Büchner funnel and wash the precipitate of 2,4-dinitrophenylhydrazone with a little water. Draw air through the funnel to dry the derivative. Place the stem of the funnel in a test tube and dissolve the precipitate in a minimum volume of chloroform, collecting the solution in the test tube. Repeat this entire procedure with each carbonyl compound, collecting all of the final solutions in the same test tube, thus giving a chloroform solution of the 2,4-dinitrophenylhydrazones of the carbonyl compounds. Suggested compounds for this experiment are acetaldehyde, acetone, camphor, and cyclopentanone. Camphor should be included in the mixture in any case, for it is the reference compound against which the migration behavior of other substances is to be measured.

Alternative Preparation. An alternative preparation uses the pure derivatives. Heat to boiling a mixture of 0.5 g of 2,4-dinitrophenylhydrazine, about 0.25 g of a carbonyl compound, and 25 ml of ethanol or methanol, cool slightly, add 0.5 ml of concentrated hydrochloric acid, and boil for 2 min. Allow the solution to cool and to stand until the 2,4-dinitrophenylhydrazone crystallizes. Filter with suction and wash with a little ethanol. Recrystallize the derivative from ethanol or methanol. Prepare in this way the crystalline 2,4-dinitrophenylhydrazones of acetaldehyde, acetone, camphor, and cyclopentanone. Make a chloroform solution containing all four derivatives.

Sample Application. Very carefully add from a pipet about 5 drops of the sample solution of 2,4-dinitrophenylhydrazones to the top of the column. It is important that the sample be distributed as evenly and as gently as possible to minimize distortion of the shape of the zone. Open the bottom end of the column and permit flow to begin. When the sample solution has passed into the packing, carefully add a few milliliters of 40% chloroform eluent from a pipet, again exercising caution to prevent channeling of the packing by the force of flowing solvent. When this solvent has passed into the column, the tube may be filled with eluent to carry out the development. Typical flow rates are 0.25 to 0.30 ml/min.

The sample can be added in a very narrow initial zone with the following alternative technique. Cut a small disk of heavy filter paper slightly smaller in diameter than the inner diameter of the chromatographic tube. With a pin punch several dozen small holes in the paper. Apply about 5 drops of the chloroform solution of 2,4-dinitrophenylhydrozones to the disk, allowing the solvent to air-dry after each drop. In this way a large amount of sample can be deposited on the paper. Very carefully lower the impregnated paper disk onto the filter paper protecting the top of the prepared chromatographic column. With a pipet run a few milliliters of 40% chloroform eluent onto the column to start the development. Proceed as described above.

Identification of the Zones. The development should be continued for about an hour or until the bands are well separated; they should not be eluted from the column. Measure the R_C value for each zone, and note its color. (If the extemporaneous method of sample preparation was used, a band of excess reagent may appear in addition to the sample bands.) In order to establish the identity of the compound in each zone it will be necessary to repeat the separation, leaving out one component of the mixture each time. Prepare a table listing the parent carbonyl compound, the color of its chromatographic zone, and its R_C value.

Experiment 17.2. Separation of Aspirin, Acetophenetidin, and Caffeine by Thin-Layer Chromatography

INTRODUCTION

Aspirin, acetophenetidin (phenacetin), and caffeine are often used in combination as an antipyretic analgesic preparation (APC). Their detection and identification in such preparations is important, and thin-layer chromatography provides a simple solution to this analytical problem [15].

The procedure of Gänshirt and Malzacher [16] has been adapted for this experiment. The very simple plate preparation method of Lees and DeMuria [17] is employed. The zones are revealed with an acidic permanganate spray reagent [18], which oxidizes the sample compounds with resulting decoloration of the permanganate.

APPARATUS AND REAGENTS

Coplin Jar (vertical slide staining jar). If a Coplin jar is not available, a perfectly satisfactory substitute (though a less convenient one) can be prepared from beakers as described below.

Spray Bottle. All-glass spray bottles are commerically available. Details for the construction of an equivalent apparatus have been published [15].

Silica Gel G for thin-layer chromatography. This adsorbent contains the binder and is ready for use.

Developer Solvent. Mix absolute methanol, glacial acetic acid, diethyl ether, and benzene in the proportions 1 : 18 : 60 : 120 (by volume).

Spray Reagent. Prepare 0.1 *N* potassium permanganate in 0.05 *N* sulfuric acid.

Sample Solutions of aspirin, acetophenetidin, and caffeine, separately and in mixture, in chloroform should be prepared to contain 5–10 mg/ml.

PROCEDURES

Preparation of Plates. Clean eight microscope slides (25 × 75 mm) in chromic acid-sulfuric acid cleaning solution, rinse thoroughly with distilled water, and dry. Tape the slides with masking tape, in sets of four, end to end on a board, overlapping the long edges of the slides with tape by about 3 mm.

Prepare a smooth slurry of 3 g of silica gel G and 6 ml of water by triturating well in a mortar. Pour about half of the slurry on the first slide of one of the sets. With a thick glass rod placed perpendicular to the long side of the slides spread the slurry into a smooth layer. The rod should be slid, not rolled, along the tape; the thumbs provide a wall along the edges to prevent the slurry from flowing off the slides. The thickness of the layer is determined by the thickness of the tape.

A somewhat more conveniently used slide may be prepared by taping the slides as above, and adding two strips of masking tape, each about $\frac{1}{16}$ in. wide, to divide the glass surface into three longitudinal strips of equal width. These strips of tape are easily cut with a straightedge and a razor blade.

After the gel has air-dried, carefully remove the tape. Place the slides on a watch glass and dry them in an oven at 100°C for 1 hr. Store the prepared slides in a desiccator; they may be conveniently held in a slotted microscope slide box.

Application of Sample. Apply two or three samples about $\frac{1}{2}$ in. from one end of slide. If the slide has been prepared with three strips of gel separated by clear glass it is very easy to apply three sample spots to each slide. The spotting is conveniently done with fine pipets drawn from melting point tubes. The sample spot should be no more than 3 mm in diameter, and its size may be limited by repeatedly applying small amounts of solution to the spot, permitting each increment to dry before the next addition. Air-dry the sample spots.

Development of the Chromatogram. Into a Coplin jar pour enough developer to contact the bottom edge of the slide but not so much that the solvent will touch the sample spots. Carefully lower the slide, sample spots down, into the solvent, and place the cover on the Coplin jar. After the solvent front has advanced about 50 mm (which will take about 15 min) carefully scratch the surface of the slide to indicate the position of the solvent front, remove the slide from the jar, and allow it to air-dry. Place it in an oven for a few minutes to remove the organic solvent.

If Coplin jars are not available an entirely satisfactory chamber can be prepared with beakers. Fix a short piece of Scotch tape to the back of the upper end of the slide (the end opposite the sample spots). Extend this tape with another short piece of tape, contacting the adhesive faces of the two lengths so that the resulting extension has an adhesive side facing away from the slide.

Suspend the slide in a 250 ml beaker so that the bottom edge is about $\frac{1}{8}$ in. above the bottom of the beaker; the slide is supported by the Scotch tape stuck to the outside of the beaker. Now carefully add, down a glass rod, enough of the developer solvent to cover the bottom $\frac{1}{8}$ in. of the slide. Immediately cover the beaker with an inverted 600 ml beaker or with a watch glass, and treat the slide as described previously.

Location of Zones. Place the dried slide across two glass rods on a large plate of glass. Spray the slide with the acidic potassium permanganate solution, using a spray bottle to deliver a fine mist. Heat the slide in an oven for a few minutes.

The zones will appear as yellowish-green spots on a violet background. The zone for caffeine is very faint and sometimes may be more easily observed by viewing it from the back side, that is, through the glass.

Calculate the R_f values for the three pure substances. Perform several such determinations and evaluate the mean and standard deviation for each R_f value. Chromatograph a known mixture of these three substances, and locate the position of each compound by comparison with the known R_f values.

Unknown Mixture. Obtain from your instructor a solution containing aspirin, acetophenetidin, or caffeine, or any mixture of these. Determine by TLC the identity of the components in your sample. It is advisable to chromatograph known samples side by side with the unknown for the reason given earlier in this chapter.

Experiment 17.3. Separation of Barbiturates by Paper Chromatography

INTRODUCTION

The solvent system used in this paper chromatographic separation of barbituric acid derivatives is adapted from the work of Macek [19]. The system is not capable of separating all the commonly used barbiturates, but it is very effective in resolving certain two, three, and four component mixtures. Suggested mixtures for study are: (1) phenobarbital, mephobarbital, butabarbital, and amobarbital; (2) diallylbarbituric acid, hexobarbital, cyclopentylallylbarbituric acid, and pentobarbital. Other barbiturates that migrate in this solvent system are secobarbital, aprobarbital, and barbital.

APPARATUS AND REAGENTS

1:1 Benzene-Chloroform Solvent. Mix equal volumes of benzene and chloroform, and saturate the mixed solvent with formamide by shaking some formamide with the solvent in a separatory funnel. This formamide-saturated mixed solvent should be prepared fresh daily, since aged solvent leads to slightly different R_f values.

20% Formamide Solution. Dilute 20 ml of formamide to 100 ml with acetone.

0.0025% Fluorescein Solution. Dissolve 2.5 mg of soluble fluorescein in a little water. Add about 3.5 ml of concentrated ammonium hydroxide and dilute to 100 ml with water.

Ultraviolet Lamp. A short wavelength mercury lamp (emitting the 2537 Å line) is required.

Whatman No. 4 Paper, cut in 2 × 20 cm strips. This paper is available in rolls 2 cm wide.

Developing Tank. The ascending technique is recommended because the necessary apparatus is simple and inexpensive. A rectangular jar measuring 10 × 10 × 21 cm is a satisfactory developing chamber, though other arrangements can be improvised. A cover is formed by taping together three pieces of cardboard to give a square cover with two slits, through which the strips of paper will be vertically hung; the strips are supported by passing pins or toothpicks through their upper ends.

PROCEDURES

Preparation of Paper. Draw a line with pencil across a paper strip about 3 cm from the lower end. Dip the entire strip into the 20% formamide solution and hang it to air-dry for 5–10 min or until the acetone has evaporated.

Sample Application. With a fine capillary drawn from a melting point tube apply a solution of a barbiturate (10–15 mg/ml in chloroform) in a small spot centered on the pencil line. The size of the spot can be limited by making several additions of solution, allowing the solvent to evaporate after each addition. Air-dry the spot.

Treat several strips in this way, applying different barbiturates to each strip. After some preliminary studies of R_f values have been completed, make up two, three, and four component mixtures and apply these samples to paper strips.

Development of the Chromatogram. Immerse the lower end of the paper strip into the formamide-saturated benzene-chloroform solvent contained in the developing chamber. The surface of the solvent should not be permitted to touch the sample spot. If the strip does not hang vertically it can be weighted at the lower end with a thumbtack or paper clip. Suspend the paper as suggested above or by any other suitable means.

After the solvent front has progressed about 12 cm beyond the starting line (which will take 35–40 min), remove the strip from the chamber and mark the position of the solvent front with a soft pencil or ballpoint pen.

Location of the Zones. Hang the developed strip in an 80°C oven for 15 min. Remove it from the oven and thoroughly spray it with fluorescein solution. Look at the strip, in a dark place, by the light of a mercury lamp emitting 2537 Å radiation. (Wear glasses while looking at this light, and do not look at the lamp directly.) The barbiturate zones will appear as blue spots against a greenish-yellow fluorescent background. Outline each zone with soft pencil or ballpoint pen to provide a permanent record. Calculate R_f values for each barbiturate.

Unknown Mixtures. Obtain a mixture of barbiturates from your instructor. Prepare a solution and chromatograph it alongside strips containing known samples. From a comparison of R_f values for the knowns and unknowns, specify the possible barbiturates in your sample.

Experiment 17.4. Separation of Aminopyrine and Antipyrine by Liquid–Liquid Column Chromatography

INTRODUCTION

This experiment permits the separation and quantitative determination of aminopyrine, **1**, and antipyrine, **2**. Both these compounds are soluble in water and in most of the common organic solvents. Aminopyrine ($pK_a = 5.0$) is a stronger base than antipyrine ($pK_a = 1.5$).

C_6H_5 / N / $O=$ / $N-CH_3$ / $(CH_3)_2N-$ / $-CH_3$

1

C_6H_5 / N / $O=$ / $N-CH_3$ / $-CH_2$

2

The chromatographic system employs Celite 545, a diatomaceous earth, as the solid support and a pH 6.5 buffer as the internal phase. The external phase is a chloroform-hydrocarbon mixture. In most column partition chromatography it is desirable to saturate the mobile phase with respect to the aqueous stationary phase before using it as the eluent, in order to prevent the stationary phase from being stripped from the column. In the system used here this preliminary saturation is unnecessary because the internal phase is very insoluble in the mobile phase.

The aminopyrine-antipyrine separation is conveniently followed by non-aqueous acid-base titration of the eluate with acetous perchloric acid. Aminopyrine is fairly basic and yields a good end point under the conditions described. Antipyrine is too weakly basic to give a sharp end point, but satisfactory results are obtainable by titrating all samples to the same color. The relatively large sample size specified is needed to consume appropriate volumes of the titrant for accurate measurement. If a more sensitive analytical method were available, the sample size could be made much smaller

The separation is quite sensitive to the pH of the internal phase [20].

APPARATUS AND REAGENTS

Chromatographic Column. The design shown in Fig. 17.11 is satisfactory. The barrel of the column is a glass tube 45 cm long and 20 mm in diameter. The lower end is fitted with several internal spurs to support a plug of glass wool; a short length of 6–8 mm glass tubing is fused below the constriction. A close-fitting glass plunger is used to pack the column.

pH 6.5 Buffer. Mix 60 ml of 0.1 *M* monosodium phosphate and 40 ml of 0.1 *M* dipotassium phosphate.

10% Chloroform in Skellysolve C. Dilute 20 ml of chloroform to 200 ml with Skellysolve C.

40% Chloroform in Skellysolve C. Dilute 40 ml of chloroform to 100 ml with Skellysolve C.

0.02 N Acetous Perchloric Acid. Pipet exactly 20.0 ml of standard 0.1 *N* perchloric acid (see Experiment 2.1) into a 100 ml volumetric flask and dilute to volume with glacial acetic acid. Calculate the normality.

p-Naphtholbenzein (PNB) Indicator. See Experiment 2.1.

PROCEDURES

Packing the Column. Stir 20 g of Celite 545 into about 100 ml of 10% chloroform solvent. Add, with stirring, 20 ml of pH 6.5 buffer and form a smooth slurry.

Clamp the column in a vertical position and close the lower end with a cork. Place a pledget of glass wool above the constriction. Now add the slurry to the column in increments, packing it firmly with the glass plunger after each addition. After a few grams of slurry has been packed into the column remove the cork and allow the solvent to flow through the column while packing the rest of the slurry. After all of the slurry has been added, push a circle of filter paper down the column to remove particles of solid clinging to the walls of the column. Allow the solvent to drain to within 2–3 mm of the top of the packing, and close both ends with corks. The column is now ready for use.

A flow rate of about 10 ml/4 min is satisfactory. This can be controlled by the firmness with which the column is packed and by the height of the organic phase above the column.

Application of Sample. Accurately weigh 15–30 mg each of antipyrine and aminopyrine into a 50 ml beaker. Dissolve this sample in 1 ml of pH 6.5 buffer. Add 1 g of Celite 545 to the solution and thoroughly mix. The resulting powder will appear dry or slightly moist. Quantitatively transfer this powder to the column and pack it firmly with the plunger. Place a circle of filter paper over the sample.

Development of the Chromatogram. Place a 10 ml graduated cylinder under the column and remove the cork. Immediately add some 10% chloroform eluent to the top of the column, being careful not to disturb the packing. Continue to add the eluent to the column. When 10 ml of the eluate has been collected place a second graduate under the column, continuing development with 10% chloroform.

Transfer each 10 ml fraction of eluate to a 50 ml Erlenmeyer flask, add about 10 ml of glacial acetic acid and several drops of *p*-naphtholbenzein indicator solution, and titrate to a green color with standard 0.02 *N* perchloric acid, using a 10 ml buret.

After the first compound has been eluted completely from the column (after about the eighth fraction), change the eluent to 40% chloroform and continue the development until the second compound has been completely eluted. The solvent level should not be permitted to pass below the surface of the packing at any time.

Make a plot of volume of titrant consumed per fraction against the number of the fraction (or the eluate volume). Draw a smooth curve through the points, as in Fig. 17.12. Calculate the total volume of titrant consumed by each compound (remembering to subtract an appropriate blank, or base line, value from the titration result for each fraction). In order to calculate the percent recoveries it is necessary to know which compound emerged first. This could be determined by chromatographing a mixture in which the two compounds are present in greatly differing amounts (on a molar basis). On this column it has been determined that aminopyrine is eluted first. Calculate the percent recovery of each compound.

Unknown Sample. Determine the composition of an unknown mixture of aminopyrine and antipyrine. The column packed for the first analysis may be reused if, after its first use, it is flushed with about 100 ml of the 10% chloroform solvent. Report the weights of aminopyrine and antipyrine per gram (if the sample is a solid mixture) or per milliliter (if it is a solution).

Experiment 17.5. Analysis of Salt Solutions by Ion Exchange

APPARATUS AND REAGENTS

Column. A glass chromatographic column 15 mm in diameter and 40 cm long will be satisfactory. These dimensions are not critical. The column should have a stopcock at its lower end.

Ion-Exchange Resin. Polystyrene-divinylbenzene sulfonic acid cation exchange resin in the hydrogen ion form, 20–50 mesh. Dowex 50 is suitable, as is any similar resin.

Salt Solutions. Accurately prepare 100 ml solutions, approximately 0.1 *N*, of each of four salts, such as potassium chloride, sodium chloride, sodium acetate, potassium sulfate, etc.

0.01 M Sodium Fluoride. Accurately prepare 100 ml of approximately 0.01 *M* NaF.

0.1 N Sodium Hydroxide and 0.1 N Hydrochloric Acid. Prepare and standardize as in Experiments 1.1 and 1.2. Prepare 0.02 *N* NaOH by quantitative dilution of the 0.1 *N* solution.

Mixed Indicator. Dissolve 40 mg of methyl red and 60 mg of bromcresol green in 100 ml of 95% ethanol.

PROCEDURES

Preparation of the Column. Seat a plug of glass wool firmly at the bottom of the column, and fill the column with water. Slurry about 10 g of swollen resin in water, and pour this into the column, allowing the beads to settle into a homogeneous bed.

If the resin is in the sodium form it must be placed in the hydrogen form. Slowly pass about 200 ml of 1 *N* HCl through the column. Follow this with distilled water until the effluent is no longer acidic.

Using the exchange capacity data supplied by the manufacturer, calculate the approximate total capacity of the column.

Determination of Total Salt. Run the water level in the column down to the top of the resin bed. Accurately pipet 5.0 ml of 0.1 *N* potassium chloride onto the top of the column, with as little disturbance of the resin bed as possible. Place a 250 ml Erlenmeyer flask under the column and open the stopcock. After the sample enters the resin bed, follow it with 50 ml of distilled water, and collect 55 ml of effluent. The flow rate can be 3–5 ml/min.

Add phenolphthalein indicator to the flask and titrate with standard 0.1 *N* NaOH. Calculate the percent recovery in terms of potassium chloride. Repeat this experiment with several other salts.

Prepare a solution of known concentrations of KCl and HCl. Titrate one aliquot of this solution directly to determine the hydrochloric acid content. Pass another aliquot through the ion-exchange column and titrate the effluent to determine the sum of KCl and HCl concentrations. Calculate the potassium chloride content of the sample by difference.

Although the column breakthrough capacity can be determined, it is simpler to regenerate the resin when an appreciable fraction (say, 0.5) of the total capacity has been utilized.

Obtain three unknown solutions from your instructor. Titrate an aliquot of each with sodium hydroxide to determine the acid concentration. Pass another aliquot through the resin column as with the known solutions, and titrate with alkali. Report the acid and salt concentrations of the solutions.

Determination of Fluorides. Accurately pipet 10.0 ml of 0.01 *N* sodium fluoride onto the resin bed. Collect the column effluent as before, washing the column with 75 ml of water. Add mixed indicator and titrate with 0.02 *N* NaOH to the light sky-blue color. Calculate the percent recovery of sodium fluoride.

Obtain a sample of stannous fluoride from the instructor. Accurately prepare a 0.01 *N* solution in water. If the solution is turbid, filter it and use the clear solution for analysis. Pipet a 10.0 ml aliquot onto the resin column, and carry out the analysis as in the preceding paragraph. Calculate the percent purity of the stannous fluoride sample.

References

1. Martin, A. J. P. and R. L. M. Synge, *Biochem. J.*, **35,** 1358 (1941).
2. Giddings, J. C., *Dynamics of Chromatography*, Part I, Marcel Dekker, New York, 1965.
3. Kirkland, J. J., *J. Chromatogr. Sci.*, **9,** 206 (1972).
4. Samuelson, O., *Ion Exchange Separations in Analytical Chemistry*, John Wiley, New York, 1963.
5. Bly, D. D., *Science*, **168,** 527 (1970).

6. Kirkland, J. J., (ed.), *Modern Practice of Liquid Chromatography*, Wiley-Interscience, New York, 1971.
7. Hadden, N., F. Baumann, F. MacDonald, M. Munk, R. Stevenson, D. Gere, F. Zamaroni, and R. Majors, *Basic Liquid Chromatography*, Varian Aerograph, Walnut Creek, California, 1971.
8. Brown, P. R., *High Pressure Liquid Chromatography*, Academic Press, New York, 1973.
9. Consden, R., A. H. Gordon, and A. J. P. Martin, *Biochem. J.*, **38,** 224 (1944).
10. Heftmann, E., *Chromatography*, 2nd ed., Reinhold, New York, 1967.
11. Sherma, J. and G. Zweig, *Paper Chromatography and Electrophoresis*, Vol. II, Academic Press, New York, 1971.
12. Macek, K., *Pharmaceutical Applications of Thin-Layer and Paper Chromatography*, Elsevier, Amsterdam, 1972.
13. Connors, K. A., *Anal. Chem.*, **46,** 53 (1974).
14. Schwartz, D. P., O. W. Parks, and M. Keeney, *Anal. Chem.*, **34,** 669 (1962).
15. Connors, K. A. and S. P. Eriksen, *Am. J. Pharm. Educ.*, **28,** 161 (1964).
16. Gänshirt, H. and A. Malzacher, *Arch. Pharm.*, **293,** 925 (1960).
17. Lees, T. M. and P. J. DeMuria, *J. Chromatogr.*, **8,** 108 (1962).
18. Cerri, O. and G. Maffi, *Boll. Chim. Farm.*, **100,** 951 (1962).
19. Macek, K., *Arch. Pharm.*, **293,** 545 (1960).
20. Connors, K. A., *Am. J. Pharm. Educ.*, **20,** 384 (1964).

FOR FURTHER READING

Smith, R. V., "A Brief History of Chromatographic Methods," *Am. J. Pharm. Educ.*, **35,** 252 (1971).

Determann, H., *Gel Chromatography*, Springer-Verlag New York, New York, 1968.

Snyder, L. R., *Principles of Adsorption Chromatography*, Marcel Dekker, New York, 1968.

Snyder, L. R. and J. J. Kirkland, *Introduction to Modern Liquid Chromatography*, Wiley-Interscience, New York, 1974.

Clarke, E. G. C. (ed.), *Isolation and Identification of Drugs*, The Pharmaceutical Press, London, 1969.

Zweig, G. and J. Sherma (eds.), *Handbook of Chromatography*, Vols. I and II, CRC Press, Cleveland, 1972.

Karger, B. L., L. R. Snyder, and C. Horvath, *An Introduction to Separation Science*, Wiley-Interscience, New York, 1973.

Problems

1. A column was prepared with 10 ml of water and 15 g of silicic acid; chloroform was the external phase. The retention volume of a fat-soluble dye was 35 ml on this column. A mixture of substances A, B, and C gave retention volumes of 120 ml, 175 ml, and 290 ml, respectively, on this column. Calculate the partition coefficients and R values of A, B, and C in the system.

2. Some carboxylic acids were chromatographed on a partition column with water as the internal phase. The peaks showed serious tailing. In order to reduce this tailing, would you buffer the internal phase to a pH greater than or less than the typical pK_a of the acids?

3. Suggest three ways in which the mobile phase volume V_M of a liquid-liquid partition column could be determined.

4. Outline procedures for the quantitative analysis of each substance in these mixtures: (*a*) oxalic acid, fumaric acid, and malic acid; (*b*) nicotinamide and nicotinic acid; and (*c*) sodium bromide, phenobarbital, and diphenylhydantoin.

5. A partition column was packed with 5 g of silicic acid and 5 ml of aqueous buffer solution; chloroform was the mobile phase. Three compounds, X, Y, and Z, with partition coefficients $K_X = 10^{-4}$, $K_Y = 1.0$, and $K_Z = 2.0$, were chromatographed on this column. Compound X had a retention volume of 8.5 ml. What were the retention volumes of Y and Z?

6. A partition column was packed with 10 ml of water and 10 g of silicic acid; the mobile phase was benzene. The retention volume of a fat-soluble dye was 12.0 ml on this column. Two compounds with partition coefficients of 1.0 and 2.5 in the water/benzene system were chromatographed.

(*a*) What is the mobile phase volume of the column?

(*b*) What were the retention volumes of the two compounds?

7. Two compounds, with partition coefficients of 10 and 20, had chromatographic retention volumes of 175 and 325 ml, respectively. What are the mobile and stationary phase volumes of the partition chromatographic column?

8. Derive an equation giving the number of plates required to resolve ($R_s = 1$) two compounds A and B having R values R_A and R_B.

9. Find the relationship between R and k', and give the range of R corresponding to the optimal k' range of 1 to 10.

10. Show that for a Freundlich isotherm a straight line is obtained when log X is plotted against log C_M. To what quantity is the slope of this line equal?

11. Show that for a Langmuir isotherm a plot of $1/X$ against $1/C_M$ is linear. Give the values of the slope and intercept.

12. Derive the relationship between the distribution coefficient D (expressed in amounts) and the coefficient K (expressed in concentrations). Show the equivalence of Eqs. 17.9 and 17.34.

13. Which solute will be eluted first when a mixture of chymotrysin and sodium sulfate is chromatographed on a gel column?

14. Two compounds, A and B, were subjected to paper chromatography. Let X = distance from the initial spot to the center of the zone, Y = distance from initial spot to solvent front, and w = width of the zone (in the direction of travel). These results were found:

$$X_A = 10.0 \text{ cm} \qquad w_A = 1.0 \text{ cm}$$

$$X_B = 8.5 \text{ cm} \qquad w_B = 0.9 \text{ cm}$$

$$Y = 12.5 \text{ cm}$$

(*a*) Calculate the R_f values.

(*b*) Calculate the chromatographic resolution.

Have the compounds been separated satisfactorily?

15. Suppose two compounds with partition coefficients of 1.0 and 2.0 are separated by LLC on a column 1 m long for which $V_M = 20$ ml and $V_S = 10$ ml.

(*a*) Predict the retention volumes.

(*b*) What will be the average width (in milliliters of eluate) of the zones when they have been separated according to the conventional criterion?

(*c*) Calculate the average number of plates required to achieve this separation.

(*d*) What is the value of H for this column?

16. (*a*) In terms of the generalized constants of the van Deemter equation, Eq. 17.24, derive an equation giving the flow velocity at which H is minimal.

(*b*) With this result, calculate the minimum value of H.

17. The following data were obtained for the elution of two zones from a column 40.0 cm in length with a flow rate of 1.5 ml/min.

Time (min)	Eluate Composition	Time (min)	Eluate Composition
16	0.05	25	0.2
17	0.2	26	0.1
18	1.4	27	0.4
19	6.0	28	1.9
20	9.5	29	4.4
21	10.0	30	5.2
22	9.4	31	4.3
23	6.1	32	2.1
24	1.2	33	0.4

(*a*) Give the retention times and volumes.

(*b*) Calculate the plate height and the number of plates on the column, using the first zone eluted.

(*c*) Calculate the resolution.

18 GAS CHROMATOGRAPHY

18.1 Principles of Gas Chromatography

When a gas is used as the mobile phase in a chromatographic system, the technique is called gas chromatography (GC). Gas chromatography is always carried out in a column, since the mobile phase must be contained. In gas-liquid chromatography (GLC) the stationary phase is a liquid, and the process is a form of partition chromatography; in gas-solid chromatography (GSC) a solid surface is the stationary phase, so this is adsorption chromatography. Martin and Synge [1], in their first paper on partition chromatography, pointed out that it should be feasible to separate volatile substances by partition chromatography with a gaseous mobile phase. This suggestion was not acted upon for several years; finally James and Martin [2], in 1952, demonstrated that GLC can be a powerful separation technique.

Theory. Separations in GC are based on the same principles as are other forms of chromatographic separations. Solutes migrate through the chromatographic system at rates determined by their affinities for the stationary phase. Resolution is a function of differential zone migration rates, tending to separate the zone centers, and of zone broadening processes that tend to merge the zones. In GC the mobile phase (the *carrier gas*) is an inert gas, so the distribution coefficient is determined solely by the solute's affinity for the stationary phase. (In liquid chromatography both the mobile and stationary phases control the distribution coefficient.)

Because of the fundamental similarities between GC and LC, it is not necessary to redevelop the principles and theory already presented for the LC systems in Chapter 17. All of Section 17.2 is applicable to GC, though some of the quantities may be interpreted differently (the partition coefficient, for example), and the parameters may have different values (especially the diffusion coefficient in the mobile phase).

In GC the solute can move through the column only when it is in the gaseous state. We therefore consider the relationship of the vapor pressure of a solute to the concentration of the solute in a liquid solvent (which in GC is the stationary phase.) If the solution is ideal, this relationship is Raoult's law,

Eq. 18.1, where p^0 is the vapor pressure of the pure solute, x is the mole fraction of solute in the solution,* and p is the vapor pressure of solute over the solution.

$$p = xp^0 \tag{18.1}$$

Real solutions do not obey this equation, but an analogous relationship, Henry's law, can be written as

$$p = \gamma x p^0 \tag{18.2}$$

Here γ is the activity coefficient, which is itself a function of x. At very low concentrations, however, the activity coefficient is essentially constant, and we have

$$\frac{x}{p} = \frac{1}{\gamma p^0} = \text{constant} \tag{18.3}$$

The quantity x/p has the nature of a partition coefficient, and it is the factor controlling selectivity in GC. Rather than work with x/p itself, we define the partition coefficient by

$$K = \frac{\text{g of solute per g of liquid phase}}{\text{g of solute per cm}^3 \text{ of gas phase}} \tag{18.4}$$

An important result of Eq. 18.3 is that the affinity of the solute for the stationary phase in GC depends upon the vapor pressure *and* upon the activity coefficient of the solute. This latter dependence means that it is possible to separate solutes that have identical vapor pressures if their activity coefficients are different in the GC stationary phase.

In Eq. 17.25 the chromatographic resolution was defined as $R_s = \Delta d/w$, where Δd is the distance between adjacent zone centers and w is the average zone width (see also Fig. 17.7). Eq. 17.27, a relationship between resolution and parameters of the solute and column, was then developed. This equation relates R_s to three terms, which measure column efficiency, selectivity, and capacity. The optimization of chromatographic conditions is based on this relationship and independent consideration of the several terms. Some of these factors are treated in Sections 17.2, 17.4, and 18.2.

Retention Parameters. A typical GC chromatogram is a tracing of recorder response (which is a function of solute concentration in the eluate) as a function of time (or distance on the recorder chart paper), as in Fig. 18.1. The *retention time* t_R is the time (in min) required to elute the zone maximum, measured from the time of sample injection. The *flow rate* F_a is the mobile phase flow rate (in ml/min), measured at the column outlet at room temperature. The

* The mole fraction of a solute is the ratio of the number of moles of solute to the total number of moles in the solution.

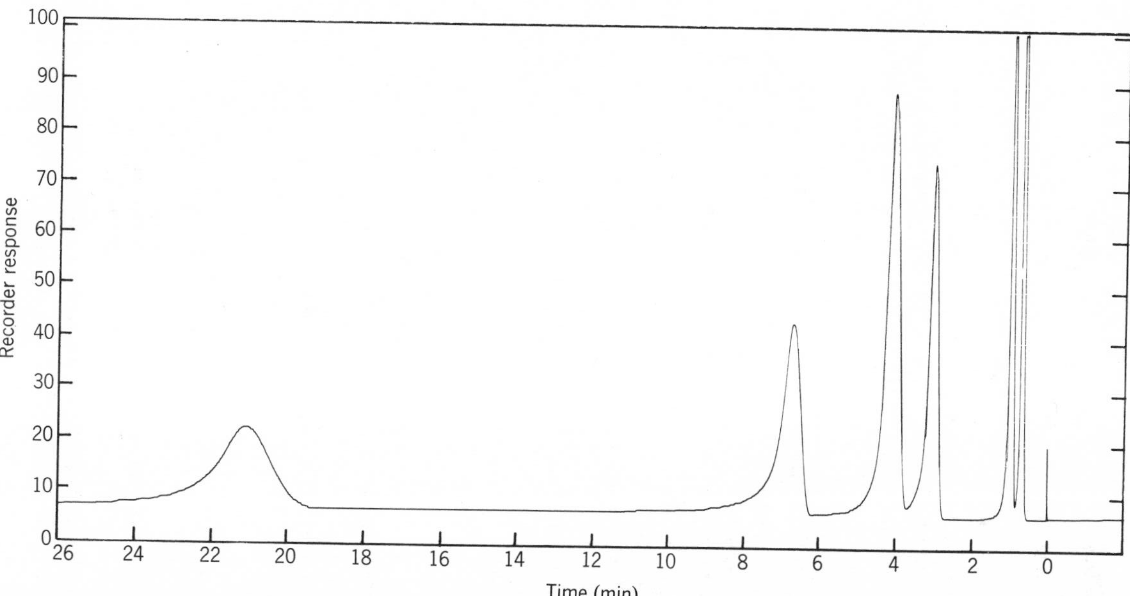

Fig. 18.1. Gas chromatographic separation of a mixture of aldehydes. Peaks in order of elution: isobutyraldehyde, paraldehyde, 2-furaldehyde, benzaldehyde, salicylaldehyde, cinnamaldehyde. Column temperature 200°C, carrier gas flow rate 18 ml/min.

flow rate inside the column, F_c, will differ from F_a if the column temperature T_c differs from the ambient temperature T_a. The relation between these quantities is $F_c = F_a(T_c/T_a)$, where the temperatures are on the absolute temperature scale. Since the correction from F_a to F_c is not universally used, it is best to state clearly if this adjustment has been made.

Eq. 18.5 now gives the *experimental retention volume* V_R:

$$V_R = F_c t_R \tag{18.5}$$

Similarly the mobile phase volume of the column, V_M, is given by $V_M = F_c t_M$, where t_M is the retention time for a substance that is not retained by the column. V_M is sometimes called the dead volume or gas holdup; it is the minimum volume of carrier gas that must be displaced before a solute peak can be eluted.

A significant practical difference between GC and LC is that in the former the mobile phase is compressible. This means that a pressure drop exists through the column, and therefore that the gas flow rate varies along the column. The retention volume must be corrected for this effect. The pressure drop correction factor j is given by

$$j = \frac{3}{2} \cdot \frac{(P_i/P_o)^2 - 1}{(P_i/P_o)^3 - 1} \tag{18.6}$$

where P_i and P_o are the inlet and outlet pressures. Then the *corrected retention volume* $V_R{}^0$ is given by $V_R{}^0 = jV_R$. $V_R{}^0$ is widely used as a measure of solute retention, and since it is related to solute partition coefficient it is helpful for compound identification.* The retention volume is also a function of column parameters, so several related quantities are sometimes used to express retention behavior. The *adjusted retention volume* V_R' is given by $V_R' = V_R - V_M$. Applying the pressure drop correction to V_R' gives the *net retention volume*, $V_N = jV_R'$. All these retention volumes still depend on the amount of stationary phase, so to eliminate this parameter we divide V_N by the weight of stationary phase on the volumn. This is usually done by calculating the *specific retention volume* V_g:

$$V_g = \frac{T_a V_N}{T_c W_S} \tag{18.7}$$

This quantity is not corrected to column temperature. It is common to calibrate the flow meter at 0°C, so that $T_a = 273$°K. Notice that the temperature correction originally applied to F_a has been canceled in calculating V_g, and Eq. 18.7 can be put in the equivalent form $V_g = jF_a(t_R - t_M)/W_s$. V_g is related to K by the flow rate temperature correction.

* With the definition of K from Eq. 18.4, $V_R{}^0 = V_M{}^0 + KW_s$, where W_s is the weight of stationary phase on the column.

The reproducibility of any of these retention parameters depends upon the reproducibility of the chromatographic conditions. In order to eliminate this dependence it is advantageous to work with the *relative retention* r, defined as a ratio of retention volumes such that multiplicative factors cancel. For two solutes A and B chromatographed on the same column, the relative retention r_{AB} is given by

$$r_{AB} = \frac{V_{N,A}}{V_{N,B}} = \frac{V'_{R,A}}{V'_{R,B}} = \frac{V_{g,A}}{V_{g,B}} = \frac{t_{R,A} - t_M}{t_{R,B} - t_M} \tag{18.8}$$

Note that the relative retention is not given by the ratios of V_R or $V_R^{\,0}$, since these contain the additive factor V_M. Relative retentions are often calculated for a series of compounds with one member of the series serving as a standard (the denominator in Eq. 18.8).

18.2 Practice of Gas Chromatography

Instrumentation. Figure 18.2 shows the essential components of a gas chromatograph. A high-pressure source of mobile phase (the carrier gas) and an associated valve to control the pressure are connected to the column, which may be coiled as indicated to accommodate a greater length in a small space. The sample is injected into the gas stream at the sample port. After emerging from the column, the effluent stream passes through the detector, which compares its composition with that of the pure carrier gas and feeds an

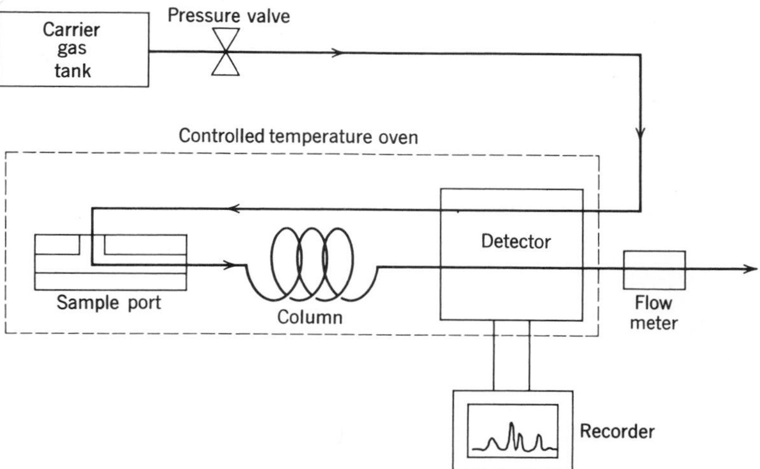

Fig. 18.2. Schematic diagram of a gas chromatograph.

electrical signal proportional to the difference between the eluate and eluent contents to a recorder. The recorder traces out the differential chromatogram; the horizontal axis, representing time, is proportional to the eluate volume if the flow rate is constant. The flow rate of the eluate is measured and the eluate is usually allowed to pass into the atmosphere. In some chromatographs provision is made for collecting the eluate so the sample components can be isolated. The sample port, column, and detector are enclosed in an oven whose temperature can be closely controlled.

The carrier gas, which is chemically inert, usually is nitrogen or helium. The column is constructed of glass or metal tubing, usually $\frac{1}{8}$ or $\frac{1}{4}$ in. in diameter and several feet in length. The stationary phase must be nonvolatile at the temperatures to be used in the separation, and, of course, it must possess suitable selectivity for the mixture to be separated; that is, the partition coefficients of the components must be different.

The sample is injected as a solution. A portion (1–50 μl) is injected into the gas stream with a syringe. It is important that the sample be small and that it be injected as a narrow zone in order to minimize the width of the elution peaks. The injection port is heated so that the sample is immediately vaporized and swept into the column by the carrier gas.

Several kinds of detectors are used. The thermal conductivity (TC) detector is based on the principle that heat is lost from a hot wire situated in a gas at a rate dependent upon the nature of the gas. The wire, immersed in the gas stream, is heated electrically. The resistance of the wire is a function of its temperature, which in turn is a function of the thermal conductivity of the gas. Therefore, by measuring the electrical resistance of the wire, the thermal conductivity of the effluent gas can be measured. As the gas composition is varied from that of pure carrier gas by the elution of a solute, the thermal conductivity varies, and this change can be recorded. In practice it is simpler to measure the difference in thermal conductivity between the effluent stream and the pure carrier gas; for this comparative measurement the carrier gas is diverted through the detector before being fed into the column (see Fig. 18.2).

With the flame ionization detector (FID) the effluent stream is fed into a small hydrogen flame. The solutes in the eluate are burned in the flame, by which process ions are produced. The flame is positioned between two electrodes across which a dc potential is applied. The current carried between these electrodes by the flame is proportional to the concentration of organic compounds in the eluate; the electrical signal is amplified and recorded as with the thermal conductivity cell.

The electron capture detector (ECD) is also based on a gas ionization process, but the carrier gas, rather than the solute, is ionized. The ionization of the carrier gas (N_2) occurs by beta decay of tritium (^3H) or ^{63}Ni, with the formation of electrons. A steady background current is developed. When a solute molecule containing strongly electronegative atoms enters the eluate stream, the electrons are "captured" by the solute, resulting in a decrease of the background current. This change in current is the signal displayed on the chromatogram. The ECD is very responsive to halogen-containing molecules and some other electronegative species, so it finds wide use in pesticide analysis. Other detectors have been developed that are particularly responsive to phosphorus compounds.

The mass spectrometer can serve as a detector on a gas chromatograph. This GC-MS combination provides a powerful means for identifying compounds, the GC ensuring that the compound is separated from closely related species, and the MS giving a unique spectrum of the substance.

Of the detectors described here, TC and MS are universal, in that they will respond to all compounds; the FID will respond to all organic compounds, the ECD only to electronegative molecules or atoms. The TC detector responds to (approximately) microgram amounts of sample, the MS and FID to nanogram quantities, and the ECD to picograms.*

Optimizing Separation Conditions. The analyst seeks acceptable resolution (usually corresponding to the criterion $R_s = 1$) in the minimum time. Theoretical considerations can guide the choice of column parameters. Since the zone velocity $= Rv$, where v is the mobile phase flow velocity, and since column length $L =$ zone velocity $\times\ t_R$,

$$t_R = \frac{L}{vR} = \frac{L}{v}\left(1 + \frac{KW_s}{V_M}\right) \qquad (18.9)$$

The retention time for a solute is directly proportional to column length and inversely proportional to mobile phase flow velocity. Equation 18.9 also shows how t_R is related to the partition coefficient and to the stationary and mobile phase parameters W_s and V_M. Decreasing the amount of stationary phase on the column (the column "loading") will decrease the retention time.

The most important part of the gas chromatograph is the column, which exerts its influence on retention as shown by Eq. 18.9. Two kinds of columns are used in GC: packed columns, analogous to those in LLC, in which the liquid stationary phase is adsorbed to the surface of a solid support; and capillary columns, which have the stationary phase coated on the interior wall of the column itself. Packed columns usually use finely powdered diatomaceous earth as the solid support, with stationary phase loadings of 1–10%. The value of the partition coefficient is determined by the chemical characteristics of the stationary phase. Usually a stationary phase is selected whose polarity is similar to the polarity of the molecules to be separated. This is because an appreciable affinity of the solutes for the stationary phase is

* One nanogram (ng) $= 10^{-9}$ g; one picogram (pg) $= 10^{-12}$ g.

required if selectivity is to be achieved. Column materials are commercially available to meet all ordinary separation requirements.

The primary effects of column temperature are manifested through its effect on the partition coefficient. An increase in temperature will decrease K (see Eq. 18.4) by increasing solute vapor pressure. According to Eq. 18.9 the retention time will thereby decrease. However, resolution will be degraded by a higher temperature, since selectivity can only be achieved as a consequence of differential affinities for the stationary phase, and at higher temperatures the solutes spend less time in the stationary phase. Choice of column temperature is therefore a compromise between speed and resolution. If the resolution, for a given set of conditions, is more than adequate, it is possible to sacrifice some resolution in order to gain speed.

The longer the time a solute spends on a column, the wider the zone will be, for reasons developed in Section 17.2. Figure 18.1 shows this effect. The retention time can be decreased, as discussed above, through the parameters appearing in Eq. 18.9. For a multicomponent mixture, whose separation requires a long period of time, improved results often are achieved by gradually increasing the column temperature during the course of the separation. With this technique of *programmed-temperature* GC the partition coefficients are altered gradually so that the strongly retarded zones are made to elute earlier than they would in isothermal GC. Their retention times are decreased and their peaks are narrowed.

Quantitative Analysis. GC is primarily a method of resolving mixtures of compounds, but the resulting chromatogram also contains information that allows a quantitative determination to be made, and quantitative analysis by GC is now a routine procedure. The key fact is that the area under a peak in the chromatogram is proportional to the amount of solute contained in the eluted zone. A quantitative analysis involves measuring this area and establishing the proportionality.

The peak area can be estimated in several ways. The simplest technique is to measure the peak height, since for a symmetrical peak that can be approximated by a triangle, the height is proportional to the area. This method is fast and precise, but its accuracy is dependent upon the extent to which peak shape remains unchanged as the sample size is changed. Another approach is to estimate the area as the product of peak height and peak width at one-half the peak height; this method also approximates the peak as a triangle. The area under a peak can be measured by carefully cutting the peak out of the chart paper with scissors and weighing the paper; the weight will be proportional to the area of paper if the paper thickness is constant. Some recorders are fitted with mechanical integrators that automatically determine area as the peak is traced on the chromatogram. In automated GC systems the area may be determined by a computer.

By one of these techniques it is possible to measure the area, or a quantity proportional to the area, under a peak on the chromatogram. This quantity must next be converted to the amount, or percentage, of the component in the sample. Three different approaches can be used.

1. Calibration by External Standard. This approach is exactly analogous to the method of establishing a working curve or standard curve in spectroscopy. A series of samples containing varying known amounts of the substance of interest are chromatographed under identical conditions. A plot of peak height or area against sample size will give a linear calibration plot. Then an unknown sample can be analyzed by chromatographing it under the same conditions and reading the amount of component from the calibration plot. The weakness of this method is its requirement that all chromatographic conditions be the same for the standards and the sample.

2. Calibration by Internal Standard. The limitation noted above can be overcome with an internal standard, which is a substance added to the sample. The internal standard must be completely resolved from other sample components, it should have a retention time close to the solute(s) being determined, and it must not be present in the normal sample mixture. The technique is to prepare a standard curve by chromatographing known weight ratios of the standard and the sample component. A plot is made of the ratio A(component)/A(standard) against W(component)/W(standard), where A is peak area and W is weight. Then an unknown sample can be determined by adding a known weight of standard to the sample, chromatographing the mixture, measuring the peak area ratio, and reading the weight ratio from the plot. Since all quantities appear as ratios, the internal standard method compensates for changes in chromatographic conditions as long as they affect the standard and the sample component equally.

3. Area Normalization. Suppose a sample contains components X, Y, and Z, and that the GC detector response is the same for all components, on a molar basis. Then the percentage of component X in the sample is equal to the percentage of total area on the chromatogram due to X, that is,

$$\%X = 100 \times \frac{\text{Area}(X)}{\text{Area}(X) + \text{Area}(Y) + \text{Area}(Z)}$$

If the response factors are different for the several components, corrections must be applied.

Applications. The great sensitivity and specificity of GC are its outstanding characteristics. The separation of members of homologous series is often a routine problem, and many isomeric substances can be separated. Microgram samples suffice for the analysis because of the high sensitivity of the detectors.

In fact, very small samples are especially desirable because they provide narrow zones and thus permit the high resolving power of the method to be fully utilized.

Many thousands of compounds have been chromatographed [3]. Fairly volatile compounds are obvious samples for GC, and these are handled easily. Less obvious applications have been made to high melting solids that are not ordinarily though of as volatile. For many such compounds LC may be an alternative approach, but GC is quite effective. A general approach to the problem of gas chromatographing nonvolatile compounds is to convert them to more volatile derivatives. This involves transforming very polar groups, such as —OH, COOH, and —NH_2, to less polar groups like —OCOR and —NHCOR. For example, the naturally occurring amino acids, which cannot themselves be gas chromatographed, can be separated as their *N*-trifluoroacetyl methyl esters:

$$\underset{\displaystyle NH_2}{R\text{—}\overset{}{CH}\text{—}COOH} \xrightarrow[HCl]{MeOH} \underset{\displaystyle NH_2}{R\text{—}CH\text{—}COOCH_3} \xrightarrow{(F_3CCO)_2O} \underset{\displaystyle NHCOCF_3}{R\text{—}CH\text{—}COOCH_3} \qquad (18.10)$$

Another important derivative in GC is the silyl derivative, silyl referring to the trimethylsilyl group, $(CH_3)_3Si$—. The active hydrogen of —OH, COOH, —NH_2, —SH, etc., can be replaced by the silyl group to give more volatile derivatives. Several silylating agents are used; all of them have the general formula $(CH_3)_3Si$—X, where X is a good leaving group. Equation 18.11 shows the formation of a silyl ether from a hydroxy compound.

$$R\text{—}OH + (CH_3)_3Si\text{—}Cl \xrightarrow{-HCl} R\text{—}OSi(CH_3)_3 \qquad (18.11)$$

Figure 18.3 shows the GC separation of several high-melting anticonvulsants as their dimethyl derivatives, formed by a technique in which the reaction is carried out on the GC column. After emergence of the solvent and reagent, the first two peaks are breakdown products of phenobarbital. The next major peaks in order are phenobarbital, alphenal, primadone, diphenylhydantoin, and *p*-methyl diphenylhydantoin.

Experiment 18.1. Gas Chromatographic Determination of Alcohol

APPARATUS

Gas Chromatograph. Any gas chromatograph should be satisfactory, since the conditions required are very moderate. Inexpensive chromatographs with thermal conductivity detection are available.

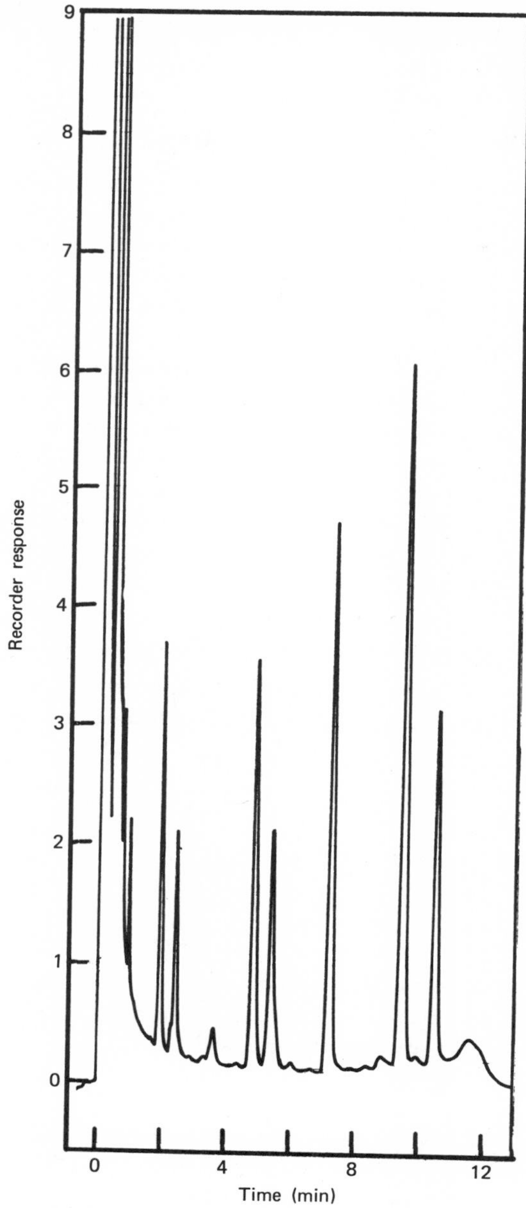

Fig. 18.3. Programmed-temperature GC separation of some dimethylated anticonvulsant drugs. Column: 3% OV 17 on chromosorb W, 6 ft glass, $\frac{1}{8}$ in. i.d.; temperature, 125–275°C at 8°/min; carrier, N_2 at 40 ml/min; FID.

Column. A satisfactory column is $\frac{1}{8}$ in. o.d., 5 ft long, 8% Carbowax on 90-100 mesh Anakrom ABS.

Syringe. Capable of injecting 5–10 μl; the Hamilton 701-N is satisfactory.

PROCEDURE

Preparation of Standard Curve. Prepare a series of aqueous solutions of ethanol to contain 5–15% (v/v) of ethanol. Inject 5 μl samples into the gas chromatograph, record the chromatograms, calculate peak area, and make a plot of peak area against alcohol concentration. The area can be calculated as the product of peak height and peak width at one-half the peak height.

Appropriate conditions are carrier gas (helium) flow rate, 60 ml/min; injector port temperature, 150°C; column temperature, 100°C.

Analysis of an Elixir. Inject a 5 μl sample of acetaminophen elixir, using the same conditions as for the preparation of the standard curve. Calculate the peak area and determine the alcohol content of the elixir by means of the standard curve.

This procedure can be used to determine the alcohol in other elixirs also. The internal standard technique, using acetone as the standard, can be used instead of the working curve method.

Experiment 18.2. Gas Chromatographic Determination of Glutethimide

Glutethimide, **1**, is a sedative drug whose concentration in blood or urine can be determined by GC. In this experiment aqueous solutions of gluteth-

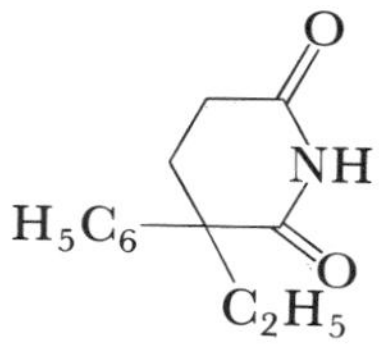

O
NH
H_5C_6
O
C_2H_5

1

imide are analyzed; the initial extraction of the drug with dichloromethane is somewhat more involved when plasma is extracted [4]. *p*-Dimethylaminobenzaldehyde is used as an internal standard.

APPARATUS

Gas Chromatograph. A chromatograph equipped with a flame ionization detector is necessary.

Column. A $\frac{1}{4}$ in. o.d., 6 ft column packed with 3% OV-225 on Chromosorb W is conditioned at 250°C for 72 h and silylated with periodic injections of Silyl 8 (Pierce Chemical Co). Nitrogen is the carrier gas. After heavy use the column is reconditioned overnight and resilylated.

PROCEDURES

Preparation of Standard Curve. Prepare a series of solutions in dichloromethane to contain 25–200 μg/ml of glutethimide, each solution also containing 100 μg/ml of *p*-dimethylaminobenzaldehyde. Inject 1 μl of each solution into the gas chromatograph. Measure the peak height ratios (glutethimide/internal standard) and make a plot of peak height ratio against the ratio weight of glutethimide/weight of standard.

The chromatographic conditions are: carrier gas flow rate, 40 ml/min; column temperature, 200°C; detector and injector temperature, 250°C. The retention times of the standard and the glutethimide are 2 and 5 min, respectively.

Analysis of Glutethimide Sample. Obtain an aqueous solution of glutethimide from your instructor. Pipet 1.0 ml of this solution into a separatory funnel or a glass-stoppered test tube. Add 5.0 ml of dichloromethane and extract the glutethimide. Pipet 2.0 ml of the dichloromethane layer into a test tube, add 0.1 ml of a stock solution of *p*-dimethylaminobenzaldehyde (100 μg/ml in dichloromethane), and evaporate the solvent under a gentle stream of dry nitrogen in a hood. Dissolve the residue in 10–15 drops of dichloromethane and inject 1–2 μl of this solution into the gas chromatograph.

Calculate the peak height ratio and determine the ratio weight of glutethimide/weight of standard from the standard curve. This quantity refers to the ratio for the dichloromethane extract. Calculate the weight of glutethimide (per ml) in this extract by multiplying by the weight of standard (per ml), since

$$\text{weight ratio} = \frac{\mu\text{g glutethimide/ml}}{\mu\text{g standard/ml}}$$

In this experiment the extract contained 5.0 μg/ml of standard. The original concentration of glutethimide in the aqueous sample was five times its concentration in the extract, because 1.0 ml of sample was extracted with 5.0 ml of dichloromethane.

References

1. Martin, A. J. P. and R. L. M. Synge, *Biochem. J.*, **35,** 1358 (1941).
2. James, A. J. and A. J. P. Martin, *Biochem. J.*, **50,** 679 (1952).
3. Zweig, G. and J. Sherma (eds.), *Handbook of Chromatography*, Vols. I, II, CRC Press, Cleveland, Ohio, 1972.
4. Cohen, J. L. and R. T. Koda, *J. Chem. Educ.*, **51,** 133 (1974).

FOR FURTHER READING

Clarke, E. G. C. (ed.), *Isolation and Identification of Drugs*, The Pharmaceutical Press, London, 1969.

Littlewood, A. B., *Gas Chromatography*, 2nd ed., Academic Press, New York, 1970.
Martin, A. J. P., "Historical Background," in *Gas Chromatography in Biology and Medicine*, R. Porter (ed.), J. and A. Churchill, London, 1969, pp. 2–10.
Giddings, J. C., *Dynamics of Chromatography*, Part I, Marcel Dekker, New York, 1965.
Heftmann, E. (ed.), *Chromatography*, 2nd ed., Reinhold Publishing, New York, 1967.
McNair, H. M. and E. J. Bonelli, *Basic Gas Chromatography*, 5th ed., Varian Corp., Walnut Creek, Calif., 1969.

Problems

1. Calculate the resolution of 2-furaldehyde and benzaldehyde in Fig. 18.1.
2. Show how α and $(\alpha - 1)/\alpha$ can be determined for a pair of solutes with retention times t_A and t_B, if the gas holdup is t_M.
3. The relative retentions of codeine, heroin, methadone, morphine, and propoxyphene are 1.00, 1.89, 0.55, 1.16, and 5.9, respectively, and t_R is 6.00 min for codeine on a 2% SE-30 column at 215°C. Calculate the retention times for the other compounds.
4. Calculate the number of plates from the elution peak for cinnamaldehyde in Fig. 18.1.
5. Estimate the retention times of the solutes in Fig. 18.1. Look up their boiling points and make a plot of bp against log t_R. Predict the retention time of *m*-anisaldehyde on this column.

Summary: Part Three

The unifying concept through the last three chapters has been the description of solute distribution between two phases as an equilibrium:

$$\text{Solute in phase 1} \rightleftharpoons \text{Solute in phase 2}$$

The equilibrium constant characterizing this reaction has been called a partition coefficient or distribution coefficient.

Because of the operation of this equilibrium, any *batch* process (exemplified by simple solvent extraction) is not a very efficient means of separation. Another example of a batch treatment would be the addition of a quantity of a cation exchange resin in the H^+ form to a solution of sodium chloride with the purpose of exchanging all the solution counterions. This is evidently impossible, because the selectivity of Na^+ for the resin is not sufficiently greater than that of H^+; at equilibrium, therefore, an appreciable concentration of sodium ion will remain in solution. This is the limitation of every batch process. As noted in Chapter 16, the batch treatment must be repeated to achieve quantitative displacement of the solute from one phase to the other, and this is an inefficient use of resources.

The inefficiency of multiple batch processes is overcome by manipulating the phase contacting techniques to produce a *cascade* process. Countercurrent distribution is a perfect example of a cascade process. This discontinuous cascade method was then refined into a continuous cascade, chromatography, with extremely efficient use being made of the fundamental distribution equilibrium. The success of cascade processes is based on an experimental arrangement that permits the migration of all components in the direction of flow of the developer fluid. The components migrate at rates determined by the equilibrium constants of their distribution equilibria, and, if these constants differ appreciably, the components can be separated.

The separation techniques described in Chapters 16–18 are not the only ones of importance, and a few more methods will be briefly outlined.

Distillation. The resolution of mixtures of volatile liquids by distillation is not widely employed as an analytical procedure, but distillation is of great utility as a purification technique. Briefly, separation by distillation is based on the difference in composition of a liquid mixture and its vapor phase in equilibrium with it. For a two component mixture, the vapor will contain a larger fraction of the more volatile component than does the liquid. If, therefore, the vapor is collected and condensed, it yields a mixture enriched in the more volatile component. If the treatment is repeated many times, by each time vaporizing the condensate of the preceding stage, eventually an essentially pure sample of the more volatile component will be recovered. Each equilibrium stage in this multistep distillation is called a theoretical plate.

This cumbersome operation is simplified considerably by passing the vapor through a column designed to provide a large degree of contact between the rising vapors and the condensate produced from the vapor throughout the length of the column. Thus the separate liquid-vapor equilibria of the preceding paragraph are incorporated into a continuous column, with a plate being considered a portion of the column in which the change in liquid composition is the same as the change produced by one stage in the discontinuous, true-equilibrium process. The length of column corresponding to the plate is the height equivalent to a theoretical plate, which is a term already familiar from chromatographic theory (Chapter 17). In fact, Martin and Synge accounted for the behavior of their partition columns by borrowing and adapting the plate concept of fractional distillation. Typical fractional distillation columns provide a large surface area for vapor-liquid contact by means of internal spurs in the glass column (Vigreux column) or with a packing of small, shaped pieces of inert material. The column packings may be hollow cylinders, rings, helices, saddles, or beads. These columns may contain 10–40 plates/m of column length.

Purification of solvents is nearly always accomplished by distillation. If the atmospheric boiling point is fairly high, it is advisable to carry out the distillation under reduced pressure, because this decreases the boiling temperature and therefore reduces the extent of decomposition during the heating necessary to vaporize the liquid.

Distillation is analytically important in a few instances. The Kjeldahl method for nitrogen (Chapter 19) can be carried out with a quantitative distillation of ammonia from a solution of nonvolatile alkali. Fractional distillation has been an important method of analysis of petroleum fractions, but gas-liquid chromatography is replacing distillation in this analysis.

A form of distillation that is of some importance in clinical analysis is *microdiffusion analysis*, in which a volatile substance passes from a solution in which its vapor pressure is appreciable to another in which its pressure is negligible, the diffusional transfer taking place through the intervening air. The technique, which is very simple in practice, can be illustrated with the analysis of ammonia. A small aliquot (ca. 1 ml) of the acidic aqueous ammonia solution is placed in a small vessel contained in a vaportight chamber. Into a second vessel in the chamber is pipetted 1 ml of standard hydrochloric acid. Then the ammonia solution is made basic with potassium carbonate. The free ammonia diffuses from the basic solution into the acidic solution. After the "distillation" is complete, the excess HCl is back-titrated with standard alkali. Microdiffusion analysis is applicable to very small-scale quantitative determinations.

Sublimation is another distillation process. Some solids vaporize without first passing into the liquid state; this direct vaporization of a solid is sublimation. A few solids can be readily purified by sublimation; the technique is not used as a quantitative method, however.

Dialysis. Dialysis is a separation method based on the molecular sieve properties of membranes. In a typical application of the method, a solution containing two solutes of greatly different molecular size is segregated from a pure water phase by a membrane permeable to the smaller molecule but impermeable to the larger one. Under the influence of the concentration gradient between the phases, the smaller solute diffuses through the membrane until its concentration becomes nearly equal in the diffusate (the solution into which the solute is diffusing) and the dialyzate (the original solution). If the diffusate is replaced periodically with pure water, eventually a complete separation of the two solutes will be achieved. This technique is used to desalt protein solutions, although for this purpose it is being replaced by gel filtration.

Dialysis can be practiced as a batch process, as just described, or it can be turned into a continuous method by conducting the dialyzate and the diffusate past the membrane in a continuous manner.

Membranes suitable for dialysis separations have been made of cellophane and nitrocellulose. The average pore diameter of the membrane determines its applicability for a given separation. Nitrocellulose membranes can be prepared with a variety of pore sizes. Each membrane is actually characterized by a pore size distribution, rather than pores of only one diameter, and this distribution of sizes is a limiting factor on the ability of dialysis membranes to separate molecules of slightly different sizes.

Precipitation. The student of inorganic analysis is familiar with separations by precipitation as they are utilized in classical gravimetric analysis. Chloride ion, for example, can be quantitatively removed from solution by adding an excess of silver nitrate, leading to the formation of the insoluble silver chloride. The description of solubility behavior of slightly soluble salts was reviewed in Chapter 3.

The conventional manner of forming a precipitate is to add a solution of the precipitating reagent to the sample solution. This technique produces local excesses of reagent, often leading to precipitates that are voluminous and hard to handle, and may even cause entrainment of soluble components in the crystals of precipitate (this is called coprecipitation). A superior precipitate is formed if the precipitating agent can be slowly generated within the solution rather than added all at once. This technique, which is called homogeneous precipitation, can be illustrated by the precipitation of metal oxides by raising the solution pH. This is accomplished homogeneously by adding urea to the solution and heating to cause hydrolysis of the urea.

$$H_2NCONH_2 + H_2O \rightarrow CO_2 + 2NH_3$$

The ammonia released increases the hydroxide concentration by the acid-base reaction $NH_3 + H_2O \rightleftharpoons NH_4 + OH^-$, causing the controlled precipitation of the metal oxide.

Among the most valuable precipitating agents are the organic precipitants, some of which are highly specific. An important precipitant, which forms insoluble chelates with nearly all metal ions, is 8-hydroxyquinoline (oxine).

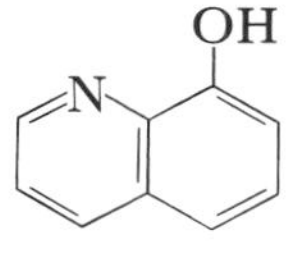

The pH of the medium is important in controlling the precipitation of oxinates, and proper selection of pH permits some selectivity of precipitating action. A more specific agent is sodium tetraphenylboron, $Na(C_6H_5)_4B$, which precipitates potassium ion in a form suitable for gravimetric determination. This precipitant also forms precipitates with protonated amines.

Dimethylglyoxime,

$$\begin{array}{l} CH_3\text{—}C\text{=}NOH \\ \qquad\;\; | \\ CH_3\text{—}C\text{=}NOH \end{array}$$

is extremely specific, forming an insoluble chelate with nickel but, under suitable conditions, with no other metals.

Organic compounds may be isolated from mixtures as insoluble compounds or complexes. As with inorganics, the precipitate may be dried and weighed, or it may be converted to another form for analysis. Some precipitating agents form colored precipitates that can be isolated and then dissolved in an organic solvent for colorimetric analysis. A widely applicable precipitant of amines is ammonium tetrathiocyanodiammonochromate, $NH_4Cr(NH_3)_2(SCN)_4 \cdot H_2O$, which is known as Reinecke's salt. The precipitate formed by reaction between Reinecke's salt and an amine is called a reineckate. Many alkaloids can be determined gravimetrically or colorimetrically as their reineckates.

Part Four: Elemental Analysis

Since every pure chemical substance is composed of one or more elements, with the proportion of each element having a definite value in each compound, evidently any substance can be quantitatively measured in terms of its elemental composition. For example, urea, NH_2CONH_2, contains 20.00% carbon, 6.71% hydrogen, and 46.65% nitrogen. If a sample is known to contain no nitrogen-containing compound other than urea, it can be analyzed for its nitrogen content, and its urea content then can be calculated directly. This is an example of *elemental analysis* (also called ultimate analysis). The great generality of elemental analysis is apparent in the first sentence of this paragraph. A corollary is that elemental analysis is relatively nonspecific. In the example just given, for instance, it is most unlikely that the impurity in an impure urea sample could be assumed to be devoid of nitrogen. Nevertheless, elemental analysis is an indispensable tool in many phases of analytical and organic chemistry. Some of its uses are described in Part Four.

Much of the elemental analysis being carried out today is conducted on a purely routine basis as a support activity for organic chemists; this pertains particularly to carbon, hydrogen, and nitrogen analyses. During the early part of this century elemental analysis was systematized and microscale techniques were developed, largely by Pregl and Emich. These methods are used to determine the elemental composition of new compounds.

Although more than 100 elements are known, the analysis of only a few of these is of broad pharmaceutical concern. Chapters 19 and 20 treat some of these elements.

19 NONMETALS

19.1 Carbon and Hydrogen

These elements are always determined simultaneously. The sample is subjected to total oxidation, all of its carbon and hydrogen being converted into carbon dioxide and water, respectively. From the weights of CO_2 and H_2O the percentages of C and H in the sample are calculated [1].

These analyses are carried out routinely on a microscale with a few milligrams of sample. A microbalance capable of weighing to 10^{-6} g is essential. The apparatus with which the combustion is conducted consists essentially of a combustion tube to contain the sample and appropriate catalysts, a furnace to heat the combustion tube, a source of oxygen with suitable pressure-controlling equipment, and absorption tubes to trap the water and carbon dioxide.

The combustion tube contains silver, platinum, copper oxide and lead chromate, and lead peroxide. The sample is heated in the presence of these substances in a stream of oxygen. The silver removes halogens and sulfur oxides from the vaporized sample. The platinum aids in the complete combustion of some resistant compounds. The copper oxide-lead chromate mixture is an oxidizing agent. The lead peroxide removes oxides of nitrogen from the vapor. As the combusted vapors, consisting of CO_2 and H_2O, leave the combustion tube, they are passed into an absorption tube of magnesium perchlorate (Dehydrite), which removes all of the water. The vapors then pass into a tube of sodium hydroxide absorbed on asbestos (Ascarite), which removes all of the carbon dioxide. The absorption tubes are weighed before and after the combustion, thus providing the weights of CO_2 and H_2O produced by the sample.

The success of the carbon-hydrogen microanalysis is dependent upon close attention to details of execution. The acceptable accuracy of the method is $\pm 0.3\%$ (absolute) of the theoretical percentages of C and H.

19.2 Nitrogen

The Dumas Method. This method is based on the quantitative conversion of organically bound nitrogen to nitrogen gas when heated in the presence of copper and cupric oxide as catalysts [2]. The cupric oxide catalyzes the breakdown of the organic sample to nitrogen and nitrogen oxides. In the presence of copper the nitrogen oxides are reduced to nitrogen. The overall reactions are

$$\text{Organic N} \xrightarrow{\text{CuO}} CO_2 + H_2O + N_2 + \text{N oxides}$$

$$\text{N oxides} \xrightarrow{\text{Cu}} N_2$$

The reaction is conducted at about 700°C in a tube containing the catalysts and the weighed sample. An atmosphere of carbon dioxide is maintained during the reaction, and when the combustion is complete the nitrogen gas is swept from the tube with a stream of CO_2. The combined gases are passed through a 50% potassium hydroxide solution, which removes all of the CO_2. The volume of the pure nitrogen gas is measured in a gas microburet (called a nitrometer or azotometer). With the volume, pressure, and temperature of the nitrogen known, its weight and therefore the percent of nitrogen in the sample can be calculated.

The Dumas method is applicable to most types of organic compounds, but some substances may give low results; pyrimidines, sulfonamides, and semicarbazides do not release stoichiometric amounts of N_2 with the conventional treatment. Compounds with *N*-methyl groups may yield low results. Usually quantitative recoveries are achieved if copper acetate and potassium chlorate are added to the combustion mixture.

Nitrogen analysis by the Dumas procedure is routinely carried out on the micro scale, with enough sample being taken to produce 0.3–0.4 ml of nitrogen gas.

The Kjeldahl Method. In 1883 Kjeldahl introduced the analytical method for organically bound nitrogen that bears his name.* The technique involves digestion of the compound in sulfuric acid, each nitrogen atom in the original molecule producing one molecule of ammonia. The ammonia is then analyzed in any convenient way. Many variations of the method have been suggested to reduce the digestion time, to extend the applicability of the technique to difficultly decomposed compounds, and to simplify the final analytical step [3]. Some of these points will be considered briefly.

Potassium sulfate is commonly added to the sulfuric acid digestion mixture in order to raise the boiling point and therefore to reduce the digestion time. It has been found that if the ratio of salt to acid is too high the excessive temperature attained may result in a loss of ammonia. Baker [4], who has studied some of the reaction variables, suggests that the optimum salt concentration is 1.0–1.5 g of potassium sulfate per milliliter of sulfuric acid. The boiling point of such a solution is in the range 365–388°C.

* The *j* is silent.

The action of a catalyst is required to achieve quantitative decomposition of most organic compounds in a reasonable time. The salts of many metals, especially of mercury, selenium, and copper, have been used for this purpose. Although many of these catalysts are satisfactory, it seems that none is superior to mercury [4], which is usually used as the oxide or sulfate.

Early in the digestion of many substances the mixture discolors, in some cases charring to a dark brown. Frothing may occur. As the heating is continued, the color will disappear, the solution finally becoming colorless; this is known as "clearing." It has been demonstrated that clearing, which is presumably a sign of the conversion of the carbonaceous material into carbon dioxide or other small molecules, does not necessarily coincide with complete conversion of the nitrogen into ammonia. It is therefore necessary, in general, to prolong the digestion beyond the clearing point. Very easily decomposed substances, such as unsubstituted amides, may quantitatively release all of their nitrogen even before clearing has occurred.

The Kjeldahl procedure is suitable for the quantitative determination of nitrogen in relatively labile compounds such as amides and amines. Azo compounds, some heterocyclic rings, and nitroso and nitro groups are often found to be resistant to complete decomposition under Kjeldahl conditions. Special treatment (for example, preliminary reduction of nitro groups) often enables these refractory substances to be analyzed.

After the Kjeldahl digestion is complete, the ammonia must be analyzed. The digestion mixture contains sulfuric acid, potassium sulfate, a catalyst, and ammonium sulfate. Some methods of ammonia analysis can be carried out directly on this mixture, whereas others require separation of the ammonia from the other components.

In the conventional Kjeldahl procedure the digestion is followed by neutralization of the sulfuric acid with sodium hydroxide. This frees the ammonia, which is removed from the mixture by steam distillation. In steam distillation the solution to be distilled is not subjected to direct heat; instead an externally generated current of steam is fed into the solution. The steam then passes out of the solution, carrying with it the volatile ammonia, and is condensed and collected as in any distillation. The distillate from the Kjeldahl mixture is received in a known volume of standard hydrochloric acid solution. The excess acid is back-titrated with standard alkali to give a measure of the ammonia content. For each ammonia molecule found in the distillate, one nitrogen atom was present in the sample. A variation of this method uses a solution of boric acid to receive the ammonia from the steam distillation; the concentration of boric acid need not be known. The ammonia is fixed in solution as ammonium borate, which can be titrated directly as a base with a standard HCl solution; this titration is a displacement of the weak acid boric by the strong acid HCl. The advantage of the boric acid procedure over the method described in the preceding paragraph is its use of only one instead of two standard solutions. Typical Kjeldahl procedures with steam distillation of the ammonia, followed by acid-base titration, are described in detail in the *United States Pharmacopeia* and the *National Formulary*.

Ammonia produced in the Kjeldahl digestion on a microscale may be recovered from the digestion mixture by microdiffusion (see p. 430) and then analyzed by acid-base titration or by colorimetry as described subsequently.

For very low concentrations of ammonia, as are obtained by steam distillation of small samples, the final analysis may be made more accurately by colorimetry than by titration. The most important colorimetric analysis of ammonia involves the formation of a yellow to brownish colloidal dispersion upon reaction with Nessler's reagent, which is an alkaline solution of potassium mercuric iodide. Standard solutions of ammonia are subjected to the same reagent, and the absorbance, at about 410 nm, of the unknown is compared with the standards.

Another colorimetric assay for ammonia, which is very sensitive, utilizes a phenol-sodium hypochlorite reagent. In alkaline solution ammonia produces a blue color with this reagent, with the absorbance being proportional to the ammonia concentration.

It is possible to eliminate the distillation step and to determine the ammonia directly in the digestion mixture. Evidently an acid-base titration is not feasible because of the overwhelming excess of sulfuric acid in the mixture. Redox titrations have been applied, however, and the most successful of these involves titration of the ammonia with hypobromite [5, 6]. The ammonia is quantitatively oxidized, in basic medium, according to

$$2NH_3 + 3OBr^- \rightarrow N_2 + 3H_2O + 3Br^- \qquad (19.1)$$

Since hypobromite solutions are not very stable, it is convenient to employ a standard solution of sodium or calcium hypochlorite [7], and to generate hypobromite in situ by incorporating an excess of bromide ion in the titration solution.

$$OCl + Br^- \rightarrow OBr^- + Cl^-$$

Because reaction 19.1 is a relatively slow reaction, it is not feasible to titrate ammonia directly to the end point with hypochlorite. Instead, an excess of hypochlorite is added and time is allowed for the reaction to occur. Then an excess of standard arsenious oxide solution is added, and the titration is completed with hypochlorite; this end point can be detected visually. The final reaction is

$$2OBr^- + As_2O_3 \rightarrow As_2O_5 + 2Br^- \qquad (19.2)$$

The entire titration can be shown diagrammatically as follows, where the lengths of the lines represent numbers of milliequivalents.

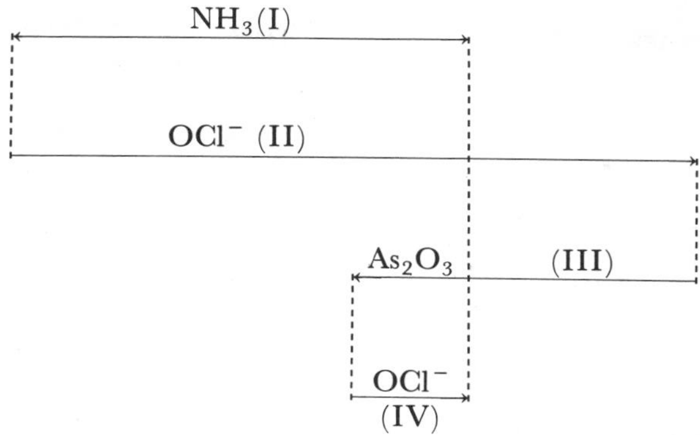

Evidently (I) = (II) + (IV) − (III). In practice it is necessary to carry out a blank determination with the same reagents, the blank titration volume being subtracted from the sample volume.

This titration is used in the Kjeldahl determination described in Experiment 19.1. Tartrazine is employed as the visual indicator [6]. Although the color change is from yellow to colorless, it is quite sharp. The arsenite-hypochlorite titration must be carried out in mildly alkaline solution, and bicarbonate is used to control the pH.

A modification of this titration involves addition of an excess of hypochlorite, as above; after oxidation of the ammonia is complete, potassium iodide is added. The liberated iodine is titrated with standard thiosulfate to give a measure of the excess hypochlorite.

EXAMPLE 19.1. Calculate the weight of nitrogen equivalent to each ml of 0.0500 *N* hypochlorite consumed in the determination of ammonia by the hypochlorite-arsenite method.

According to reaction 19.2, 2 moles of OBr^- (and therefore of OCl^-) are equivalent to 1 mole of As_2O_3. Since the equivalent weight of As_2O_3 is equal to one-fourth its molecular weight, then for hypochlorite EW = MW/2. From reaction 19.1, 6 equivalents (3 moles) of OBr^- react with 2 moles (6 equivalents) of ammonia; thus for ammonia EW = MW/3. Therefore 1 equivalent of NH_3 is 5.68 g, which corresponds to 4.67 g of nitrogen. One milliliter of 0.05 *N* NaOCl therefore corresponds to 0.05 meq or 0.2335 mg of nitrogen.

19.3 The Halogens

Analysis of the halide content of halide and hydrohalide salts provides a rapid indication of purity. The method is, of course, not very specific. For example, it is inadvisable to analyze ephedrine hydrochloride merely by titrating the chloride with silver nitrate, because the sample may contain another chloride salt. When analysis of halide salts is desirable, the halide usually can be released for analysis simply by dissolving the salt in water or acid.

Halogen-containing organics in which the halogen atom is covalently bonded to the organic structure require more drastic treatment to release the halogen for analysis. In the Carius method the halogen compound is sealed in a combustion tube with silver nitrate and nitric acid and the tube is heated for several hours. The organic material is decomposed according to the reactions

$$\text{Organic X} \rightarrow H_2O + CO_2 + X_2$$
$$X_2 \xrightarrow{AgNO_3} 2AgX$$

The tube is opened and the insoluble silver halide is weighed.

Another method utilizes fusion of the sample with sodium peroxide in a heavy-walled container called a Parr bomb. Halogens are converted into their sodium salts, which can be analyzed by conventional methods.

The Schöniger oxygen-flask combustion technique is a simple and rapid method for halogen analysis. The organic compound is wrapped in filter paper and clamped in platinum gauze. The assembly is lighted and immediately placed in a closed flask filled with oxygen. After the combustion is complete the gases are absorbed in a suitable liquid, and this solution is analyzed.

The organically bound halogen having been transformed into halide ion, it is usually determined by precipitation titration with silver nitrate. The end point can be detected visually (see Chapter 3), potentiometrically (Chapter 6), or amperometrically (Chapter 7). If the sample contains more than one of the halogens chlorine, bromine, and iodine, the mixture can be titrated amperometrically, or the anions can be separated by ion-exchange chromatography prior to analysis. Gravimetric determination of halides as their silver salts, though more time-consuming than titration, is capable of greater accuracy.

Sulfur and phosphorus can also be determined by the Carius, Schöniger, and Parr methods, the sulfur and phosphorus being converted to sodium sulfate and sodium phosphate, respectively. Sulfate is determined by titration with barium ion. Phosphate can be determined gravimetrically as the insoluble ammonium phosphomolybdate.

Experiment 19.1. Kjeldahl Determination of Nitrogen without Distillation [8]

INTRODUCTION

The digestion conditions employed in this experiment have been selected in accordance with the studies of Baker [4]. The ammonia analysis is the hypochlorite-arsenite titration described earlier.

Most nitrogen-containing organic compounds are suitable samples for this analysis. Amines, amides, carbamates, and many heterocyclics are determinable. Suggested samples are urea, acetamide, caffeine, and urethane.

REAGENTS

0.05 N Arsenious Oxide. Dissolve exactly 1.2363 g of dried primary standard As_2O_3 in 10–20 ml of 1 *N* sodium hydroxide. Add 1 *N* hydrochloric acid or sulfuric acid until the solution is neutral or slightly acid. Then dilute to exactly 500.0 ml with distilled water.

0.01 N As_2O_3. Pipet 20.0 ml of 0.05 *N* As_2O_3 into a 100 ml volumetric flask and dilute to volume with water.

Tartrazine Indicator. Prepare a 0.05% aqueous solution of tartrazine (Colour Index No. 19,140, 2nd ed.).

0.05N Sodium Hypochlorite. Dilute 40 ml of 5.25% sodium hypochlorite (Clorox or a similar bleach) to 1 liter with water. Standardize this solution as follows: pipet 20.0 ml of 0.05*N* As_2O_3 into an Erlenmeyer flask. Add about 1 g each of sodium bicarbonate and potassium bromide and 5 drops of tartrazine indicator solution. Titrate from a 25 ml buret with the 0.05 *N* NaOCl until the indicator color begins to fade. Add 5 more drops of tartrazine and titrate to the end point (marked by the yellow to colorless transition), which is sharp. (Shortly beyond the end point the solution turns yellow again due to the excess hypobromite, but with ordinary care this should cause no confusion.) Perform a blank titration and subtract the blank volume from the standardization volume.

Store the standard hypochlorite solution in a dark bottle or otherwise protect it from light [8].

PROCEDURES

Sample Size. If a 25 ml buret is to be used in the titration, for optimum results take a sample containing 4–5 mg of nitrogen. Thus if the compound contains 5% N, take about 80 mg; 10% N, 40 mg; 15% N, 30 mg; 20% N, 20 mg; etc.

Digestion. Accurately weigh the sample into a 30 ml Kjeldahl flask. Add 50–100 mg of yellow mercuric oxide, 4 g of potassium sulfate, and 3 ml of concentrated sulfuric acid. Try to wet all of the organic compound with the acid so that none of it will be volatilized in the heating process.

Clamp the flask in a slanting position (pointing away from you!) in a hood. Heat the flask with an open flame, heating gently until the solids go into solution. Then heat more vigorously, maintaining a gentle boiling state; try to avoid loss of white fumes from the flask. The solution may discolor; continue heating until clearing occurs. Labile compounds such as unsubstituted amides and ureas will be decomposed at this point; other compounds require an additional 10–15 min of digestion. Heating should be continued at least until the rapid evolution of bubbles characteristic of the initial phases of digestion has ceased.

Excessive application of heat will cause loss of ammonia, probably by driving off sulfuric acid and thus raising the boiling point. If the solution, after clearing, develops a pale yellow color, it probably has been heated too severely, and ammonia has been lost.

Carry out a blank determination in exactly the same way, omitting only the sample.

Allow the solution to cool for a few minutes. Carefully run some distilled water into the flask to dilute the solution and prevent it from forming a solid cake. If a cake does form, add water and use heat to dissolve it. Quantitatively transfer the contents of the flask, with the aid of water, to a 250 ml Erlenmeyer flask. The solution should be perfectly clear at this point.

Titration. Carefully neutralize the sulfuric acid with solid sodium bircarbonate. Near the neutralization point yellow mercuric oxide may be visible, and when neutralization is complete effervescence will no longer occur. Add about 1 g of $NaHCO_3$ in excess. Add about 2 g of potassium bromide and wash down the sides of the flask with water.

Titrate with standard 0.05 N NaOCl until a small excess (0.5–1 ml) of titrant has been added, as indicated by a permanent greenish-yellow color. Allow the solution to stand 3–5 min. Pipet exactly 10.0 ml of 0.01 N As_2O_3 into the solution. Add 5 drops of tartrazine and continue titrating with NaOCl until the indicator color begins to fade. Add 5 more drops of indicator and titrate to the end point. Carry out the titration of the blank in exactly the same way.

Calculation. Convert the total volume of standard NaOCl used in the sample titration to the equivalent volume of 0.0500 N NaOCl. Similarly convert the blank volume. Subtract the blank volume of 0.05 N NaOCl from the sample volume of 0.05 N NaOCl. The remainder represents sodium hypochlorite consumed in the titration of the sample. Each ml of 0.0500 N NaOCl is equivalent to 0.2335 mg of nitrogen (see Example 19.1). Calculate the percent of nitrogen in the sample compound, and compare your result with the theoretical value.

Unknown Sample. Obtain a pure sample of a nitrogen-containing organic compound from your instructor, who will tell you its approximate percentage of nitrogen. Determine the nitrogen content of your sample compound by the Kjeldahl method.

References

1. Ingram, B. and M. Lonsdale, *Treatise on Analytical Chemistry*, I. M. Kolthoff and P. J. Elving (eds.) Part II, Vol. II, Wiley-Interscience, New York, 1965, p. 297.

2. Gustin, G. M., *ibid.*, p. 408.
3. Ogg, C. L., *ibid.*, p. 457.
4. Baker, P. R. W., *Talanta*, **8,** 57 (1961).
5. Belcher, R. and M. K. Bhatty, *Mikrochim. Acta*, **1956,** 1183.
6. Belcher, R., *Anal. Chim. Acta*, **4,** 468 (1950).
7. Kolthoff, I. M. and V. A. Stenger, *Ind. Eng. Chem. Anal. Ed.*, **7,** 79 (1935).
8. Cohen, J. L. and K. A. Connors, *Am. J. Pharm. Educ.*, **29,** 245 (1965).

Problems

1. A 16.42 mg sample of a nitrogen-containing organic compound was subjected to the conventional Kjeldahl analysis. Before the ammonia was steam distilled, 20.0 ml of 0.020 *N* HCl was placed in the receiver. After the distillation, 8.4 ml of 0.020 *N* NaOH was required to back-titrate the excess acid. Calculate the percent of nitrogen in the sample.

2. A 37.25 mg sample of a nitrogen-containing compound was analyzed by the Kjeldahl method with hypochlorite titration, as in Experiment 19.1. 17.60 ml of 0.0580 *N* NaOCl was consumed in the sample titration (2.00 ml of 0.05 *N* As_2O_3 was used in the back-titration), and 1.97 ml of 0.0580 *N* NaOCl was used in the blank determination. What is the percentage of nitrogen in the sample compound?

3. Suggest three different ways in which a sample of phenobarbital could be quantitatively analyzed. Compare these methods with respect to their sensitivity, specificity, and ease of performance.

4. A sample known to contain only barbital and lactose assayed as 6.09% nitrogen by the Kjeldahl method. What percent of the sample is barbital?

20 METALS

As trace constituents, impurities, or contaminants, many metals may require determination in pharmaceutical samples. The USP and NF may specify an upper limit for the heavy metals content of pharmaceutical materials; classical precipitation tests are used to establish this level. For the quantitative determination of traces of metals, several of the physical methods discussed in Part Two provide excellent approaches; these include visible absorption spectroscopy of metal-ligand complexes, polarography, atomic absorption spectroscopy, activation analysis, and emission spectroscopy.

When a metal is the active ingredient of a pharmaceutical it is usually present in substantial amounts. It may occur as an inorganic salt or as an organometallic compound. Usually the metal is freed from such combinations and is then determined as the element [1]. It is clear that, although this approach may simplify the determination of the element in the sample, it provides no information about the nature of the molecule in which the metal was present in the original sample.

Many metals have direct pharmaceutical use. These include aluminum, calcium, magnesium, sodium, and potassium in compounds used as antacids; mercury, silver, lead, and iron, both as inorganic and organic compounds; and some elements formerly more widely used than at present, such as arsenic and gold. This chapter will outline some standard analytical methods for a few important metals.

20.1 Mercury

Both inorganic and organic mercurials are used in pharmacy. Some of them, of which mercuric chloride, phenylmercuric benzoate, and merbromin are examples, are antiseptics. Others have diuretic properties; meralluride, mercumatilin, and mersalyl are examples of mercurial diuretics. Theophylline is often incorporated in preparations containing mercurial diuretics.

Mercury is an extremely toxic substance, and its poisonous effects are cumulative. Because of its considerable volatility, mercury metal should always be stored in a tightly closed container, and any spilled mercury should be cleaned up promptly.

Sample Preparation. The mercury compounds used in pharmacy have the general structure R—Hg—R′, where one but not both of the bonds may be a carbon-mercury bond. Usually the first step in the analysis of a mercurial is the conversion of the mercury by reduction to the free metal or by oxidation to mercury (II). For many mercurials, especially the inorganics, this pretreatment merely involves solution in nitric acid.

Reductions are commonly carried out with zinc. The product of the reaction is a solution of excess zinc and the free mercury (this solution is called a zinc amalgam). Zinc and acetic acid or zinc and hydroxide are common reducing media for this reaction [1]. After reduction is complete, the amalgam is dissolved in acid (thus converting the mercury metal to mercuric ion) and the mercury is determined by one of the methods to be considered in the next section. Other reducing agents that have found some use are glycerin, monoethanolamine, and diethanolamine.

Combustion methods can be used to free the mercury. The compound is burned in the presence of oxygen, lead oxide, or lead peroxide. The mercury vapor is collected and determined.

The most widely applicable degradative treatment for mercurials is wet oxidation, in which the sample is refluxed in an oxidizing mixture, freeing the bound mercury and placing it in the Hg^{2+} form. A sulfuric acid-nitric acid mixture is used in most of the official assays. Sulfuric acid-hydrogen peroxide and nitric acid-potassium permanganate mixtures have been utilized.

Thiocyanate Titration. The most popular mercury assay is a direct titration of mercuric ion in nitric acid solution with standard thiocyanate, with ferric ion added as an indicator. This titration is already familiar as the Volhard titration of silver (Experiment 3.1). The method is very accurate, but certain precautions must be observed [2]. The end point color is caused by the formation of ferric thiocyanate, which is brownish-red. However, the dissociation constant of mercuric thiocyanate is sufficiently large that before the true equivalence point is reached, the solution contains a high enough concentration of thiocyanate to produce a faint color with ferric ion. This means that the end point is premature. This effect is diminished as the temperature is lowered and it is negligible at 15°C.

Chloride and bromide interfere in the thiocyanate titration of mercury, because these anions form slightly dissociated complexes with mercuric ion. Phosphate also interferes. Halides and phosphate can be separated from mercury by precipitating the mercury as the sulfide and removing the HgS by filtration. The mercuric sulfide is treated by the wet oxidation procedure to prepare it for titration with thiocyanate [2].

Silver obviously interferes in the Volhard titration of mercury. Silver can be removed by precipitation with excess hydrochloric acid. The chloride must then be removed before titration.

The thiocyanate solution can be standardized against pure mercury, mercuric oxide, or silver nitrate. Note that the product of the Volhard silver determination is AgSCN (a 1:1 product), while in the mercury analysis a 1:2 product, $Hg(SCN)_2$, is formed.

Colorimetry. Mercuric ion forms a colored complex with dithizone (diphenylthiocarbazone, **1**). This molecule is capable of keto-enol tautomerization,

$$S{=}C\begin{matrix} \diagup NH{-}NH{-}C_6H_5 \\ \diagdown NH{-}NH{-}C_6H_5 \end{matrix}$$

1

with the keto form favored in acid solution. The color of the mercury-dithizone complex is dependent upon the tautomeric form of the dithizone. Usually the complex is formed at pH 1–3, the acidity being adjusted with sulfuric acid rather than hydrochloric acid because of the strong complexing tendency of chloride ion.

The experimental technique is simple. The acidified solution of mercuric ion is shaken with a chloroform solution of dithizone. The mercury-dithizone complex, which is soluble in organic solvents, is extracted into the chloroform layer. The absorbance of the solution at about 500 nm, which is due to the complex, is measured and compared with a standard curve prepared with known mercury samples. Alternatively, the absorbance at 620 nm may be measured; this is a measure of the excess dithizone.

The mercury-dithizone color is unstable, being sensitive to light. The color is stabilized by acetic acid. Some metals interfere in this method, and must be absent or present in low concentration. Copper, silver, gold, and bismuth are among these. Most interference by metals can be eliminated with the addition of EDTA and thiocyanate.

The dithizone method is applicable to amounts of mercury in the range 0.001–0.2 mg. A somewhat more sensitive method utilizes di-β-naphthylthiocarbazone; the procedure with this reagent is similar to the dithizone method. Several other colorimetric methods have been suggested for mercury [2].

Other Methods. Although the thiocyanate titration and dithizone colorimetric procedures account for most mercury analyses, other methods are available. Some of these are preferable, in special circumstances, to the conventional techniques. A few of these will be outlined briefly. (This treatment is very incomplete.)

Mercuric ion can be determined gravimetrically as mercuric sulfide. An advantage over the thiocyanate titration is that chloride and bromide do not interfere. Other heavy metals interfere. In another gravimetric procedure the mercury is subjected to reduction, it is volatilized, and the free mercury is collected on gold foil, on which it is weighed. A related microscale method involves isolation of the mercury as mercuric sulfide, combustion in a capillary tube in the presence of lead chromate and magnesium carbonate, and condensation of the mercury metal in a cool part of the tube. The condensate is collected into a globule, and the diameter of the globule is measured under a microscope [3]. If the amount of mercury is small, the globule will be spherical, and from the diameter of the globule and the density of mercury its weight can be calculated. This method is applicable to 0.01–2000 μg.

Many redox titrimetric analyses have been developed. Most of these involve reduction to mercury metal. A direct titration with a reducing agent (for example, Ti^{3+} or Cr^{2+}) is possible. Alternatively, the mercury is reduced with Sn^{2+} or arsenite, followed by titration of the excess reducing agent with a suitable oxidant. A third route utilizes reduction of the mercuric sample to mercury metal and subsequent oxidimetric titration of the metal. In the Rupp method the reduction is carried out in an alkaline formaldehyde solution containing iodide ion; the $HgI_4{}^{2-}$ complex is reduced to the metal. The mercury is dissolved in an excess of standard iodine solution (again to give $HgI_4{}^{2-}$) and the excess iodine is back-titrated with thiosulfate.

Mercuric ion can be titrated with EDTA, and several other complexing agents (of which thiocyanate is the most useful) have provided analytical methods.

Occasionally it is necessary to determine mercurous mercury. This may be accomplished by oxidizing the mercury (I) to mercury (II) and then applying one of the methods already discussed. If it is desired to analyze the sample as mercury (I), or to determine mercury (I) in the presence of mercury (II), a simple procedure is to precipitate it with an excess of chloride. The mercuric ion will form the soluble $HgCl_4{}^{2-}$ complex, whereas the mercurous ion will produce the insoluble Hg_2Cl_2 (calomel). The chloride can be separated and weighed, or it can, after separation, be oxidized to mercury (II) and determined as described earlier.

A very simple assay of mercury (I) involves its oxidation with an excess of standard iodine solution. The excess iodine is back-titrated with thiosulfate. This iodometric assay is described in Experiment 20.2.

20.2 Iron

Both ferrous and ferric iron, in the form of their salts, are employed in pharmacy. Some important redox assays of these species were considered in Chapter 5.

Ferrous ion can be titrated with permanganate (Experiment 5.1), dichromate, or ceric ion. For most samples the titration can be carried out directly. If the sample is suspected of containing both ferrous and ferric ion, and the total iron content is desired, the redox titration may be preceded by a zinc reduction, which ensures that all of the ion is in the ferrous state.

Ferric ion can be determined iodometrically by adding excess iodide.

$$2Fe^{3+} + 2I^- \rightarrow 2Fe^{2+} + I_2$$

The iodine released is titrated with thiosulfate. Another redox method utilizes reduction of Fe^{3+} to the ferrous form, followed by redox titration as described in the preceding paragraph.

Ferric ion forms a stable EDTA complex, and it can be determined complexometrically. Gravimetric procedures for Fe^{3+} have been based on its precipitation as ferric oxide or as ferric 8-hydroxyquinolate (ferric oxinate).

Spectrophotometry may be used for low concentrations of ferric ion; in the presence of perchloric acid ferric ion exhibits an absorption maximum at 240 nm. Many colorimetric methods are available [2]. Ferric ion gives a color with thiocyanate that is suitable for quantitative analysis. Several ligands with the grouping shown in **2** are effective colorimetric reagents for ferrous iron.

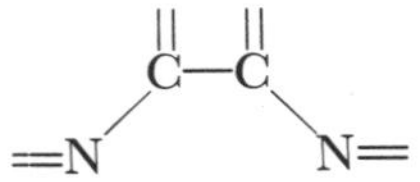

2

The most widely used of these are 1,10-phenanthroline (**3**) and 2,2′-bipyridyl (**4**). These ligands form chelates with iron with the stoichiometry $FeL_3{}^{2+}$.

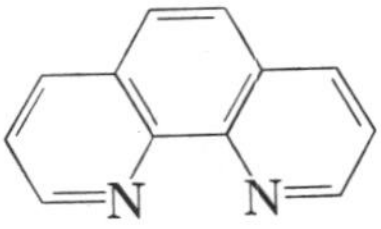

3

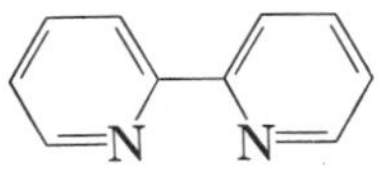

4

Experiment 20.3 describes the colorimetric measurement of iron with 1,10-phenanthroline.

20.3 Calcium

Many pharmaceuticals contain calcium salts as active ingredients, the calcium often being the pharmacologically useful portion of the salt. Calcium may be precipitated as its oxalate. (Magnesium does not interfere, if not present in excessive amounts, because magnesium oxalate is soluble under the usual precipitation conditions.) The calcium oxalate is removed by filtration, dissolved in acid, and titrated with potassium permanganate. This used to be the official assay method for calcium salts.

The preferred assay method now is a direct complexometric titration of the calcium with EDTA, as described in Chapter 4. The indicator of choice is hydroxynaphthol blue.

Experiment 20.1. Thiocyanate Titration of Mercury (II)

INTRODUCTION

Many labile mercury compounds do not require drastic oxidative treatment prior to titration with thiocyanate. Simple dissolution of such mercury compounds in the nitric acid medium converts the mercury to the titratable mercuric ion. Most compounds containing the mercury-carbon bond are more refractory and must be subjected to rigorous conditions to free the mercury. Compounds with the structure **5**, such as mersalyl and meralluride, undergo the facile elimination shown and do not require drastic degradation prior to titration [4].

$$\underset{\mathbf{5}}{-\overset{\overset{\displaystyle OR}{|}}{\underset{|}{C}}-\overset{|}{\underset{|}{C}}-HgX} + HX \longrightarrow ROH + \gt C{=}C\lt + HgX_2 \qquad (20.1)$$

REAGENTS

0.1 M Potassium Thiocyanate (or Ammonium Thiocyanate). Prepare and standardize this solution as described in Experiment 3.1. *Ferric ammonium sulfate* solution is also described in Experiment 3.1.

PROCEDURES

Known Samples. Among the compounds that can be titrated directly are mercuric acetate, mercuric oxide, and mercuric succinimide. Accurately weigh a sample equivalent to 0.1–0.3 g of mercury. Dissolve the sample in 10 ml of 6 N nitric acid and dilute to about 100 ml with distilled water. Cool the solution to below 15°C, add 1 ml of ferric ammonium sulfate solution, and titrate, with strong shaking, with 0.1 M thiocyanate to a permanent reddish-brown color. Calculate the percent purity of the sample. Perform at least three analyses. Calculate the mean and standard deviation of your results.

Mersalyl, meralluride, and mercurophylline can be analyzed similarly [4]. The compound is dissolved in 10 ml of water and 10 ml of sulfuric acid is added, dropwise, to the cooled solution with frequent shaking. The titration is made as above.

Unknown Sample. Obtain a sample of a mercurial from the instructor, who will tell you its identity. Analyze it for its mercury content by the thiocyanate titration. Report the percent of mercury and the percent of mercurial compound in your sample.

If your sample consists of tablets of the mercurial, weigh a counted number of not fewer than 20 tablets and grind them to a powder, with a mortar and pestle. Accurately weigh a portion of the powder equivalent to about 300 mg of the mercurial compound, and analyze this sample as indicated. Calculate the weight of mercurial per tablet.

Experiment 20.2. Iodometric Titration of Mercury (I)

INTRODUCTION

Oxidation of mercurous salts (mercurous chloride, for example) with iodine occurs readily with the production of mercury (II), which, in the presence of potassium iodide, forms the complex potassium mercury iodide [5].

$$Hg_2Cl_2 + I_2 + 6I^- \rightarrow 2HgI_4^{2-} + 2Cl^-$$

REAGENTS

0.1 N Iodine, 0.1 N Sodium Thiosulfate, and starch indicator solution; see Experiment 5.2.

PROCEDURES

Analysis of Calomel. Accurately weigh about 300 mg of dried mercurous chloride (calomel) into a glass-stoppered Erlenmeyer flask. Add 35 ml of standard 0.1 *N* iodine and 1 g of potassium iodide. Stopper the flask and shake until the solid dissolves. Back-titrate the excess iodine with standard 0.1 *N* thiosulfate. Calculate the percent purity of the calomel. Carry out at least three determinations.

Unknown Sample. Obtain a sample of calomel tablets from your instructor. Weigh and finely powder a counted number of at least 20 tablets. Accurately weigh a portion of the powder equivalent to about 300 mg of calomel into a beaker, mix with about 50 ml of water, filter the mixture, and wash the residue on the filter with water. Discard the filtrate.

Transfer the filter paper and residue to a glass-stoppered Erlenmeyer flask, add 35 ml of 0.1 *N* iodine and 1 g of potassium iodide, and continue the analysis as described above for calomel. Calculate the average weight of calomel per tablet.

Experiment 20.3. Colorimetric Determination of Iron (II)

INTRODUCTION

In this analysis the solution of iron is treated with hydroquinone to reduce any Fe (III) to Fe (II). Many divalent metals interfere by themselves forming complexes with the reagent; Zn, Cu, Ni, and Co should not be present at levels higher than 10 ppm. Chloride and sulfate do not interfere, but phosphate should not exceed 20 ppm.

Beer's law is obeyed by the iron complex, and the color is very stable.

REAGENTS

1,10-Phenanthroline Solution. Prepare a 0.25% solution of 1,10-phenanthroline in water, warming to dissolve. Keep the solution in the dark and discard it if a color develops.

Sodium Citrate Solution. Dissolve 250 g in 1 liter of water.

Hydroquinone Solution. Prepare a 1% solution in water.

Standard Iron Solution. Accurately weigh about 30 mg of ferrous sulfate monohydrate, transfer it quantitatively to a 1 liter volumetric flask with the aid of water, and dilute to volume. Calculate the iron concentration in milligrams of iron per milliliter.

PROCEDURE

Preparation of Standard Curve. Accurately pipet 2, 4, 6, 8 and 10 ml aliquots of the standard iron solution into 25 ml volumetric flasks. To each flask add 1 ml of hydroquinone solution and 2 ml of phenanthroline solution. Add enough sodium citrate solution to bring the solution pH to about 3.5. (This can be determined by prior testing on a portion of the standard solution, using pH indicator paper.) Allow the solutions to stand for an hour above 20°C.

Dilute the solutions to volume and measure the absorbance in a 1 cm cell against a reagent blank prepared in the same way, omitting only the iron. Make a Beer's law plot.

Unknown Sample. Obtain a solution containing iron from your instructor. Pipet a portion of the solution estimated to contain 0.02–0.1 mg of iron into a 25 ml volumetric flask, and treat it as described for the standards. Report the concentration of iron (in mg/ml) in your unknown solution.

References

1. Medwick, T., *Pharmaceutical Analysis*, T. Higuchi and E. Brochmann-Hanssen (eds.), Interscience, New York, 1961.
2. Sandell, E. B., *Colorimetric Determination of Traces of Metals*, 3rd ed., Interscience, New York, 1959.
3. Coetzee, J. F., *Treatise on Analytical Chemistry*, Part II, Vol. 3, I. M. Kolthoff and P. J. Elving (eds.), Interscience, New York, 1961, p. 231.
4. Theimer, E. E. and P. Arnow, *J. Am. Pharm. Assoc. Sci. Ed.*, **44,** 381 (1955).

Problems

1. Suggest analytical procedures suitable for the quantitative determination of each substance in these mixtures.

(*a*) Mercuric chloride, sodium chloride, and phenol in aqueous solution.

(*b*) Calomel and mercurophylline.

2. One milliliter of exactly 0.1 *N* potassium thiocyanate consumed in the titration of mercury is equivalent to how many milligrams of mercury?

3. A 0.5250 g sample of mercuric oxide was dissolved in nitric acid and titrated with 0.1025 *M* potassium thiocyanate, 45.50 ml being consumed. What was the percent purity of the sample?

Part Five: Functional Group Analysis

A "functional group" is an atom or group of atoms that exhibits a characteristic chemical reactivity. Hydroxy groups, amino groups, halogen atoms—these are examples of functional groups. All molecules (within rather wide limits) containing a certain functional group undergo the reactions characteristic of that group. Upon this observation* is based the powerful analytical approach called *functional group analysis*.

Functional group methods consist of two parts: (1) the chemical reaction or reactions that the sample compound is made to undergo; and (2) the final measurement (the "finish"), which is usually quantitative. Sometimes these two components are merged together, as in a simple titration, but usually they are discrete operations. In earlier chapters we have already discussed some functional group analyses, such as acid-base titrations, spectrophotometry after preparing a colored derivative, and gas chromatography of volatile derivatives.

Functional group analyses can be discussed by considering this general reaction:

$$\text{Sample} + \text{Reagent} \rightleftharpoons \text{Product A} + \text{Product B}$$

Two general phenomena control the analytical usefulness of the reaction. One of these is *equilibrium*, or the extent to which the reactants form products when equilibrium has been attained. The equilibrium constant is a measure of this, and a large equilibrium constant is obviously desirable. The equilibrium properties of many analytical reactions have been described in several earlier chapters.

The second controlling feature is the *rate* of reaction. The rate must be great enough to meet the practical requirements of analytical speed. Several

* This "observation" is really a truism, for it is just a restatement of our definition of a functional group.

conditions (temperature, catalyst, solvent) can be altered to increase reaction rate.

If the analytical reaction possesses satisfactory rate and equilibrium properties, it can be used to determine the sample compound by adding an excess of the reagent. After the reaction is "complete" (that is, after equilibrium is achieved), the quantitative finish is made by (1) determining the amount of unreacted reagent, which can be subtracted from the total reagent added to yield the amount of sample; (2) determining the amount of product A; or (3) determining the amount of product B. These measurements may themselves require further reactions. The finish can be made with methods already discussed, such as titrimetry, spectrophotometry, polarimetry, refractometry, polarography, fluorimetry, or chromatographic detection.

Sometimes functional group analysis is carried out by physical methods, that is, without the occurrence of a chemical reaction. Spectroscopic methods are, in a sense, functional group detectors. Nuclear magnetic resonance is a good example of a technique capable of detecting functional groups; uv and ir spectroscopy are also effective. In this part of the book, however, we will concentrate on functional group analysis as it has been defined here. The organization is by functional group. Each of these chapters is a brief presentation of a few of the many analytical methods available. References are given to more complete discussions.

21 HYDROXY COMPOUNDS

Many compounds used in pharmacy contain the hydroxyl group. These substances can be analyzed by taking advantage of the characteristic reactions of this group, and in this chapter the important functional group methods for hydroxy compounds will be described.

The chemical behavior of the hydroxy group is markedly affected by the structure of the rest of the molecule. This variation in chemical reactivity leads to the use of different methods for the analysis of the several types of compound. The substances to be considered are alcohols (primary, secondary, and tertiary), glycols, enols, and phenols. The discussion will be organized in terms of analytical methods, but the applicability of the methods to these classes of compounds will be pointed out. In Section 21.4 the determination of water, which is unique, is described.

21.1 Acylation (Esterification) Methods

Principles. A widely applicable analysis for hydroxy groups is based on their reaction to form esters. The esterification reaction involves replacement of the hydroxy hydrogen with an acyl group. The general reaction is

$$R{-}OH + R'COOH \rightleftharpoons R'COOR + H_2O$$

This particular reaction is not a suitable analytical reaction for two reasons: (1) the reaction between an alcohol and a carboxylic acid is too slow; and (2) the equilibrium is unfavorable. Both limitations are removed by using suitable combinations of solvent, temperature, catalyst, and acylating agent. A carboxylic acid is not a very potent acylating agent, and the analytically useful agents must be more reactive than the parent acid. Acid chlorides and acid anhydrides are used. The acylation reactions with these acylating agents are written:

$$R{-}OH + R'COCl \rightarrow R'COOR + HCl \qquad (21.1)$$

$$R{-}OH + (R'CO)_2O \rightarrow R'COOR + R'COOH \qquad (21.2)$$

A typical procedure involves addition of excess acid anhydride to the hydroxy sample. After the esterification is complete, the unreacted anhydride is hydrolyzed and the total acid in the solution is titrated with standard alkali. Then a blank determination is carried out by adding the same amount of anhydride to the solvent, but with the sample omitted. The anhydride is hydrolyzed and the acid is titrated. The blank will consume more alkali than the sample. The difference between the equivalents of alkali consumed by the blank and by the sample is equal to the number of equivalents of hydroxy group in the sample. A more detailed treatment of the calculation is given in Experiment 21.1. Acylation methods with spectrophotometric finishes are given in Section 21.3.

The results of hydroxyl group determinations can be expressed in several ways. The "percent hydroxyl" of the sample can be reported by converting equivalents of hydroxyl to weight of hydroxyl (1 eq OH = 17.01 g). The equivalent weight of the compound, with respect to acylable groups, is another way to express the analytical result. When the number of OH groups per molecule is known, the purity of a compound can be calculated in the usual way. All these methods are used when analyzing relatively pure compounds or samples of definite composition. Many hydroxy-containing samples, especially fats and oils, are complex mixtures, and a "percent purity" based on a hydroxy determination would be meaningless. For such samples it is common to report a "hydroxyl value"; the *hydroxyl value* is the number of milligrams of potassium hydroxide equivalent to the hydroxyl content of 1 g of sample. It is unnecessary to use KOH in the actual analysis, for one can convert equivalents of hydroxy to milligrams of KOH. The hydroxyl value is also called the hydroxyl number.

EXAMPLE 21.1. Calculate the theoretical hydroxy equivalent weight, percent hydroxyl, and hydroxyl value of methanol.

Evidently the hydroxy equivalent weight is equal to the molecular weight, or 32.04, since there is only one OH group per molecule. The percent hydroxyl is simply $17.01/32.04 \times 100 = 53.08\%$ OH. To calculate the theoretical hydroxyl value of methanol we find the number of equivalents per gram, which is $1/32.04 = 0.0312$ eq/g. Multiplying by the milligrams of KOH per equivalent of KOH we get (0.0312 eq/g) (56110 mg/eq) = 1751 mg/g as the theoretical hydroxyl value.

Nucleophilic Catalysis. In order to increase the rate of the acylation reaction, a catalyst is often added to the reaction mixture. A classical procedure uses pyridine as the catalyst. Pyridine functions as a nucleophilic catalyst; that is, it attacks a carbon atom of low electron density (the acyl carbon), giving an intermediate acylpyridinium ion, as in

$$(R'CO)_2O + C_5H_5N \rightleftharpoons R'{-}\overset{O}{\overset{\|}{C}}{-}\overset{+}{N}C_5H_5 + R'{-}COO^- \qquad (21.3)$$

The anhydride $(R'CO)_2O$ is more reactive than the acid R′COOH because the anhydride has a better "leaving group." In general, the less basic X^- is in RCOX, the more reactive the compound will be.

Now the acylpyridinium ion, which is the actual acylating agent, is itself attacked by the nucleophilic hydroxy compound to form an unstable tetrahedral intermediate, which breaks down to regenerate the pyridine and produce the ester. The sum of reactions 21.3–21.5 gives the overall esterification reaction 21.2.

$$R'{-}\overset{O}{\overset{\|}{C}}{-}\overset{+}{N}C_5H_5 + R{-}OH \rightleftharpoons R'{-}\underset{OR}{\overset{OH}{C}}{-}\overset{+}{N}C_5H_5 \qquad (21.4)$$

$$R'{-}\underset{OR}{\overset{OH}{C}}{-}\overset{+}{N}C_5H_5 \longrightarrow R'COOR + C_5H_5N + H^+ \qquad (21.5)$$

Obviously the catalyst in this reaction cannot be a primary or secondary amine, for these substances would be acylated; pyridine fits this requirement for the reaction catalyst. Moreover, the acylpyridinium ion is more reactive than the acid anhydride from which it is formed, which is why the reaction rate is increased by its appearance. The additional requirement that the acylpyridinium ion be sufficiently stable to exist in concentrations large enough to achieve an appreciable rate of reaction with the alcohol is met by this catalyst. These several properties of pyridine make it a very favorable catalyst for acylation reactions. It is also a good solvent for the reaction, and by combining with the acidic by-product of the acylation it displaces the equilibrium toward the products. Even though pyridine is a good catalyst, it is still necessary to heat the reaction mixture to achieve a reasonable reaction rate. A faster rate is obtained by using *p*-dimethylaminopyridine (DMAP), **1**, as the catalyst, as in Experiment 21.3.

$$NC_5H_4{-}N(CH_3)_2$$

1

After the acylation of the hydroxy compound is complete, the excess anhydride is hydrolyzed by adding water to the system. This hydrolysis is catalyzed by pyridine in accord with reactions 21.3, 21.4, and 21.5, where H_2O is to be written instead of R—OH.

Acetic anhydride, $(CH_3CO)_2O$, is the usual acylating agent. This compound is sufficiently reactive to give short reaction times, and the acetyl group is small enough to esterify hydroxy groups that are adjacent to rather bulky groups. A disadvantage of acetic anhydride is that it reacts (nonstoichiometrically) with aldehydes, which therefore must be absent from samples of hydroxy compounds that are to be analyzed with this reagent. Most primary and secondary alcohols are determinable by the acetic anhydride-pyridine method, the temperature and time of reaction depending on the structure of the alcohol. Tertiary alcohols and highly substituted phenols cannot be analyzed with this method, though many mono- and disubstituted phenols can. Primary and secondary amines and thiols can be analyzed by this procedure (see Experiment 24.1).

Acetyl chloride has found some use; it is more reactive than acetic anhydride. Phthalic anhydride, **2**, is less reactive than acetic anhydride; its use is advantageous when the sample may contain aldehydes, which do not react with it.

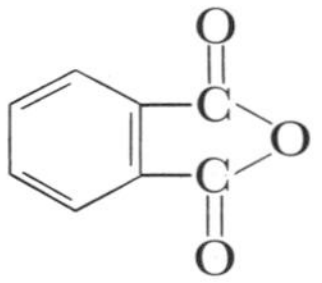

2 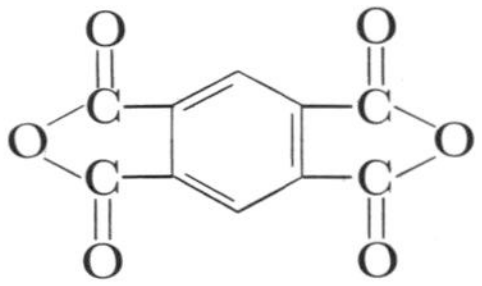 **3**

Pyromellitic dianhydride (PMDA), **3**, is a better acylating agent. These cyclic anhydrides can be used to determine alcohols in the presence of phenols, apparently as a consequence of their capabilities for intramolecular catalysis [2].

Small amounts of water do not interfere in these acylation methods (remember that after the acylation reaction is complete, water is added to the system) except by using up some of the reagent.

Acid Catalysis. Fritz and Schenk [3] introduced an acylation procedure utilizing perchloric acid as the catalyst. The solvent is ethyl acetate, and the acylating agent is acetic anhydride. The mechanism is believed to involve the formation of the acetylium ion,

$$(Ac)_2O + HClO_4 \rightleftharpoons (Ac)_2OH^+ + ClO_4^-$$

$$(Ac)_2OH^+ \rightleftharpoons HOAc + Ac^+$$

$$Ac^+ + R\text{—}OH \rightleftharpoons AcOR + H^+$$

where Ac^+ represents the acetylium ion, CH_3CO^+. Acylations with this system are much more rapid than are pyridine-catalyzed esterifications. A somewhat milder reagent is provided by combining acetic anhydride, perchloric acid, and pyridine. The acylation in this procedure probably proceeds via the acetylpyridinium ion as described in reactions 21.3–21.5, with the perchloric acid aiding the formation of this ion.

Primary and secondary alcohols, enols, and phenols can be determined quantitatively by the perchloric acid method. The pyridine-perchloric acid reagent does not acylate tertiary alcohols, so primary and secondary alcohols can be analyzed in the presence of tertiary alcohols with this reagent. The ethyl acetate reagent, because of its high reactivity, is subject to numerous interferences. Ketones and aldehydes interfere in this system.

The perchloric acid-catalyzed acylation method is described more fully in Experiment 21.1.

21.2 Other Titrimetric Methods

Titration of Acidic Hydroxyl Groups. Alcohols are very weak acids because of the acid-weakening inductive effect of electron release that can be ascribed to alkyl groups. Very few alcohols can be titrated as acids.

The situation is different with phenols. The relatively marked acidic properties of these compounds can be partly ascribed to resonance stabilization of the anion by delocalization of the negative charge. These effects are discussed in Chapter 1, and Table 1.5 gives pK_a values for some monosubstituted phenols. Although these compounds are too weakly acidic to be accurately titrated in aqueous medium, their titration in nonaqueous systems is possible. Chapter 2 describes the principles and practice of these titrations. Acid-base titration is a good means for determining phenols in the presence of other acylable compounds, especially alcohols and amines.

A methylene group situated between two keto groups is subject to an electron deficiency because of the electron-withdrawing properties of the carbonyl groups. Acetylacetone is an example of this structure. This compound is capable of keto-enol tautomerization, in which a proton shifts from the methylene carbon to one of the carbonyl oxygens. The enol form is relatively

$$\underset{\textit{keto form}}{CH_3\overset{\overset{O}{\|}}{C}—CH_2—\overset{\overset{O}{\|}}{C}CH_3} \rightleftharpoons \underset{\textit{enol form}}{CH_3\overset{\overset{OH}{|}}{C}=CH—\overset{\overset{O}{\|}}{C}CH_3}$$

acidic (pK_a for acetylacetone is 8.2) and these compounds can be titrated as acids under the same conditions described for phenols. The position of the keto-enol equilibrium is irrelevant in the acid-base titration, because as the enol form is titrated the equilibrium will shift until all of the compound has been titrated.

Periodic Acid Oxidation of 1,2-Glycols. Polyhydroxy compounds can be determined by acylation, but a more specific analytical method is available for many of these compounds. A 1,2-dihydroxy compound (ethylene glycol is the simplest example) is oxidized to two aldehyde fragments by periodic acid.

$$R{-}\underset{}{\overset{OH}{\overset{|}{C}H}}{-}\overset{OH}{\overset{|}{C}H}{-}R' + HIO_4 \longrightarrow RCHO + R'CHO + H_2O + HIO_3 \tag{21.6}$$

Each primary hydroxy group produces formaldehyde. Glycerol consumes 2 moles of periodic acid, yielding 2 moles of formaldehyde and 1 mole of formic acid. Several modifications of the method have been described [1, 4, 5].

$$\begin{matrix} CH_2OH \\ | \\ CHOH \\ | \\ CH_2OH \end{matrix} + 2HIO_4 \longrightarrow 2CH_2O + HCOOH + H_2O + 2HIO_3$$

All these involve reaction of the glycol with excess periodic acid followed by determination of excess periodic acid or by analysis of a reaction product. In a typical procedure, potassium iodide is added after the oxidation is complete. The liberated iodine is titrated with thiosulfate. Both periodate, IO_4^-, and iodate, IO_3^-, oxidize iodide to iodine, but they produce different amounts per mole. Therefore the difference in thiosulfate consumed between a blank and the sample is related to the amount of periodic acid used in oxidizing the glycol. The details of this procedure will be found in Experiment 21.2.

Glycerol can be determined in the presence of other glycols by periodic acid oxidation because formic acid is produced. Titration with standard alkali then determines the amount of glycerol.

A few compounds other than alcohols with adjacent hydroxy groups may consume periodic acid under the conditions of this analysis. Amino alcohols and hydroxy ketones are possible interferences. Simple alcohols and phenols do not interfere, so the periodic acid oxidation is a good way to analyze glycols in the presence of alcohols.

Bromination of Phenols. Phenol can be quantitatively brominated in the *ortho* and *para* positions:

$$C_6H_5{-}OH + 3Br_2 \longrightarrow Br{-}C_6H_2Br_2{-}OH + 3HBr$$

A few other phenols, among them resorcinol and some *p*-alkyl phenols, also undergo bromination, though they are not tribrominated [1]. This reaction forms the basis for a quantitative analysis of phenol. Since bromine solutions are unstable, a solution of potassium bromate and potassium bromide is utilized; when this solution is acidified, bromine is produced according to the equation

$$BrO_3^- + 5Br^- + 6H^+ \rightarrow 3Br_2 + 3H_2O$$

After the bromine substitution reaction with the phenol is complete, potassium iodide is added and the liberated iodine is titrated with thiosulfate.

This method is characteristic of the aromatic ring rather than of the phenolic hydroxy group. Aromatic amines undergo the same reaction and therefore interfere in this analysis. Unsaturated compounds interfere by adding bromine.

21.3 Spectrophotometric Methods

Phenols. The aromatic ring of phenols is responsible for fairly strong absorption of radiation in the uv region, and this forms the basis of direct uv spectrophotometric determination of phenols. Ring substitution and ionization can markedly alter the absorption properties.

Some sensitive colorimetric methods are available for phenol determination. The color produced when a phenol is treated with ferric ion is characteristic of this class of compound, and may be used for quantitative analysis. Salicylic acid can be determined, for example in body fluids, by measuring the purple color produced by a solution of ferric nitrate in nitric acid.

Phenols couple with diazonium salts to yield colored dyes; the chemistry of diazotization and coupling was presented in Experiment 8.1. In that experiment, which illustrated the colorimetric analysis of aromatic amines, the *sample* was diazotized and then coupled with a reagent. In the present instance, the *reagent* is diazotized and coupled with the sample (the phenol). Coupling occurs *para* to the phenolic group unless this position is occupied, in which case coupling will take place in the ortho position. Equations 21.7 and 21.8 show the reactions that occur in the determination of phenol using diazotized sulfanilic acid as the reagent.

$$HO_3S\text{—}C_6H_4\text{—}NH_2 \xrightarrow[HCl]{HNO_2} HO_3S\text{—}C_6H_4\text{—}N_2^+ \qquad (21.7)$$

$$HO_3S\text{—}C_6H_4\text{—}N_2^+ + C_6H_5\text{—}OH \longrightarrow$$

$$HO_3S\text{—}C_6H_4\text{—}N{=}N\text{—}C_6H_4\text{—}OH \qquad (21.8)$$

Several colorimetric methods are based on coupling of a reagent to a phenol under the influence of an oxidizing agent. Equations 21.9 and 21.10 show two of these reactions; compound **4** is 3-methyl-2-benzothiazolinone hydrazone (MBTH) and **5** is 4-aminoantipyrine. All these colorimetric methods require

$$\textbf{4} \; (\text{C=N—NH}) + C_6H_5OH \xrightarrow{(NH_4)_4Ce(SO_4)_4} \text{C=N—N=}C_6H_4\text{=O} \qquad (21.9)$$

$$\textbf{5} \; (C_6H_5\text{—N}, CH_3\text{—N}, NH_2, CH_3) + C_6H_5OH \xrightarrow{K_3Fe(CN)_6} \text{N=}C_6H_4\text{=O} \qquad (21.10)$$

the preparation of a standard curve (Beer's law plot) with known concentration of the compound being determined.

Alcohols. Since alcohols show no significant absorption in the uv and visible regions, all colorimetric methods for these compounds require their conversion to an absorbing derivative. Primary and secondary alcohols undergo acylation by 3,5-dinitrobenzoyl chloride in pyridine solution to form the corresponding 3,5-dinitrobenzoate esters; the mechanism of this reaction was discussed earlier. These esters appear to form colored quinoidal ions in basic medium, and the intensity of the color can be measured to provide an analysis of the original amount of alcohol. Phenols do not give stable colors with this method.

A similar but simpler spectrophotometric method is based on pyridine-catalyzed acylation of an alcohol with *p*-nitrobenzoyl chloride; the resulting ester absorbs strongly in the ultraviolet, and after removal of the pyridine and excess acid chloride by solvent extraction, the ester concentration is measured spectrophotometrically [6].

Trace amounts of 1,2-glycols are analyzed by oxidizing them with periodate (see Section 21.2) and then developing a color by reacting the formaldehyde produced with chromotropic acid (1,8-dihydroxynaphthalene-3,5-disulfonic acid), which is a specific reagent for formaldehyde. Only 1,2-glycols with at least one primary hydroxy group are determinable by this method.

21.4 Determination of Water

Although it is a single compound rather than a class of compounds, water deserves special treatment because knowledge of the moisture content of an analytical sample is usually required. Water in liquid samples is regarded as either a diluent or an impurity, depending upon the sample. The water contained in solids may be classified as either free or bound water; free (unbound) water is moisture adsorbed on the surface of the solid, and bound water is water of crystallization ("water of hydration"). Free water is therefore to be regarded as an impurity, whereas bound water, although it is in effect a diluent, is really a part of the crystal structure.

The determination of the amount or concentration of water in a sample is not to be confused with "water analysis," which is the determination of the concentrations of the inorganic and organic substances that always are found in samples of water. This latter study is of great importance in the chemical industry, sanitary engineering, geochemistry, oceanography, and other fields in which water is an important medium.

The determination of water is sometimes called *aquametry* [7, 8].

The Karl Fischer Titration. In 1935 Karl Fischer described a specific titrimetric method for the determination of water [9]. The reagent, which has since become known as the Karl Fischer reagent, is a solution of iodine, sulfur dioxide, and pyridine in methanol. The reaction with water appears to take place in two steps:

$$C_5H_5N{\cdot}I_2 + C_5H_5N{\cdot}SO_2 + C_5H_5N + H_2O \rightarrow 2C_5H_5N{\cdot}HI + C_5H_5N{\cdot}SO_3$$

$$C_5H_5N{\cdot}SO_3 + CH_3OH \rightarrow C_5H_5NH^+SO_4CH_3^-$$

Pyridine serves some important functions not immediately obvious from these equations. The first reaction is reversible, and pyridine forces the position of equilibrium far to the right by combining with the HI produced. Pyridine also increases the stability of the reagent by forming charge-transfer complexes with iodine and sulfur dioxide, thus reducing the vapor pressures of these volatile substances.

According to the stoichiometric equations, the composition of the reagent should be, on a molar basis, $1I_2:1SO_2:1CH_3OH:3C_5H_5N$. However, numerous side reactions among these substances can occur, thus depleting the reactants, and Karl Fischer reagent is usually prepared as a solution of iodine, sulfur dioxide, and pyridine in methanol, the approximate molar ratios being $1I_2:3SO_2:10C_5H_5N$. The effective strength of the reagent is therefore limited by the iodine content. The observed strength (which is expressed in milligrams of water equivalent to 1 ml of reagent) is always less than the theoretical strength because of the consumption of iodine by the side reactions mentioned above. Freshly prepared Karl Fischer reagent has a strength about 80% of the theoretical, but this rapidly falls to about 50% in 1 month and 40% in 3 months [7]. Typical strengths of Karl Fischer reagent for macroscale titrations are in the range 3–6 mg H_2O/ml reagent.

Karl Fischer reagent is standardized by titrating known quantities of water. Liquid water is a satisfactory standard, though its small equivalent weight is a disadvantage. Crystalline hydrates have been proposed as primary standards because they have high equivalent weights and are nonvolatile. Such a standard should meet several criteria [10]: (1) it should be commercially available in reagent grade purity and should contain the theoretical water content; (2) it must release its water quantitatively for reaction with Karl Fischer reagent in methanolic solution, and must not undergo side reactions with the reagent; (3) it should be stable and should not adsorb atmospheric moisture under ordinary laboratory storage conditions; and (4) its water content should be accurately determinable by an independent method. Many substances have been tested and found unsatisfactory. For example, sodium acetate trihydrate is hygroscopic at high humidity and efflorescent at low humidity. The official compendia specify sodium tartrate dihydrate as the primary standard [10]. The theoretical water content of this substance is 15.66%. It has been reported recently that sodium tartrate dihydrate contains about 0.3% of occluded water in addition to the water of crystallization, and the recommendation was made that this substance not be used as a primary standard [11].

The end point in a Karl Fischer titration can be located in several ways. Active Karl Fischer reagent contains iodine and is colored deep reddish-brown. "Spent" reagent (that is, reagent exhausted by reaction with water) is canary yellow. It is therefore possible to titrate water in a sample (which is usually dissolved in methanol, pyridine, or dioxane) to a visual end point. Before the end point the solution is yellow, and after the end point the first excess of active reagent imparts the characteristic reddish iodine color to the solution. Although the end point is not very sharp, it is quite reproducible when a blank comparison solution is employed. This technique is utilized in Experiment 21.4.

A photometric Karl Fischer titration can be carried out by measuring the absorbance of the titration solution at 525 nm, at which wavelength active reagent absorbs light but spent reagent does not, as titrant is added to the solution [12]. A plot is made of absorbance versus titrant volume. Before the end point the absorbance remains close to zero, but after the end point it increases linearly with volume. The end point is marked by the intersection of the two straight lines. Photometric titration provides greater sensitivity and precision than can be achieved with visual detection of the end point.

Electrometric location of the end point is preferred to the visual method by many analysts when many routine samples are to be analyzed because it is susceptible to semiautomated operation. Two platinum electrodes are used. A potential is applied across these electrodes until a galvanometer in the circuit registers zero deflection when the electrodes are immersed in the solution.* When the end point is reached the first small excess of iodine in the solution causes a relatively large current to flow, with a resultant large deflection of the galvanometer needle. This form of electrometric titration has been called the "dead-stop" end point method, because the solution is merely titrated until the galvanometer needle is sharply deflected; no point-by-point measurements are taken. The dead-stop technique is nothing more than a relatively crude amperometric titration (see Chapter 7).

Electrometric titration is applicable on the macro and micro scales. It is readily adapted to routine use, and commercial apparatus is available that can terminate the titration automatically.

The Karl Fischer titration is the method of choice for the determination of water in most kinds of samples. The sample is dissolved in methanol, pyridine, or dioxane, and is titrated to the visual or electrometric end point with standardized Karl Fischer reagent. Precautions must be taken to exclude atmospheric moisture from the titrant and from the sample solution. A blank titration is necessary to correct for water in the solvent. If the water is released from the sample only with difficulty, a back-titration may be used; an excess of Karl Fischer reagent is added, and the unreacted reagent is back-titrated with standard water-in-methanol solution. The Karl Fischer titration usually gives both the free and bound water in a sample.

Most classes of organic compounds do not interfere [8]. Water can be titrated in the presence of acids, alcohols, phenols, ethers, hydrocarbons, anhydrides, amines, amides, halides, sulfides, and many other substances. Materials that consume iodine interfere; thiols and ascorbic acid are examples of substances that interfere quantitatively, so a separate analysis often will permit a correction to be applied. Carbonyl compounds interfere by forming

* Although the two electrodes may appear to be identical, one of them will adopt the role of "reference" electrode and the other will become the "indicator" electrode.

acetals and ketals with methanol, releasing water in the process. This interference is eliminated by converting the carbonyl compound to the cyanohydrin by addition of hydrogen cyanide.

Carboxylic acids are capable of esterification with methanol; this condensation reaction produces water and may invalidate the determination. Such condensation reactions are promoted by excess Karl Fischer reagent, which of course functions as a powerful desiccant. The use of pyridine or dioxane as the titration medium will limit esterification reactions.

Distillation. Many pairs of liquids have been discovered that cannot be resolved into the pure components by distillation because of the occurrence of "constant-boiling" mixtures of the components. The fractional composition of such a constant-boiling mixture depends upon the pressure, showing that the mixture is not a compound. Nevertheless, a binary solution with the composition of the constant-boiling mixture will distill as if it were a single substance, that is, without change in boiling point or composition. Such a constant-boiling mixture is called an azeotrope. An example is provided by chloroform (atmospheric boiling point 61.2°C) and acetone (bp 56.1°C), which form an azeotrope, at atmospheric pressure, with bp 64.4°C and chloroform content 78.5% (by weight).

This phenomenon has been used to advantage for separating water from other components of a mixture. Water and toluene form an azeotrope with bp 84.1°C; the azeotrope contains 19.6% water. Since these two liquids are practically immiscible, the condensed distillate separates into two layers. The volume of the aqueous (lower) phase is measured to give a direct measure of the water content of the sample. Toluene is the customary organic liquid, though others have been used.

The apparatus is shown in Fig. 21.1. *A* is a 500 ml flask into which is placed about 200 ml of toluene and a weighed portion of sample estimated to contain 2–4 ml of water. The receiving tube *D*, which is graduated to 5 ml in 0.1 ml divisions, is filled with toluene through the condenser *C*. The flask is heated and the toluene is slowly distilled. The vapors rise into the condenser, and the distillate falls into the receiver, where it separates into two phases. The heavier water displaces the toluene, which returns to the distilling flask via tube *B*. The distillation is prolonged (sometimes for several hours) until all of the water has been collected in *D*. Beads of water adhering to the walls of the condenser are dislodged, and finally the volume of water in the receiver is read.

This method is clearly applicable only if the sample does not contain other volatile substances that could affect the apparent volume of water in the receiver. Thus the presence of ethanol in the sample would lead to an erroneously high result.

The toluene distillation method is applicable to crude drugs, to many ointments, and to other complex mixtures that might not be amenable to analysis by Karl Fischer titration.

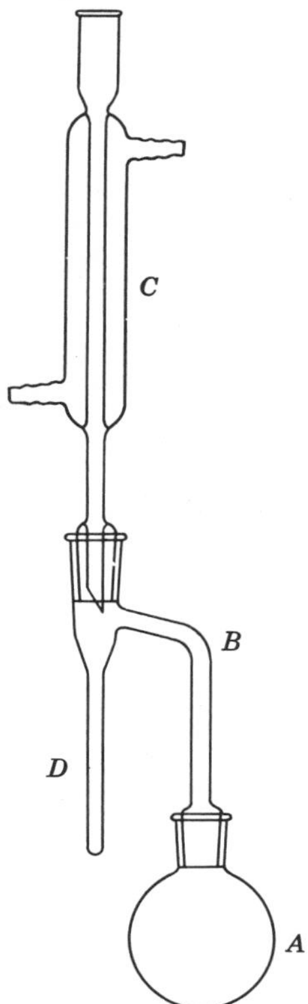

Fig. 21.1. Apparatus for water determination by the toluene distillation method.

Oven Drying. Perhaps the simplest method for the determination of water in solids is oven drying at atmospheric pressure and 100–150°C until constant weight is attained. The loss in weight of the sample is attributed to the loss of water. In order for this method to be valid there must be no volatile substances other than water in the sample, and the sample compound must be stable under the conditions of the drying treatment. Both free and bound water can be measured. It is necessary to ascertain for each compound the appropriate temperature and period of drying required to drive off all water. Some hydrated compounds are very resistant to complete expulsion of water by oven drying.

If the sample compound is heat labile, oven drying may still be applicable if the pressure is reduced. This of course has the effect of lowering the boiling point of water, so a lower temperature may be utilized for the drying process. Vacuum ovens are available for this purpose. Other means are commonly employed in the laboratory for drying under reduced pressure. A "drying pistol" (also called an Abderhalden pistol) is a glass apparatus designed to permit the sample to be enclosed in an evacuated chamber, which is bathed in the vapor of a refluxing liquid. The temperature of the sample chamber is established by the selection of the boiling liquid. The vacuum is provided by a conventional rotary oil vacuum pump. If drying under reduced pressure at room temperature is sufficient for complete removal of the water, a vacuum desiccator is the simplest apparatus for the purpose. A desiccant is placed in the bottom of the desiccator to absorb moisture; among the best desiccants are anhydrous magnesium perchlorate (Dehydrite), anhydrous calcium sulfate (Drierite), and phosphorus pentoxide. A vacuum pump establishes the vacuum. If the sample contains a considerable amount of water, a sustained pumping action is desirable to exhaust the desiccator of water vapor. An acetone-dry ice trap should be interposed between the desiccator and the pump to prevent passage of water into the pump or of chemical vapors from the pump oil into the desiccator. When the sample contains only traces of moisture it may be satisfactory merely to develop a vacuum in the desiccator and then to seal it until the desiccant has absorbed all of the water.

It is important to appreciate the nature of the drying process under the influence of reduced pressure. This process can be described as an approach to equilibrium. Equilibrium is attained when the partial pressure of water is the same everywhere in the system. Thus in the initial stages of a drying by desiccation the partial pressure of water vapor over the sample is far greater than it is over the desiccant, so the water passes ("distills") from the sample to the desiccant. With this picture of the desiccation process it becomes apparent that cooling a hot oven-dried sample preparatory to weighing is a potential source of error. If the sample is drier than the desiccant, water will pass from the desiccant to the sample. This is why a very efficient desiccant should be used.

The use of a water aspirator as a pump to achieve reduced pressure in a vacuum desiccator is seen to be a questionable practice. The partial pressure of water in the entire system will tend to approach the vapor pressure of water at the temperature of the water in the aspirator. Effective drying cannot be expected under these conditions.

Experiment 21.1. Determination of Hydroxy Compounds by Perchloric Acid-Catalyzed Acetylation

INTRODUCTION

The basis of this method was explained earlier (Section 21.1). The procedure involves the addition of the sample to a reagent containing acetic anhydride and perchloric acid. After acylation is complete, the excess anhydride is hydrolyzed and the total acetic acid is titrated with standard alkali. A blank determination is carried out. Since each mole of unreacted anhydride yields 2 moles of acetic acid, whereas each mole of reacted anhydride yields only 1 mole of acetic acid, the difference between the blank and sample titration volumes is directly related to the amount of hydroxy group in the sample. The following diagram may make this clearer. The lengths of the lines represent numbers of moles or equivalents, as appropriate. Successive steps in the procedure are described by successive lines (proceeding from top to bottom). Evidently meq of ROH = meq of KOH in the blank determination − meq of KOH in the sample determination, or meq of ROH = $N(V_B - V_S)$, where N is the normality of the potassium hydroxide. Sample determination:

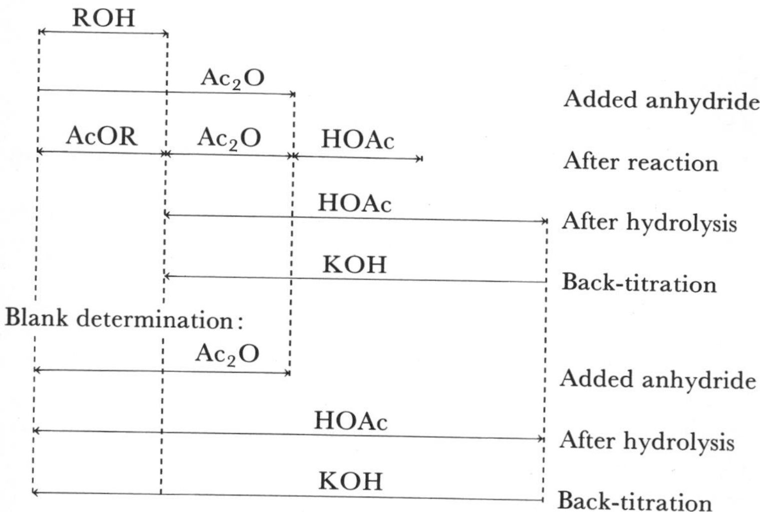

If all of the anhydride were consumed in the acylation of the sample, then V_S would equal $V_B/2$. This is an undesirable result, because it indicates that insufficient anhydride was present to react with all of the sample. If V_S is not at least 60% of V_B, it is wise to repeat the analysis with a smaller sample.

Pyridine is added after the acylation step to catalyze the hydrolysis of the excess anhydride. Fritz and Schenk [3] suggested ethyl acetate as the solvent for the acylating agent, but the resulting solution often discolors, becoming dark enough to obscure the visual end point. Replacement of the ethyl acetate by 1,2-dichloroethane provides some improvement [13]. A straw-colored reagent is quite satisfactory.

Most alcohols and phenols are acylated in 5 min at room temperature with the procedure described in this experiment. A semimicro procedure has also been developed [14]. Other acylable compounds, in particular amines and thiols, interfere in this method. In fact, the same assay procedure can be employed in the analysis of amines and thiols.

REAGENTS

2 M Acetic Anhydride. Add 3.2 ml of 60% perchloric acid to 150 ml of 1,2-dichloroethane (ethylene dichloride) in a 250 ml glass-stoppered flask. Pipet 8 ml of reagent grade acetic anhydride into the flask and permit it to stand at room temperature for at least 30 min. Cool to 5°C and add 42 ml of cold acetic anhydride. Keep the flask at 5°C for 1 hr, then allow the solution to warm to room temperature. This reagent is stable for about 2 weeks.

Pyridine-Water Solution. Mix 40 ml of water and 120 ml of reagent grade pyridine.

Phenolphthalein Solution. See Experiment 1.1. Fritz and Schenk suggest a mixed indicator of cresol red and thymol blue [3], but phenolphthalein is satisfactory.

0.55 N Potassium Hydroxide. Dissolve 35.2 g of potassium hydroxide in 70 ml of cooled, freshly boiled water. Dilute to 1 liter with absolute methanol and store in a polyethylene bottle. Standardize the solution against potassium bipthalate as described in Experiment 1.1, remembering to weigh out samples whose size is appropriate to the solution normality and the buret capacity (see Appendix A).

PROCEDURES

Known Sample. Select a typical monohydroxy compound (for example, ethanol, isopropanol, *n*-butanol, phenol, etc.) for analysis. Accurately weigh 4–6 meq of the compound into a dry glass-stoppered 125 ml Erlenmeyer flask and pipet exactly 5.0 ml of the acetic anhydride reagent into the flask. Shake the mixture to dissolve the sample. Allow the solution to stand about 5 min to complete the acylation. (See Appendix A for suggestions on weighing volatile samples.)

Add 1–2 ml of water to the flask, shake the mixture, then add 10 ml of the pyridine-water solution and allow to stand 5 min to hydrolyze the excess anhydride. Add phenolphthalein indicator and titrate to the end point with standard 0.55 *N* potassium hydroxide, using a 50 ml buret.

Carry out a blank determination with exactly the same procedure and reagents. Calculate the percent recovery of the hydroxy compound as outlined above.

If the sample is highly colored, an indicator titration may be impossible. In such a circumstance the assay can be performed with potentiometric determination of the end point, using a pH meter with glass and saturated calomel electrodes.

Unknown Sample. Obtain a sample of a pure hydroxy compound from your instructor. Determine the hydroxy content of the compound, and report your results as the following three equivalent quantities: (1) equivalent weight with respect to acylable groups; (2) hydroxy value; (3) percent hydroxy groups. Alternatively your sample may be a solution of a hydroxy compound, and you can then report the concentration of the solution.

Since the accuracy in this assay method depends equally upon the accuracy of the blank and sample titrations, it is advisable to carry out several blank determinations.

Experiment 21.2. Determination of 1,2-Glycols by Periodic Acid Oxidation

PRINCIPLE

The chemical basis of this method has been described in Section 21.2. The glycol is added to a periodic acid solution. Another portion of periodic acid solution, identical with the sample solution except that the glycol is omitted, is designated the blank. After the oxidation is complete, excess potassium iodide is added to each solution. The liberated iodine is titrated with standard thiosulfate. Let us first consider the blank titration. The periodic acid oxidizes iodide to iodine according to the equation:

$$2H^+ + HIO_4 + 2I^- \rightarrow HIO_3 + I_2 + H_2O \qquad (21.11)$$

However, the iodic acid produced is itself capable of oxidizing iodide:

$$5H^+ + HIO_3 + 5I^- \rightarrow 3I_2 + 3H_2O \qquad (21.12)$$

The overall result is that each mole of periodic acid yields 4 moles (8 equivalents) of iodine.

Now consider the sample titration. After the oxidation of the glycol is complete the solution contains excess periodic acid plus 1 mole of iodic acid for each 1,2-dihydroxy unit that was oxidized (Eq. 21.11). Therefore each HIO_4 leads to $4I_2$ and each HIO_3 leads to $3I_2$, with the overall result that each 1,2-dihydroxy unit in the sample results in a decreased production of 1 mole (2 eq) of iodine relative to the blank titration. That is, 1 mole of a 1,2-dihydroxy unit corresponds to a decrease in thiosulfate consumption of 2 eq, so the equivalent weight of a single 1,2-dihydroxy unit is equal to one-half its molecular weight, on the basis of the final titration reaction.

It has been observed that, if a compound possesses n consecutive adjacent hydroxy groups, $n - 1$ moles of periodic acid will be consumed in the oxidation. Therefore $n - 1$ dihydroxy units actually are oxidized, and the equivalent weight of the sample compound is equal to $1/2(n - 1)$ times its molecular weight. For ethylene glycol, $n = 2$ and EW = MW/2; for glycerol, $n = 3$ and EW = MW/4; and for mannitol, $n = 6$ and EW = MW/10. It is on this basic that the volumetric factors in published procedures have been calculated.

According to the preceding reasoning, if the glycol sample consumes all of the periodic acid, the volume of thiosulfate consumed in the sample titration will be 75% of that consumed in the sample titration. If the observed sample volume is less than about 80% of the blank volume, it is therefore advisable to repeat the analysis with a smaller sample of glycol in order to be sure that an excess of periodic acid is present.

Among the compounds that can be analyzed by this assay are ethylene glycol, propylene glycol, glycerol, monoglyceride esters, mannitol, and dextrose.

REAGENTS

Periodic Acid Solution. Dissolve 5 g of periodic acid in 200 ml of distilled water. Dilute this solution to 1 liter with glacial acetic acid. This reagent should be protected from light.

Potassium Iodide Solution. Dissolve 20 g of reagent grade potassium iodide in enough water to make 100 ml.

0.1 N Sodium Thiosulfate. Prepare and standardize as described in Experiment 5.2.

PROCEDURES

Known Sample. Accurately weigh 0.5–1 meq of a pure 1,2-glycol or polyhydroxy compound into a 250 ml glass-stoppered Erlenmeyer flask. Pipet exactly 100.0 ml of periodic acid solution into the flask, shake to dissolve the sample, and allow to stand $\frac{1}{2}$ hr at room temperature. To another flask (the blank) also add 100.0 ml of periodic acid solution.

Add 20 ml of potassium iodide solution to each flask. Titrate the iodine in each flask with standard 0.1 N sodium thiosulfate, using starch solution as an indicator. If V_B and V_S are the volumes of thiosulfate required to titrate the blank and the sample, respectively, then $N(V_B - V_S)$ is equal to the milliequivalents of dihydroxy compound in the sample, where N is the normality of the thiosulfate. Calculate the percent recovery of the sample.

Unknown Sample. Obtain from your instructor a sample of a pure liquid or solid compound containing at least one pair of adjacent hydroxy groups. Accurately weigh a sample and carry out a quantitative periodic acid oxidation as described above. If the sample titration volume is not at least 80% of the blank titration volume, repeat the analysis with a smaller sample. Carry out 3 assays. Calculate the equivalent weight with respect to oxidizable glycol units. Report the mean, standard deviation, and 95% confidence limits of your equivalent weight.

Experiment 21.3. Determination of Hydroxy Compounds by 4-Dimethylaminopyridine-Catalyzed Acetylation

INTRODUCTION

The mechanism of catalysis by 4-dimethylaminopyridine (DMAP) is probably as shown for pyridine in Section 21.1. In this experiment pyridine is used as the solvent. Since DMAP is a much more powerful catalyst than is pyridine, DMAP accounts for most of the catalysis in this system [15]. The calculation is identical with that of Experiment 21.1.

REAGENTS

DMAP Solution. Dissolve 2 g of 4-dimethylaminopyridine in enough reagent grade pyridine to make 100 ml.

Acetic Anhydride Solution. Mix 10 ml of reagent grade acetic anhydride with 40 ml of pyridine. This solution must be prepared fresh daily.

Phenolphthalein Solution. See Experiment 1.1.

0.5 N Sodium Hydroxide. Dilute 30 ml of saturated sodium hydroxide solution to 1 liter with freshly boiled water. Store the solution in a polyethylene bottle. Standardize it against potassium biphthalate (see Experiment 1.1 and Appendix A).

PROCEDURES

Known Sample. Accurately weigh 20–30 meq of a hydroxy compound (e.g., ethanol, propanol, phenol, etc.) and dissolve it in enough pyridine to make 10.0 ml. (Use a 10 ml volumetric flask.)

Pipet 1.0 ml of this sample solution into a 50 ml Erlenmeyer flask. Add 5.0 ml of DMAP solution followed by exactly 2.0 ml of acetic anhydride solution, and mix well. Stopper the flask tightly and immerse the body of the flask in a water bath at about 55–60°C (the exact temperature is not critical). Carry out a blank determination in exactly the same way, omitting only the sample.

After 15–20 min remove the flasks from the water bath, add 25 ml of water to each, and allow them to cool to room temperature. If the solution is not homogeneous, add 5 ml of *n*-butanol. Add 3 drops of phenolphthalein solution, and titrate with standard 0.5 *N* NaOH, using a 25 ml buret. Carry out several determinations of both the sample and the blank.

Calculate the percent recovery of the sample hydroxy compound.

Unknown Sample. A solution of isopropyl alcohol will be furnished. Taking 1.0 ml samples, determine its concentration using the procedure described above. Report the result as mean concentration in mg/ml.

Experiment 21.4. Karl Fischer Titration of Water

REAGENTS

Karl Fischer Reagent. A commercial reagent is recommended.

Standard Water Solution. Weigh a dry 100 ml volumetric flask and its stopper. Pipet about 1 ml of water into the flask, put the stopper in place, and reweigh. Dilute to volume with reagent grade absolute methanol.

The same lot of methanol must be used for the standard solution and subsequent blank and sample titrations, because the water content of methanol may vary from lot to lot.

PROCEDURES

Standardization of Karl Fischer Reagent. Standardize the reagent against the standard water solution.

Pipet 25.0 ml of the absolute methanol into a dry 100 ml volumetric flask. Titrate with Karl Fischer reagent, contained in a 25 ml buret and protected with a drying tube, until the appearance of the characteristic iodine color of the active reagent. The end point is marked by a definite and permanent reddish color. Stopper the flask and retain it for end point color comparisons. This is the blank titration. It indicates the volume of reagent equivalent to the water contained in 25.0 ml of absolute methanol.

Pipet 15.0 ml of absolute methanol and 10.0 ml of the standard water solution into another dry 100 ml volumetric flask. (Volumetric flasks are good titration flasks because their long, narrow necks limit absorption of atmosperhic moisture during the titration.) Titrate to the end point with Karl Fischer reagent. Match the color of the blank solution as closely as possible. Titrations should be carried out quickly to avoid the introduction of significant amounts of moisture from the air.

Subtract the blank titration volume from the standardization volume and calculate the titer of the Karl Fischer reagent. Express the result as milligrams of water equivalent to 1 ml of reagent.

Karl Fischer reagent should be restandardized daily.

Determination of Water of Hydration. Accurately weigh about 250 mg of hydrated sodium acetate into a dry 100 ml volumetric flask. Add 25.0 ml of absolute methanol and dissolve the salt. Titrate the water with standardized Karl Fischer reagent. Subtract the appropriate blank volume and calculate the percentage of water in the sample. Calculate the formula of the hydrate.

Unknown Samples. (1) Obtain a solid or liquid sample from your instructor. This may be a water-in-methanol solution or a substance with a known water content. Determine the concentration of water in your sample by Karl Fischer titration. (2) A pure sample of a hydrated salt will be provided. Dissolve an accurately weighed portion in absolute methanol and titrate with

Karl Fischer reagent. Calculate the percent of water contained by the salt, and calculate its equivalent weight (that is, the weight of sample that contains 1 mole of water.)

References

1. Siggia, S., *Quantitative Organic Analysis via Functional Groups*, 3rd ed., John Wiley and Sons, New York, 1963.
2. Connors, K. A., *Reaction Mechanisms in Organic Analytical Chemistry*, Wiley-Interscience, New York, 1973, pp. 597–601.
3. Fritz, J. S. and G. H. Schenk, *Anal. Chem.*, **31,** 1808 (1959).
4. Mehlenbacher, V. C., *Org. Anal.*, **1,** 1 (1953).
5. Critchfield, F. E., *Organic Functional Group Analysis*, Macmillan, New York, 1963, Chap. 5.
6. Scoggins, M. W., *Anal. Chem.*, **36,** 1152 (1964).
7. Mitchell, J., Jr. and D. M. Smith, *Aquametry*, Interscience, New York, 1948.
8. Mitchell, J., Jr., *Treatise on Analytical Chemistry*, I. M. Kolthoff and P. J. Elving (eds.), Part II, Vol. I, Interscience, New York, 1961, pp. 69–206.
9. Fischer, K., *Z. Angew. Chem.*, **48,** 394 (1935).
10. Neuss, J. D. M., G. O'Brien, and H. A. Frediani, *Anal. Chem.*, **23,** 1332 (1951).
11. Beasley, T. H., Sr., H. W. Ziegler, R. L. Charles, and P. King, *Anal. Chem.*, **44,** 1833 (1972).
12. Connors, K. A. and T. Higuchi, *Chemist-Analyst*, **48,** 91 (1959).
13. Magnuson, J. A. and R. J. Cerri, *Anal. Chem.*, **38,** 1088 (1966).
14. Schenk, G. H. and J. S. Fritz, *Anal. Chem.*, **32,** 987 (1960).
15. Connors, K. A. and K. S. Albert, *J. Pharm. Sci.*, **62,** 845 (1973).

FOR FURTHER READING

Veibel, S., *The Determination of Hydroxyl Groups*, Academic Press, New York, 1972.

Cheronis, N. D. and T. S. Ma, *Organic Functional Group Analysis by Micro and Semimicro Methods*, Interscience, New York, 1964.

Ashworth, M. R. F., *Titrimetric Organic Analysis*, Part II, Interscience, New York, 1965.

Problems

1. Give the theoretical percent hydroxyl, the hydroxyl value, and the equivalent weight of each of these compounds; ethanol; phenol; cetyl alcohol; and 1,3-dihydroxypropane.

2. 0.3910 g of phenol was analyzed by the perchloric acid-catalyzed acetylation method. The sample determination required 36.85 ml of 0.6368 *N* NaOH, and the blank determination consumed 43.00 ml. What is the purity of the phenol?

3. Give practical analytical methods for the quantitative determination of each component in these mixtures.
   (*a*) Phenol, sodium benzoate, and mercuric chloride
   (*b*) Ethanol and propylene glycol
   (*c*) Pyridine, methanol, and acetic acid

4. Show that the hydroxyl value of a sample as determined by the acylation procedure is given by the formula

$$\text{Hydroxyl value} = \frac{56.11N(V_B - V_S)}{\text{g of sample}}$$

where the symbols have the meanings assigned earlier in this chapter.

5. The following data were obtained in the course of identifying a widely used analgesic drug:

(*a*) uv absorption maximum at 248 nm in methanol solution; molar absorptivity 1.7×10^3 at this wavelength.

(*b*) Solution showed no detectable optical rotation.

(*c*) Elemental analysis gave 9.28% as the nitrogen content.

(*d*) Titration with sodium methoxide in nonaqueous medium gave equivalent weight 150.8.

(*e*) When dissolved in glacial acetic acid and titrated with perchloric acid, no titrant was consumed.

(*f*) Quantitative acetylation gave equivalent weight 151.6.

Propose a structure consistent with all the data (including the pharmacology).

6. Twenty tablets of salicylamide, $C_7H_7NO_2$, MW 137.5, weighed 8.250 g. They were powdered and a portion weighing 0.940 g was analyzed by acylation with acetic anhydride. The normality of the NaOH was 0.450. The blank consumed 42.00 ml and the sample consumed 31.00 ml. Calculate the average weight of salicylamide per tablet.

7. 0.5404 g of water was dissolved in methanol to make 50.0 ml. 5.0 ml of this solution was added to 20.0 ml of methanol and titrated with Karl Fischer reagent, 9.50 ml being consumed. 25.0 ml of the same methanol consumed 0.80 ml of reagent. Calculate the titer of the Karl Fischer reagent.

8. 0.2310 g of a sample was dissolved in 10.0 ml of methanol and was titrated with the Karl Fischer reagent of Problem 7. 2.40 ml of reagent was required to titrate the water in the sample. What percent of water did the sample contain?

9. Calculate the theoretical water content of borax, $Na_2B_4O_7 \cdot 10H_2O$.

10. If a sample of sodium tartrate dihydrate contains 0.3% (absolute) occluded water, what will be the percentage error (relative) in the standardization of Karl Fischer reagent against this sample?

22 CARBONYL COMPOUNDS

The analysis of aldehydes, **1**, and ketones, **2**, will be treated in this chapter. Several derivatives of carbonyl compounds, which can be readily converted to the corresponding carbonyl compound, also will be considered. These are acetals, **3**, ketals, **4**, vinyl ethers, **5**, and imines (Schiff bases), **6**. Classes **3–6**

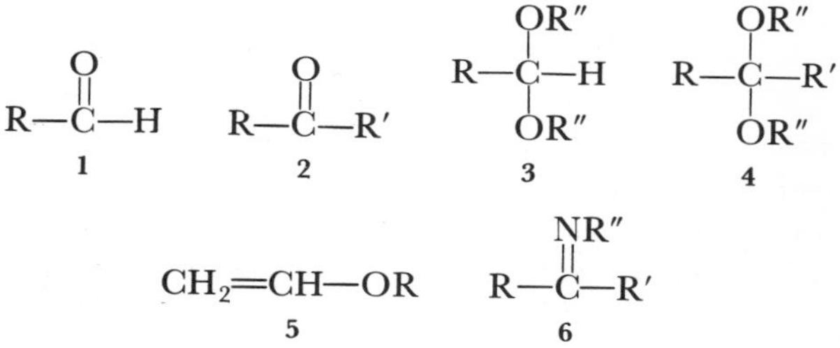

$$\underset{\mathbf{1}}{R-\overset{\overset{O}{\|}}{C}-H} \qquad \underset{\mathbf{2}}{R-\overset{\overset{O}{\|}}{C}-R'} \qquad \underset{\mathbf{3}}{R-\overset{\overset{OR''}{|}}{\underset{\underset{OR''}{|}}{C}}-H} \qquad \underset{\mathbf{4}}{R-\overset{\overset{OR''}{|}}{\underset{\underset{OR''}{|}}{C}}-R'}$$

$$\underset{\mathbf{5}}{CH_2{=}CH-OR} \qquad \underset{\mathbf{6}}{R-\overset{\overset{NR''}{\|}}{C}-R'}$$

can be hydrolyzed to the parent carbonyl under acid conditions. The resulting

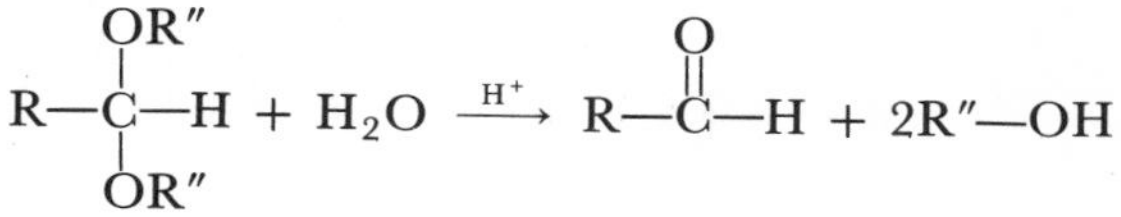

$$R-\overset{\overset{OR''}{|}}{\underset{\underset{OR''}{|}}{C}}-H + H_2O \xrightarrow{H^+} R-\overset{\overset{O}{\|}}{C}-H + 2R''-OH \qquad (22.1)$$

$$R-\overset{\overset{OR''}{|}}{\underset{\underset{OR''}{|}}{C}}-R' + H_2O \xrightarrow{H^+} R-\overset{\overset{O}{\|}}{C}-R' + 2R''-OH \qquad (22.2)$$

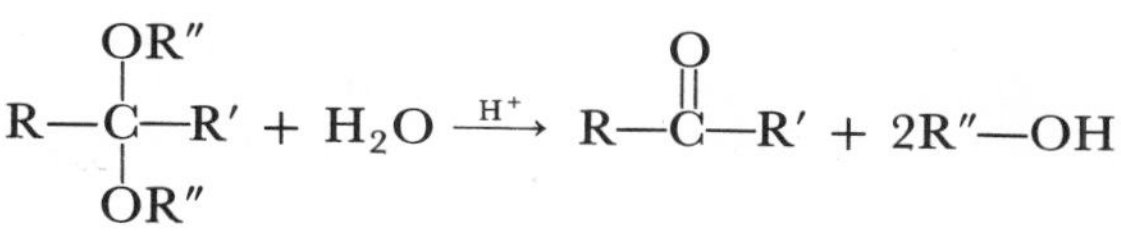

$$CH_2{=}CH-OR + H_2O \xrightarrow{H^+} CH_3CHO + ROH \qquad (22.3)$$

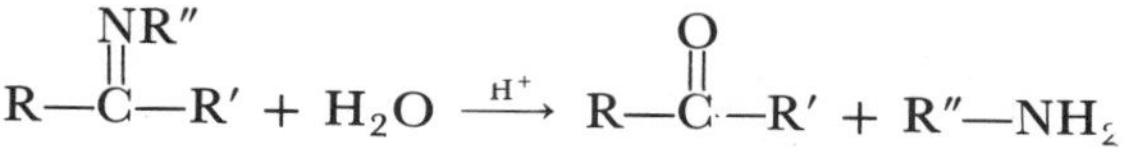

$$R-\overset{\overset{NR''}{\|}}{C}-R' + H_2O \xrightarrow{H^+} R-\overset{\overset{O}{\|}}{C}-R' + R''-NH_2 \qquad (22.4)$$

carbonyl is analyzed as described in this chapter. Those carbonyl methods that utilize an acidic medium cause these hydrolyses to occur directly, and therefore can be used to determine acetals, ketals, etc. without modification.

22.1 Methods Based on Condensation Reactions

The most characteristic reaction of carbonyl compounds is addition across the C=O double bond, initiated by nucleophilic attack on the carbonyl carbon. When the attacking nucleophile has two protons, water is subsequently lost, as shown in Eq. 22.5. Such a reaction is called a condensation. Several condensation reactions provide good analytical methods for carbonyls.

$$\text{>C=O} + H_2X \rightleftharpoons \text{>C(OH)(XH)} \rightleftharpoons \text{>C=X} + H_2O \qquad (22.5)$$

Oximation. The product of the condensation of an aldehyde or ketone with hydroxylamine, NH_2OH, is called an oxime. Oximation is specific acid-

$$R{-}\overset{\overset{\displaystyle O}{\|}}{C}{-}R' + NH_2OH \rightleftharpoons R{-}\overset{\overset{\displaystyle N{-}OH}{\|}}{C}{-}R' + H_2O \qquad (22.6)$$

catalyzed (that is, catalyzed by hydronium ion in aqueous solution) and general acid-catalyzed (catalyzed by all other acidic species, namely, undissociated weak acids). The mechanism probably involves an increase in the electrophilicity of the carbon-oxygen double bond by protonation or hydrogen bonding with an acid catalyst, followed by attack of the nucleophilic molecule NH_2OH. Water is then lost from the tetrahedral intermediate to give the oxime. Since the reaction is acid-catalyzed, the rate of reaction

$$R{-}\overset{\overset{\displaystyle O}{\|}}{C}{-}R' + HA \rightleftharpoons R{-}\overset{\overset{\displaystyle O{-}{-}{-}HA}{\|}}{C}{-}R' \qquad (22.7)$$

$$R{-}\underset{\delta^+}{\overset{\overset{\displaystyle \delta^- O{-}{-}{-}HA}{\|}}{C}}{-}R' + NH_2OH \rightleftharpoons R{-}\underset{\underset{\displaystyle NH{-}OH}{|}}{\overset{\overset{\displaystyle OH}{|}}{C}}{-}R' + HA \qquad (22.8)$$

$$R{-}\underset{\underset{\displaystyle NH{-}OH}{|}}{\overset{\overset{\displaystyle OH}{|}}{C}}{-}R' \rightleftharpoons R{-}\overset{\overset{\displaystyle N{-}OH}{\|}}{C}{-}R' + H_2O \qquad (22.9)$$

increases as the pH is decreased. On the other hand, a lower pH decreases the fraction of hydroxylamine in the unprotonated, nucleophilic form, which should decrease the reaction velocity (the pK_a of hydroxylamine is 6.0).

The net result is that the rate of oximation exhibits an optimal pH at which it is maximized; at higher and lower pH the rate decreases.*

Equation 22.6 appears to provide a basis for a good analytical method; an excess of hydroxylamine could be added to the sample, and after oximation is complete the excess NH_2OH could be titrated with acid. Unfortunately, free hydroxylamine is very unstable, being oxidized by oxygen. This method is therefore not feasible. Instead the oximation reaction is carried out with hydroxylamine hydrochloride, which is very stable. Each mole of oxime

$$R{-}\overset{\overset{\displaystyle O}{\|}}{C}{-}R' + NH_2OH{\cdot}HCl \rightleftharpoons R{-}\overset{\overset{\displaystyle N{-}OH}{\|}}{C}{-}R' + H_2O + HCl \qquad (22.10)$$

formed results in the production of 1 mole of hydrochloric acid, which can be titrated with standard alkali to give a measure of the carbonyl in the sample.

This method has three limitations. First, reaction 22.10 is an equilibrium and for many carbonyls the position of equilibrium is not favorable; that is, at equilibrium an appreciable fraction of the sample is in the carbonyl form. Another way to express this is by saying that the reaction does not "go to completion" for all carbonyl compounds.

The second limitation is that the final analytical measurement, the titration of HCl with NaOH, is complicated by the presence of a second acid, the excess hydroxylammonium chloride, which consumes alkali immediately following titration of the HCl. The result is a diminished sharpness of the end point. This can be overcome by carrying out a potentiometric titration, though this is time-consuming. A visual titration is feasible, though at some sacrifice in precision. Experiment 22.1 describes this technique.

Another restriction on the use of this method is slowness of the reaction rate for the oximation of many compounds, especially carbonyl compounds with bulky groups. The oximation reaction is often conducted at reflux to increase the reaction velocity.

Modifications of the oximation method have utilized nonaqueous solvents; the purpose of these alterations has been to increase the reaction rate, shift the equilibrium position for analytical use, and improve the sharpness of the end point. Thus the reaction has been carried out in glacial acetic acid with hydroxylammonium acetate as the reagent; after oximation the excess reagent was titrated with acetous perchloric acid [2]. This procedure requires a potentiometric titration. A different approach utilizes hydroxylamine

* This explanation is oversimplified. Actually the pH maximum in the rate is the result of a change in rate-determining step. At low pH the attack of the nucleophile on the carbonyl compound (Eq. 22.8) is rate-determining, but at higher pH the dehydration of the intermediate (Eq. 22.9) becomes rate-determining [1].

hydrochloride in methanol-isopropanol with a base, dimethylaminoethanol, added to consume HCl as it is produced. The excess base is titrated with perchloric acid. In this procedure a visual end point can be detected [3]. Schenk [4] has reviewed the development of oximation methods.

Both aldehydes and ketones are determined in hydroxylamine methods. Acetals, ketals, and vinyl ethers are easily hydrolyzed under the acidic conditions of most of these methods, and so these compounds can also be analyzed in this way. Of course this means that acetals and ketals are interfering substances in the oximation analysis of aldehydes and ketones.

Hydrazone Formation. The product of the condensation reaction between a carbonyl compound and a hydrazine is called a hydrazone. Of the many

$$R-\overset{\displaystyle O}{\overset{\|}{C}}-R' + R''NHNH_2 \rightleftharpoons R-\overset{\displaystyle N-NHR''}{\overset{\|}{C}}-R' + H_2O \qquad (22.11)$$

volumetric analyses that have been based upon this reaction, apparently the most successful employs unsymmetrical dimethylhydrazine, $(CH_3)_2N-NH_2$, as the reagent [5]. The reaction is carried out with excess reagent. The excess is back-titrated with standard acid, using a potentiometric titration.

The hydrazones of aromatic aldehydes are practically nonbasic, so the method as described is suitable for the analysis of these compounds. The hydrazones of aliphatic aldehydes are noticeably basic, although less basic than dimethylhydrazine, so the potentiometric titration curve shows successive breaks representing the titration first of the excess reagent and then of the product. The hydrazones of ketones are quite basic and cannot be potentiometrically distinguished from the reagent. Therefore when this method is applied to a ketone the titration merely yields the total amount of reagent initially added.

Because of these varied responses, the dimethylhydrazone method is not applicable to the determination of ketones, but aldehydes can be analyzed. Moreover, aromatic (but not aliphatic) aldehydes can be determined in the presence of ketones. Another advantage of this method follows from the basic medium in which the reaction is conducted, for acetals and ketals are not hydrolyzed under alkaline conditions. Thus these compounds do not interfere in the analysis of aldehydes by this method.

$$RR'C=O + H_2NNH-C_6H_3(NO_2)_2 \longrightarrow RR'C=NNH-C_6H_3(NO_2)_2 + H_2O \qquad (22.12)$$

An accurate gravimetric analysis of aldehydes and ketones is based on their conversion to the corresponding 2,4-dinitrophenylhydrazones. 2,4-Dinitrophenylhydrazones are insoluble, colored, crystalline derivatives. They are easily isolated and weighed, and the high molecular weight of the hydrazone permits the analysis of relatively small samples. A sample containing about 4×10^{-4} mole of carbonyl is adequate for the analysis [5]. The hydrazone formation is carried out in acid solution (so acetals and ketals also can be determined in this way), and the mixture is filtered through a tared filter, which is then weighed. Pharmaceutical preparations of ketosteroids can be assayed with this technique. The method is quite specific, with most classes of compounds presenting no interference.

When alkali is added to a solution of a 2,4-dinitrophenylhydrazone, a wine red color is produced, probably as a result of resonance delocalization of the negative charge resulting from removal of a proton. This color provides

$$R{-}CH{=}N{-}N^{-}{-}C_6H_3(NO_2)_2 \longleftrightarrow R{-}CH{=}N{-}N{=}C_6H_3(NO_2){=}NO_2^{-}$$

a very sensitive spectrophotometric assay for aldehydes and ketones. The hydrazone is formed in acid solution, the mixture is made basic, and the absorbance is measured at 480 nm against a blank treated in the same way. The molar absorptivities of the 2,4-dinitrophenylhydrazones of practically all monocarbonyl compounds are essentially identical, with $\epsilon = 2.72 \times 10^4$.

This colorimetric method has been applied to the determination of traces of carbonyls in aqueous solutions and in organic solvents. A chromatographic separation of carbonyls as their 2,4-dinitrophenylhydrazones is described in Experiment 17.1.

Condensations with Active Methylene Compounds. Equation 22.13, which is analogous to Eq. 22.5, shows a carbonyl condensation in which the attacking nucleophile is a carbon atom. This carbanion can be derived from a molecule

$$>C{=}O + {-}\bar{C}H{-} \longrightarrow {-}C(O^{-}){-}CH{-} \longrightarrow {-}C(OH){-}CH{-} \longrightarrow >C{=}C< \qquad (22.13)$$

possessing a methylene group flanked by two electron-withdrawing groups. Many important reactions fit this general pattern. Very often highly conjugated products, which absorb visible light, are formed, and these reactions are used to detect (e.g., in spot tests or on TLC plates) or to determine (spectrophotometrically) aldehydes and ketones. Some of the reagents that have been used in this way are dimedon, **7**; thiobarbituric acid, **8**; 4-nitrophenylacetonitrile,

9; and malononitrile, **10**. The first two reagents react with aldehydes and the last two give colors with quinones.

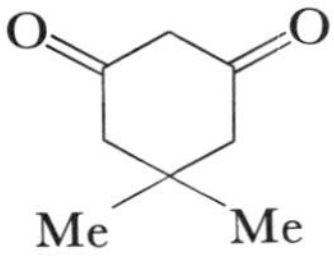

O O

Me Me

7

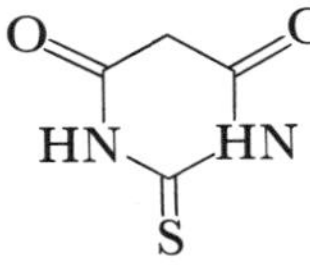

O O

HN HN

S

8

$O_2N-C_6H_4-CH_2-CN$

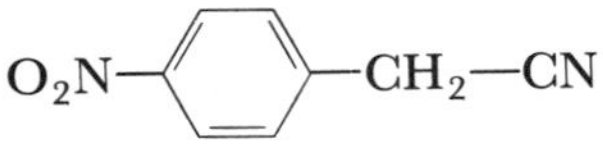

9

$CH_2(CN)_2$

10

22.2 Other Methods

Bisulfite Addition. Bisulfite adds across the carbonyl double bond. A

$$R-\overset{\overset{\displaystyle O}{\|}}{C}-R' + HSO_3^- \rightleftharpoons R-\underset{\underset{\displaystyle SO_3^-}{|}}{\overset{\overset{\displaystyle OH}{|}}{C}}-R' \qquad (22.14)$$

carbon to sulfur bond is formed. Aldehydes undergo this reaction readily. Methyl ketones and alicyclic ketones also add bisulfite, though rather slowly, and bulkier ketones are even less reactive. Only aldehydes ordinarily can be determined in this way.

Bisulfite is quite unstable, so the preferred procedure utilizes an excess of sodium sulfite, Na_2SO_3, to which is added, just prior to the sample introduction, a known volume of standard sulfuric acid. After the addition reaction is complete, the excess bisulfite is back-titrated to sulfite with alkali. The large excess of sulfite helps to maintain the addition equilibrium far to the right as the excess bisulfite is titrated [5].

Oxidation Methods. Aldehydes can be oxidized to the corresponding carboxylic acid; ketones do not undergo this reaction. Silver oxide is the oxidizing agent in one such method.

$$R-CHO + Ag_2O \rightarrow RCOOH + 2Ag$$

In one procedure the reagent is prepared by mixing silver nitrate and sodium hydroxide solutions; the precipitated silver oxide is dissolved by forming an ammonia complex. (This solution is called Tollen's reagent.) This reagent is unstable, and the decomposed solution may explode violently, so it should always be discarded after use.

An aldehyde is determined by adding an excess of Tollen's reagent. The appearance of a silver mirror or brown turbidity is a sign of reaction. After the oxidation is complete, the excess silver is determined by titration with potassium iodide. An improved reagent has been developed that employs *tert*-butylamine rather than ammonia as the complexing agent [5].

Acids, acetals, and ketones do not interfere in this method. Halides, of course, must be absent from the sample.

Another approach to the silver oxide method involves oxidation of the aldehyde with solid Ag_2O. The analysis is completed either by titrating the acid produced with standard alkali or by redissolving the unreacted silver oxide and titrating it with thiocyanate.

A solution of potassium mercuric iodide will oxidize aldehydes.

$$\text{R—CHO} + K_2HgI_4 + 3KOH \rightarrow RCOOK + Hg + 4KI + 2H_2O$$

The reagent composition is critical, and the recommended preparation is referred to as "mercural reagent" to distinguish it from Nessler's reagent [5]. The sample is added to the mercural reagent and oxidation is allowed to occur. Agar is then added to disperse the mercury metal. Iodine is added to oxidize the mercury, and the excess iodine is back-titrated with standard thiosulfate. A blank determination is carried out, and the difference in titration volumes between the blank and sample is a measure of the aldehyde content of the sample.

Most acids, ketones, esters, acetals, alcohols, and ethers do not interfere in this method.

Experiment 22.1. Determination of Carbonyl Compounds by Oximation

INTRODUCTION

The principle of the oximation method has been discussed in Section 22.1. There it was pointed out that incomplete conversion of the carbonyl to the oxime is a limitation of the method. Most aldehydes and unhindered ketones can be determined however. It is advisable always to carry out test analyses on a pure sample before applying this method to a new compound, in order to establish its applicability.

The procedure involves adding an accurately weighed sample containing about 2 meq of carbonyl to about 9 meq of hydroxylamine hydrochloride in aqueous solution. If the sample is not fully soluble in the aqueous medium, 20% of ethanol is incorporated. Because most carbonyls are quite volatile, the reaction is carried out in tightly closed flasks; volumetric flasks are convenient for this purpose.

The time required for the reaction to reach its equilibrium position of course depends upon the structure of the sample compound and upon the temperature of the solution. For reactive compounds (for example, acetone, acetaldehyde, formaldehyde) 15 min at room temperature is sufficient. Slower reacting carbonyls may require 15–30 min at 60–70°C. There seems to be no harm in extending the reaction time beyond the period required to reach equilibrium.

After reaction is complete, bromphenol blue indicator is added and the solution is titrated with standard alkali. The end point color change is not abrupt, so it is not possible to titrate accurately to the color change. Rather a blank solution is prepared with 7 meq of hydroxylamine hydrochloride in the same volume as the sample solution at the end point. The color of the sample solution is matched to that of the blank. With care and some experience a precision of 0.5–1.0% can be achieved. If desired, potentiometric detection of the end point can be employed.

Among the compounds that can be successfully analyzed are acetone, formaldehyde, acetaldehyde, methyl ethyl ketone, benzaldehyde, cyclopentanone, and vanillin. Acetophenone does not react completely, but it is found that if the titration is carried out very slowly until a permanent end point color is obtained, the equilibrium will be drawn completely to the right, and quantitative recoveries are attainable. This is not entirely satisfactory, however, for it is a laborious procedure (the titration takes about one-half hour). Camphor cannot be determined by the oximation procedure given here.

REAGENTS

0.3 N Hydroxylamine Hydrochloride. Dissolve about 21 g of reagent grade hydroxylamine hydrochloride (hydroxylammonium chloride) in water to make 1 liter.

0.1 N Sodium Hydroxide. Prepare and standardize as in Experiment 1.1.

Bromphenol Blue Solution. Prepare a 2% solution of bromphenol blue in ethanol.

PROCEDURES

Sample Treatment. Add 30 ml of 0.3 *N* $NH_2OH{\cdot}HCl$ and 20 ml of water to a 50 ml volumetric flask. Apply silicone stopcock grease to the stopper, and place it in the flask. Accurately weigh the stoppered flask and its contents. From a dropper or a pipet deliver about 2 meq of acetone into the flask, being careful not to touch the grease with the sample. Immediately stopper the flask tightly and reweigh it. The exact weight of the sample is obtained by difference. Mix the solution and allow it to stand for 15 min at room temperature.

Quantitatively transfer the solution, with the aid of 20 ml of water, to an Erlenmeyer flask. Add 1 drop of bromophenol blue solution and titrate with standard 0.1 *N* NaOH until the light blue color denoting the end point exactly matches the color of the blank.

Blank Treatment. Into a flask of the same size as the one used for the sample place 23 ml of 0.3 *N* $NH_2OH \cdot HCl$, 67 ml of water, and 1 drop of bromphenol blue solution. Titrate with 0.1 *N* NaOH to the light blue color. The indicator will pass through several shades of blue, and it is not particularly important which shade is selected as the end point. What is important is that the sample be titrated until its color exactly matches that of the blank. The two solutions should be placed side by side, with a light background, to facilitate the comparison.

The blank titration volume should be about 0.5 ml.

Calculation. Subtract the blank titration volume from the sample titration volume, and multiply by the normality of the alkali to find the number of milliequivalents of HCl produced in the oximation reaction. This is equal to the milliequivalents of acetone present in the sample. Calculate the percent purity of the acetone.

Unknown Sample. Obtain from your instructor a sample of a carbonyl compound. Analyze the sample by the oximation method and report the percent purity or the percent carbonyl (C=O) in the sample, as the instructor directs.

If the compound is not water soluble, prepare the sample mixture with 30 ml of reagent, 10 ml of water, and 10 ml of ethanol. It is essential that ethanol be included in the blank also. Since it is important that the blank and sample solutions have approximately the same concentration of hydroxylamine hydrochloride at the end point, try to adjust the sample size so that it contains close to 2 meq of carbonyl.

If your sample contains vanillin, which is a volatile solid, the preferred manner of preparing the sample is to add the sample to the dry, tared flask, reweigh, and immediately add the reagent.

References

1. Jencks, W. P., *J. Am. Chem. Soc.*, **81,** 475 (1959).
2. Higuchi, T. and C. H. Barnstein, *Anal. Chem.*, **28,** 1022 (1956).
3. Fritz, J. S., S. S. Yamamura, and E. C. Bradford, *Anal. Chem.*, **31,** 260 (1959).
4. Schenk, G. H., *Organic Functional Group Analysis*, Pergamon Press, Oxford, 1968, Chap. 1.
5. Siggia, S., *Quantitative Organic Analysis via Functional Groups*, 3rd ed., John Wiley and Sons, New York, 1963, Chap. 2.

Problems

1. 0.350 g of methyl ethyl ketone was treated with excess hydroxylamine hydrochloride and the liberated HCl was titrated with 27.60 ml of 0.1205 *N* NaOH; a blank consumed 0.45 ml of the alkali. Calculate the percent purity of the sample.

2. (*a*) Calculate the molecular weight increase resulting from the formation of the 2,4-dinitrophenylhydrazone of acetone.

(*b*) One gram of acetone will produce what weight of its 2,4-dinitrophenylhydrazone?

(*c*) One milliter of an aqueous solution of acetone was reacted with 2,4-dinitrophenylhydrazine and the resulting hydrazone was collected and dried. It weighed 0.5950 g. What was the acetone concentration in the sample solution?

3. Devise practical methods for the quantitative analysis of these mixtures.

(*a*) Acetone, isopropyl alcohol, and isopropylamine

(*b*) Benzaldehyde and acetophenone

4. Design an experimental approach that would establish the optimum pH in the oximation method for carbonyls.

5. A solution of formaldehyde was assayed by the oximation method of Experiment 22.1. 0.2693 g of sample was treated with hydroxylamine hydrochloride and the liberated HCl was titrated with 30.15 ml of 0.1109 *N* NaOH. The blank consumed 0.48 ml of alkali. Calculate the percentage of formaldehyde in the sample solution.

6. Identify the nucleophilic carbon atoms in the reagents **7–10**.

23 CARBOXYLIC ACIDS AND THEIR DERIVATIVES

The carboxylic acid function, RCOOH, is found in many molecules used in pharmacy. Carboxylic acid esters, RCOOR′, may be regarded as the condensation product of an acid and an alcohol or phenol. Amides, RCONHR′, are condensation products of acids and amines. Imides, RCONHCOR, have two acid functions condensed with an amine. Acid chlorides, RCOCl, and acid anhydrides, $(RCO)_2O$, are condensation products of two acids. The function RCO— is called an acyl group. A key difference between the reactions of carbonyl compounds (Chapter 22) and carboxylic acid derivatives is that the latter have relatively good leaving groups bonded to the acyl group. As a result they tend to undergo reactions fitting the general equation

$$\mathrm{RCOX + HY \rightarrow RCOY + HX}$$

This is therefore variously called an acyl transfer reaction, an acylation of HY by the acylating agent RCOX, or a substitution on the acyl carbon. In contrast, carbonyls usually undergo addition reactions.

These carboxylic functional groups provide convenient and pertinent "handles" with which to analyze the compounds containing them—convenient because the groups undergo some very characteristic and straightforward reactions, and pertinent because the pharmaceutical significance of such compounds is, in many instances, directly related to the presence of these groups.

23.1 Acid-Base Titrimetry

Carboxylic Acids and Their Salts. Most carboxylic acids have pK_a values in the range 3–6, and are therefore strong enough to be titrated accurately in aqueous solution with visual detection of the end point. The theory and practice of such titrations, and the relationships of chemical structure to acid strength, were discussed in Chapter 1. Potentiometric titration (Chapter 6) is recommended when titrating weaker acids, and is always advisable when developing a titrimetric analysis of an acid of unknown strength.

Since many carboxylic acids are but slightly soluble in water, it is common practice to use ethanol-water mixtures as titration media. The same titration principles apply in these solvent systems. However, the pH meter standardized against the aqueous standard buffers have no absolute significance, though they are valid in relative terms. For example, a "pH" of 4.0 determined in this way in 75% ethanol cannot be interpreted to mean that $[H^+] = 10^{-4}\ M$ in this solution, but it does mean that $[H^+]$ in this solution is 10 times its value in a similar solution of "pH" 5.0. It is usually preferable to record potential in millivolts rather than in apparent pH units when titrating in mixed solvents.

The salts of carboxylic acids are of course weak bases; their base strength is readily calculated from the pK_a of the conjugate acid: $pK_b = pK_w - pK_a$. Since most carboxylic acids have pK_a values in the range 3–6, their salts have pK_b values of 8–11. They are therefore very weakly basic, and their titration with strong acid is feasible only in fairly concentrated solution. Visual end point detection is preferably achieved by matching the indicator color in the titration solution to the color of a reference solution prepared to have the same composition.

The purity of an acid is often expressed in terms of its *neutralization equivalent*, which is simply its equivalent weight with respect to titration with strong base. Another quantity sometimes used, especially in characterizing fats and other complex mixtures, is the *acid number* (acid value), which is defined as the number of milligrams of potassium hydroxide required to neutralize the free acid in 1 g of sample.

These substances can also be titrated in nonaqueous solvents, as described in Chapter 2. Because carboxylic acids are strong enough to be accurately titrated in water, there is little advantage (other than their better solubility behavior) in analyzing them by nonaqueous titrimetry. Nevertheless, this is a perfectly feasible method and it is very accurate. The alkali methoxide and tetraalkylammonium hydroxide titrants are used in combination with neutral or basic solvents.

The analysis of carboxylate salts is greatly facilitated by titration as bases in nonaqueous media. Few of these compounds are sufficiently basic to be conveniently titrated in water, but in acidic solvents they behave as strong bases. For nearly all such analyses the solvent to be preferred is glacial acetic acid, with acetous perchloric acid as the titrant. Indicators are suggested in Chapter 2. Potentiometric titration may be utilized (see Experiment 2.1).

Amides. Amides are very weak bases, relative to amines, because of the electron-withdrawing ability of the acyl group (see Eqs. 2.9 and 2.10).

Amides can be titrated as bases in acetic anhydride as the solvent [1]. Potentiometric titration is used to detect the end point.

Imides. With the introduction of two acyl groups on a molecule of ammonia, the electron density on the nitrogen atom is reduced to a level permitting the remaining hydrogen to dissociate; that is, imides are weak acids (see Eq. 2.11). They can be titrated effectively in nonaqueous media with techniques given in Chapter 2. Many important drugs are cyclic imides; these include glutethimide (see Experiment 18.2), the hydantoins, and the barbituric acid derivatives (structures **1** and **2** in Chapter 2).

23.2 Saponification of Esters

Principles. A carboxylic ester can be hydrolyzed to its constituent acid and alcohol (or phenol).

$$\mathrm{RCOOR' + H_2O \rightarrow RCOOH + R'OH}$$

As the basis for an analytical method this reaction, as written, is not satisfactory, because the equilibrium may not lie sufficiently far to the right and because the hydrolysis in pure water is too slow. The reaction is catalyzed by acid and by base, however, thus allowing the kinetic limitation to be overcome. Moreover, in alkaline solution the acid produced is converted to the conjugate base, and this secondary reaction shifts the equilibrium completely to the right. For these reasons the hydrolysis of an ester, as a means for analyzing it, is always carried out in strong alkali. The reaction is written

$$\mathrm{RCOOR' + OH^- \rightarrow RCOO^- + R'OH} \tag{23.1}$$

and the process is referred to as *saponification* (soap making) because soaps, which are alkali salts of fatty acids, are made by hydrolyzing the glyceryl esters of fatty acids in a lye solution.

The analytical method involves the addition of a known excess volume of standard alkali to the ester sample, heating if necessary to ensure complete hydrolysis, and back-titration of the excess alkali with standard acid; by using phenolphthalein or a similar indicator, the end point of the back-titration represents the titration of all excess alkali but of none of the carboxylate salt. Each ester group consumes one hydroxide, so the titration data permit calculation of the ester groups in the sample. If a blank determination is made, it is not necessary to know the normality of the alkali; the reasoning behind this calculation is presented in Experiment 23.1.

The analytical results can be presented in terms of sample purity or weight of ester. Another quantity frequently employed, especially when characterizing new compounds, is the *saponification equivalent*, which is the equivalent weight with respect to saponifiable groups. A sample with a poorly defined composition may be described by its *ester value;* this is the number of milligrams of potassium hydroxide required to saponify the esters in 1 g of sample. The ester value is a convenient quantity to describe fats and oils, which are mixtures of glyceryl esters. The *saponification value* is the number of milligrams of potassium hydroxide required to neutralize the free acids and saponify the esters in a 1 g sample.

Mechanism of Ester Hydrolysis. Functional group methods of analysis are usually developed empirically, and for their normal application an intimate knowledge of the reaction characteristics in these methods is not necessary. Such detailed knowledge could, however, lead to more efficient assay methods and a rational selection of reaction conditions [2]. It is from this practical point of view that we shall consider the mechanism of the alkaline hydrolysis of esters.

Much study of this reaction has led to the following formulation of the mechanism [3]:

$$\mathrm{R{-}\overset{\overset{\delta^-}{O}\,\|}{\underset{\delta^+}{C}}{-}OR' + OH^- \rightleftharpoons R{-}\overset{O^-}{\underset{OH}{C}}{-}OR'}$$

$$\mathrm{R{-}\overset{O^-}{\underset{OH}{C}}{-}OR' \longrightarrow R{-}\overset{O}{\overset{\|}{C}}{-}OH + R'O^-}$$

$$\mathrm{R'O^- + H_2O \rightleftharpoons R'OH + OH^-}$$

$$\mathrm{RCOOH + OH^- \rightleftharpoons RCOO^- + H_2O}$$

In the first step, the strong nucleophile hydroxide ion attacks the electrophilic carbonyl carbon, in a reversible reaction, to give a tetrahedral intermediate. This intermediate can break down to the products. The subsequent acid-base equilibria are very fast and do not affect the rate of the overall hydrolysis reaction, which is controlled by the first two steps. The sum of these four reactions gives the saponification reaction, Eq. 23.1.

Note that an ester can conceivably be cleaved at either of two places, as shown in structure **1**. Cleavage at the bond labeled Ac is called acyl-oxygen

$$\mathrm{R{-}\overset{O}{\overset{\|}{C}}\underset{Ac}{\vdots}O\underset{Al}{\vdots}R'}$$

1

cleavage, and that at the other point is alkyl-oxygen cleavage. Nearly all esters undergo alkaline hydrolysis with acyl-oxygen cleavage, as shown in the sequence of reaction steps above. (If the alkyl group can separate off as a relatively stable carbonium ion, R'^{+}, then alkyl-oxygen cleavage is possible, and the above mechanism does not apply.)

Several predictions can be made, on the basis of this mechanistic scheme, concerning the reactivity of esters.

1. The introduction of electronegative (electron-withdrawing) groups into R and R′ will increase the rate of alkaline hydrolysis by reducing the electron density at the carbonyl carbon and thus favoring attack by the incoming nucleophile. This effect should be more pronounced with a group introduced into the acyl function (R) than in the alkyl function (R′), because R is in direct linkage with the carbonyl group, while R′ is "buffered" from it by the alkyl oxygen. Electron-donating groups in R and R′ will decrease the reaction rate by increasing the electron density at the carbonyl group. Actual charges will be especially effective in aiding or hindering the approach of the hydroxide ion.
2. Bulky R and R′ groups will decrease the rate of hydrolysis by interfering with the attacking nucleophile.
3. An acyl function that can interact with the carbonyl group by direct resonance conjugation (for example, an aromatic ring) will tend to stabilize it and thus decrease the reactivity of the ester.
4. The greater the stability of the "leaving group," $R'O^-$, the more readily the intermediate will break down into products instead of returning to the reactants. The stability of $R'O^-$ is measured by the pK_a of the conjugate acid R′OH, because the stronger R′OH is as an acid, the weaker $R'O^-$ is as a base, and therefore the greater its stability, in the present sense.

Extensive investigations have shown that the rate of alkaline ester hydrolysis can be described by

$$\text{Rate} = k[\text{ester}][\text{OH}^-] \tag{23.2}$$

where the brackets signify molar concentration, k is a constant of the system called the rate constant, and the rate is expressed in moles of ester hydrolyzed per liter per second. The units of k are liters per mole per second. It is a relatively easy matter to evaluate k, and rate constants for the alkaline hydrolysis of some esters are listed in Table 23.1. The rate constant is a sensitive function of solvent and temperature.

Table 23.1 also includes the *relative rates* of hydrolysis, that is, the rates relative to the ethyl acetate rate, which was arbitrarily taken as unity. These figures give quantitative expression to the qualitative conclusions presented

TABLE 23.1
Rates of Alkaline Hydrolysis of Some Esters[a,b]

Ester	10^2k (liter/mole-sec)	Relative Rate
Ethyl acetate	4.65	1.00
Benzyl acetate	6.99	1.50
p-Nitrobenzyl acetate	13.7	2.95
Phenyl acetate	57.6	12.4
p-Nitrophenyl acetate	805	173
Methyl benzoate	0.901	0.194
Ethyl benzoate	0.287	0.062
Methyl *p*-nitrobenzoate	64.0	13.8
Ethyl *p*-nitrobenzoate	24.4	5.25
Ethyl *p*-aminobenzoate	0.0084	0.0018

[a] At 25°C in 56% (w/w) acetone-water.
[b] Data from *Tables of Chemical Kinetics*, Circular of the National Bureau of Standards 510, (1951); Supplement 1 (1956).

earlier. Compare, for example, the relative rates of ethyl and methyl benzoates. The methyl ester hydrolyzes 3.1 times faster than the ethyl ester; the decrease in reactivity on passing from methyl to ethyl may be ascribed to the greater inductive effect of electron release of the ethyl group. The methyl ester of any acid hydrolyzes two to three times faster than the corresponding ethyl ester.

The electron-withdrawing capability of benzyl relative to ethyl probably accounts for the small increase in reactivity of benzyl acetate over ethyl acetate. The much greater reactivity of phenyl acetate is probably due to the greater stability of the leaving group—phenols are much stronger acids than are alcohols—as proposed in point 4 above. The potent effect of an electron-withdrawing substituent is shown nicely by several pairs of rates in Table 23.1. The ratios of the rate constants for the *p*-nitro substituted and unsubstituted members of some esters are as follows:

$$\frac{p\text{-Nitrobenzyl acetate}}{\text{Benzyl acetate}} \qquad 2.0$$

$$\frac{p\text{-Nitrophenyl acetate}}{\text{Phenyl acetate}} \qquad 14$$

$$\frac{\text{Methyl } p\text{-nitrobenzoate}}{\text{Methyl benzoate}} \qquad 71$$

$$\frac{\text{Ethyl } p\text{-nitrobenzoate}}{\text{Ethyl benzoate}} \qquad 85$$

These four ratios are in accord with the earlier statements. Thus the electronegative nitro group increases the reactivity of benzyl acetate by a factor of two. The same group enhances the reactivity of phenyl acetate by 14-fold because of its much greater effect on the stability of the leaving group; alternatively this marked effect could be ascribed to a resonance interaction with the carbonyl group, increasing its positive character as in **2**. Probably

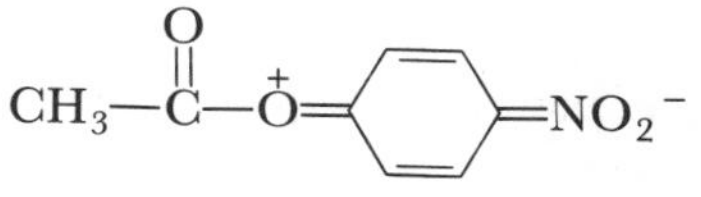

$$CH_3-\overset{\overset{\displaystyle O}{\|}}{C}-\overset{+}{O}{=}\langle\text{ring}\rangle{=}NO_2^-$$

2

both effects are operative. Comparing a *p*-nitrobenzoate with the corresponding benzoate, we find a rate enhancement of about 80-fold; this is consistent with the expectation that a variation in the acyl portion should have a more profound effect than the same variation in the alkyl portion of the ester. The similarity of the rate effect for the methyl and ethyl esters indicates that in similar circumstances a particular group can be expected to cause similar effects.

The effect of an electron-donating group is, as expected, inhibitory, as suggested by the rates of hydrolysis of ethyl benzoate and ethyl *p*-aminobenzoate (benzocaine). The electron density at the carbonyl carbon probably is greatly increased by a contribution to the resonance hybrid by structure **3**.

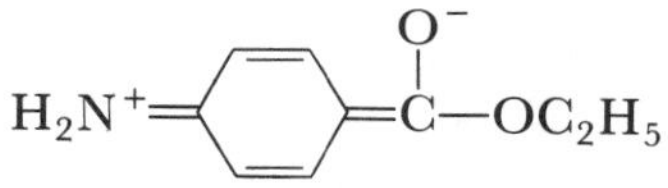

$$H_2N^+{=}\langle\text{ring}\rangle{=}\overset{\overset{\displaystyle O^-}{|}}{C}-OC_2H_5$$

3

The effect of structure on reactivity can be described quantitatively [2, 4], but such a treatment is beyond the scope of this chapter. From estimates of relative reactivity obtained with the kind of reasoning demonstrated here, one may anticipate special problems before they arise. The usual difficulty in saponification analyses is an incomplete hydrolysis of the sample. When the structure of the ester suggests very refractory behavior toward hydrolysis, suitable modification of the reaction conditions can be made.

Saponification Conditions. Water has a limited usefulness as the solvent in a saponification because few esters are soluble in water. For this reason alcohols are usually employed as the reaction medium, methanol, ethanol, or the propanols being satisfactory. Potassium hydroxide is preferred to sodium hydroxide because it is more soluble in these solvents.

The rate of the saponification reaction is shown by Eq. 23.2 to be directly proportional to the alkali concentration. This relationship suggests that the rate can be increased to any convenient value simply by increasing the alkali concentration. Within limits this is true, but it must be remembered that reasonable analytical accuracy requires that an appreciable fraction of the added alkali be consumed in the saponification. In practice, the initial alkali concentration is usually taken as 0.1, 0.5, or 1 N, depending upon the resistance to hydrolysis and the sample size.

The rate constant k in Eq. 23.2, and therefore the rate of the reaction, is a function of temperature. The rates of chemical reactions increase as the temperature increases, so the rate of saponification can be increased simply by raising the temperature of the solution. As a rough approximation, the rate may be expected to double for a 10° (C) rise in temperature. The reaction is carried out under reflux conditions, so the boiling point of the solution sets the upper limit to the attainable temperature. Amyl alcohol or diethylene glycol are preferred solvents for the saponification of very resistant esters because of their high boiling points. The increase in rate achieved by selecting a solvent with a higher boiling point is partly offset by the decrease in rate observed when the solvent polarity is decreased. In fact, with the single limitation of its poor capability as a solvent for esters, water is a very good solvent for saponification assays. Dimethyl sulfoxide (DMSO) is an excellent saponification solvent [5, 6].

Lactones, which are internal esters with the general structure **4**, are quite

$$\begin{array}{lcl} CH_2 & \text{---} & C{=}O \\ | & & | \\ (CH_2)_n & \text{---} & O \end{array}$$

4

labile and seldom require special treatment. They may even be titrated directly with alkali, the hydrolysis occurring rapidly at room temperature, as if they were in the unesterified form. Acid anhydrides and acid halides are also hydrolyzed readily and can be analyzed by alkaline hydrolysis.

23.3 The Ferric Hydroxamate Colorimetric Method

Although saponification provides a satisfactory analysis of macro, semi-micro, and micro *amounts* of esters, it is not satisfactory for the analysis of very low *concentrations* of esters. Some compounds containing the ester group absorb ultraviolet light strongly, and their solutions can be determined spectrophotometrically, but such absorption is a characteristic not of the ester function but of the rest of the molecule. A colorimetric method has been developed for carboxylic acid derivatives in general. This analysis is based on reaction with hydroxylamine to form hydroxamic acids. Equation 23.3

illustrates the reaction with an ester as the sample compound. Hydroxamic

$$\mathrm{R{-}\overset{\overset{\displaystyle O}{\|}}{C}{-}OR' + NH_2OH \rightleftharpoons R{-}\overset{\overset{\displaystyle O}{\|}}{C}{-}NHOH + R'OH} \qquad (23.3)$$

acids form a red-violet complex with ferric ion; the intensity of the color is proportional to the concentration of complex and therefore to the original ester concentration. The color produced on adding ferric ion to a hydroxamic acid appears to be due to a 1:1 complex (at least under the usual analytical conditions). Equation 23.4 has been suggested to describe this complex formation [7]. A solution of a hydroxamic acid prepared in the course of an

$$\mathrm{RCONHOH + Fe^{3+} \rightleftharpoons \left[\begin{array}{c} R{-}C{-}NH \\ \| \quad\;\; | \\ O \quad\; O \\ \diagdown \; \diagup \\ Fe \end{array}\right]^{2+} + H^+} \qquad (23.4)$$

analysis contains a large excess of hydroxylamine, which contributes to the instability of the ferric hydroxamate color by effecting, in an irreversible reaction, the reduction of ferric ion to ferrous ion [7].

$$2NH_2OH + 2Fe^{3+} \rightarrow 2Fe^{2+} + N_2O + 2H^+ + 2H_2O$$

In an unbuffered system the hydrogen ion produced soon inhibits further reduction. This decrease of pH has a deleterious effect on the color intensity, however, by shifting equilibrium 23.4 toward the left. The consequence of these two effects is that at some intermediate pH the color intensity should be maximal. This occurs at pH 1.4 for the ferric complexes of acethydroxamic acid and benzhydroxamic acid. Color stability of ferric hydroxamate solutions has been studied by Notari and Munson [8], who find that the stability is controlled primarily by the ratio $[Fe^{3+}]/[NH_2OH]$, which should be at least 5.

The reaction of hydroxylamine with an ester is another example of nucleophilic attack at the carbon-oxygen double bond. This reaction is base-catalyzed, and the mechanism is fairly complex [9, 10]. Esters, anhydrides, acid halides, amides, imides, lactones, and thiol esters give hydroxamic acids with an alkaline hydroxylamine reagent. Carboxylic acids themselves do not react under these conditions, so they do not interfere in the analysis of their derivatives; this is often an advantage of the method. Under analytical conditions the molar absorptivity of the ferric hydroxamate complex at its absorption maximum (520–540 nm) is about 1.1×10^3; the method is therefore not highly sensitive, but its generality makes it valuable. Details of the procedure are given in Experiment 23.2.

Although carboxylic acids do not form hydroxamic acids in alkaline solution, they do react in acidic solution and under the influence of nickel ion as a catalyst [11]. Acids have been determined by first converting them to the acid halide and then forming the hydroxamic acid. Alcohols have been analyzed by esterifying them and subjecting the esters to this assay. Acid hydrazides, $RCONHNH_2$, which cannot be determined with an alkaline hydroxylamine reagent, undergo conversion catalyzed by nickel [12].

23.4 Other Methods

Oxidimetric Methods. Oxalic acid and its salts can be quantitatively oxidized by titration in acidic medium with potassium permanganate; this titration was described in Chapter 5. This method is also applicable to esters of oxalic acid. Formic acid can be oxidized with alkaline permanganate. Esters of malic, citric, and tartaric acids have been titrated with permanganate. All these methods are rather limited in their applicability.

The alkali metal salts of carboxylic acids can be analyzed by a simple combustion procedure that converts the salt to the carbonate [13]. The sample, contained in a platinum boat, is ignited until all carbon traces have been burned off. The alkali carbonate is dissolved in excess standard acid, and the solution is back-titrated with alkali.

Active Hydrogen Methods. Many functional groups contain hydrogen that is reactive to Grignard reagents, RMgX. For example, alcohols react with methyl magnesium iodide to yield methane.

$$ROH + CH_3MgI \rightarrow CH_4 + ROMgI$$

This process can be thought of as an acid-base reaction, the weak acid ROH reacting with the strong base CH_3MgI to produce the very weak acid methane. According to this point of view any substance that is an appreciably stronger acid than methane will react with CH_3MgI to give methane. The hydrogen atoms that are exchanged in this reaction are called active hydrogens. Obviously carboxylic acids possess active hydrogen, as do alcohols, phenols, thiols, amines, amides, and activated methylene compounds. All these substances can be determined by reaction with excess methyl magnesium iodide and measurement of the resulting methane in a gas buret. Each gram-atom of active hydrogen provides 1 mole of methane. This active hydrogen method is known as the Zerewitinoff determination. It is evidently not very specific. Water is a particularly troublesome interference.

Numerous functional groups consume the Grignard reagent stoichiometrically, in an addition reaction, but produce no methane. Among these are aldehydes, ketones, esters, and nitriles. Esters consume 2 moles of Grignard reagent per mole, according to the overall reaction

$$RCOOR' + 2CH_3MgI \longrightarrow R\text{—}\overset{\displaystyle OMgI}{\overset{|}{C}}\text{—}(CH_3)_2 + R'OMgI$$

Compounds that add the Grignard reagent are determined by reacting them with excess reagent, adding aniline or alcohol to decompose the excess CH_3MgI, and measuring the volume of methane. Carboxylic acids exhibit special behavior with the Grignard reagent; 1 mole of reagent reacts with the active hydrogen to produce 1 mole of methane, and another mole reacts in

$$RCOOH + 2CH_3MgI \longrightarrow CH_4 + R\text{—}\overset{\displaystyle CH_3}{\overset{|}{C}}\text{—}(OMgI)_2$$

an addition. Acids can be analyzed either by measuring the methane evolved or by determining the excess reagent [4].

Lithium aluminum hydride, $LiAlH_4$, a powerful reducing agent, also has been employed in active hydrogen determinations. With this reagent molecular hydrogen is produced; the volume of H_2 gives a measure of the active hydrogen in the sample. Carboxylic acids react as shown.

$$4RCOOH + 3LiAlH_4 \rightarrow LiAl(OCH_2R)_4 + 2LiAlO_2 + 4H_2$$

As with the Grignard reagent, the nonspecificity of the lithium aluminum hydride reaction is a major disadvantage.

Reduction of Amides. A fairly general method for amides involves their reduction to the amine with lithium aluminum hydride, the carbonyl group being reduced to a methylene group [15].

$$RCONH_2 \xrightarrow{LiAlH_4} RCH_2NH_2$$

The amine is steam distilled into acid, and the excess acid is back-titrated with standard alkali. Many unsubstituted, monosubstituted, and disubstituted amides have been analyzed with this procedure. Succinimide can be determined successfully, but urea cannot be analyzed. Although many substances react with lithium aluminum hydride (that is, all active hydrogen compounds), thus consuming the reagent, very few of these lead to the production of volatile bases. Nitriles and aliphatic nitro compounds give amines on reduction with $LiAlH_4$, and these compounds will interfere with amide determination by this technique.

Hydrolysis of Amides. Any amide or imide can be determined by the Kjeldahl method (Chapter 19), but this is not properly classed as a functional group method because it is general for most nitrogen-containing compounds. Amides can be determined by saponification, as for esters, but the method is not widely used because amides are relatively resistant to hydrolysis. Unsubstituted amides ($RCONH_2$) and carbamates ($ROCONH_2$) have been analyzed by subjecting them to alkaline hydrolysis and then measuring the resulting ammonia by one of the methods described in Section 19.2.

The penicillins are both amides and β-lactams, as shown by the general structure **5**. The several kinds of penicillins vary in the nature of the R group. Penicillin can be inactivated by hydrolytic cleavage of the lactam ring under the catalytic influence of alkali or the specific enzyme penicillinase. The product is penicilloic acid, **6**. Although the intact penicillin molecule does

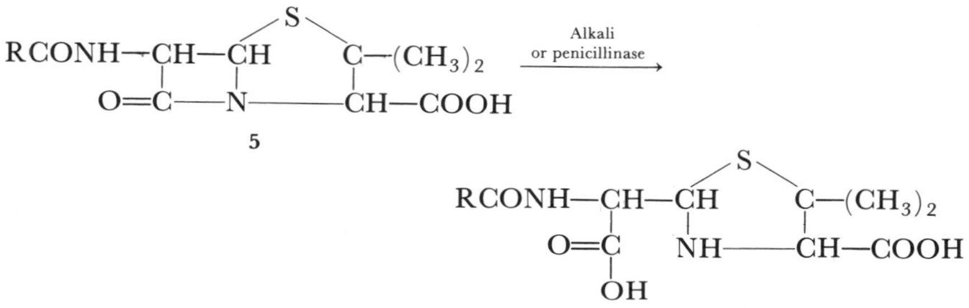

```
                     S
                   /   \
RCONH—CH—CH          C—(CH3)2        Alkali
       |   |          |          or penicillinase
     O=C——N——————————CH—COOH     ———————————————→

           5
                                      S
                                    /   \
                   RCONH—CH—CH            C—(CH3)2
                          |   |           |
                        O=C   NH——————————CH—COOH
                          |
                          OH
                                     6
```

not consume iodine, penicilloic acid does. An iodometric assay takes advantage of this behavior [16]. The following steps are involved: two identical aliquots of an aqueous solution of the penicillin are transferred to separate flasks. To one, the sample, is added sodium hydroxide or penicilinase; after a waiting period an excess of iodine solution is added. The excess iodine is back-titrated with thiosulfate. To the other, the blank, iodine is added directly, without the initial inactivation step; the iodine is back-titrated with thiosulfate. The difference in the volumes of iodine solution consumed is related to the penicillin content of the aliquot.

The blank determination and the inactivation step make the method quite specific, and it is an excellent assay for total penicillins in a pharmaceutical sample. The stoichiometry of the iodine consumption is dependent upon the reaction conditions (in particular, on the pH and the concentration of iodide in the iodine solution), however, so a theoretical stoichiometry cannot be assumed in calculating the analytical results. About 8 equivalents of iodine are consumed per mole of penicillin; the exact equivalence must be ascertained by analyzing a pure sample of penicillin under the same conditions used for the unknown. The procedure is used in Experiment 23.3.

Experiment 23.1. Quantitative Saponification of Esters

PRINCIPLE

The theory of the saponification method was discussed in Section 23.2. It appeared from that discussion that it is only necessary to add excess standard

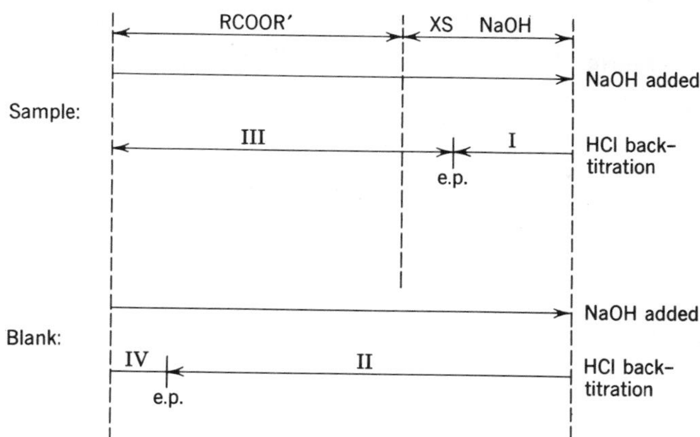

Fig. 23.1. Titration diagram for an ester saponification with blank determination.

alkali, reflux to complete the saponification, and back-titrate with acid. The difference between equivalents of alkali added and equivalents of acid taken in the back-titration is equal to the equivalents of ester in the sample. This procedure is, in fact, adequate for most samples. It can be refined, however, by including a blank determination.

The simple procedure just outlined assumes that alkali is consumed only by the ester. This may not be a valid assumption, especially if the alkali concentration is rather low or if the period of reflux is long, for alkali can be consumed by the glass surface of the reaction vessel and by carbon dioxide absorbed from the atmosphere. These sources of error are minimized by performing a blank analysis. The nature of the determination, and the calculations required, are seen easily with the aid of the titration diagram in Fig. 23.1 of the type introduced in Appendix A and used in Chapters 19 and 21. The lengths of the lines are proportional to milliequivalents of reactants.

If no alkali were consumed by extraneous materials, then milliequivalents of ester would equal III. This, however, is not so. Instead we find, by inspection of the diagram,

$$\text{Meq ester} = \text{III} - \text{IV}$$

which accounts for the consumption of alkali by substances other than the ester. In order to calculate III and IV, the volumes and normalities of both the alkali and acid are required.

An alternative, and simpler, calculation is available. Referring to the titration diagram we note that

$$\text{Meq ester} = \text{II} - \text{I}$$

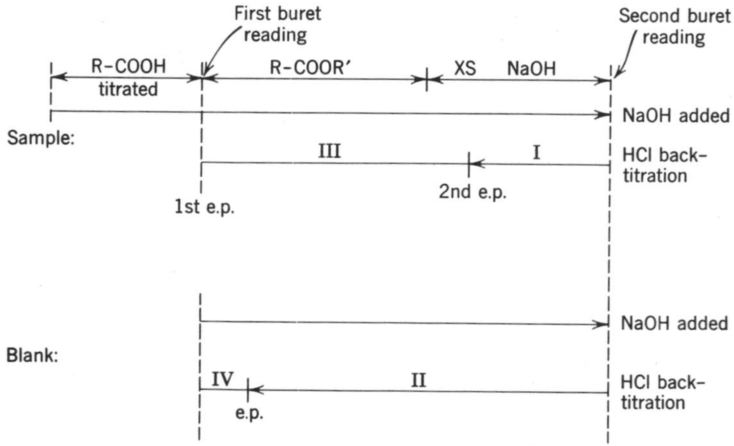

Fig. 23.2. Titration diagram for an ester saponification with blank determination and preliminary titration of free acid groups.

The quantities II and I can be calculated from a knowledge of the volumes and the normality of the acid used in the back-titrations; the normality of the alkali is unnecessary as long as the same volume of the same alkali solution is used in the sample and in the blank determinations. (In effect, the blank determination is equivalent to a standardization of the alkali under the conditions of the assay.)

If the sample contains, besides an ester, some free carboxylic acid, which may be present as a product of partial ester decomposition or may be a part of the ester molecule, a further refinement is necessary to correct for consumption of alkali by this component. Aspirin, **7**, is an important example of an ester molecule with an associated acid function. Samples of aspirin may also contain some acetic acid as a consequence of hydrolysis of the ester group.

COOH

$-OCOCH_3$

7

Aspirin can be analyzed according to the diagram in Fig. 23.1 with the exception that a preliminary titration of the free carboxyl group is made; consumption of alkali by this group is thus eliminated from the calculation. Figure 23.2 shows the manner of this determination. Some of the notes in the diagram will be explained later. Again the amount of ester is given by either of the relations

$$\text{Meq ester} = \text{III} - \text{IV}$$

or

$$\text{Meq ester} = \text{II} - \text{I}$$

In this experiment procedures will be given for a simple ester (for example, ethyl acetate) and for an ester that also possesses a carboxylic acid group (aspirin). Your instructor will ask you to perform one or the other of these determinations.

REAGENTS

0.1 N Hydrochloric Acid and 0.5 N Hydrochloric Acid. Prepare and standardize these solutions as described in Experiment 1.2.

0.1 N Sodium Hydroxide and 0.5 N Sodium Hydroxide. These solutions need not be standardized.

The 0.1 *N* reagents are used in the aspirin assay, the 0.5 *N* reagents in the ethyl acetate assay.

Phenolphthalein Solution. See Experiment 1.1.

PROCEDURES

Known Ethyl Acetate Sample. Accurately weigh about 1.5 g of ethyl acetate in a stoppered weighing bottle. Transfer the sample quantitatively, with the aid of a little water, to a 250 ml Erlenmeyer flask with a $\frac{24}{40}$ $\mathfrak{T}$ joint. Add exactly 50.0 ml of 0.5 *N* sodium hydroxide, fit a $\frac{24}{40}$ $\mathfrak{T}$ water-cooled condenser to the flask, and heat it on a water bath for 1 hr. Allow the solution to cool, add phenolphthalein indicator solution, and titrate the excess alkali with standard 0.5 *N* HCl.

Carry out a blank determination with the same quantity of alkali, omitting only the sample. Calculate the weight of ethyl acetate from the volumes of standard acid used in the sample and blank determinations. Calculate the purity of the ethyl acetate sample.

Unknown Sample. Obtain from your instructor a pure sample of an ester whose identity will be unknown to you. Using the procedure outlined for the ethyl acetate assay, determine the saponification equivalent of your ester.

Known Aspirin Assay. Accurately weigh about 500 mg of aspirin into a 250 ml Erlenmeyer flask with $\frac{24}{40}$ $\mathfrak{T}$ joint. Dissolve the sample in about 20 ml of cool alcohol (15–20°C), add phenolphthalein indicator, and immediately titrate to the end point with 0.1 N NaOH. Record the buret reading. Add to the titrated solution a volume of the 0.1 *N* NaOH equal to that consumed in the titration plus about 15 ml more. Record this second buret reading.

Fit a reflux condenser to the flask and connect a drying tube containing Ascarite to the top of the condenser. Heat the flask for 15 min, with frequent agitation, on a boiling water bath. Cool the solution to room temperature and back-titrate the excess alkali with standard 0.1 *N* HCl.

Perform a blank titration by using a volume of the 0.1 *N* NaOH equal to that between the two buret readings in the sample determination. Omit the aspirin, but otherwise repeat the procedure. Refer to the titration diagram in Fig. 23.2 for an appreciation of the volume relationships. Calculate the weight of aspirin found and the percent purity of the aspirin. Compare your result with the official requirement.

Analysis of Aspirin Tablets. Obtain a sample of aspirin tablets from the instructor. Weigh and finely powder, without loss, a counted number of at least 20 tablets. Accurately weigh a portion of the powder equivalent to about 500 mg of aspirin and analyze it exactly as described above. Calculate the average weight of aspirin per tablet.

Some aspirin tablets may contain a substance (for example, a binder or lubricant) that causes the phenolphthalein to decompose, thus rendering the second visual end point indistinct. There are two ways to overcome this undesirable effect if it should occur: (1) carry out a potentiometric back-titration; or (2) titrate one portion of the powdered sample with NaOH to the phenolphthalein end point, and use this value to calculate the volume of NaOH that would be consumed by another portion to be subjected to saponification. Add the appropriate volume of alkali to the sample portion, omitting phenolphthalein, and carry out the reflux. After the solution has cooled, add indicator and back-titrate with acid.

Experiment 23.2. Colorimetric Determination of Pilocarpine by the Ferric Hydroxamate Method

PRINCIPLE

The chemistry of the ferric hydroxamate method for carboxylic acid derivatives is discussed in Section 23.3. In this experiment pilocarpine, **8**, which is a lactone, is determined. The same procedure can be used for other

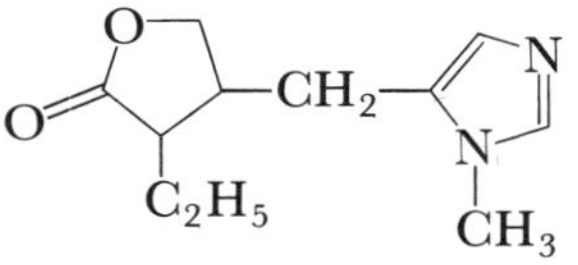

O, O, CH_2, N, N, C_2H_5, CH_3

8

carboxylic acid derivatives, but longer reaction times at the elevated temperature may be required.

REAGENTS

Hydroxylamine Solution. Dissolve 17.38 g of hydroxylamine hydrochloride in enough water to make 100 ml. This solution is 2.5 *M* in hydroxylamine.

Sodium Hydroxide Solution. Dissolve 10.80 g of sodium hydroxide in enough water to make 100 ml. This solution is 2.7 *M* in sodium hydroxide.

Ferric Perchlorate Solution. Dissolve 196.5 g of ferric perchlorate hexahydrate, $Fe(ClO_4)_3 \cdot 6H_2O$, and 21.7 ml of 60% perchloric acid in enough water to make 100 ml. This solution is 1.7 *M* in ferric perchlorate and 0.8 *M* in perchloric acid. (Ferric chloride can be used instead of the perchlorate, but it produces a higher blank absorbance.)

Pilocarpine Stock Solution. Dissolve 122 mg of pilocarpine hydrochloride in enough water to make 100 ml. This solution is 0.005 *M* in pilocarpine.

PROCEDURES

Preparation of Standard Curve. Prepare five solutions according to the following schedule (the numbers represent milliliters):

Hydroxylamine Solution	NaOH Solution	Pilocarpine Solution	Water
2.0	2.0	0	6.0
2.0	2.0	1.0	5.0
2.0	2.0	2.0	4.0
2.0	2.0	3.0	3.0
2.0	2.0	4.0	2.0

All volumes should be delivered by pipet or buret. Stoppered test tubes or 25 ml volumetric flasks are convenient vessels. The solution containing no pilocarpine is the reagent blank.

Loosely stopper the containers and place them in a water bath at about 75°C. After 4 min remove them and cool in an ice-water bath. Bring the contents to room temperature and add 15.0 ml of ferric perchlorate solution to each vessel. Store the flasks in the dark (or wrap them in aluminum foil) and after 30 min measure the absorbance of each solution, at 530 nm in a 1 cm cell, against the reagent blank as the reference. Make a Beer's law plot of absorbance against the pilocarpine concentration in the final solution. Calculate the molar absorptivity of the ferric hydroxamate complex.

Unknown Solution. From your instructor obtain a sample of a pilocarpine solution. If this is an ophthalmic solution it must be diluted 20-fold before analysis. Prepare one or more reaction solutions exactly as in the preparation of the standard curve. For best results carry out the unknown analysis at the same time as the standard curve preparation.

With the absorbance of the unknown sample determine, from the standard curve, the unknown concentration. Convert this, with the appropriate dilution factors, to the concentration of pilocarpine in the original sample solution. Report this result in w/v percent (g/100 ml).

Experiment 23.3. Iodometric Determination of Penicillin

PRINCIPLE

This method is discussed in Section 23.4. In order to achieve reproducible results it is important to pay close attention to procedural details, such as protecting iodine solutions from light and ensuring identical reaction times for the blank and sample.

The potency of a penicillin sample can be expressed in USP pencillin units. One USP unit is the antibiotic activity of 0.6 μg of USP sodium penicillin G reference standard, so 1 mg of this substance is equivalent to 1667 units. The equivalent potency of other pencillins is related to this by their molecular weights; thus 1 mg of potassium penicillin G is equivalent to 1595 units.

REAGENTS

Buffer Solution. Dissolve 60 g of potassium biphthalate and 80 ml of 1.0 *N* NaOH in enough water to make 1 liter.

Iodine Solution. Dissolve 1.3 g of iodine and 8.3 g of potassium iodide in enough water to make 1 liter. This solution, which does not have to be standardized, should be stored in the dark. It is about 0.01 *N* in iodine and 0.05 *N* in potassium iodide.

0.01 N Sodium Thiosulfate. Dissolve 2.5 g of $Na_2S_2O_3{\cdot}5H_2O$ and 2–3 g of borax in enough freshly boiled water to make 1 liter. The solution is standardized against iodine produced by reacting a known amount of dichromate with excess iodide. Accurately weigh about 2 g of dried reagent grade potassium dichromate. Add this plus 2 g of sodium bicarbonate and 10 g of potassium iodide to a 250 ml volumetric flask, dissolve all solutes in water, and dilute to volume. Immediately titrate 25.0 ml aliquots with the thiosulfate solution, adding a few drops of starch indicator shortly before the end point. Calculate the normality of the thiosulfate solution.

The dichromate-iodide solution should be used within 15 min of its preparation. The equivalent weight of potassium dichromate is 49.04 in this standardization.

Starch Indicator Solution. Make a paste of 1–2 g of soluble starch in a few milliliters of cold water. Add this to 100 ml of boiling water containing 1 g of boric acid. This solution is best prepared fresh daily.

PROCEDURES

Standard Determination. Accurately weigh about 25 mg of a pure sample of sodium or potassium penicillin G into a 50 ml volumetric flask, dissolve it in water, and dilute to volume. The entire analysis should be completed within one hour of preparing this solution. This may require careful scheduling.

Two 5.0 ml aliquots, labeled B and S, are pipetted into separate 125 ml glass-stoppered Erlenmeyer flasks. Five milliliters of buffer solution and 15.0 ml of iodine solution are added to the flask containing B. The flask is stoppered and placed in the dark for 15 min. At the end of this time the excess iodine is titrated with standard 0.01 *N* thiosulfate, starch solution being added as the indicator shortly before the end point.

To aliquot S is added 1.0 ml of 1 *N* NaOH and the flask is allowed to stand 20 min at room temperature. Then 5 ml of buffer solution and 15.0 ml of iodine solution are added, and the solution is placed in the dark for 15 min; it is then titrated with 0.01 *N* thiosulfate.

If A is the number of milliequivalents of iodine consumed by the penicillin in the 5 ml aliquot, then $A = N(V_B - V_S)$, where N is the normality of the thiosulfate and V_B and V_S are the volumes (in ml) of thiosulfate consumed in the blank and sample titrations. If w g of penicillin with molecular weight M was contained in the 5 ml aliquot, then the number of equivalents of iodine consumed per mole of penicillin is $MA/1000w$.

Another way to express the standard result is to calculate the factor F, which is the number of milliliters of 0.01 *N* iodine consumed by 1.0 mg of the standard penicillin. In terms of the above symbols, $F = A/10w$.

Unknown Sample. Obtain from your instructor a sample of penicillin G of unknown potency. Accurately weigh a portion equivalent to about 25 mg of penicillin and dissolve it in enough water to make 50.0 ml. Take 5.0 ml aliquots and assay them exactly as described for the standard.

The purity of the sample can be calculated on a chemical basis, using the empirical result from the standard determination relating equivalents of iodine consumed to amount of penicillin. Alternatively the potency of the sample, in USP units per milligram, can be calculated from the relationship

$$\text{Potency of unknown} = \text{Potency of standard} \times \frac{N(V_B - V_S)_{\text{unknown}}}{10F} \tag{23.5}$$

where F was determined in the assay of the standard penicillin.

References

1. Wimer, D. C., *Anal. Chem.*, **30,** 77 (1958).
2. Connors, K. A., *Reaction Mechanisms in Organic Analytical Chemistry*, Wiley-Interscience, New York, 1973.
3. Bender, M. L., *Mechanisms of Homogeneous Catalysis from Protons to Proteins*, Wiley-Interscience, New York, 1971.
4. Hammett, L. P., *Physical Organic Chemistry*, 2nd ed., McGraw-Hill, New York, 1970.
5. Vinson, J. A., J. S. Fritz, and C. A. Kingsbury, *Talanta*, **13,** 1973 (1966).
6. Vinson, J. A. and E. K. Hocker, *J. Chem. Educ.*, **46,** 245 (1969).
7. Aksnes, G., *Acta Chem. Scand.*, **11,** 710 (1957).

8. Notari, R. E. and J. W. Munson, *J. Pharm. Sci.*, **58,** 1060 (1969).
9. Jencks, W. P., *J. Am. Chem. Soc.*, **80,** 4581, 4585 (1958).
10. Notari, R. E., *J. Pharm. Sci.*, **58,** 1069 (1969).
11. Connors, K. A. and J. W. Munson, *Anal. Chem.*, **44,** 336 (1972).
12. Munson, J. W. and K. A. Connors, *J. Pharm. Sci.*, **61,** 211 (1972).
13. Siggia, S., *Quantitative Organic Analysis via Functional Groups*, 3rd ed., John Wiley, New York, 1963, Chap. 3.
14. Cheronis, N. D. and T. S. Ma, *Organic Functional Group Analysis by Micro and Semimicro Methods*, Interscience, New York, 1964, pp. 409–423.
15. Siggia, S. and C. R. Stahl, *Anal. Chem.*, **27,** 550 (1955).
16. Connors, K. A., Chap. VI in *Pharmaceutical Analysis*, T. Higuchi and E. Brochmann-Hanssen (eds.), Interscience, New York, 1961.

FOR FURTHER READING

Tiwari, R. D. and J. P. Sharma, *The Determination of Carboxylic Functional Groups*, Pergamon Press, Oxford, 1970.

Wimer, D. C., "Amides and Related Compounds," Chap. 9 in *Analytical Chemistry of Nitrogen and its Compounds*, Part 1, Wiley-Interscience, New York, 1971.

Hall, R. T. and W. E. Shaefer, "Determination of Esters," *Org. Anal.*, **2,** 19 (1954).

Veibel, S., "Carboxyl and Derived Functions," in *Treatise on Analytical Chemistry*, Part II, Vol. 13, I. M. Kolthoff and P. J. Elving (eds.), Interscience, New York, 1966, pp. 223–299.

Problems

1. 1.296 g of a purified ester was refluxed in 50.0 ml of a sodium hydroxide solution. The resulting solution was back-titrated to the phenolphthalein end point with 22.50 ml of 0.180 *N* HCl. A blank determination required 57.00 ml of 0.180 *N* HCl. What is the saponification equivalent of the ester?

2. 1.000 g of a sample of phenyl benzoate was refluxed for 30 min in 50.0 ml of 0.100 *N* NaOH. The excess alkali was back-titrated with 17.5 ml of 0.105 *N* HCl, but the end point was overrun, so the excess acid was finally back-titrated with 2.5 ml of the 0.100 *N* NaOH. Calculate the percent purity of the phenyl benzoate sample.

3. An unknown substance is titrated potentiometrically and is found to have $pK_a = 3.0$ and neutralization equivalent 143; it appears to be monobasic. A quantitative hydrolysis experiment gave as its saponification equivalent 145. It is optically inactive and contains no nitrogen or halogens. The compound exhibits fairly strong ultraviolet absorption around 250 nm. Write a possible structure for this compound. Is it possible to assign the structure unambiguously with this information?

4. Propose practical assay methods that will permit the quantitative determination of each component in these mixtures.
   (*a*) Ethyl benzoate, benzoic acid, and ethanol
   (*b*) Salol and aspirin
   (*c*) Salicylic acid and salicylamide

5. Draw the structure of the product resulting from the reaction of hydroxylamine with pilocarpine, **8**.

6. Derive Eq. 23.5.

7. 0.5350 g of salol (phenyl salicylate) was assayed by the saponification method as follows: 25.00 ml of 0.2150 *N* NaOH was added to the sample, and it was refluxed. After cooling, the sample was back-titrated with 28.40 ml of 0.1080 *N* HCl. A blank was carried out in the same way, 47.70 ml of the 0.1080 *N* HCl being required. Calculate the percent purity of the sample.

8. A drug (*A*) had the following properties:

(1) Melting point 128–131°

(2) Pharmacological activity: vitamin

(3) 20 mg of A was added to 5 ml of dilute sodium hydroxide solution and boiled; the odor of ammonia was obvious.

(4) Uv absorption: λ_{max} 261.5 nm, log ϵ_{max} 3.7

(5) 305.0 mg of *A* was dissolved in glacial acetic acid and titrated to the end point with 0.100 *N* perchloric acid; 24.95 ml was consumed.

(6) Compound *A* was added to dilute sodium hydroxide solution, which was boiled. After cooling, the solution was made acid with hydrochloric acid. A white precipitate, compound *B*, was produced.

Compound *B* had these properties:

(7) Mp 234–237°

(8) Pharmacological activity: vitamin

(9) 425.0 mg of *B* was dissolved in water and titrated with 34.50 ml of 0.100 *N* sodium hydroxide to the phenolphthalein end point.

Another drug *C* had these properties:

(10) Mp 22–24°C

(11) Pharmacological activity: central stimulant

(12) Drug *C* was boiled in sodium hydroxide solution; an odor of diethylamine was perceptible.

(13) 400.0 mg of *C* was titrated with 0.100 *N* perchloric acid in acetic acid, 22.45 ml being consumed.

(14) Compound *C* was boiled in dilute sodium hydroxide, cooled, and the solution acidified with hydrochloric acid. Compound *B* precipitated out.

Give possible structures of compounds *A*, *B*, and *C*.

9. For an ester known to follow Eq. 23.2, hydrolysis was essentially complete in 1 hr at pH 10.5. At what pH will the reaction proceed to the same degree of completion in 30 min?

10. Propose a mechanism for the base-catalyzed hydrolysis of an amide. Why are amides more resistant to hydrolysis than are esters?

11. How could you analyze the following tablet formulation?

Salicylanilide

Acetaminophen

Aspirin

12. Devise a good approach to the quantitative analysis, using functional group methods, of a mixture of salicylic acid, methyl salicylate, salicylamide, and salicylaldehyde.

24 AMINES

In this chapter the common functional group methods for primary amines (RNH_2), secondary amines (R_2NH), tertiary amines (R_3N), and their salts, and of quaternary ammonium compounds ($R_4N^+X^-$) are described. Many compounds useful in pharmacy contain amino groups. The alkaloids received their class name because of their basicity (alkaloid ≡ "like alkali"), which is a characteristic of the alkaloid amino function. The antihistamines are amines. Sulfonamide drugs contain an amino group, apart from the sulfonamide function, and this amino group provides a convenient analytical approach. Many more amine drugs can be named. Their analysis is obviously of great importance, and the characteristic chemical behavior of the amino function may be utilized for the analytical purpose.

24.1 Acid-Base Titration of Amines and their Salts

Aliphatic amines are basic enough to titrate with a strong acid in aqueous solution. Although the feasibility of the titration depends on the concentration of the base as well as upon its strength, the rough generalization can be given that accurate titration is possible with visual end point detection if the pK_a is 8 or greater (pK_b is 6 or smaller).* This limit can be extended by another pK unit by means of potentiometric detection of the end point. The theory and practice of these titrations were discussed in Chapter 1, where it was noted that aliphatic amines are usually strong enough, whereas aromatic amines are too weak, to titrate in aqueous solution.

Many pharmaceutically important alkaloids are titratable in aqueous solution [1]. With these substances, as with many other amines, their low solubility in water leads to the use of hydroalcoholic solvents. Alcohol does not markedly affect the sharpness of the end point break of neutral bases; this behavior will be accounted for shortly.

* Recall that $pK_a + pK_b = pK_w$ for a conjugate pair, so it is necessary to specify only pK_a or pK_b. "pK_a of an amine" really means the pK_a of its conjugate acid. The higher the pK_a (smaller K_a), the weaker the conjugate acid is, and therefore the stronger the compound is as a base.

It has been discovered [2] that titrations of very weak bases such as aromatic amines may be carried out in aqueous concentrated neutral salt solutions. Thus aniline can be accurately titrated in 8 *M* sodium iodide solution. Visual or potentiometric end point detection may be applied. The pH of the titration solution is similar in water and in the salt solution prior to the end point, but after the end point the pH in the salt solution is much lower than that in water at identical concentrations of hydrogen ion. This means that the activity of the strong acid is greater in a concentrated salt solution than in water. This effect can be accounted for qualitatively with the assumption that a large fraction of the water in a concentrated salt solution is tied up as hydration shells by the salt anions and cations; this water is not available to the acid, whose effective concentration is therefore much higher than its nominal concentration.

Titration of salts of amines (for example, amine hydrochlorides) with alkali in aqueous solution may be regarded as the titration of a weak acid with a strong base. The same considerations apply, with respect to titration feasibility, as in the titration of neutral acids. Thus the salts of aniline and of pyridine are easily titrated, whereas those of the aliphatic amines are too weakly acidic for accurate titration in aqueous solution. The addition of alcohol to the titration medium can be helpful in sharpening titration end points for these substances. The acid-base equilibrium between the acid and the neutral base forms of the amine may be written, taking methylamine as an example,

$$CH_3NH_3^+ \rightleftharpoons H^+ + CH_3NH_2$$

As the titration medium is changed from pure water to pure ethanol, the dielectric constant drops from 79 to 24. This change has little effect on the K_a of a cationic acid like $CH_3NH_3^+$, however, because no separation of charges occurs when it dissociates. Actually the pK_a of a cationic acid increases by about 1 unit on passing from water to ethanol, probably because ethanol is a weaker base than water [3]. The feasibility of the titration is governed by the titration equilibrium:

$$CH_3NH_3^+ + OH^- \rightleftharpoons CH_3NH_2 + H_2O$$

The equilibrium constant for this reaction is obviously $1/K_b = K_a/K_s$, where K_b is the base dissociation constant of methylamine and K_s is the autoprotolysis constant of the solvent. In water, therefore, the equilibrium constant for the titration reaction is about 2.4×10^3, whereas in ethanol this constant is about 2.4×10^7. Changing the solvent has made the titration perfectly feasible. Usually a hydroalcoholic medium is selected because of its desirable solubility properties.

The advantageous effect of alcohol on the titration behavior of amine salts is to be contrasted with its negligible effect on the titration characteristics of the neutral amines. The titration reaction is, for methylamine,

$$CH_3NH_2 + H^+ \rightleftharpoons CH_3NH_3^+$$

and its equilibrium constant is $1/K_a$. This value is, according to the preceding paragraph, little affected by the solvent change, so no analytical advantage ensues from adding alcohol to the titration medium.

The titration of amines in nonaqueous systems is a very favorable method of analysis. More experience has been gained with glacial acetic acid as a nonaqueous titration medium than with any other solvent. Acetic acid levels all bases whose pK_a values (in H_2O) are 4 or greater to the strength of the solvent anion. Most amines fall into this category, and these bases are readily titrated with visual detection of the end point, as explained in Chapter 2 and Experiment 2.1. Those amines with pK_a (H_2O) values in the range 2–4 cannot be titrated visually in acetic acid, but potentiometric titration of these bases is successful. Many heterocyclic amines and substituted aromatic amines fall into this class.

Differentiation of mixtures of amines by potentiometric titration is often feasible in a neutral solvent like acetonitrile or nitromethane. These solvents do not level bases, so inherent differences in base strength may be exploited for a differentiating titration. In very general terms it may be estimated that if the strengths of two bases differ by at least 3.5 pK units they may be differentiated by potentiometric titration in acetonitrile or nitromethane [4].

Amine salts can be titrated as acids in nonaqueous media, but since it is usually the amine portion of the molecule that is of pharmaceutical interest, it is this part that should be analyzed. This cannot be accomplished by direct titration with acid, because the amine is already protonated. The method proposed by Pifer and Wollish [5] provides a convenient solution to this problem. The amine salt is reacted with excess mercuric acetate, which frees the amine for titration:

$$2RNH_3X + Hg(OAc)_2 \rightarrow HgX_2 + 2RNH_2 + 2HOAc$$

Quaternary ammonium halides also can be analyzed in this way. The mercuric acetate procedure is utilized in Experiment 2.1.

24.2 Acylation of Primary and Secondary Amines

The reaction of a primary or secondary amine with an acylating agent results in the formation of an amide. Taking acetic anhydride as the acylating agent,

$$(CH_3CO)_2O + RNH_2 \rightarrow CH_3CONHR + CH_3COOH \quad (24.1)$$

$$(CH_3CO)_2O + RR'NH \rightarrow CH_3CONRR' + CH_3COOH \quad (24.2)$$

Obviously tertiary amines, which possess no replaceable hydrogen, do not undergo this reaction.

The mechanism of this reaction is identical with that already described for the acylation of hydroxy compounds (Section 21.1), and the experimental techniques are the same for amines and hydroxy compounds. Amines usually react faster than alcohols and phenols. Perchloric acid-catalyzed acylation is described in Experiment 21.1, and *p*-dimethylaminopyridine-catalyzed acylation in Experiment 21.3. The classical pyridine-catalyzed procedure is given in Experiment 24.1.

A mixture containing an alcohol and an acylable amine can be analyzed for both components by carrying out an acylation, thus giving the sum of the two, and then titrating the amine in another portion of the sample. The alcohol is found by difference. This functional group approach to mixture analysis can be applied to mixtures of amines and, indeed, to mixtures of many classes of organic compounds.

Other finishes can be combined with an acylation reaction. Thus amines can be converted to their cinnamides by acylation with *trans*-cinnamic anhydride:

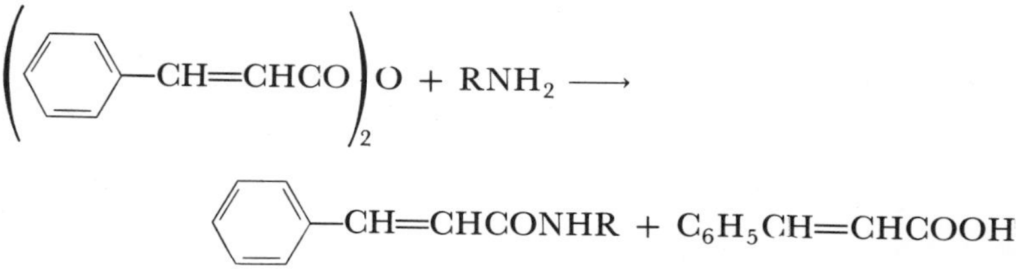

$$(C_6H_5\text{—}CH{=}CHCO)_2O + RNH_2 \longrightarrow$$

$$C_6H_5\text{—}CH{=}CHCONHR + C_6H_5CH{=}CHCOOH \qquad (24.3)$$

The amide is separated from the other reaction components by solvent extraction, and is measured by ultraviolet spectrophotometry [6]. A fluorometric method for amines reacts them with 1-dimethylaminonaphthalene-5-sulfonyl chloride, **1** (dansyl chloride), to give fluorescent sulfonamides.

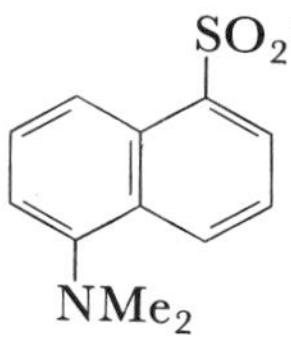

SO_2Cl

NMe_2

1

Amines can be acylated with trifluoroacetic anhydride, $(CF_3CO)_2O$, and the resulting trifluoroacetamides separated by gas chromatography [7].

24.3 Diazotization of Primary Aromatic Amines

Nitrous acid reacts with the primary aromatic amine group to produce a diazonium salt.

$$ArNH_2^+ + HNO_2 + HCl \rightarrow ArN_2^+Cl^- + 2H_2O \qquad (24.4)$$

The diazonium ion can be coupled to another aromatic molecule to produce a dye suitable for colorimetric measurement. This diazotization-coupling method for primary aromatic amines is discussed in detail in Experiment 8.1.

The diazotization reaction can serve as an analytical process via a direct titration of the amine with nitrous acid. Since nitrous acid solutions are unstable, the analysis is carried out by titrating an acidic solution of the primary aromatic amine with a sodium nitrite solution. The end point is detected with an "external" indicator; after the end point a drop of the titration solution produces a blue color on starch-iodide paste. Internal indicators have also been used [8, 9].

Nitrite titration is an important method in pharmaceutical analysis because most sulfonamide drugs are primary aromatic amines, and this is the official assay method for many of these compounds. The general structure of the sulfonamides containing the primary amine group is $H_2N—C_6H_4—SO_2NHR$. The experimental details will be found in Experiment 24.2.

Other amines will interfere with this method by consuming nitrous acid. Secondary amines form the *N*-nitroso derivatives; this reaction may be employed for the direct nitrite titration of some secondary amines [10]. Aliphatic amines produce nitrogen gas upon reaction with nitrous acid; this reaction has some value for the analysis of amino groups.

24.4 Other Methods

Methods Based on Imine Formation. Primary amines undergo condensation with carbonyls, as in Eq. 24.5, to give *imines* (Schiff bases).

$$RNH_2 + R'CHO \rightleftharpoons R'CH{=}NR + H_2O \qquad (24.5)$$

Some titrimetric methods are based on this reaction. Two of the reagents that have been used are salicylaldehyde, **2**, and 2,4-pentanedione, **3** (shown in the enol form). The carbonyl compound is reacted with the amine in pyridine

$$\underset{\mathbf{2}}{\text{(2-hydroxybenzaldehyde: } C_6H_4(CHO)(OH))} \qquad \underset{\mathbf{3}}{CH_3—\overset{\overset{O}{\|}}{C}—CH{=}\overset{\overset{OH}{|}}{C}—CH_3}$$

solvent. After imine formation is complete the excess carbonyl compound, which is acidic, is back-titrated with standard alkali methoxide solution. The method is applicable to aliphatic primary amines, alcoholamines, and amino acids, but aromatic amines cannot be determined.

Imine formation is employed to advantage in the alkalimetric titration of amino acids. These compounds exist largely in the zwitterion form in aqueous solution, and the titration reaction is

$$^{+}H_3NRCOO^- + OH^- \rightleftharpoons H_2NRCOO^- + H_2O$$

This direct titration is not very successful because of the appreciable basicity of the free amine form H_2NRCOO^-. This can be overcome by adding formaldehyde to the titration solution. As the amine is formed it reacts with the formaldehyde to form an imine, which is a very much weaker base than is the amine.

$$CH_2O + H_2NRCOO^- \rightleftharpoons H_2C{=}NRCOO^- + H_2O$$

The titration therefore proceeds as if the zwitterion were a much stronger acid than it really is. This technique is called the *formol titration.*

The same principle applies in the alkalimetric titration of ammonium salts in the presence of formaldehyde, though the product of the ammonia-formaldehyde reaction is hexamethylenetetramine (methamine, **4**) rather than an imine. This product is much weaker than is ammonia itself, so the titration reaction proceeds favorably.

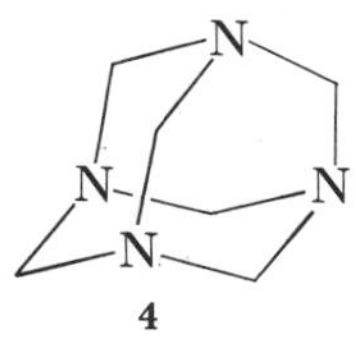

4

A colorimetric method for primary aliphatic amines utilizes their reaction with salicylaldehyde to form imines. The imine from this condensation is treated with cupric ion, which forms a cupric-imine complex. The complex is extracted from aqueous solution into *n*-hexanol. The copper in the hexanol solution is determined colorimetrically by reaction with *N,N*-di(hydroxyethyl)dithiocarbamic acid [4].

Methods Based on Nucleophilic Aromatic Substitution. In an important type of reaction an amine, functioning as a nucleophile, displaces a halide ion from an aromatic compound. Analytically the most important method based on this reaction uses 1-fluoro-2,4-dinitrobenzene (FDNB), **5**, as the reagent. The

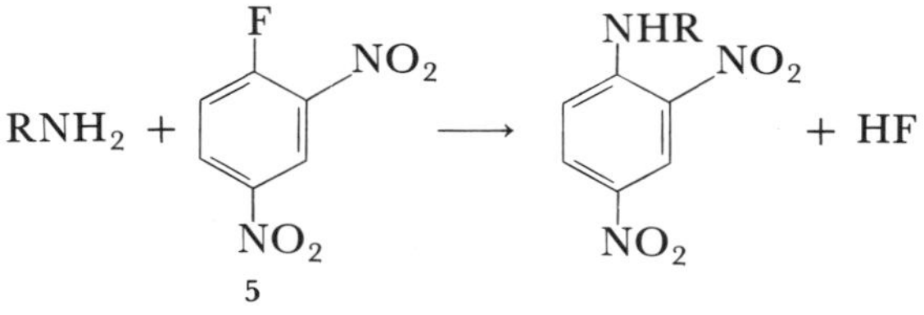

$$\mathrm{RNH_2} + \text{[2,4-dinitrofluorobenzene, } \mathbf{5}\text{]} \longrightarrow \text{[N-substituted 2,4-dinitroaniline (NHR, } NO_2, NO_2\text{)]} + \mathrm{HF} \tag{24.6}$$

resulting dinitrophenylamines can be determined spectrophotometrically [11]. Many more amine methods have been based on nucleophilic substitution [12]. Compound **6**, 9-chloroacridine, undergoes this reaction and is an effective analytical reagent for primary aromatic amines [13]; the finish is spectrophotometric.

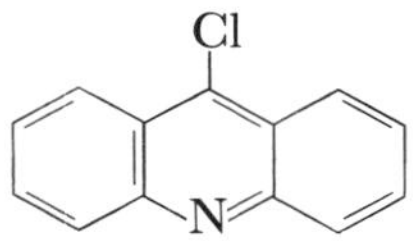

[9-chloroacridine structure: Cl, N]

6

Ion-Pair Extraction. Many amines and quaternary ammonium compounds can be determined in aqueous solution by forming a salt or ion pair between the positively charged nitrogen compound and a negatively charged dye or indicator molecule, extracting this ion pair into an organic solvent, and measuring the concentration of extracted dye spectrophotometrically [14]. Typical dyes are bromcresol purple, bromthymol blue, bromcresol green, and methyl orange. This technique is called the ion pair extraction or acid dye method. It is based on these requirements: (*a*) a stoichiometric ion pair is formed from the positively charged nitrogen compound and the negatively charged dye molecule; (*b*) this ion pair is quantitatively extracted into the organic phase; and (*c*) the uncombined dye molecule (which is added in excess) is not extracted into the organic phase.

The pH of the aqueous phase is critical to the success of the method. Since uncombined dye must not be extractable, and since to form the ion pair the dye must be in its anion form, the pH will usually be near or above the pK_a of the acid dye. On the other hand, the amine compound must be positively charged, so the pH must be acidic enough to protonate the amine. Quaternary ammonium compounds are charged at all pH's. Because of this property, it is possible to extract and determine quaternary ammonium compounds and amines in the presence of each other by suitable pH control [15, 16].

Small amounts of polar organic solvents incorporated into the organic phase can influence markedly the partition behavior of the ion pair [17]. The ion-pair phenomenon has also been used to manipulate partition behavior in the separation of amine drugs by liquid chromatography [18. 19].

Experiment 24.1. Determination of Primary and Secondary Amines by Pyridine-Catalyzed Acetylation

INTRODUCTION

Refer to Chapter 21 for a discussion of the theory of this method. The calculation required is identical with that used in Experiment 21.1. Many variations of this technique have been proposed; in this experiment the procedure of Ogg, Porter, and Willits [20] is presented. Although the method was developed for hydroxy determinations, it is directly applicable to amine analysis. Amines are acylated under relatively mild conditions; 15 min at room temperature will be adequate for the quantitative acetylation of most amines [21].

n-Butanol is added to the reaction mixture prior to titration to keep the solution homogeneous.

REAGENTS

Acetylating Reagent. Mix 10 ml of reagent grade acetic anhydride with 30 ml of reagent grade pyridine. Prepare this reagent fresh daily.

Mixed Indicator. Mix 1 part of 0.1% aqueous solution of cresol red neutralized with sodium hydroxide and 3 parts of 0.1% thymol blue neutralized with sodium hydroxide.

0.5 N Alcoholic Sodium Hydroxide. Dilute 30 ml of saturated aqueous sodium hydroxide solution to 1 liter with ethanol or methanol. Standardize this solution against primary standard potassium biphthalate, using the mixed indicator. If the standard solution throws down a precipitate on standing, it will be necessary to restandardize. Protect the solution from unnecessary exposure to the atmosphere.

PROCEDURES

Known Sample. Accurately weigh 2–4 meq of an amine (for example, *n*-butylamine, morpholine, aniline, etc.) into a glass-stoppered 250 ml Erlenmeyer flask. Pipet exactly 3.0 ml of acetylating reagent into the flask and swirl to dissolve the sample. Stopper the flask and allow the solution to stand at room temperature for about 15 min. Treat a blank in exactly the same way, omitting the sample.

Add 5 ml of water to each flask, mix well, and allow to stand 10 min to hydrolyze the excess acetic anhydride. Add 10 ml of *n*-butanol and 3 drops of mixed indicator to each flask and titrate with standard 0.5 *N* sodium hydroxide to the gray color. Match the sample and blank colors.

Calculate the weight of amine found and the percent purity of the amine.

Unknown Samples. Your instructor will give you either a pure amine whose identity is unknown to you or a solution of a known amine in pyridine, the concentration of the amine being unknown to you. Analyze the sample by pyridine-catalyzed acetylation, and report either the equivalent weight of the amine (for a pure sample) or its concentration (for a solution).

Experiment 24.2. Nitrite Titration of Primary Aromatic Amines

The chemistry of this method is discussed in Section 24.3 and Experiment 8.1. The instability of nitrous acid solutions has been pointed out. It is desirable to avoid high local concentrations of nitrous acid in the titration solution, so the solution should be well stirred. The official assay method for many sulfonamide drugs specifies nitrite titration at reduced temperature to minimize loss of nitrous acid. Most workers now agree that the titration can be carried out at room temperature without loss of the acid [22].

REAGENTS

0.1 M Sodium Nitrite. Dissolve about 7 g of sodium nitrite in 1 liter of distilled water. Standardize this solution against reagent grade sulfanilic acid that has been dried at 105°C for 4 hr. The standardization procedure is identical with the assay procedure described below.

Starch-Iodide Paste. To 100 ml of boiling water contained in a 250 ml beaker add a solution of 0.75 g of potassium iodide in 5 ml of water, then 2 g of zinc chloride dissolved in 10 ml of water, and then, while the solution is boiling, stir in a smooth suspension of 5 g of potato starch in 30 ml of cold water. Continue to boil the mixture for 2 min, then cool it. Store in a closed container in a refrigerator.

PROCEDURES

Bulk Sulfonamide Sample. Accurately weigh about 500 mg of a sulfonamide with a free amino group (for example, sulfanilamide, sulfamerazine, sulfadiazine, etc.) into a beaker. Add 20 ml of concentrated hydrochloric acid and 50 ml of water to dissolve the sample. The solution may be cooled prior to titration by the addition of 25 g of crushed ice, but this is not essential. Titrate the solution with standard 0.1 *M* sodium nitrite, keeping the buret tip immersed in the solution. As the end point is neared, titrate slowly. The end point is marked by the immediate appearance of a blue color when a glass rod dipped into the titration solution is streaked on a smear of starch-iodide paste. When the titration is complete, the end point color is reproducible after the mixture has been allowed to stand for 1 min. Calculate the percent purity of the drug.

Do not mistake a slowly developing blue color on the paste for the immediate color indicative of the true end point. The slow color development observed before the end point is caused by air oxidation of the iodide in the acidic medium.

Sulfonamide Tablets. Obtain a sample of sulfonamide tablets. Weigh a counted number of at least 20 tablets, reduce them to a powder, and accurately weigh a portion of the powder equivalent to about 500 mg of active ingredient. Analyze this sample by nitrite titration. Perform this analysis in triplicate. Calculate the average weight of the sulfonamide per tablet.

References

1. Kolthoff, I. M. and V. A. Stenger, *Volumetric Analysis*, Vol. II, 2nd ed., Interscience, New York, 1947, Chap. IV.
2. Critchfield, F. E. and J. B. Johnson, *Anal. Chem.*, **30,** 1247 (1958).
3. Bell, R. P., *The Proton in Chemistry*, Cornell University Press, Ithaca, New York, 1959, Chap. IV.
4. Critchfield, F. E., *Organic Functional Group Analysis*, Macmillan, New York, 1963, Chap. 2.
5. Pifer, C. W. and E. G. Wollish, *Anal. Chem.*, **24,** 300 (1952).
6. Hong, W. H. and K. A. Connors, *Anal. Chem.*, **40,** 1273 (1968).
7. Hirtz, J. and A. Gerardin, *Ann. Pharm. Fr.*, **27,** 581 (1969).
8. El-Sebai, A. I., Y. Beltagy, and R. Soliman, *Pharmazie*, **26,** 615 (1971).
9. Szekely, E., A. Bandel, and M. Flitman, *Talanta*, **19,** 1429 (1972).
10. Siggia, S., *Quantitative Organic Analysis via Functional Groups*, 3rd ed., John Wiley and Sons, New York, 1963, Chap. 11.
11. Dubin, D. T., *J. Biol. Chem.*, **235,** 783 (1960).
12. Connors, K. A., *Reaction Mechanisms in Organic Analytical Chemistry*, Wiley-Interscience, New York, 1973, pp. 274–283.
13. Stewart, J. T., T. D. Shaw, and A. B. Ray, *Anal. Chem.*, **41,** 360 (1969).
14. Higuchi, T. and J. I. Bodin, Chap. VIII in *Pharmaceutical Analysis*, T. Higuchi and E. Brochmann-Hanssen (eds.), Interscience, New York, 1961, pp. 413–418.
15. Auerbach, M. E., *Ind. Eng. Chem. Anal. Ed.*, **15,** 492 (1943).
16. Mukerjee, P., *Anal. Chem.*, **28,** 870 (1956).
17. Higuchi, T., A. Michaelis, T. Tan, and A. Hurwitz, *Anal. Chem.*, **39,** 974 (1967).
18. Doyle, T. D. and J. Levine, *Anal. Chem.*, **39,** 1282 (1967).
19. Rader, B. R., *J. Pharm. Sci.*, **62,** 1148 (1973).
20. Ogg, C. L., W. L. Porter, and C. O. Willits, *Ind. Eng. Chem. Anal. Ed.*, **17,** 394 (1945).
21. Hillenbrand, E. F., Jr. and C. A. Pentz, *Org. Anal.*, **3,** 163 (1956).
22. Woods, J. T. and G. H. Schneller, Chap. V in *Pharmaceutical Analysis*, T. Higuchi and E. Brochmann-Hanssen (eds.), Interscience, New York, 1961.

Problems

1. Each milliliter of 0.100 M $NaNO_2$ consumed in the titration of sulfamethazine is equivalent to how many milligrams of sulfamethazine?

2. A mixture of benzocaine (ethyl *p*-aminobenzoate) and procaine (*N,N*-diethylaminoethyl *p*-aminobenzoate) is to be separated by column partition chromatography. Suggest three ways in which the course of the separation may be followed—that is, three methods of analyzing the eluate.

3. A local anesthetic was believed to have one of these structures:

I. $(CH_3)_2N—C_6H_4—COOCH_2OCH_3$

II. $H_2N—C_6H_4—COOCH_2CH_2N(CH_3)_2$

III. $(C_3H_7)HN—C_6H_4—COOC_2H_5$

The compound gave these analytical results: saponification equivalent, 207.7; equivalent weight with respect to acylation, 207.3. When reacted with nitrous acid and then with *N*-(1-naphthyl)ethylenediamine a pink color was produced. These data suggest that which structure is the correct one?

4. Devise a method for the analysis of a mixture containing ethylamine, triethylamine, ethanol, and acetic acid.

5. Postulate a reasonable mechanism for imine formation.

6. An antitubercular drug gave the following analytical results:

(*a*) Mp 150–151°C

(*b*) uv absorption in ethanol solution:

λ_{max} 206 nm, log ϵ 4.30
λ_{max} 237 nm, log ϵ 3.92
λ_{max} 280 nm, log ϵ 4.14
λ_{max} 304 nm, log ϵ 4.17

(*c*) 0.250 g dissolved in acid solution was titrated to a starch-iodide end point with 16.05 ml of 0.10 *N* $NaNO_2$.

(*d*) 0.500 g dissolved in water was titrated to a phenolphthalein end point with 32.2 ml of 0.10 *N* NaOH. The pH was 3.25 when 16.1 ml of titrant had been added.

(*e*) Acylation with an acetic anhydride reagent gave an equivalent weight of 75.9 with respect to acylable groups.

Postulate a structure consistent with all data (including the pharmacology).

7. Twenty sulfanilamide tablets, total weight 10.105 g, were powdered. A 595.0 mg portion was assayed by the sodium nitrite method, 28.16 ml of 0.10 *M* $NaNO_2$ being consumed. Calculate the average weight of sulfanilamide per tablet.

8. An unidentified drug, which we will call compound *A*, had these experimental characteristics:

(*a*) It could be extracted into chloroform from aqueous alkaline solution but not from aqueous acid solution.

(*b*) 1.18 g of *A* was added to excess KOH and the solution was refluxed. After cooling it was back-titrated with 0.50 *N* HCl, 12.50 ml being consumed. A blank treated in exactly the same way consumed 22.50 ml of 0.50 *N* HCl.

(*c*) An acidic solution of *A* was treated with sodium nitrite and then with the Bratton-Marshall reagent; a pink color formed immediately.

(*d*) In acidic solution *A* has λ_{max} 290 nm.

(*e*) *A* gave a positive ferric hydroxamate test.

(*f*) Upon injection *A* has local anesthetic action.

(*g*) When *A* was refluxed in alkali and the cooled solution was acidified, a solid compound (*B*) precipitated from solution. Compound *B* had these characteristics:

(1) *B* gave a positive test with the Bratton-Marshall reagent.

(2) *B* had λ_{max} 289 nm.

(3) B gave a negative ferric hydroxamate test.

(4) B could be extracted into chloroform from aqueous acid solution but not from alkaline solution.

(5) Potentiometric titration of B showed that it had an acidic group of pK_a 2.38 and a basic group with pK_b 9.11. Titration with base gave an equivalent weight of 137.

Deduce chemical structures of A and B that are consistent with all the data.

25 OTHER CLASSES OF COMPOUNDS

25.1 Compounds Containing the Alkoxyl Group

The alkoxyl group is represented by —OR, where R is alkyl. This group appears in alcohols, esters, acetals, ketals, and ethers. With the exception of ethers, all these compounds have been discussed in earlier chapters. We shall now consider the analysis of the alkoxyl group as it occurs in ethers. The methoxyl ($—OCH_3$) and ethoxyl ($—OC_2H_5$) groups are most often encountered, frequently in the form of ring-substituted methyl or ethyl phenyl ethers. The methoxyl group occurs widely in natural products.

Ethers are cleaved by hydriodic acid to convert the alkoxyl group into the corresponding alkyl iodide:

$$CH_3OC_2H_5 + 2HI \rightarrow CH_3I + C_2H_5I + H_2O$$

$$CH_3OC_6H_5 + HI \rightarrow CH_3I + C_6H_5OH$$

This reaction forms the basis for the alkoxyl group determination. The alkyl iodide is quantitatively determined to give a measure of the original alkoxyl group. The analysis of the alkyl iodide may be accomplished in several ways.

In a gravimetric determination [1] the methyl or ethyl iodide is reacted with silver nitrate to yield, after suitable treatment, a precipitate of silver iodide that is collected and weighed. A titrimetric analysis is preferred by many. The alkyl iodide is oxidized by bromine to iodic acid, HIO_3. An excess of iodide is added, and the liberated iodine is titrated with standard thiosulfate. The reactions are, in sequence:

Cleavage of ether: $ROCH_3 + HI \rightarrow ROH + CH_3I$

Oxidation of alkyl iodide: $CH_3I + Br_2 \rightarrow CH_3Br + IBr$;

$IBr + 2Br_2 + 3H_2O \rightarrow HIO_3 + 5HBr$

Addition of iodide: $HIO_3 + 5I^- + 5H^+ \rightarrow 3I_2 + 3H_2O$

Titration of iodine: $I_2 + 2S_2O_3{}^{2-} \rightarrow 2I^- + S_4O_6{}^{2-}$

Nonaqueous titrimetry has been applied to this problem [2]. The alkyl iodide produced by reaction of the ether with HI is flushed, by means of a stream of nitrogen, into a pyridine solution. The alkyl iodide reacts with pyridine to form an alkylpyridinium iodide:

$$RI + C_5H_5N \rightarrow C_5H_5NR^+I^-$$

The alkylpyridinium iodide acts as a weak acid in the pyridine medium, whereas the excess hydriodic acid (which also is carried over by the stream of nitrogen) is a strong acid. A potentiometric titration, with tetrabutylammonium hydroxide titrant, differentiates these two acids. The amount of alkylpyridinium iodide is equivalent to the amount of alkoxyl group in the sample.

Methoxyl and ethoxyl groups are readily determined by these methods. Propoxyl and butoxyl groups can be analyzed, but they are not often encountered. Aliphatic esters can be determined with this procedure for alkoxyl groups.

Gas chromatography provides an effective finish for alkoxyl group determinations [3]. The alkyl iodides are produced as described above, and are then separated and measured by GC. This is applicable also to mixtures of alkoxyl compounds.

25.2 Alkenes and Alkynes

Many types of unsaturation have been encountered in preceding chapters; and in this section we consider carbon-carbon unsaturation. Compounds containing the carbon-carbon double bond are called alkenes or, in earlier terminology, olefins, and those containing the triple bond are alkynes or acetylenes. Aromatic unsaturation, which is chemically quite distinct from aliphatic unsaturation, will not be included here.

The kind and degree of chemical reactivity conferred on a molecule by carbon-carbon unsaturation depend upon the local molecular structure. Several types of unsaturated compounds, which differ appreciably in their chemical behavior, occur widely in natural and synthetic products:

R—CH═CH—R′	Isolated double bond
R—CH═CH—CH═CH—R′	Conjugated diene
R—CH═CH_2	Vinyl unsaturation
R—CH═CH—X	α,β-unsaturation (X is an electron-withdrawing group)
R—C≡CH	Terminal alkyne

Most analytical methods for unsaturated compounds are based on the addition of suitable reagents to the unsaturated bond according to the general overall reaction:

$$\text{—CH=CH— + X—Y} \rightarrow \text{—CHX—CHY—}$$

Polgar and Jungnickel [4] have given a thorough review of alkene analyses.

Addition of Halogens to Alkenes. In polar solvents the addition of halogens across the carbon-carbon double bond proceeds by an ionic mechanism. This reaction has been carefully studied. It appears that the double bond acts as a nucleophile in the initial step of the reaction, with the attacking agent being a halogen cation. A three-membered ring is formed. This structure is then attacked by a halide ion. The mechanism is illustrated with the bromination of ethylene. *Trans* addition is observed because the attacking halide ion

$$Br_2 \rightleftharpoons Br^+ + Br^-$$

$$CH_2{=}CH_2 + Br^+ \longrightarrow \underset{\underset{+}{Br}}{CH_2\text{——}CH_2}$$

$$\underset{\underset{+}{Br}}{CH_2\text{——}CH_2} + Br^- \longrightarrow CH_2Br\text{—}CH_2Br$$

approaches from the relatively unencumbered "back" side of the ring.

Electron-withdrawing groups adjacent to the double bond would be expected to reduce the electron density at the unsaturated carbons and therefore to reduce the reactivity, since the addition reaction is mediated by an electrophilic attack. Thus we find that *trans*-cinnamic acid, $C_6H_5CH{=}CHCOOH$, adds bromine much more slowly than does sytrene, $C_6H_5CH{=}CH_2$.

Mixed halogens, such as iodine chloride (ICl), present another possibility in their addition to a nonsymmetrical alkene. Since chlorine is more electronegative than iodine, the expected manner of ionization is

$$ICl \rightleftharpoons I^+ + Cl^-$$

with I^+ being the initial attacking agent. The resulting intermediate will then be attacked by chloride to give the product predicted on the basis that the more stable carbonium ion will be formed during the ring-opening step. (Recall that the stability of carbonium ions decreases in the order tertiary: secondary: primary.)

$$\mathrm{R{-}CH{=}CH_2 + I^+ \longrightarrow R{-}\underset{\diagdown\ I_+ \diagup}{CH{-}CH_2}}$$

$$\mathrm{R{-}\underset{\diagdown\ I_+ \diagup}{CH{-}CH_2} \rightleftharpoons R{-}\overset{+}{C}H{-}\underset{|\atop I}{C}H_2}$$

$$\mathrm{R{-}\overset{+}{C}H{-}\underset{|\atop I}{C}H_2 + Cl^- \longrightarrow R{-}\overset{Cl\atop |}{C}H{-}\underset{|\atop I}{C}H_2}$$

The relative reactivities of several halogens in alkene addition (in acetic acid solution) are I_2, 1; IBr, 3×10^3; Br_2, 10^4; ICl, 10^5; and BrCl, 4×10^6. Chlorine is even more reactive. From the analytical point of view, high reactivity is desirable, which eliminates iodine as a good reagent, and reasonable stability of the reagent solution is necessary, which eliminates chlorine. Bromine, iodine chloride, and iodine bromide are the halogenating agents useful for the analysis of alkenes.

Substitution by halogens is an undesirable side reaction that may occur under analytical conditions. It is obvious that consumption of reagent by a substitution reaction (that is, replacement of hydrogen by halogen) will vitiate the analytical results.

Bromine may be employed in carbon tetrachloride or acetic acid solution. The instability of free bromine solutions is a disadvantage; bromine is readily lost by volatilization. This loss of bromine may be reduced by dissolving the bromine in an aqueous or methanolic solution of potassium bromide, forming the nonvolatile tribromide ion. Another approach utilizes a standard solution of potassium bromate in excess potassium bromide. This solution, which is very stable, liberates an equivalent amount of bromine when it is acidified. Bromination methods employing these solutions involve the addition of the alkene to an excess of the brominating reagent. After the addition reaction is complete, excess potassium iodide is added. The iodine liberated from oxidation of iodide by unreacted bromine ($Br_2 + 2I^- \rightarrow I_2 + 2Br^-$) is titrated with standard thiosulfate. A blank determination is performed. The difference between blank and sample titration volumes corresponds to the equivalents of double bond in the sample. Bromination methods are quite satisfactory for compounds containing isolated double bonds. α,β-Unsaturated acids cannot be analyzed, but their salts can; this difference in behavior is explicable in terms of the mechanistic information given earlier.

Iodine monochloride dissolved in acetic acid (Wijs' solution) is a standard reagent for the determination of the unsaturation content of fats and oils. This solution is prepared by passing chlorine gas into a solution of iodine. Iodine bromide is preferred by some analysts as a halogenating agent; the reagent (Hanus' solution) is prepared by dissolving appropriate amounts of iodine and bromine in glacial acetic acid. The volumetric measurement of the extent of reaction is carried out just as described in the preceding paragraph for bromine reagents.

The results of a halogenation analysis can be expressed in several ways. If the sample consists of a compound of known composition, the percent purity of the sample can be calculated as in any similar analytical situation; 1 mole of halogenating reagent reacts with 1 "mole" of double bond. Sometimes the structure of the compound is unknown, but the sample is pure; then the analysis of unsaturation may be a key step in the identification of the compound. The results in such an instance are expressed either as the equivalent weight of the compound (with respect to halogen addition), or as percent of double bond, where the group weight of the double bond is 24.02.

Fats and oils are mixtures of indefinite composition, so they cannot reasonably be characterized by a "percent purity" or "equivalent weight." The results of unsaturation analyses of these compounds often are given as iodine numbers. The *iodine number* is the number of grams of iodine consumed by 100 g of the sample. This quantity can be calculated even though iodine is never used as the actual agent in the additional reaction. A *bromine number* is defined, in an analogous way, as the number of grams of bromine consumed by 100 g of sample.

EXAMPLE 25.1. (*a*) Calculate the theoretical iodine number of oleic acid.

Oleic acid has the structure $CH_3(CH_2)_7CH{=}CH(CH_2)_7COOH$; its molecular weight is 282.5. Therefore 1 mole of oleic acid (282.5 g) consumes 1 mole of iodine (253.8 g) by addition to the double bond. Setting up a simple proportion then gives the weight of iodine consumed by 100 g of pure oleic acid:

$$\frac{282.5}{100} = \frac{253.8}{X}$$

$$X = 89.8$$

The iodine number of pure oleic acid is 89.8.

(*b*) A 0.2590 g sample of oleic acid is assayed by the iodine monochloride (Wijs) method. The blank consumed 44.60 ml of 0.1035 N sodium thiosulfate, and the sample consumed 28.34 ml of the same titrant. Calculate the iodine number and the percent purity of the sample.

Evidently 44.60 ml − 28.34 ml = 16.26 ml of thiosulfate corresponds to the amount of iodine monochloride added to the oleic acid. This is converted to milliequivalents of ICl by utilizing the normality of the thiosulfate: (16.26 ml) (0.1035 N) = 1.683 meq of ICl added. If I_2 had been the halogenating agent, the same number of milliequivalents would have been added to the sample. We therefore may calculate that, if iodine had been used, (0.001683 eq)(126.9 g/eq) = 0.2136 g of I_2 would have been added to the 0.2590 g sample. Again using the simple proportionality incorporating the definition of iodine number:

$$\frac{0.2590}{100} = \frac{0.2136}{X}$$

$$X = 82.5$$

The iodine number of the sample is 82.5. The sample purity can be calculated directly from the experimental and theoretical iodine number: percent purity = (82.5)(100)/89.8 = 91.9%. Alternatively the titration data can be used to calculate the weight of oleic acid in the sample as the product of the equivalent weight of oleic acid and the number of equivalents of oleic acid.

It is essential to understand the reasoning in titrimetric calculations of this type. The mode of the calculation of course follows directly from the definition of iodine number. After such a computation is understood, it is permissible, and even advantageous, to put it into formula form. Thus the iodine number calculation of the preceding paragraph is represented by the formula:

$$\text{Iodine number} = \frac{(V_B - V_S)N\,(12.69)}{W}$$

where V_B = volume of thiosulfate for blank titration (ml)
V_S = volume of thiosulfate for sample titration (ml)
N = normality of thiosulfate solution
W = weight of sample (g)

Mercuric Acetate Method. Mercuric acetate adds to olefins according to the overall reaction

$$\text{—CH=CH— + Hg(OAc)}_2 \text{ + ROH} \longrightarrow \underset{\text{OR}}{\text{—CH}}\text{—}\underset{\text{HgOAc}}{\text{CH}}\text{— + HOAc}$$

where R can be hydrogen or an alkyl group. Several assay methods have been formulated on the basis of this reaction. In one of these procedures the addition reaction is carried out with an excess of mercuric acetate. The unreacted reagent is converted to mercuric chloride by adding sodium chloride to the mixture. Finally the acetic acid produced in the addition reaction is titrated with standard alkali. Each mole of acetic acid corresponds to an equivalent of alkene in the sample. It is necessary to destroy the unreacted mercuric acetate because this compound will interfere in the titration by forming mercuric oxide.

In another modification a known volume of mercuric acetate solution is employed. After the addition reaction is complete the reaction mixture is diluted with 1 : 1 proplyene glycol-chloroform and the solution is titrated with standard hydrochloric acid in the same solvent. The excess reagent consumes 2 moles of titrant acid:

$$Hg(OAc)_2 + 2HCl \rightarrow HgCl_2 + 2HOAc$$

while the addition product consumes 1 mole:

$$\underset{\displaystyle OR}{-\overset{|}{CH}}-\underset{\displaystyle HgOAc}{\overset{|}{CH}}- + HCl \longrightarrow \underset{\displaystyle OR}{-\overset{|}{CH}}-\underset{\displaystyle HgCl}{\overset{|}{CH}}- + HOAc$$

A blank determination is made in exactly the same way. The difference in equivalents of HCl consumed in the blank and sample titrations is equal to the number of equivalents of alkene in the sample. Experiment 25.1 gives the details of this procedure.

The mercuric acetate procedure is applicable to isolated double bonds and to vinyl unsaturation. For these groups it provides a convenient and accurate method of analysis. If the alkene is branched at one of the unsaturated carbons, only the *cis* isomer can be determined. α,β-Unsaturated compounds form adducts with mercuric acetate, but these products are cleaved very readily under the usual titration conditions, so this method fails for such compounds. For example, styrene can be assayed accurately, but cinnamic acid cannot.

Other Methods for Alkenes. Although many methods have been proposed for the determination of carbon-carbon unsaturation [4], few of these are used widely. A general method is based on the catalytic hydrogenation of the double bond. The amount of hydrogen consumed in the reaction is a measure

$$\gt C=C\lt + H_2 \xrightarrow{\text{catalyst}} \gt CH-CH\lt$$

of the alkene content of the sample. The apparatus required is relatively complex. An advantage of the method is that it may be applicable when other methods are ruled out because of the presence of other interfering groups in the sample. A simplified modification of the hydrogenation method uses sodium borohydride ($NaBH_4$) as the source of hydrogen [5].

When a double bond is situated α,β to a strongly electron-withdrawing group, the nucleophilic character of the bond is greatly reduced. This is why the usual methods (halogenation and mercury acetate addition) fail for these compounds. The electrophilic strength of the β carbon in such a substance renders it susceptible to attack by a nucleophilic agent, and a satisfactory method has been developed in which morpholine, a secondary amine, adds to the double bond [6]. The excess morpholine is acetylated with acetic an-

$$\text{O}(\text{CH}_2\text{CH}_2)_2\text{NH} + \text{RCH}{=}\text{CH}{-}\text{X} \longrightarrow \text{O}(\text{CH}_2\text{CH}_2)_2\text{N}{-}\underset{\substack{|\\ \text{R}}}{\text{CH}}{-}\text{CH}_2{-}\text{X}$$

hydride in acetonitrile medium. In this system the amide is relatively neutral, and the tertiary amine is titrated with standard hydrochloric acid. This method is applicable to substances with the structure $H_2C{=}CHX$, where X is any strongly electron-withdrawing group such as —COOH, —COOR, —C≡N. When X is carbonyl or carboxylate the method fails, but these compounds can be analyzed by other methods. Esters of acrylic, fumaric, and maleic acids are readily analyzed with the morpholine procedure.

Determination of Alkynes. A fairly general method for the analysis of alkynes is based on their hydration to give ketones. This reaction is catalyzed by

$$\text{R}{-}\text{C}{\equiv}\text{C}{-}\text{R}' + \text{H}_2\text{O} \longrightarrow \text{R}{-}\overset{\substack{\text{O}\\ \|}}{\text{C}}{-}\text{CH}_2{-}\text{R}'$$

mercuric sulfate. The resulting ketone is determined by the oximation method or, for the few ketones that cannot be analyzed in this way, gravimetrically as the 2,4-dinitrophenylhydrazone [7]. The hydration reaction is carried out at reflux, with a 30–60 min reaction time being sufficient for most alkynes. The solution is neutralized, hydroxylamine hydrochloride is added, and after oxime formation is complete the liberated hydrochloric acid is titrated potentiometrically with standard alkali. This method is free from most interferences. Thus acids and bases do not interfere because of the neutralization step prior to the oximation. Olefins do not yield carbonyls upon hydration. Carbonyls themselves interfere, but can be corrected for in an analysis of a separate portion of the sample prior to hydration of the alkyne.

Terminal alkynes are of fairly common occurrence. These substances possess an active hydrogen, and can be analyzed by active hydrogen methods (Section 23.4), which are rather nonselective, however. Better methods are available. Alkynes with an acetylenic hydrogen form silver salts as shown:

$$\text{R}{-}\text{C}{\equiv}\text{C}{-}\text{H} + \text{AgNO}_3 \rightarrow \text{R}{-}\text{C}{\equiv}\text{C}{-}\text{Ag} + \text{HNO}_3$$

The resulting nitric acid is titrated with alkali, thus giving a measure of the alkyne in the sample. A similar method utilizes silver perchlorate in methanol. A double salt is formed, with the release of 1 mole of perchloric acid per mole of alkyne. The perchloric acid is titrated in the anhydrous medium with a standard solution of tris(hydroxymethyl)aminomethane.

$$\text{R}{-}\text{C}{\equiv}\text{C}{-}\text{H} + 2\text{AgClO}_4 \rightarrow \text{R}{-}\text{C}{\equiv}\text{C}{-}\text{Ag}{\cdot}\text{AgClO}_4 + \text{HClO}_4$$

25.3 Thiols, Sulfides, and Disulfides

Thiols, which have the general structure R—SH, are also known as mercaptans or sulfhydryl compounds. They are sulfur analogues of hydroxy compounds. *Sulfides* may be represented R—S—R′; these compounds are referred to as thioethers. *Disulfides* are written R—S—S—R′.

These sulfur compounds occur widely in nature, and they are often encountered in pharmaceutical samples. The generally applicable assay methods are described here.

Titrimetric Methods for Thiols. Thiols are much stronger acids than are their oxygen analogues. Ethanethiol (ethyl mercaptan, C_2H_5SH) has $pK_a = 10.5$, and for thiophenol, C_6H_5SH, $pK_a = 6.5$.

Part of this effect may be ascribed, in a very crude description, to the greater size of the sulfur atom compared with oxygen; thus the electron density is lower on sulfur and the proton can more readily leave sulfur in a thiol than oxygen in an alcohol. In fact, the thiophenol is sufficiently acidic to be titrated in aqueous solution. Nonaqueous titration is more widely applicable.

Thiols have been analyzed by acylation, as described in Chapter 21 for alcohols and Chapter 24 for amines. A possible source of error in this method is the lability of the thiolester formed in the reaction (RCOSR′); this product may be hydrolyzed during the titration with alkali.

Silver nitrate reacts with mercaptans to precipitate silver mercaptides (also called silver thiolates).

$$\text{R—SH} + \text{AgNO}_3 \rightarrow \text{R—S—Ag} + \text{HNO}_3$$

This reaction forms the basis of several accurate procedures for the analysis of thiols. A very simple assay utilizes a direct argentometric titration with potentiometric detection of the end point. A more sensitive titration can be made if the end point is located amperometrically, with the rotating platinum electrode (see Experiment 7.1). The amperometric titration is carried out in ammoniacal solution.

The silver method may be conducted by adding an excess of silver nitrate and then back-titrating the excess silver with thiocyanate (Volhard titration). Alternatively, the nitric acid produced in the reaction can be titrated with alkali to provide a quantitative measure of the thiol in the sample.

Thiols are susceptible to oxidation by many oxidizing agents. (In fact, air oxidation is a potential side reaction in all systems containing thiols.) A simple and accurate iodometric assay is based on this behavior.

$$2\text{R—SH} + \text{I}_2 \rightarrow \text{RSSR} + 2\text{HI}$$

An excess of iodine solution is added to the sample, and the unreacted iodine is back-titrated with standard sodium thiosulfate. This is an excellent method, although it is subject to interference by any substance that is oxidized by iodine.

N-Ethylmaleimide Spectrophotometric Method for Thiols. Thiols react rapidly in neutral aqueous solution with *N*-ethylmaleimide, **1**, according to the following equation.

$$\text{R—SH} + \begin{matrix}\text{CH—C=O} \\ \| \qquad \diagdown \\ \| \qquad\quad \text{N—C}_2\text{H}_5 \\ \| \qquad \diagup \\ \text{CH—C=O}\end{matrix} \longrightarrow \begin{matrix}\text{R—S—CH—C=O} \\ | \qquad \diagdown \\ | \qquad\quad \text{N—C}_2\text{H}_5 \\ | \qquad \diagup \\ \text{CH}_2\text{—C=O}\end{matrix}$$

1

The powerful nucleophile R—S$^-$ attacks the electrophilic double bond (which is in the α,β position to two electron-withdrawing groups). The product of the reaction possesses no conjugated double bonds, in contrast to the reactant, so the light absorption by *N*-ethylmaleimide (λ_{max} 300 nm, ϵ_{max} 602) decreases on reaction with thiols. The product does not absorb light at 300 nm, so the decrease in absorbance at this wavelength is directly related to the number of moles of *N*-ethylmaleimide reacted. The analytical method is quite simple [8, 9]. The absorbance of 0.001 *M* *N*-ethylmaleimide in pH 6.8 phosphate buffer is measured at 300 nm. Another solution containing the same concentration of reagent is prepared to be 0.0001–0.0009 *M* in thiol. The absorbance of this solution is measured, also at 300 nm. Applying Beer's law to each solution,

$$A_B = a_{\mathrm{NEM}} b c^B_{\mathrm{NEM}}$$

$$A_S = a_{\mathrm{NEM}} b c^S_{\mathrm{NEM}}$$

where B and S represent the blank and sample solutions, a_{NEM} is the absorptivity of *N*-ethylamaleimide (NEM), and c_{NEM} is its concentration. Subtracting these equations gives

$$c^B_{\mathrm{NEM}} - c^S_{\mathrm{NEM}} = \frac{A_B - A_S}{b a_{\mathrm{NEM}}}$$

or, since each mole of thiol in the sample consumed 1 mole of NEM,

$$c_{\mathrm{thiol}} = \frac{A_B - A_S}{b a_{\mathrm{NEM}}}$$

A notable advantage of this method is its independence of a pure sample of the thiol to establish an absorptivity or a standard curve. Only the NEM adsorbs at 300 nm, and so NEM serves as the standard substance.

This spectrophotometric procedure is applicable to thiol concentrations as low as 0.001 *M*. A modification has extended this range to about 10^{-7} *M* [10]. The thiol-NEM reaction is carried out in isopropanol solution, which is then made alkaline. An intense red color develops, presumably from an ionized form of the addition product. The absorbance of the solution is proportional to the original thiol concentration.

Sulfides and Disulfides. Sulfides can be oxidized by bromine to give sulfoxides:

$$\text{R—S—R}' + \text{Br}_2 + \text{H}_2\text{O} \longrightarrow \text{R—}\overset{\overset{\text{O}}{\|}}{\text{S}}\text{—R}' + 2\text{HBr}$$

As a basis for an analytical method this reaction is complicated by the further oxidation of the sulfoxide to the sulfone:

$$\text{R—}\overset{\overset{\text{O}}{\|}}{\text{S}}\text{—R}' + \text{Br}_2 + \text{H}_2\text{O} \longrightarrow \text{R—}\underset{\underset{\text{O}}{\|}}{\overset{\overset{\text{O}}{\|}}{\text{S}}}\text{—R}' + 2\text{HBr}$$

Since oxidation to the sulfoxide proceeds more rapidly than does the oxidation to the sulfone, it is possible to utilize the first reaction for a quantitative analysis of sulfides if appropriate measures are taken to minimize the secondary oxidation. This is accomplished by direct titration with bromine. (Actually a standard bromate-bromide solution is used, and the sulfide solution is made acidic.) Thus an excess of oxidizing agent is avoided, and sulfone production is claimed to be rendered negligible [11]. The end point is marked by the appearance of the yellow bromine color.

Disulfides also can be determined by direct bromine titration. The reaction product is either the sulfonyl bromide

$$\text{R—SS—R} + 5\text{Br}_2 + 4\text{H}_2\text{O} \rightarrow 2\text{R—SO}_2\text{Br} + 8\text{HBr}$$

or the sulfonic acid:

$$\text{R—SS—R} + 5\text{Br}_2 + 6\text{H}_2\text{O} \rightarrow 2\text{R—SO}_3\text{H} + 10\text{HBr}$$

From the analytical point of view it makes no difference which compound is produced because in either case 1 mole of disulfide reacts with 5 moles of bromine.

Another approach to disulfide analysis is based on reduction to the mercaptan followed by analysis of the mercaptan.

$$\text{R—SS—R} + 2\text{H} \rightarrow 2\text{R—SH}$$

Sodium borohydride has been used as the reducing agent. The mercaptan may be analyzed with methods discussed earlier.

Mixtures of sulfides and disulfides can be determined by bromine oxidation to give the sum of the sulfide and disulfide, followed by reduction analysis of a second sample to give the disulfide content. The sulfide is then calculated by difference. Mixtures of thiols and disulfides (which are often encountered, because oxidation of a thiol yields a disulfide) can be analyzed by determining the thiol content by any of the methods described earlier. Then a second portion of the sample is subjected to reductive treatment and the total thiol content is measured. The disulfide content is found by difference.

25.4 Isocyanates and Isothiocyanates

Isocyanates, R—N═C═O, and isothiocyanates, R—N═C═S, are important intermediates in the synthesis of pharmaceuticals and other organics. Allyl isothiocyanate, $CH_2{=}CHCH_2NCS$, is the active ingredient of mustard.

These compounds readily undergo addition reactions, and their analysis is based on this behavior. An isocyanate adds an amine, forming a substituted urea, and an isothiocyanate adds an amine to give a thiourea. The reactions with a primary amine are

$$\mathrm{R{-}N{=}C{=}O + R'{-}NH_2 \longrightarrow R{-}NH\overset{\overset{\displaystyle O}{\|}}{C}{-}NHR'}$$

$$\mathrm{R{-}N{=}C{=}S + R'{-}NH_2 \longrightarrow R{-}NH\overset{\overset{\displaystyle S}{\|}}{C}{-}NHR'}$$

Among the amines that are employed for the quantitative analysis of these compounds are *n*-butylamine, dibutylamine, and piperidine. An excess of the amine, dissolved in anhydrous dioxane or toluene, is added to the sample. After the reaction is complete, the excess amine is back-titrated with standard acid. A blank is carried out in the same way.

Experiment 25.1. Determination of Alkenes by Mercuric Acetate Addition [12]

REAGENTS

Thymol Blue Indicator Solution. Make a 0.2% solution of thymol blue in ethanol.

Mixed Solvent. Mix equal volumes of propylene glycol and chloroform.

Mercuric Acetate Reagent. Dissolve about 20 g of reagent grade mercuric acetate in 500 ml of methanol and add 1 ml of glacial acetic acid. Mix well and filter.

0.1 N Hydrochloric Acid. Dilute about 9 ml of concentrated hydrochloric acid to 1 liter with the 1 : 1 propylene glycol/chloroform mixed solvent. Standardize as follows: accurately weigh about 0.2 g of reagent grade, dried mercuric oxide. Dissolve the sample in 5 ml of glacial acetic acid with gentle heating and then evaporate nearly to dryness. Dissolve the residue in 25 ml of mixed solvent, add thymol blue indicator, and titrate with the hydrochloric acid solution. Carry out at least three titrations.

In the dissolution step HgO is converted to mercuric acetate, which is transformed into $HgCl_2$ in the titration. Write the reactions and calculate the normality of the hydrochloric acid.

PROCEDURES

Known Sample. Select a monoolefin with a terminal or isolated double bond (for example, styrene, cyclohexene, allyl alcohol, vinyl acetate). Deliver about 2 meq of compound into a tared glass-stoppered 125 ml Erlenmeyer flask and accurately weigh it. Pipet 25.0 ml of mercuric acetate reagent into the flask, dissolve the sample, and permit the solution to stand at room temperature until the addition reaction is complete. This will take 5–10 min for styrene, 10–15 min for cyclohexene, and 30 min for allyl and vinyl compounds. Add about 25 ml of the mixed solvent and some thymol blue indicator, and titrate with the standard hydrochloric acid solution. The end point color change is from yellow to pink.

Carry out a blank determination in exactly the same way, being sure to use the same volume of mercuric acetate reagent as in the sample determination. The basis of the calculation is explained in Section 25.2, and is analogous to the calculation used in Experiment 21.1. Calculate the percent purity of your sample compound.

Unknown Sample. Obtain an unknown alkene from your instructor and analyze it as above. Calculate the equivalent weight of your compound. Carry out at least three determinations and report the mean, standard deviation, and 95% confidence limits of your result.

References

1. Steyermark, A., *Quantitative Organic Microanalysis*, 2nd ed., Academic, New York, 1961, Chap. 16.
2. Cundiff, R. H. and P. C. Markunas, *Anal. Chem.*, **33,** 1028 (1961).
3. Siggia, S. (ed.), *Instrumental Methods of Organic Functional Group Analysis*, Wiley-Interscience, New York, 1972, p. 158.
4. Polgár, A. and J. L. Jungnickel, *Org. Anal.*, **3,** 203 (1956).
5. Brown, H. C., K. Sivasankaran, and C. A. Brown, *J. Org. Chem.*, **28,** 214 (1963).
6. Critchfield, F. E., G. L. Funk, and J. B. Johnson, *Anal. Chem.*, **28,** 76 (1956).
7. Siggia, S., C. R. Stahl, and R. Reinhardt, *Anal. Chem.*, **28,** 1481 (1956).
8. Roberts, E. and G. Rouser, *Anal. Chem.*, **30,** 1291 (1958).
9. Alexander, N. M., *Anal. Chem.*, **30,** 1292 (1958).
10. Broekhuysen, J., *Anal. Chim. Acta*, **19,** 542 (1958).

11. Siggia, S., *Quantitative Organic Analysis via Functional Groups*, 3rd ed., John Wiley and Sons, New York, 1963, Chap. 20.
12. Das, M. N., *Anal. Chem.*, **26,** 1086 (1954).

Problems

1. Design three different analytical methods for the quantitative determination of acetophenetidin.
2. What is the equivalent weight (in terms of its molecular weight) of an alkoxyl compound in the titrimetric iodometric analysis described in Section 25.1?

Part Six: General Topics

Chapters 26 and 27 deal with matters that either call on information presented in many other chapters (as in the determination of drugs in body tissues) or that underlie the application of specific techniques discussed earlier (for example, sampling and statistics, which are relevant to all analytical methods).

26 ANALYTICAL TOXICOLOGY

26.1 Introduction

Throughout this book the analysis of bulk samples and pharmaceutical dosage forms has been emphasized, and such samples account for much of the attention of the pharmaceutical analyst. Other kinds of samples may sometimes have to be analyzed, however. The pharmaceutical analyst may be asked to determine drugs or drug metabolites in urine, blood, or other body tissues in support of biopharmaceutical and pharmacokinetic studies. Another large area of application of drug analysis is the field of analytical toxicology, that is, the analysis of toxic substances, which may include drugs (legal and illicit), pollutants (such as pesticide residues and other environmental contaminants), and poisons in the most general sense. Analytical toxicology can be subdivided into clinical toxicology, which is practiced in support of therapy, and forensic toxicology, dealing with situations of crime or suspected crime.

A wide range of challenging analytical problems may arise in these fields. Characteristic of these problems is the scarcity of reliable information about the history of the sample, in the sense that the first goal of the analyst must be to identify the drug or toxic agent. In a clinical situation this information may be necessary to institute effective treatment, and so speed is often required. In forensic toxicology a high probability of correct identification must be assured, since a person's liberty may depend upon the result, and the analyst may have to appear in court as an expert witness and submit to unsympathetic questioning.

Quantitative information is also valuable, but its interpretation may be difficult. In poisoning cases the information desired is the identity and dosing schedule of the toxic agent, and knowledge of drug concentrations in tissues may enable the dosage regimen to be inferred. This inference is difficult, however, because so many variables are involved. These include the kinetics of absorption, distribution, metabolism, and elimination of the particular substance in the particular patient, the time, and the nature of the samples available. Much experience with specific drugs has been gained, and often fairly definite conclusions can be reached.

It will be appreciated that the amounts and concentrations of drugs in these samples are usually very small. The titrimetric methods that we found to be widely applicable in dosage form analysis are therefore of little use in analytical toxicology. Instead the more sensitive spectroscopic and chromatographic techniques are the usual methods of choice.

This chapter is a brief introduction to a few of the techniques and problems of analytical toxicology.

26.2 Isolation of Drugs

If the sample is accompanied by presumptive evidence about the possible identity of the drug, an abbreviated isolation scheme may be applicable. If speed is essential, a simple screening test on the sample (or on an extract) may be carried out to furnish information for immediate action; some of these tests will be described later. Often, however, a more systematic search must be made for the drug (or drugs). No single approach is completely general, but some procedures of wide applicability have been devised. The following isolation scheme is given by Jackson [1], but most extraction schemes are similar.

The method of isolation leads to these five classes of toxic substances:

(*a*) Volatile compounds, such as the lower alcohols, esters, aldehydes and ketones, ethers, hydrocarbons, and chlorinated hydrocarbons. These may be recoverable by distillation or gas chromatography. A useful technique is headspace GC, in which the sample (tissue, urine, blood) is placed in a closed container and heated very gently; a portion of the vapor over the sample is injected into the gas chromatograph.

(*b*) Metals, particularly the heavy metals. These can be recovered by acid digestion of the sample and isolation by classical precipitation methods. Spectroscopic methods are powerful identification tools for metals.

(*c*) Anions, such as halides, chlorate, permanganate, nitrite, nitrate, oxalate, etc. Dialysis is an effective way to isolate anions.

(*d*) Nonvolatile organic compounds. This comprises most modern drugs and other toxic substances, and is the only class that will be dealt with subsequently.

(*e*) Miscellaneous poisons, which are very water-soluble or water-insoluble at all pH values, and therefore do not fit into class *d* as it is ordinarily isolated. Proteins and glycosides are examples.

We now consider the isolation of drugs from class *d*. The general approach is solvent extraction, and the procedure can be divided into these three stages [1]:

Stage One. Removal of proteins from the sample.
This stage may not be necessary.

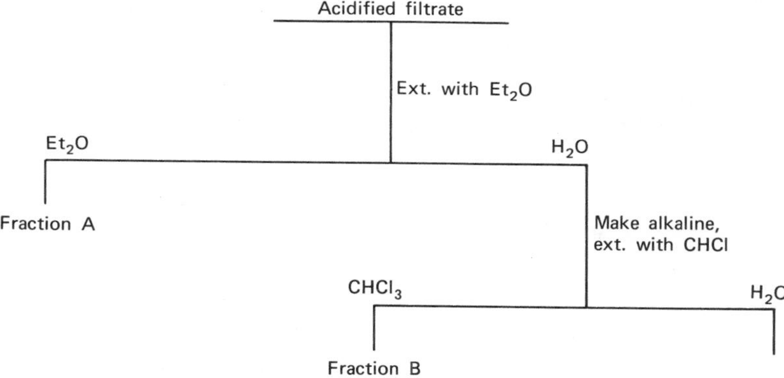

Fig. 26.1. Extraction scheme for the second stage of a general drug isolation procedure. Fraction A contains acidic and neutral drugs; fraction B contains basic drugs.

Stage Two. Separation by solvent extraction into two fractions. Fraction A will contain all acidic and neutral drugs, Fraction B all basic drugs.

Stage Three. Separation by solvent extraction of Fraction A into three subfractions:
- A1, the strongly acidic drugs*;
- A2, the weakly acidic drugs;
- A3, the neutral drugs.

The purpose of the first stage is to prepare a proteinfree acidic aqueous solution of the sample. Some samples do not require treatment to remove proteins; these include aqueous solutions, dosage forms, dilute stomach washings, and for some analyses, urine and blood. Liquid samples are acidified; solid samples are extracted with acidic water and filtered.

Samples whose protein content might interfere in subsequent extractions include urine, blood, feces, contents of the gastrointestinal tract, liver and other organs, foods, and milk. Several treatments are available to produce a proteinfree solution. The Stas-Otto procedure involves extraction with ethanol or acetone; proteins may be precipitated with tungstate or with ammonium sulfate; or the proteins may be hydrolyzed in acid. The choice of procedure will depend upon the nature of the sample and upon the analyst's experience. In any case, an aqueous filtrate, ready for treatment in Stage Two, will be the result.

In the second stage the acidified filtrate from Stage One is subjected to the extraction flow diagram shown in Fig. 26.1. It is first extracted with ether.

* In this connection "strong" and "weak" acids are defined by their extraction behavior, as explained subsequently.

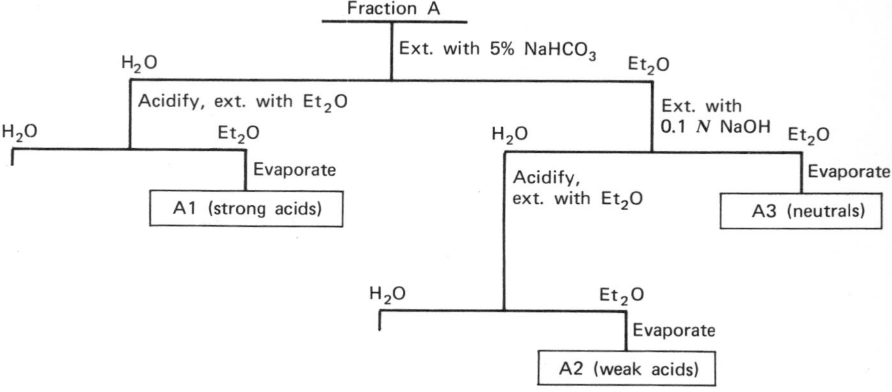

Fig. 26.2. Extraction scheme for the subdivision of fraction A (see Fig. 26.1).

The ether layer contains Fraction A, the acidic and neutral drugs. The aqueous layer, after separation of the phases, is made alkaline and is extracted with chloroform; this chloroform layer contains Fraction B, the basic drugs.

Fraction A is subdivided according to the extraction scheme of Fig. 26.2. "Strong" acids are those extracted into 5% sodium bicarbonate; these constitute fraction A1. The pH of 5% $NaHCO_3$ is 8.0; hence acids with $pK'_a < 8$ (approximately) in this medium will be extracted into this fraction. The ether phase remaining is extracted with 0.1 *N* NaOH (pH 13), removing very weak acids (A2). The neutral compounds are left in the ether (A3).

The basic premise of this isolation scheme is that charged molecules will distribute preferentially into the aqueous phase, whereas uncharged molecules will partition into the organic phase. It must be recognized that perfectly "clean" separations into different fractions will not be possible for all compounds with this general scheme. However, if specific information is available about the partition behavior of drugs in the sample, it may be possible to control the extraction (as by adjustment of pH to suit the drug pK'_a) in order to optimize the separation.

Often the isolation procedure can be simplified if only a few specified drugs are being tested for. This is the case, for example, in assays of blood for sedative drugs, or mass screening of urine samples for drugs of abuse. Many descriptions of isolation procedures are available [1–7].

If the full extraction scheme has been carried out as outlined in Figs. 26.1 and 26.2, four fractions (A1, A2, A3, B) are now at hand. Each of these may itself be a mixture of drugs, and the next step (unless evidence is available ruling out mixtures) often is to apply some form of chromatography to these fractions.

26.3 Problems in Drug Analysis

Barbiturates and Related Drugs. The 5,5-disubstituted barbituric acid derivatives have the general structure **1**. Thiobarbituric acids have the 2-oxygen

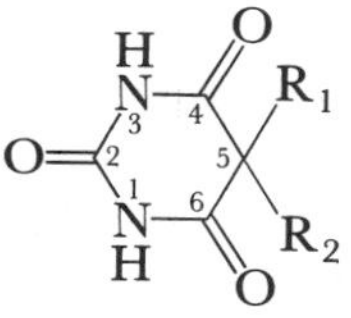

1

replaced by sulfur; in *N*-methyl barbiturates one of the nitrogens carries a methyl group. Approximately 50 barbiturates are used in therapy. They are responsible for most cases of drug overdoses.

Some chemically related compounds are conveniently considered here. Diphenylhydantoin, **2**, is an example of the hydantoins; **3** is glutethimide.

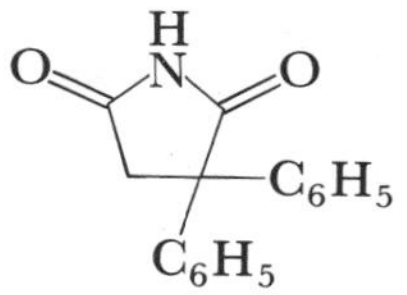

2 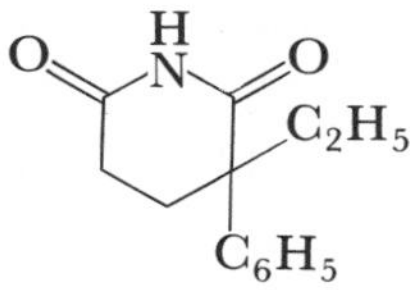 **3**

All these compounds contain the imide structure. They are therefore weak acids, and they appear in the A2 fraction upon extraction [1] (see Section 26.2). Several reviews of barbiturate analysis have been published [5, 8–10].

Some rapid tests can be applied to the extracted residue in order to check the possibility that barbiturates may be present. The best color test for barbiturates is the Parri test, in which treatment of a barbiturate with a cobalt salt and a base gives an immediate and stable pink-violet color. Chemically related compounds may give colors, but some differentiation is possible on the basis of the color, its intensity, and its stability [10]. The Parri test is not very sensitive. Another general test for barbiturates is the Zwikker reaction, the formation of colored copper-pyridine-barbiturate complexes.

Crystallographic examination, including determination of the melting point and crystal habit with the optical microscope, may be valuable if a single barbiturate has been isolated.

The uv spectra of barbiturates, and especially their dependence on ionic state (and therefore on pH) are very characteristic. Figure 8.12 shows the spectra of the three forms of barbital. All 5,5-disubstituted barbiturates have similar spectra, which can establish that a substance is a member of this class.

Small differences in the spectra of different barbiturates may permit identification.

Usually at this stage the isolated material should be subjected to some form of chromatography in order to establish the number of compounds present and to obtain purified samples. Paper, thin-layer, and gas chromatography have been used [10, 11], and liquid chromatography is being applied more widely. (Experiment 17.3 describes the separation of barbiturates by paper chromatography and Experiment 18.2 gives a GC method for glutethimide.) Retention times or R_f values will provide evidence of identity. Confirmatory data should be obtained when possible by the ir or MS examination of eluted zones. In all cases, it is essential that authentic specimens of the drugs be examined for comparison.

Once the drug has been identified, its quantitative determination is relatively simple. The isolation procedure may now be abbreviated. Spectrophotometry or column chromatography would be preferred methods for the quantitative determination of barbiturates.

Aspirin and Other Analgesics. Aspirin (acetylsalicylic acid, ASA), **4**, can be absorbed from the gastrointestinal tract as the intact molecule, but it is rapidly hydrolyzed to salicylic acid (SA, **5**) in the blood. Quantitative deter-

$$C_6H_4(COOH)(OCOCH_3) + H_2O \longrightarrow C_6H_4(COOH)(OH) + CH_3COOH$$

4 **5**

mination is often based on total SA, but for pharmacokinetic and metabolic studies it is essential to determine ASA and SA individually.

After isolation by extraction, ASA is usually found as SA. In any case, both ASA and SA will be found in the A1 fraction. SA gives a blue-violet color with ferric ion. Trinder's reagent ($HgCl_2$ and $Fe(NO_3)_3$) produces a purple color that is suitable for the quantitative determination of SA. The uv spectrum of SA is very characteristic (see Fig. 8.8), and strong absorption at about 300 nm is diagnostic for SA in a urine or blood extract.

Determinations of ASA and SA individually can be either direct or by difference. Difference methods determine SA before and after hydrolysis; the difference between these results gives the ASA. A fluorometric method illustrates this approach [12]. Only SA fluoresces. Both SA and ASA are extracted with ether. Reextraction into pH 7 phosphate buffer is followed by fluorometric measurement of SA. Another portion of the pH 7 extract is heated to hydrolyze the ASA, then total SA is measured fluorometrically.

The ratio ASA/SA in blood rapidly falls to very low values because of the facile hydrolysis of ASA in blood. The percentage error in an ASA concentration determined by difference quickly becomes unacceptable, and a direct method of analysis is to be preferred. A GC assay illustrates this approach [13]. Acidified plasma is extracted with ether, the ASA in the extract is silylated, and the silyl derivative is measured by GC after the addition of an internal standard. SA is determined fluorometrically on a separate portion of the extract.

Normal salicylate blood levels may be up to 5 mg/100 ml (5 mg%). Rheumatoid arthritic patients on continuing therapy may have levels of 25–30 mg%, and blood levels above 40 mg% are associated with toxic symptoms.

Many other analgesic drugs may be encountered. Salicylamide (**6**) and *p*-acetaminophen (**7**, APAP) are weak acids. Acetanilide (**8**) and acetophenetidin (**9**, phenacetin) are neutral drugs.

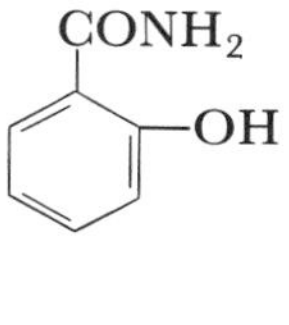

$CONH_2$ / OH

6

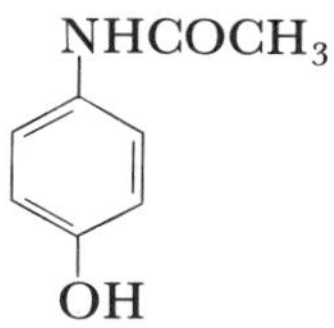

$NHCOCH_3$ / OH

7

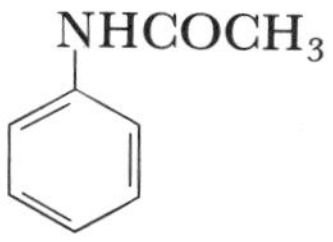

$NHCOCH_3$

8

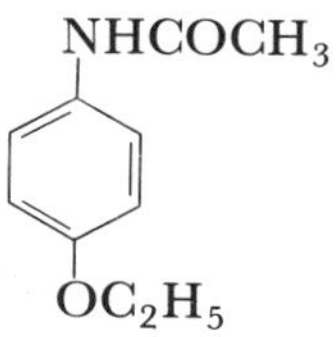

$NHCOCH_3$ / OC_2H_5

9

Renal toxicity is associated with the acetanilide-type analgesics. Acetanilide itself is seldom used now; it is quickly hydroxylated *in vivo* to *p*-acetaminophen, which is the active agent. Phenacetin has been widely used in the form of APC (aspirin-phenacetin-caffeine) tablets and capsules (see Experiment 17.1 for a TLC separation of this mixture); analgesic drugs are often used in combinations. The main metabolite of phenacetin is *p*-acetaminophen. The plasma half-life of *p*-acetaminophen appears to be an indicator of toxic effect; liver damage is expected if the half-life exceeds 4 hr. Overdosage plasma levels are 30–300 μg/ml. Much of the drug is excreted in "conjugated" forms, that is, as metabolic derivatives such as esters and ethers.

Salicylamide and *p*-acetaminophen give positive color tests with ferric ion. All the acetanilide analgesics give red colors upon hydrolysis and successive treatment with nitrous acid and the Bratton-Marshall reagent.

Tranquilizers and Antidepressants. These drugs can be classed chemically as the carbamates, the benzodiazepines, and the tricyclic antidepressants (phenothiazines, imipramines, and triptylines). A few structures will illustrate the range of substances. The carbamate group, $—OCONH_2$, which is both an amide and an ester, occurs in meprobamate, **10**, and ethinamate, **11**. The

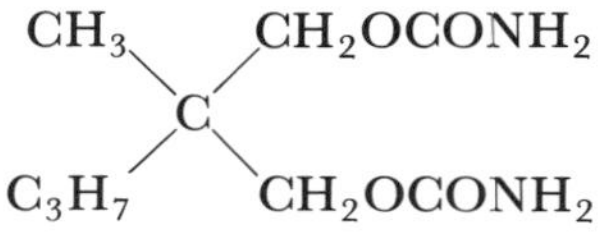

CH_3 CH_2OCONH_2 C C_3H_7 CH_2OCONH_2

10

$OCONH_2$ $—C{\equiv}CH$

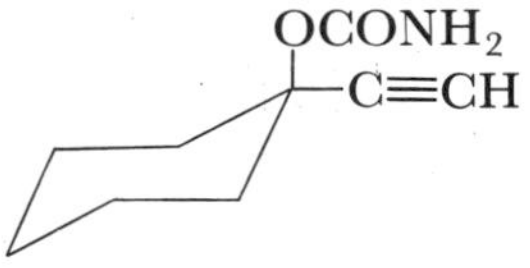

11

benzodiazepines are examplified by diazepam, **12**, and chlordiazepoxide, **13**.

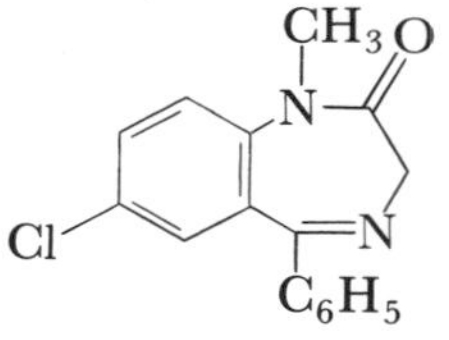

CH_3 O N Cl N C_6H_5

12

$NHCH_3$ N Cl N C_6H_5 O

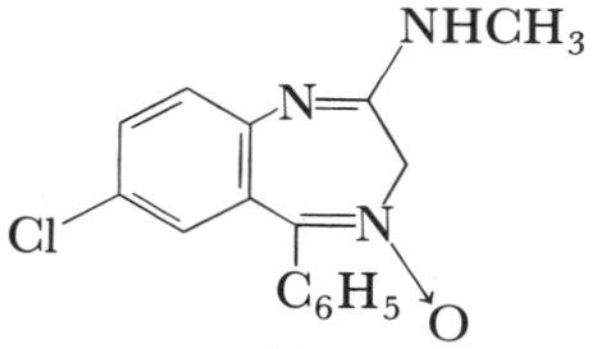

13

Tricyclic antidepressants have structures of the phenothiazine type illustrated by **14** (chlorpromazine), or imipramine (**15**), or amitryptyline (**16**).

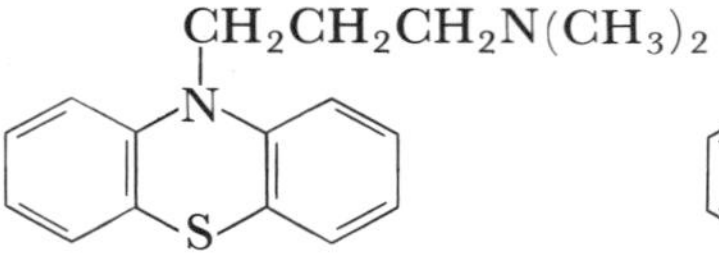

$CH_2CH_2CH_2N(CH_3)_2$ N S

14

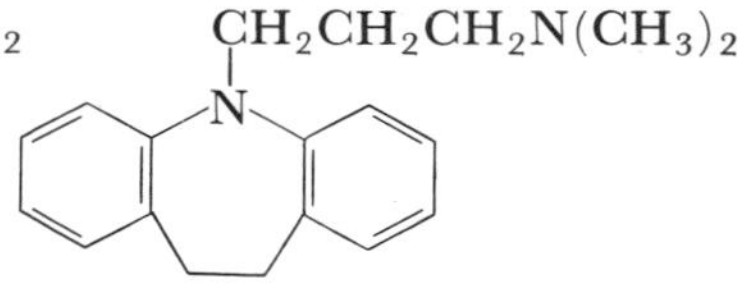

$CH_2CH_2CH_2N(CH_3)_2$ N

15

$CHCH_2CH_2N(CH_3)_2$

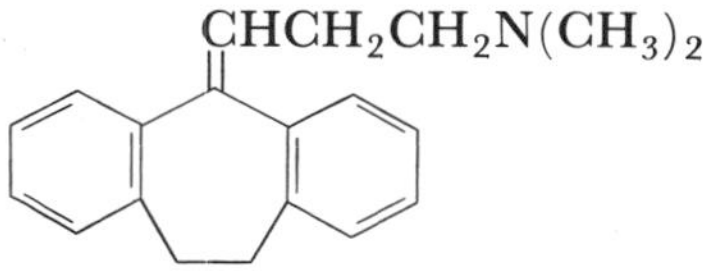

16

Many screening tests are available for the rapid detection of these drugs [11]. Some of these can be carried out directly on urine or blood. For example, FPN reagent (a mixture of ferric chloride, perchloric acid, and nitric acid) added to urine produces a variety of colors if a phenothiazine is present. Forrest reagent (potassium dichromate plus sulfuric, perchloric, and nitric acids) gives a green color when added to urine containing an imipramine drug.

Systematic analyses rely heavily on GLC, TLC, and HPLC of extracts of urine or blood. Drug metabolites and decomposition products must be considered. Thus phenothiazines are metabolized extensively to their sulfoxides. Many uv data for these compounds have been reported [14]. The phenothiazines show three maxima and two minima in their uv spectra; their sulfoxides have four maxima and three minima. The imipramines produce a blue color when oxidized and a yellow color upon treatment with sodium nitrite.

An interesting complication in the extraction of triptylines is that their hydrochloride salts are appreciably chloroform-soluble. This organic solubility of amine hydrochlorides is not unusual.

Alkaloids and Amines. The term alkaloid originally meant basic nitrogen-containing compounds of plant origin, but it now often refers to such compounds of whatever source. These substances will appear in the B fraction (Fig. 26.1). Usually chromatographic methods are applied to this fraction, after evaporation and redissolution to concentrate the solutes. A great many paper and thin-layer chromatographic systems have been described for this purpose. A general screening system has been described by Clarke [4, 11]. Paper chromatography is carried out on Whatman No. 1 paper that has been dipped in 5% sodium dihydrogen citrate and dried. The mobile phase solvent is a solution of 4.8 g of citric acid in 130 ml of water and 870 ml of *n*-butanol. After development of the chromatogram the paper is examined under uv light or sprayed with a variety of color reagents. By combining these visualization test results with R_f values tentative identification may be possible. Hundreds of basic compounds have been subjected to this procedure and the results have been tabulated [4, 11]. The same solvent system on TLC gives similar R_f values. Many chromatographic systems for specialized classes of compounds have been worked out [11, 15].

One class of alkaloids whose identification is important is the opiate narcotics. Morphine (**17**) and codeine (**18**) are the principal alkaloids of opium. The main opiate of abuse, however, is heroin, **19** (diamorphine,

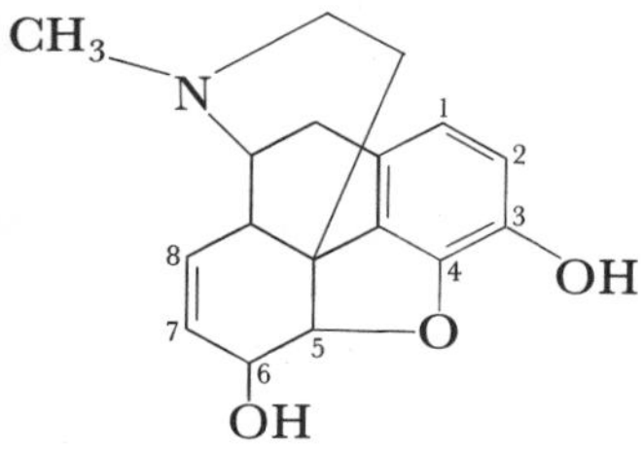

17

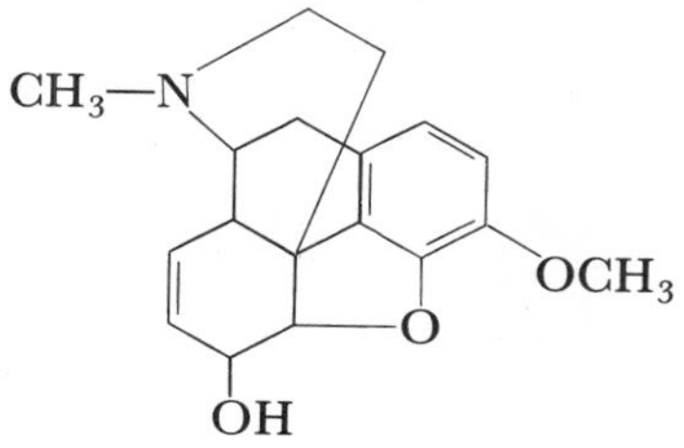

18

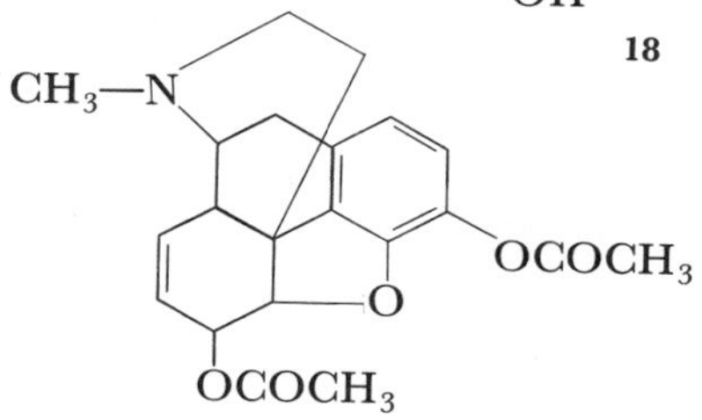

19

diacetylmorphine). Heroin is very rapidly hydrolyzed *in vivo* to 6-monoacetylmorphine and to morphine. Moreover, since heroin is made by acetylating morphine or opium extracts, usually illicitly, the product may contain the above compounds plus 3-monoacetylmorphine and 6-acetylcodeine. The analytical problem is complicated further by the slow metabolic conversion of codeine to morphine. In addition, heroin samples are usually diluted with other drugs, and the analyst may encounter barbiturates, quinine, caffeine, etc., that have been administered with the heroin.

TLC and GLC have been the methods of choice for the identification of these substances [11]. Recently immunoassay methods for morphine have been developed, and these will find important application, especially in screening for drug abuse.

Another alkaloid whose detection is required as an abused drug is lysergic acid diethylamide (LSD), **20**, the *N,N*-diethylamide of lysergic acid, an alkaloid from ergot. LSD is extracted in the basic fraction. Its instability is an

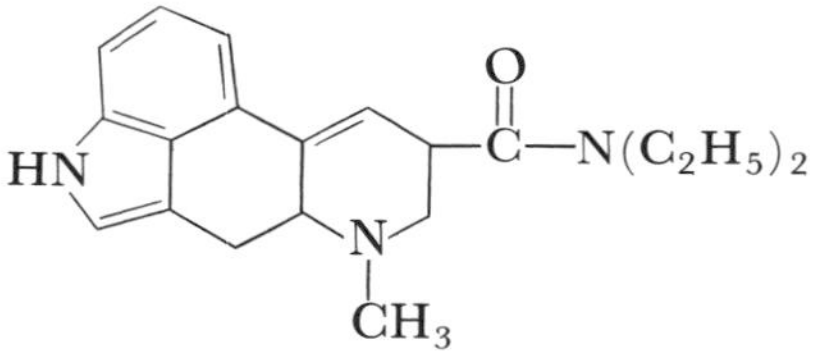

HN — O — C—$N(C_2H_5)_2$ — N — CH_3

20

analytical problem, and protection from light and air is helpful. A fast screening test for LSD, used in field kits, uses these two observations:

1. A blue fluorescence when irradiated with light of 254 nm.
2. A violet color when treated with *p*-dimethylaminobenzaldehyde and HCl.

Ergot alkaloids other than LSD respond to these tests, and a few other compounds may give them, so they are diagnostic rather than conclusive. Identification of LSD usually is based on positive results with these tests plus R_f values in several solvent systems.

The detection of LSD in illicit dosage forms can be hindered by measures taken to prevent detection. Some subterfuges include the incorporation of a violet dye to confound the screening color test with *p*-dimethylaminobenzaldehyde, and the inclusion of LSD in valid drug products. Since LSD is very active and highly toxic, it is diluted, and dosage forms may also include other psychotropic drugs.

Many other amines and alkaloids are used as drugs. Several derivatives of amphetamine, **21**, are used as stimulants, both in therapy and illegally.

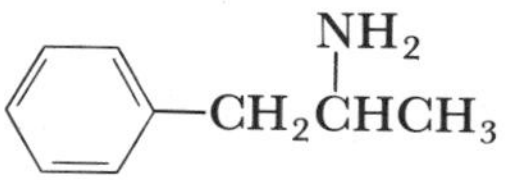

$$\text{C}_6\text{H}_5\text{–CH}_2\text{CH(NH}_2\text{)CH}_3$$

21

All the antihistamines are amines. Some of the alkaloids are routinely used in therapy. A recent analytical advance for the quantitative determination of primary amines in the picomole range (10^{-12} mole) utilizes a reaction with the reagent fluorescamine (**22**) to give a highly fluorescent product [16].

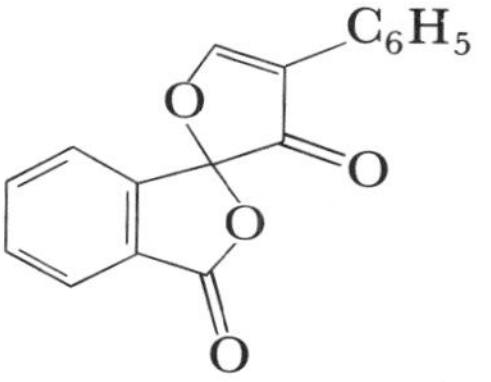

22

Cannabis. Cannabis is the dried tops of *cannabis sativa*, also called marijuana (marihuana). Great variety in appearance and chemical composition is observed depending upon geographical source. Hashish is an alcoholic extract of marijuana.

The active ingredients have structures based on **23**, which shows the most common numbering systems. All the active compounds have a double bond in

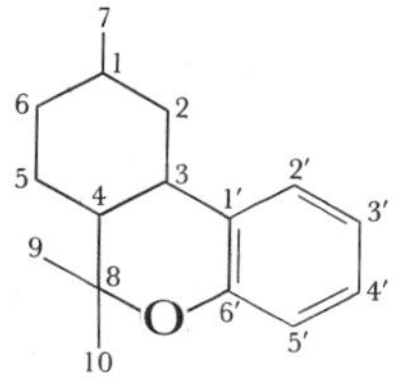

23

Monoterpenoid numbering

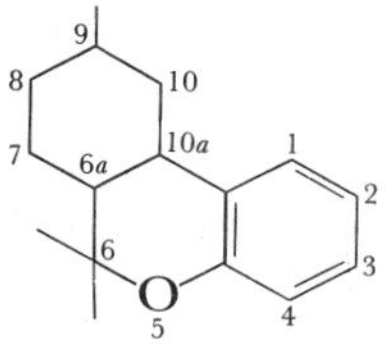

Dibenzopyran numbering

the terpene ring; these are called cannabinoids. The most important cannabinoids are shown on p. 548.

Upon heating, Δ^9-THCA(A) is converted to Δ^9-THC. Cannabinol (CBN), which is not active, has an aromatic ring in the terpene portion. Cannabidiol (CBD) is related to Δ^9-THC by cleavage of the 5,6 bond (dibenzopyran numbering).

There is considerable uncertainty about the stability of cannabis constituents. It has been claimed that solutions are unstable, yet a 43-year old

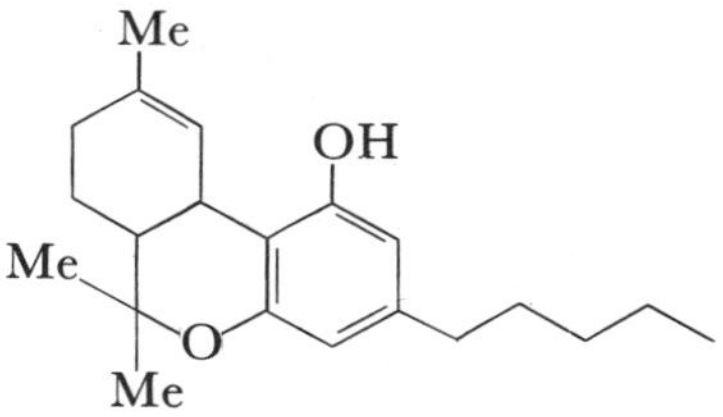

Δ^9-Tetrahydrocannabinol
(Δ^9-THC or Δ^1-THC)

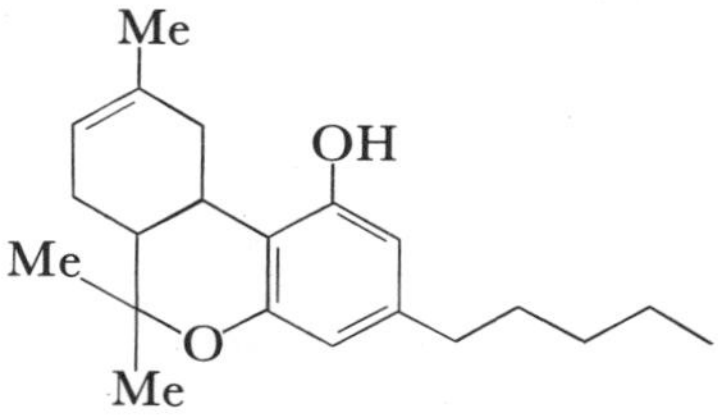

Δ^8-THC (Δ^6-THC)

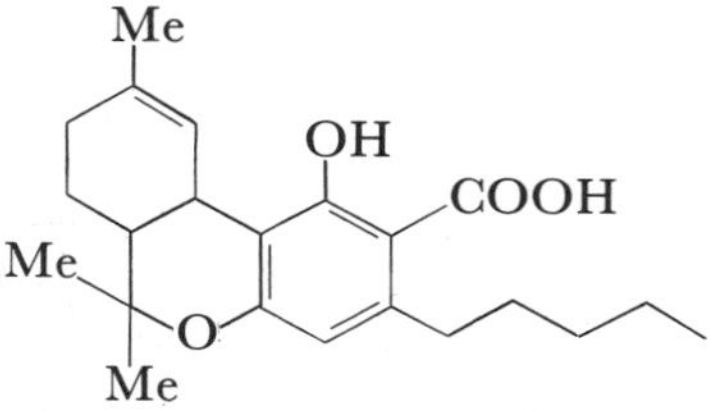

Δ^9-Tetrahydrocannabinolic acid A
[Δ^9-THCA(A)]

sample of cannabis fluid extract USP was found to contain substantial concentrations of CBD, CBN, and Δ^9-THC [17].

The identification of marijuana as a plant relies on microscopic identification of morphological structures [18]. In the absence of plant parts the constituents must be identified chemically. The usual color test for the detection of cannabinoids is the Duquenois test. This is carried out by extracting a few milligrams of sample with petroleum ether and evaporating the solvent. The residue is treated with an ethanol solution of vanillin and acetaldehyde, then with concentrated HCl. A deep blue to blue-violet color is a positive test. Shaken with chloroform, the blue-violet color is extracted into the chloroform.*

The specificity of this test has been studied [19], although the chemistry is not well understood. The minimum structural requirement seems to be the bicyclic system **24**. Some substitution of reagents can be made. The extractability into chloroform may be a consequence of the hydrophobic amyl side chain on the cannabinoids.

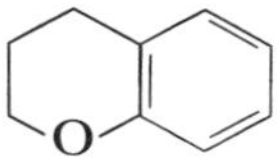

24

Ir, GLC, and fluorescence have been used to analyze cannabis for its constituents.

* When this extraction step is included, the procedure is known as the Duquenois-Levine test.

Alcohol. Alcohol (ethanol) determinations may be needed in dosage forms (see Experiment 18.1), alcoholic beverages, and in body fluids. The bulk of alcohol analyses arise in connection with traffic violations. Most methods fall into these classes: (1) oxidation methods; (2) alcohol dehydrogenase (ADH) methods; (3) gas chromatography.

The best chemical oxidation method is with potassium dichromate in sulfuric acid, the balanced reaction being

$$2Cr_2O_7^{2-} + 3C_2H_5OH + 16H^+ \rightarrow 4Cr^{3+} + 3CH_3COOH + 11H_2O$$

Each milliliter of 0.100 *N* $K_2Cr_2O_7$ consumed is equivalent to 1.15 mg of C_2H_5OH. The sample is reacted with excess standard dichromate, and the unreacted dichromate is measured either titrimetrically or spectrophotometrically. Of course any substance that can be oxidized by dichromate will interfere, so the alcohol usually must be separated from the sample (often blood) by distillation or microdiffusion.

ADH methods are based on this reaction.

$$C_2H_5OH + NAD \xrightleftharpoons{ADH} CH_3CHO + NADH$$

NAD is nicotinamide-adenine dinucleotide, a coenzyme. The reaction is reversible but is forced to completion by adding semicarbazide, $H_2NNHCONH_2$, which condenses with the acetaldehyde. The reduced coenzyme, NADH, is measured spectrophotometrically at 340 nm, where NAD does not absorb. Although ADH is fairly selective, it will give responses with higher alcohols. It is therefore essential that no alcohols be used for cleaning the skin when taking blood samples for alcohol analysis.

GC is specific for C_2H_5OH, since conditions can be found in which the alcohol retention time is significantly different from that of any conceivable interferent. Quantitative analysis by GC is easily possible.

Typical blood level values and their interpretation will be treated later. Most alcohol analyses are now made on samples of breath. Instruments are commercially available for collecting and analyzing the breath sample. The rationale for employing breath samples is that the mean ratio of alcohol in the breath to alcohol in the blood is essentially constant at 1:2100; that is, 2100 ml of alveolar ("deep-lung") breath contains the same amount of alcohol as 1 ml of blood. Of course breath samples are easier (for nonmedical personnel) to collect than blood samples. Since impairment of physical faculties can be related to blood alcohol concentration, it has become standard practice to determine alcohol in the breath, convert this to an equivalent blood level, and proceed legally on this basis [20–24].

The concentration of alcohol is expressed in several ways. The alcohol of commerce, called 95% alcohol, contains 94.9% by volume of C_2H_5OH. In alcoholic beverages the concentration is expressed in proof, which in the United States is twice the percent by volume. (In the United Kingdom proof refers to alcohol 57% by volume, and other concentrations are given as percent under or over proof.) Concentrations of alcohol in blood are expressed as mg/100 ml of blood (mg%) or as g/100 ml of blood. (%). The usual range of interest in traffic cases is about 0.05–0.15% blood alcohol.

The legal use and interpretation of alcohol analyses is based partly on scientific studies and partly on legal theory and practice [23, 24]. The legal definition of "under the influence," etc., is related to blood alcohol concentration, obtained from breath analyses; the limit above which a driver is judged to be in statutory violation has decreased progressively as more information has been obtained. States are now required to establish as the presumptive impairment limit a maximum of 0.10% blood alcohol. Some jurisdictions set this legal limit at 0.08%. It has been argued [24] that, because of uncertainties in converting the breath content to a reliable blood level, the breath analysis itself should serve as the basis for legal action.

Experiment 26.1. Isolation and Identification of Drugs in Urine

INTRODUCTION

In this experiment you will be given a sample of urine to which one or more drugs have been added. Your task is to identify the drugs. The isolation procedure described in Section 26.2 is suggested, but as you gain experience with your sample you may be able to introduce modifications.

Since your instructor can design many different problems bv adding different drugs, no general directions will be given for identification. A procedure is suggested, however, with which you can obtain experience in this kind of analysis. For a general unknown you will have to consult the literature, for example, to find recommended TLC solvents, R_f values, and color tests. The drugs that may be encountered will depend upon the time and equipment available; they could include aspirin, salicylamide, salicylic acid, *p*-acetaminophen, barbituric acid derivatives, alkaloids, etc.

APPARATUS

Separatory funnels and spot plates are needed. Equipment for TLC is essential, including spray reagents and a uv lamp for examining fluorescent chromatograms. Other valuable capabilities are GC, ir, MS, and uv spectroscopy. Fume hoods and electric hot plates must be used when evaporating organic solvents.

REAGENTS

Parri Reagents. (*a*) Prepare a 1% solution of a cobalt salt (the acetate, chloride, nitrate, or perchlorate) in methanol; (*b*) mix 2 ml of concentrated ammonium hydroxide and 20 ml of water, and dilute to 50 ml with methanol.

Ferric Reagent. Make a 5% solution of ferric chloride in water.

Bromine Water. Dissolve 1 ml of liquid bromine in 50 ml of water.

Authentic specimens of all drugs used will be available on request for comparison tests.

PROCEDURES

Known Sample. It is advisable to gain experience by working with solutions of known drugs. A procedure will be described for the isolation and identification of barbital, salicylic acid, and quinine in an aqueous solution.

Dissolve 25–30 mg of barbital, 30–40 mg of salicylic acid, and 80–100 mg of quinine hydrochloride in enough water to make 100 ml of solution. Take 25 ml of this solution and dilute it to 100 ml with water. Bring it to about pH 1 (using pH indicator paper) by the dropwise addition of concentrated HCl. Transfer to a 500 ml separatory funnel, and extract with 250 ml of ether. Separate the phases and reextract the aqueous phase with a fresh 150 ml portion of ether. Combine the ether extracts; this ether solution contains fraction A drugs.

Make the aqueous phase alkaline (pH $\approx$ 11) by adding concentrated ammonium hydroxide. Extract with 150 ml of chloroform, swirling gently to avoid emulsification. (If an emulsion forms, it can be separated by passing the chloroform layer through filter paper.) The chloroform solution contains Fraction B drugs.

Treat Fraction A as follows: evaporate the ether solution to about 100 ml in a hood. Transfer to a 250 ml separatory funnel and extract with 80 ml of 5% sodium bicarbonate. Separate the phases, transferring the ether to a beaker. Add 10–20 g of anhydrous sodium sulfate to the ether, mixing well to absorb moisture. Filter the ether solution and transfer it to a very clean evaporating dish. Gently evaporate to dryness. Redissolve the residue in 1 ml of methanol, transfer to a depression in a spot plate, and run the Parri test for barbiturates by adding a few drops of the cobalt and ammonia reagents. A positive test consists of an immediate violet color.

Returning to the aqueous phase of the preceding paragraph, carefully acidify it by adding concentrated HCl dropwise. Extract with 40 ml of ether, separate the phases, evaporate the ether to dryness redissolve the residue in 1 ml of water, and test for salicylate with the ferric reagent on the spot plate.

Now the Fraction B chloroform solution will be tested. Evaporate the chloroform to dryness, redissolve the residue in 1 ml of water, transfer to the spot plate, and add 1 drop of bromine water. After the orange color has faded to pale yellow, expose the solution to ammonia vapor by inverting a large beaker over a container of concentrated NH_4OH and placing the spot plate in this atmosphere. Quinine will produce a lime green color after several minutes.

Unknown Sample. Obtain a sample of urine that has been spiked with some drugs. Isolate and identify the drugs following a procedure like that described above. The first step is to dilute 25 ml of urine to 100 ml with water. Your instructor may give you some information limiting the number and kinds of drugs that you will have to look for. Carry out screening color tests, and follow up with chromatographic and spectroscopic methods for resolution of mixtures and identification.

References

1. Jackson, J. V., pp. 16–30 in *Isolation and Identification of Drugs*, E. G. C. Clarke (ed.), The Pharmaceutical Press, London, 1969.
2. Curry, A. S., Chap. 7 in *Toxicology: Mechanisms and Analytical Methods*, Vol. I, C. P. Stewart and A. Stolman (eds.), Academic, New York, 1960.
3. Curry, A. S., *Poison Detection in Human Organs*, 2nd ed., Charles C Thomas, Springfield, Ill., 1969.
4. Clarke, E. G. C., *Methods Forensic Sci.*, **1,** 1 (1962).
5. Schmidt, G., *Methods Forensic Sci.*, **1,** 373 (1962).
6. Turner, L. K., *Methods Forensic Sci.*, **2,** 177 (1963).
7. Hensel, E. B., *Methods Forensic Sci.*, **3,** 113 (1964).
8. Curry, A. S., Chap. 5 in *Toxicology: Mechanisms and Analytical Methods*, Vol. II, C. P. Stewart and A. Stolman (eds.), Academic, New York, 1961.
9. Connors, K. A., Chap. VI in *Pharmaceutical Analysis*, T. Higuchi and E. Brochmann-Hanssen (eds.), Interscience, New York, 1961.
10. De Zeeuw, R. A., *Prog. Chem. Toxicol.*, **4,** 59 (1969).
11. Clarke, E. G. C. (ed.), *Isolation and Identification of Drugs*, The Pharmaceutical Press, London, 1969.
12. Harris, P. A. and S. Riegelman, *J. Pharm. Sci.*, **56,** 713 (1967).
13. Rowland, M. and S. Riegelman, *J. Pharm. Sci.*, **56,** 717 (1967).
14. De-Leenheer, A., *J. Assoc. Offic. Anal. Chem.*, **56,** 105 (1973).
15. Sunshine, I., W. W. Fike, and H. Landsman, *J. Forensic Sci.*, **11,** 428 (1966).
16. Weigele, M., S. L. DeBernardo, J. P. Tengi, and W. Leimgruber, *J. Am. Chem. Soc.*, **94,** 5927 (1972).
17. Kubena, R. K., H. Barry, A. B. Segelman, M. Theiner, and N. R. Farnsworth, *J. Pharm. Sci.*, **61,** 144 (1972).
18. Thornton, J. I. and G. R. Nakamura, *J. Forensic Sci. Soc.*, **12,** 461 (1972).
19. Pitt, C. G., R. W. Hendron, and R. S. Hsia, *J. Forensic Sci.*, **1972,** 693.
20. Smith, H. W., *Methods Forensic Sci.*, **4,** 1 (1965).
21. Harger, R. N. and R. B. Forner, *Prog. Chem. Toxicol.*, **3,** 1 (1967).
22. Curry, A. S., *Advances in Forensic and Clinical Toxicology*, CRC Press, Cleveland, Ohio, 1972, Chap. 2.
23. Lovell, W. S., *Science*, **178,** 264 (1972).
24. Mason, M. F. and K. M. Dubowski, *Clin. Chem.*, **20,** 126 (1974).

FOR FURTHER READING

Sunshine, I. (ed.), *Handbook of Analytical Toxicology*, CRC Publishing Co., Cleveland, Ohio, 1969.

Sunshine, I. (ed.), *Manual of Analytical Toxicology*, CRC Publishing Co., Cleveland, Ohio, 1971.

Problems

1. In forensic toxicology, would it usually be more acceptable to make a false negative identification or a false positive?

2. (*a*) Let C_{body} and C_{blood} be concentrations of alcohol averaged over the whole body and in the blood, respectively. Then $r = C_{\text{body}}/C_{\text{blood}}$ is called the Widmark ratio; r is about 0.68 for males and 0.55 for females. If d is the density of alcohol and w is body weight (in 10^2 g units), show that $v = rwC_{\text{blood}}/d$, where v is the minimum number of milliliters of alcohol ingested.

(*b*) Why does this equation give the minimum volume ingested?

3. Predict the fraction in which each of the following drugs will be maximally found if subjected to the isolation procedure of Figs. 26.1 and 26.2: thiopental, testosterone, dextroamphetamine, atropine, phenol, benzoic acid.

4. An analgesic drug was subjected to these tests: (*a*) when treated with Fe (III) it gave a positive test (color); (*b*) when boiled in aqueous acid, then treated successively with sodium nitrite and the Bratton-Marshall reagent, a pink color developed. What was the drug?

27 THE ANALYTICAL PROBLEM

Familiarity with the principles of modern analytical techniques and skill in their application are necessary attributes of the successful pharmaceutical analyst, but they do not ensure the satisfactory solution of all the problems he may encounter. This final chapter surveys some auxiliary knowledge that can aid the analyst in selecting an analytical method, modifying it to suit the peculiarities of the sample at hand, and interpreting the raw data. Much of the information might be more logically placed in the first rather than the last chapter of this book, but it probably is more meaningful when read with the analytical background provided by preceding chapters.

27.1 Sampling

Usually the analyst is presented with a small portion of a production lot or other bulk unit, and from his analysis of this small portion a statement is made concerning the strength or purity of the bulk lot. It is obvious that the portion selected for analysis must be representative of the bulk if the analytical results are to be transferable to the unanalyzed bulk lot. The selection of a representative portion is called sampling. It is the first step in an analysis, and it is of critical importance. The theory and techniques of sampling have received much attention, the serious pitfalls are now recognized, and valid sampling techniques are available for most kinds of materials [1, 2]. Sampling of some kinds of pharmaceutical dosage forms is not yet on an entirely satisfactory basis, however.

The bulk lot is called the *population* or *universe*. This might be, for example, a tank car of ethanol, or 1000 barrels of magnesium oxide, or 1 million phenobarbital tablets. The sample is a portion of the population selected in such a way that it is representative of the population. Thus, for one of the above examples, the sample might consist of 1 liter of ethanol withdrawn from the tank car. In order to obtain a representative sample it is usually necessary to take a portion considerably larger than that required for the actual analysis. The analyst then selects a small portion, the *analytical sample*, from the sample that has been submitted to him. The acceptability of the entire population finally depends, then, on the analysis of a tiny portion that is presumed to possess the essential characteristics of the population. A homogeneous material, such as a liquid solution, readily yields a representative sample. Heterogeneous materials, however, are apt to yield biased samples to the careless sampler. Powders, granulations, vegetable drugs, ointments, emulsions, and suspensions are difficult to sample.

Powdered materials always exhibit a range of particle sizes, and the flow properties of the powder depend upon the particle size distribution. A marked segregation of the particles occurs when the powder flows, as when it is formed into a pile by pouring it from a shovel. A sample taken from the periphery of the pile would have a different particle size distribution than a sample taken at the top of the pile. If the powder were a mixture, the smaller particles might be richer in one component than would the larger particles, and samples of the types described would not be representative of the entire population. A common technique for obtaining a good sample from powdered material is by "coning and quartering." The powder is deposited on a flat surface by shovel or spatula, each successive shovelful being added to the apex of the cone built up by the previous addition. The entire cone is then formed into another cone by repetition of the process, the purpose being to mix the material. Then the cone is flattened and divided into four equal parts by forming two perpendicular diameters. The material from two diagonally opposed quarters is combined and formed into another cone, that material in the other two quarters being set aside. The coning and quartering process is continued until a sample of the requisite size is obtained.

When the population consists of discrete units, such as drums of solvent, packages of ampuls, bottles of capsules, etc., there are two general sampling approaches. In *random sampling* the population units are numbered serially. Then numbers are selected in some random manner, and the corresponding units are taken for the sample. Random selection means that all parts of the population have an equal probability of being selected. Thus bias is eliminated. A good way to select the numbered units randomly is to use a table of random numbers, which is a sequence of two- or three-digit numbers themselves arranged randomly [3]. Random sampling is an effective way to obtain unbiased, representative samples, but it is apt to be laborious and time-consuming. A more widely used technique is *systematic sampling*, in which every nth unit is selected to constitute the sample. The selection of n is of course critical, as the interval between selected units must not correspond to any periodicity in the population. Thus if a packaging machine operates on a rotary basis with 24 packages being fed onto a moving belt per turn of the rotor, evidently a very biased sample would be obtained by collecting every 24th package, for every package in the sample will then have been filled at the same point in the rotor mechanism.

In routine quality control analysis, the analyst seldom obtains his own samples. In research and developmental work he may perform the sampling function. Since it often happens that the sample (which we shall suppose is representative of the population) is larger than the analyst needs, he must subdivide it until he has a portion small enough for analysis. If the material is a solution this presents no problem; the sample is mixed thoroughly and a suitable portion is taken for assay. Heterogeneous samples are not so easily subdivided. The best guide to follow in reducing the sample to an appropriate analytical sample is the published specifications describing the product. The USP and NF often specify the manner in which an analytical sample should be taken.

Tablets, which are the most widely used dosage form, conventionally have been analyzed after preparation of the analytical sample as follows: at least 20 tablets (the manner of their selection is left to the discretion of the analyst) are counted, weighed, and reduced to a fine powder. An accurately weighed portion (the analytical sample) of the powder is taken for assay. The assay result can be converted back, by means of the weights and the number of tablets, to an average weight of drug per tablet. This quantity must fall within certain specified limits for the sample to be acceptable. This is a perfectly valid sampling approach, if the tablets are selected wisely. However, it suffers from its incapability of providing information about the variability among tablets. This information is important because a patient does not take an "average" tablet; he takes a single real tablet. Granting, therefore, that the average content of 20 tablets meets specifications, it is desirable to go beyond this and analyze the content of individual tablets. The concept of "single dose analysis" is a relatively new sampling technique that will probably be applied widely in the future because of the valuable knowledge it provides about dose-to-dose variation. Single-dose analysis presents some new problems in practical analysis, among them being the reduced analytical sample size, the increased labor because of the greater number of assays required, the setting of admissible limits for dose-to-dose variability, and of course the number of doses, and manner of their selection, needed for meaningful results [4].

27.2 Statistical Interpretation of Data

The results of a chemical analysis (or of any quantitative measurement) are usually available as a set of numbers representing replicate determinations made under (so far as is necessary and possible) identical conditions. These numbers may correspond to percentage purity, normality, weight of compound, etc. The interpretation of these raw data by the analyst answers two important questions: (1) What is the *best estimate* of the "true" value of the quantity being measured? (2) *How reliable* is this number as an estimator of the true value? The detailed study of these and related questions is the concern of a branch of mathematics called statistics. In this section we consider some of the results of mathematical statistics that are pertinent to the interpretation of analytical data. Many of the assertions made will not be justified here, and some of them are perhaps oversimplified, from the statistician's point of view; however, the treatment is adequate for most of the requirements of practical analysis.

Types of Errors. Error is associated with every measurement. Even if obvious mistakes in calculation or technique are eliminated, error remains. The analyst must reduce the magnitude of the error to an acceptable level; he can never eliminate it altogether. Errors are of two types: *systematic* or *random*.

Systematic errors, or determinate errors, are those introduced by an inadequacy in the analytical method or by poor judgment or unconscious bias on the part of the analyst. Many examples can be given to illustrate systematic error. Thus an incomplete reaction caused by an unfavorable equilibrium will introduce an error into results calculated on the basis of complete reaction. Impurities in reagents, improperly calibrated glassware and weights, a poorly seated spectrophotometer cell compartment cover that admits stray light; neglect of the temperature effect on K_w when it should be considered, color blindness leading to poorly judged visual endpoints—all these are real sources of systematic errors in analytical measurements. With very careful attention to all details of the analytical method in its development and application, systematic errors should be reducible to a negligible level. If unacceptable systematic errors remain after assiduous efforts to eliminate them, the method must be discarded as impracticable.

The estimation of systematic error is closely related to the problem of accuracy, which will be considered shortly. For the present we shall accept the notion that a "true" value of the quantity being measured exists, and that it is known to us. Then the ***absolute error*** E of a measurement is the difference between the observed, O, and true, T, values: $E = O - T$. The *relative error* is defined to be E/T. Many systematic errors are either additive or proportional. An additive error is one whose magnitude is independent of sample size; it causes a constant absolute error in a series of determinations of increasing sample weights. The partial loss of a precipitate by dissolution is an example; if the solvent volume is identical in the series of analyses, an identical weight of precipitate will be lost in each experiment. A proportional error, on the other hand, increases as the sample size increases; it often leads to a constant relative error. An incorrectly standardized titrant solution will produce a proportional error in titrations of a set of samples of increasing weights. During the development and testing stages of a new assay method, various amounts of a known sample should be tested in order to locate systematic error and to determine if the error is additive or proportional. This information may help in detecting and eliminating the source of the error.

Random errors, or indeterminate errors, remain even after all systematic errors have been eliminated. It is a familiar observation that duplicate determinations of a quantity almost never yield the same number when the maximum sensitivity of the measuring device is utilized. This variability is the manifestation of random errors. It is found that replicate observations group themselves about a most frequently observed value, with large deviations from this value being rarer than small ones. Random errors are caused by limitations inherent in the observational method. They can be minimized but not eliminated. Because of random errors some uncertainty is always associated with every measurement. The evaluation of this uncertainty requires statistical methods.

Accuracy and Precision. The statistical treatment of experimental data requires a conception of the nature of these data that is different from that usually held by the analyst. The statistician regards an experimental observation as a single member randomly selected from an infinite population of individuals characteristic of the system under consideration. Because of the operation of random errors, replicate observations, representing further random selections from the hypothetical infinite population of such observations, will not be identical, but will exhibit more or less variation, with the general type of distribution described in the preceding paragraph. If a graph is made of the value of each experimental observation on the horizontal axis against the number of times each value is observed (its frequency) on the vertical axis, a symmetrical figure will usually be produced with a maximum corresponding to the most frequently observed value. As the number of observations is increased toward the limit of infinity the figure will adopt the form of a smooth curve. Such a curve is called a frequency distribution.

Although one can imagine many possible curves with such an appearance, it is in practice found that such experimental frequency distributions can usually be closely fitted by a theoretical frequency distribution variously called the *normal distribution*, the *Gaussian distribution*, or the *normal error curve.* The equation of the normal distribution is

$$f(x) = \frac{1}{\sigma\sqrt{2\pi}} e^{-(1/2)[(x-\mu)/\sigma]2} \tag{27.1}$$

where $f(x)$ is the frequency of occurrence of the value x of the variable, and μ and σ are parameters of the population. The symbol μ represents the *population mean*, which is that value of x corresponding to the maximum in the curve. σ, the *population standard deviation*, determines the "spread" or width, of the bell-shaped curve. A graph of the normal curve is shown in Fig. 27.1. Graphically the standard deviation may be represented as the horizontal distance from the mean to either inflection point of the curve, as indicated in the figure. Approximately 68% of the area under the normal curve, and hence 68% of the members of the population, lie within 1 standard deviation of the mean, that is, in the range $\mu \pm \sigma$. About 95% of the population are included in the range $\mu \pm 2\sigma$, and over 99% in the range $\mu \pm 3\sigma$.

The infinite population of experimental observations on most of the real systems encountered by the analyst is characterized by a close adherence to the normal frequency distribution. The population mean μ, representing the most frequently occurring value of the variable, and therefore the midpoint of the symmetrically disposed observations, is regarded as the "true value" of the quantity being measured. This quantity is of course inaccessible because of our inability to perform the infinite number of analyses necessary to define the curve; in fact, the number of observations, far from being infinite, is usually in the range 3–6. These few observations are taken as representative of the infinite population. Because of the symmetrical nature of the frequency distribution, the best estimate of the population mean is the arithmetic average, or *mean*, m, of the experimental observations:

$$m = \frac{\sum x_i}{n} \tag{27.2}$$

where x_i is the value of the ith observation and n is the number of observations.

The *accuracy* of an analytical result is considered to be the closeness with which the mean m estimates the population mean μ. With this symbolism

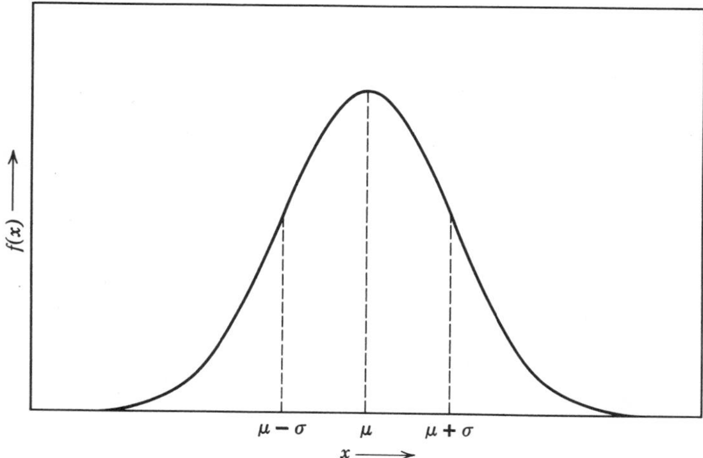

Fig. 27.1. The normal error curve with mean μ and standard deviation σ.

the earlier definition of error E becomes $E = m - \mu$. The smaller the error, the higher is the accuracy. Unfortunately, the population mean is usually unknown, so the error, and hence the accuracy, of a result cannot be evaluated. In practice the accuracy may often be gauged by comparing the mean m with a "known" value that is set by the experimenter with a standard sample. This procedure is used in assay development work, and it has been incorporated into many of the experiments in this book. In this way systematic errors can be detected. Obviously systematic errors must be absent or of negligible magnitude if satisfactory accuracy is to be obtained. The analyst should strive for a level of accuracy consistent with the use to be made of the results.

Occasionally the *median* is employed as the estimate of the population mean. The median is that value that exceeds as many values as it itself is exceeded by (for n odd). If n is even, the median is the average of the two values satisfying the same criterion. If the frequency distribution is symmetrical the population mean and median are identical. The median is not as sensitive to a widely discordant result as is the mean.

It happens that some variables are not normally distributed but even in these cases it can be shown that the means of small numbers of observations are themselves normally distributed. Thus the new population, composed of replicate means of small sets of the original population, may be treated as a normally distributed variable.

Precision is a synonym for reproducibility. It evidently is associated with the population standard deviation σ, for this quantity characterizes the width of the normal curve. The narrower the population frequency distribution (smaller σ), the higher is the precision of the measurements. As the experimental estimate of σ we take s, the *standard deviation*, which is equal to the square root of the variance V,

$$V = \frac{\sum (x_i - m)^2}{n - 1} \tag{27.3}$$

$$s = \sqrt{V} \tag{27.4}$$

where the symbols have their usual meanings. The quantity $(n - 1)$ is sometimes called the degrees of freedom, for it represents the number of independently assignable quantities necessary to fix the system once the other parameters (in this case the mean) are fixed. A small value of s is associated with high precision and a narrow distribution curve.

The variance is a fundamental statistical quantity with the convenient attribute of additivity. If the overall precision of an analytical method can be partitioned into the precision associated with several stages of the method, for example, sampling, solution preparation, instrument reading, etc., and if a variance can be calculated for each of these stages by appropriate experimentation, then the variance of the overall method is equal to the sum of the variances of its parts.

Other estimates of precision are sometimes reported, but these do not possess the theoretical significance of the standard deviation and are usually inferior to it as a measure of reproducibility. The *average deviation* or mean deviation is given by

$$\text{Average deviation} = \frac{\sum |x_i - m|}{n - 1} \tag{27.5}$$

where the absolute value of the deviation is taken to prevent the sum from going to zero. The *range*, w, is defined as the difference between the smallest and largest observations in a set. The range is a useful indication of precision when n is very small.

In analytical situations the precision is often reported on a relative basis as follows:

$$\text{Precision in percent} = \frac{100s}{m}$$

The precision in percent is also referred to as the coefficient of variation.

$$\text{Precision in parts per thousand (ppt)} = \frac{1000s}{m}$$

$$\text{Precision in parts per million (ppm)} = \frac{10^6 s}{m}$$

Sometimes the average deviation and the range are similarly expressed in a relative manner.

It must be realized that good precision in a set of observations does not ensure good accuracy, for a systematic error may lead to inaccurate results that are quite precise.

Confidence Limits of the Mean. We earlier noted that even if a population of individuals is not normally distributed, the means of several sets of observations drawn from the population will be normally distributed. It is, in fact, such means of small sets of observations that we are concerned with in practice, for the usual situation is that a small number of observations is made, a mean m and standard deviation s are calculated, and some idea of the reliability of m is desired. This could presumably be obtained with the aid of the information given earlier pertaining to the characteristics of the normal distribution. However, for small n, the distribution of the observations or their means will in general not be normal, even if the population is distributed normally. The actual distribution of the observations (or their means) in such a situation is

TABLE 27.1
Some Values of Student's t

Degrees of Freedom	P = 0.10	0.05	0.01
1	6.314	12.706	63.657
2	2.920	4.303	9.925
3	2.353	3.182	5.841
4	2.132	2.776	4.604
5	2.015	2.571	4.032
6	1.943	2.447	3.707
7	1.895	2.365	3.499
8	1.860	2.306	3.555
9	1.833	2.262	3.250
10	1.812	2.228	3.169

given by Student's t distribution,* which exhibits a wider spread than the normal curve. In Table 27.1 are listed some values for Student's t. The first column gives the degrees of freedom, which in the cases of interest is equal to $(n - 1)$. The headings of the other columns are values of P, the probability that the limits calculated may be exceeded by chance. The values in the body of the table give the distribution of t (which approaches the normal distribution as n becomes larger).

The standard deviation s is really the standard deviation of a single observation; that is, it describes the reproducibility of a single observation. Since, however, it is the mean of several observations that is the quantity of analytical importance, it is desirable to have a measure of the reproducibility of the mean. This quantity, the *standard deviation of the mean*, s_m, is calculated by

$$s_m = \frac{s}{\sqrt{n}} \tag{27.6}$$

Notice that the precision of the mean is always higher than the precision of the observations contributing to the mean.†

The analyst desires a measure of the reliability of his mean result. This measure is called the *confidence limits* of the mean, and it is calculated with the aid of Student's t distribution. Suppose a set of n observations has been made. The mean m, the standard deviation s, and the standard deviation of the mean s_m are calculated. It is desired to know the limits within which a chosen percentage of additional means of n observations will fall. These confidence

* Student was the pen name of W. S. Gosset, a British statistician and chemist.

† Both the standard deviation [5] and the standard deviation of the mean [6] are sometimes referred to as the "standard error." Because of the possibility for confusion this term probably should not be used.

limits are given by

$$m \pm ts_m$$

where t is read from Table 27.1, the appropriate column being selected. The technique and interpretation of this calculation are best demonstrated with an example.

EXAMPLE 27.1. The following numbers are the percent recoveries in seven identical nonaqueous titrations of a urea sample: 98.4, 100.2, 99.3, 101.7, 97.4, 98.2, and 100.8.

(*a*) Calculate the mean, standard deviation, and standard deviation of the mean for the set of analyses.

It is best to arrange the work in tabular form as shown. The mean is given by Eq. 27.2, $m = 696.0\%/7 = 99.4\%$. The variance is $14.34\%^2/6 = 2.39\%^2$, so the standard deviation is 1.55% and the standard deviation of the mean is 0.61%.

Titration, i	Percent Recovery (x_i)	$(x_i - m)$	$(x_i - m)^2$
1	98.4	−1.0	1.00
2	100.2	0.8	0.64
3	99.3	−0.1	0.01
4	101.7	2.3	5.29
5	97.4	−2.0	4.00
6	98.2	−1.2	1.44
7	100.8	1.4	1.96

(*b*) Find 95% and 99% confidence limits for the mean. The 95% confidence limits would usually be written $P = 0.05$, thus letting P represent the fraction of further means that will be expected to fall outside the range specified. For $P = 0.05$, and 6 degrees of freedom, we find from Table 27.1 that $t = 2.447$. The confidence limits ($P = 0.05$) are therefore $m \pm ts_m$ or $99.4 \pm 2.447(0.61)\% = 99.4 \pm 1.5\%$. This means that if many additional sets of seven titrations were performed, about 95% of the means of such sets would be expected to fall within the range 97.9–100.9% (the confidence interval).

For $P = 0.01$, $t = 3.707$. The confidence limits ($P = 0.01$) are $99.4 \pm 2.2\%$. Obviously the limits are wider at $P = 0.01$ than at $P = 0.05$, for we have used the same information but have required that a larger fraction of additional means will fall within specified limits.

Rejection of Doubtful Results. Occasionally it happens that one observation in a set appears to be widely discordant. The question arises whether or not one

TABLE 27.2
Q Rejection Ratios[a]

n	$Q_{0.90}$
3	0.94
4	0.76
5	0.64
6	0.56
7	0.51
8	0.47
9	0.44
10	0.41

[a] From Ref. 7.

is justified in rejecting the doubtful result. This decision involves two kinds of risk. On the one hand, there is the risk of rejecting a result that really belongs to the set. Remember that an infrequent large deviation from the mean is to be expected, if the population of observations from which one is, in effect, randomly withdrawing individuals is normally distributed. In fact, about 1 observation out of every 20 may be expected to deviate from the mean by at least $2s$.

On the other hand is the risk of retaining a result that really should be rejected. It is necessary to adopt a compromise position in which one risk is balanced against the other. Many criteria have been suggested as a basis for this decision. The following procedure is suggested by Dean and Dixon [7]: (1) first examine carefully the data leading to the discordant result. If a definite error is located the result must be rejected. (2) If no error is found, apply the Q rejection test explained below. If the Q test permits rejection of the doubtful result, the remaining values may be used for calculation of the mean, etc. (3) If the Q test does not permit rejection of the result, it should be retained. The median of the set may be taken, rather than the mean, as an estimate of the true value, because the median is less influenced by a divergent value. It may be advisable to obtain additional results.

The Q test is performed by subtracting the doubtful result from its nearest neighbor and dividing this difference by the range. The resulting ratio, called Q, is compared with the ratio in Table 27.2 for the appropriate number of determinations. If Q exceeds the tabulated ratio, the questionable value may be rejected with 90% probability that its rejection is justified.

EXAMPLE 27.2. The following values were obtained in the standardization of a sodium hydroxide solution. Can the doubtful value (which is evidently

0.1008) be rejected? Normality found = 0.1013, 0.1015, 0.1008, 0.1012, 0.1012, 0.1014.

$$Q = \frac{0.1012 - 0.1008}{0.1015 - 0.1008} = \frac{4}{7} = 0.57$$

Q exceeds 0.56 (Table 27.2); hence the questionable value may be rejected with a probability of about 90% that this is the proper action.

27.3 The Analytical Literature

Bibliography of Analytical Sources. Few analyses are so simple and foolproof in execution that the analyst can carry them out extemporaneously, without reference to printed accounts. Selection of optimum conditions, possible interferences, sensitivity and selectivity, accuracy, and precision are all factors pertinent to the performance of an assay that must be known to the analyst before he begins laboratory operations. Vast amounts of such information are available in the literature, and the skilled analyst will learn to find it and profit by it. There are several kinds of analytical literature.

Introductory textbooks of quantitative analysis: every chemical and pharmaceutical library contains many quantitative analysis texts. The fundamentals of theory, calculations, and analytical experimentation are treated in these books, with the emphasis being placed on classical volumetric and gravimetric inorganic analysis.

Textbooks of qualitative inorganic analysis: these texts present identification schemes for inorganic cations and anions based primarily on separation by precipitation, followed by individual color or precipitation tests.

Textbooks of qualitative organic analysis: the subject treated by these books is the identification of organic compounds. Mixtures are separated by distillation and solvent extraction, and the isolated components are identified (characterized) by a comparison of their physical and chemical properties with those of authentic samples. Melting and boiling points, and the melting points of crystalline derivatives of the unknown substance, have been the strongest basis for characterization in the past. The present trend is to emphasize spectroscopic methods, especially uv, ir, MS, and nmr.

Textbooks of quantitative organic analysis: Two instructive volumes are*:

Fritz, J. S. and G. S. Hammond, *Quantitative Organic Analysis*, John Wiley and Sons, New York, 1957.

Siggia, S. and H. J. Stolton, *An Introduction to Modern Organic Analysis*, Interscience, New York, 1956.

* None of the bibliographical listings in this section pretends to be exhaustive. A few representative books, in English, are mentioned to provide the student with a place to begin looking.

Textbooks of pharmaceutical analysis:

Jenkins, G. L., A. M. Knevel, and F. E. DiGangi, *Quantitative Pharmaceutical Chemistry*, 6th ed., McGraw-Hill, New York, 1967.

Beckett, A. H. and J. B. Stenlake, *Practical Pharmaceutical Chemistry*, 2nd ed., Athlone Press, London, Part I, 1968; Part II, 1970.

Gearien, J. E. and B. F. Grabowski, *Methods of Drug Analysis*, Lea and Febiger, Philadelphia, 1969.

Chatten, L. G. (ed.), *Pharmaceutical Chemistry*, Marcel Dekker, New York, Vol. I, 1966; Vol. II, 1969.

Advanced textbooks of analytical chemistry:

Meites, L. and H. C. Thomas, *Advanced Analytical Chemistry*, McGraw-Hill, New York, 1958.

Laitinen, H. A., *Chemical Analysis*, McGraw-Hill, New York, 1960.

Handbooks: the following are of general value.

Handbook of Chemistry and Physics, 54th ed., Chemical Rubber Publishing Co., Cleveland, 1973.

Handbook of Analytical Chemistry, L. Meites (ed.), McGraw-Hill, New York, 1963.

The Merck Index, 8th ed., Merck and Co., Rahway, N.J., 1968.

The Chemist's Companion, A. J. Gordon and R. A. Ford, Wiley-Interscience, New York, 1972.

There are, in addition, several specialized works dealing with chromatography, spectroscopy, etc.

Standard compendia:

Pharmacopeia of the United States of America, 19th revision, United States Pharmacopeial Convention, Washington, D.C., 1975.

The National Formulary, 14th ed., American Pharmaceutical Association, Washington, 1975.

These two volumes set official standards for drugs in the United States. The pharmacopeias of other countries and the compilations of allied fields provide further analytical information.

British Pharmacopoeia, Pharmaceutical Press, London, 1973.

Official Methods of Analysis of the Association of Official Agricultural Chemists, 9th ed., Association of Official Agricultural Chemists, Washington, D.C., 1960.

Official Standardized and Recommended Methods of Analysis, S. C. Jolly (ed.), Society for Analytical Chemistry, Cambridge, 1963; Supplement, 1967.

The Givaudan Index, 2nd ed., Givaudan-Delawanna, Inc., New York, 1961.

Food Chemicals Codex, Publication 1406, National Academy of Sciences—National Research Council, Washington, D.C., 1966.

Reference works on pharmaceutical analysis:

Higuchi, T. and E. Brochmann-Hanssen (eds.), *Pharmaceutical Analysis*, Interscience, New York, 1961.

Garratt, D. C. (ed.), *The Quantitative Analysis of Drugs*, 3rd ed., Chapman and Hall, London 1964.

Clarke, E. G. C. (ed.), *Isolation and Identification of Drugs*, The Pharmaceutical Press, London, 1969.

Hashmi, M.-U.-H., *Assay of Vitamins in Pharmaceutical Preparations*, John Wiley and Sons, New York, 1973.

Review series:

Organic Analysis, Interscience, New York, Vol. 1, 1953; Vol. 2, 1954; Vol. 3, 1956; Vol. 4, 1960.
Advances in Analytical Chemistry and Instrumentation, C. N. Reilley (ed.), Vol. 1, Interscience, New York, 1960.
Analytical Profiles of Drug Substances, K. Florey, (ed.), Vol. 1, 1972, Vol. 2, 1973, Academic Press, New York.
Encyclopedia of Industrial Chemical Analysis, F. D. Snell, C. L. Hilton, and L. S. Ettre (eds.), Wiley-Interscience, New York, Vol. 1, 1966.

The above are continuing series.

Kolthoff, I. M. and P. J. Elving (eds.), *Treatise on Analytical Chemistry*, Interscience, New York (first volume 1959).
Wilson, C. L. and D. W. Wilson (eds.), *Comprehensive Analytical Chemistry*, Elsevier, Amsterdam (first volume 1959).

These are multivolumed treatises covering the entire field of analytical chemistry.

Monographs. A monograph is, in the present sense, a book-length account of a single subject or area of study. It is pointless to list illustrative titles here; the reader interested in a special topic in analysis will be able to locate pertinent monographs in the library subject card index. Many monographs have been cited in this book, and the student may find it illuminating to look into some of these.

Periodicals. All the types of literature described above are *secondary sources;* that is, the information contained in them has been collected from a source closer to its discovery; it has perhaps been abstracted and interpreted, and has then been presented in the form of a text, review, or monograph. The *primary source* from which the information was taken is the periodical literature. This consists of thousands of scientific journals that publish research papers reporting original investigations. Each broad area of scientific and humanistic study has journals devoted to its progress. A few journals publish articles from many fields. Most journals, however, are rather specialized, dealing with a narrow aspect of one of the sciences, for example. Much of this mass of literature is not of direct use to the analyst, although he should always be ready to adopt any approach that will help him solve his analytical problems. A few journals of special interest to the analyst are listed here. Their titles indicate their area of specialization in many instances. Some of the more general journals are included because they often publish material, such as absorption spectra and dissociation constants, that can be put to analytical use. If the language of the articles is not English it is specified after the title. Conventional abbreviations are indicated in boldface.

Acta Chemica **Scand**inavica (Eng., Fr., Ger.)
American **J**ournal of **Pharm**aceutical **Educ**ation

Analytical **Biochem**istry
Analytical **Chem**istry (formerly Industrial and Engineering Chemistry, Analytical Edition)
Analytica **Chim**ica **Acta** (Eng., Fr., Ger.)
Analytical **Lett**ers
Analusis
Analyst
Annales **Pharm**aceutiques **Fr**ancaises (Fr.)
Archives of **Biochem**istry and **Biophy**sics
Archiv der **Pharm**azie (Ger.)
Arzneimittel-**Forsch**ung (Ger.)
Biochemistry
Biochemical Journal
Biochemical **Pharmacol**ogy
Biochimica et **Biophys**ica **Acta**
Bollettino **Chim**ico **Farm**aceutico (Ital.)
Chemist-Analyst
Chemical and **Pharm**aceutical **Bull**etin (**Tokyo**) (Eng., Ger.)
Chromatographia
Clinical **Chem**istry
Collection of **Czech**oslovak **Chem**ical **Commun**ications (Eng., Ger., Russ.)
Drug Standards (discontinued; formerly Bulletin of the National Formulary Committee)
Farmaco (Ital.)
Journal of **Agr**icultural and **Food Chem**istry
Journal of the **Am**erican **Chem**ical **Soc**iety
Journal of the **Am**erican **Oil Chem**ists' **Soc**iety
Journal of the **Assoc**iation of **Off**icial **Anal**ytical **Chem**ists (formerly Journal of the Association of Official Agricultural Chemists)
Journal of **Biol**ogical **Chem**istry
Journal of **Chem**ical **Educ**ation
Journal of the **Chem**ical **Soc**iety
Journal of **Chromatogr**aphy
Journal of **Chromatogr**aphic **Sci**ence (formerly Journal of Gas Chromatography)
Journal of **Clin**ical **Invest**igation
Journal of **Med**icinal **Chem**istry
Journal of **Org**anic **Chem**istry
Journal of **Pharmacol**ogy and **Exp**erimental **Ther**apeutics
Journal of **Pharm**acy and **Pharmacol**ogy (formerly Quarterly Journal of Pharmacy and Pharmacology)

Journal of **Pharm**aceutical **Sci**ences (formerly Journal of the American Pharmaceutical Association, Scientific Edition)
Journal of **Physi**cal **Chem**istry
Microchemical Journal
Mikrochimica Acta (Eng., Fr., Ger.)
Molecular **Pharmacol**ogy
Nature
Pharmaceutica **Acta Helv**etiae (Eng., Fr., Ger., Ital.)
Pharmazie (Ger.)
Recueil des **Trav**aux **Chim**iques des Pays-Bas (Eng., Fr.)
Science
Talanta
Zeitschrift fur **Anal**ytische **Chem**ie (Ger.)

Abstract Journals. The location of a desired article or bit of information in the vast chemical literature is made possible by abstract services, which publish brief summaries of scientific articles together with detailed indexes to subjects and authors. *Chemical Abstracts* is the most complete of these services. *Analytical Abstracts* limits its coverage to papers of analytical interest.

Alerting Services. In order to help the reader locate articles of interest in very recent issues of journals, some "alerting services" have been developed. Some of these are periodicals that print the contents pages of other journals, and some provide computer-generated indexes to help find articles. *Chemical Titles* and *Current Contents* are two useful services.

Using the Literature. The information sought determines the manner in which a search of the literature is conducted. Although in principle it is not necessary to resort to printed accounts at all, in practice this is the most efficient way to approach the solution of a problem. It is very expensive and time-consuming, and totally unnecessary, to carry out research on a problem that someone else has already solved. If the problem is general or very fundamental in nature, an explanation may be answered by monographs. If the analyst needs to know how to analyze a given drug, the reference volumes and official compendia probably will provide sufficient information. Often further leads to the periodical literature will be obtained from these preliminary searches. The method suggested in this paragraph is nonsystematic, but it suffices to supply the needed information at small cost in time and effort for nearly all analytical problems.

Occasionally *all* of the published work on a compound, a method, or an area of study must be compiled. A systematic attack is necessary. The subject index of *Chemical Abstracts* is the starting point for the search. All likely subject headings are investigated in the index, and promising entries are pursued in the abstracts section. At this stage notes should be made of all articles that seem pertinent; the title of the article, journal name and volume number, page, year, the *Chemical Abstracts* reference itself, authors' names, and a brief statement of the content of the paper should be recorded. Index cards of 4 × 6 in. size are convenient. The next stage involves perusal of the original articles when the journals are available.

Modern methods of photocopying make it simple to acquire the full article for leisurely study away from the library. Often a few notes can be made in the library, abstracting the needed information from the article. Another way to obtain copies of recent papers is to write to the author, requesting a reprint.

The references cited within these articles may lead to more papers that were overlooked in the *Chemical Abstracts* search. Eventually a nearly complete record will be obtained of published work relating to the subject. We can never be sure that we have located all references, but this approach is fairly effective. A thorough literature search is a laborious undertaking. Modern computer methods are being devised to make literature searching easier, faster, and more thorough, but the individual reader is not yet obsolete.

27.4 The "Method of Choice"

It will have become clear from the 26 chapters preceding this one that any compound can be analyzed in many ways. Each physical property, each chemical reaction, provides a potential analytical approach. Many of these possible approaches have proved to be fruitful ones, with the result that a battery of assay methods is available for practically every type of compound. How does the analyst select the "best" method for the problem at hand?

The analytical problem will fall into one of these three classes: (1) it may be essentially identical with a problem already solved, and the earlier analytical technique is therefore directly applicable; (2) it may be related to an earlier problem, and the prior technique then may require some modification before it can be successfully applied; or (3) it may be a new problem, one never before encountered or solved. Then original analytical research will be required to develop a satisfactory analytical method. Even if a problem fits into the first class a decision must be made, for many methods will appear, at first glance, to be applicable. Several factors must be taken into account, however, and in effect the analyst must ask himself the following questions when evaluating an analytical method with a specific use in mind.

1. *Does this method possess the requisite sensitivity?* Suppose the problem is to determine the exact concentration of an aqueous solution containing about 10^{-4} *M* fumaric acid. Although titration of an aliquot with standard alkali

immediately presents itself as a suitable method, the very low concentration is a prohibitive factor. Ultraviolet spectrophotometry might be applicable; it would be necessary to determine, by experiment or from the literature, the absorption spectrum of fumaric acid and how it is affected by pH before this method could be adopted.

2. *Is this method sufficiently selective for direct use without interference by other components in the sample?* Although tablets of barbituric acid derivatives can be assayed by titration of the powdered tablet with a strong base in nonaqueous media, the analysis is vitiated by stearic acid, which may be present in the tablet formulation as a lubricant. The analyst must be alert to such complications. When they occur, it is necessary either to adopt another method free of the interference (for example, ultraviolet spectrophotometry in the present instance) or to employ a separation technique to remove the desired component from the interfering substance.

3. *Are the accuracy and precision attainable with this method commensurate with the information desired?* If, for example, it is required to determine the purity of a high-grade sample of benzoic acid to within 0.01%, it is pointless to subject the sample to a phase solubility analysis, which is capable only of about ±0.5% accuracy. Instead a titration with standard alkali, with extreme care being taken in all phases of the analysis, may yield results of the desired accuracy. Another aspect of this question is encountered when the analytical method is much more accurate than is necessary. This might happen when the sampling error is (say) 5% and the analytical error is 0.1%; then the overall error is controlled by the sampling step, and it is wasteful of time and effort to strive for analytical accuracy far beyond the limit already set by the sampling operation.

4. *Are the reagents and equipment required in this method available or obtainable at reasonable cost?* The economics of analysis is important. Although one always selects the best method, if two comparable assays are available the one that costs less should be chosen. In determining cost the use of instruments, and their maintenance and depreciation, are factors to be considered.

5. *Is the time required to carry out this method acceptable?* The time factor can be broken down into "operator time" and "elapsed time." Operator time is the time actually spent by the analyst per analysis, and elapsed time is the total time consumed from receipt of sample to reporting the analytical result. For some assays the elapsed time is greater than the operator time because of waiting periods (for refluxing, dissolution, etc.) that do not require the operator's attention. During these periods he can perform other tasks, such as preparing additional samples for analysis. It is quite possible that the elapsed time per analysis may be prohibitive if only one or a few samples are to be analyzed, but if very many samples are to be assayed the time per analysis may be reasonable.

When modification of a known analytical method seems necessary before it can be applied, the preceding questions must be asked at each stage of the proceedings. Often the adjustment is minor in scope, though very important to the success of the analysis. Suppose it is desired to determine the ethyl ester of *p*-methoxybenzoic acid by the quantitative saponification technique, a method that has been in daily use in the same laboratory for the determination of ethyl benzoate. The only modification that may be needed will be to alter the time of reflux to be sure saponification is complete. This is easily established by running a series of analyses in which the reflux time is varied in order to find the minimum time required. Such minor adjustments must often be made by the analyst, but they should always be based on sound principles and must always be tested in the laboratory before they are accepted. Among the alterations that will sometimes improve assay performance are a suitable change of indicator; use of potentiometric or other instrumental means instead of visual detection of titration end points; shift in working wavelength in spectrophotometric analysis for greater selectivity or sensitivity; change of solvent composition or pH to alter spectral properties or solubility; change in reaction time to maximize extent of principal reaction or to minimize extent of side reactions; and change in catalyst type or concentration.

It often happens that minor alterations in a known procedure fail to produce a successful analytical method for the problem confronting the analyst. A fresh approach is then called for, and the development of new analytical methods is an important aspect of chemical research. Research is hard work and it is notoriously inefficient, but besides being necessary it is fun. It is worth noting that all the analytical methods described in this or any other book required original research by their developers, who enjoyed their work.

References

1. Tomlinson, R. C., Chap. 3 in *Comprehensive Analytical Chemistry*, Vol. IA, C. L. Wilson and D. W. Wilson (eds.), Elsevier, Amsterdam, 1959.
2. Walton, W. W. and J. I. Hoffman, Chap. 4 in *Treatise on Analytical Chemistry*, Part I, Vol. I, I. M. Kolthoff and P. J. Elving (eds.), Interscience, New York, 1959.
3. Wilson, E. B., Jr., *An Introduction to Scientific Research*, McGraw-Hill, New York, 1952, Sec. 10.3.
4. Flann, B., *J. Pharm. Sci.*, **63,** 183 (1974).
5. Wood, E. C., Chap. 4 in *Comprehensive Analytical Chemistry*, C. L. Wilson and D. W. Wilson (eds.), Elsevier, Amsterdam, 1959.
6. Boas, M. L., *Mathematical Methods in the Physical Sciences*, John Wiley and Sons, New York, 1966, p. 716.
7. Dean, R. B. and W. J. Dixon, *Anal. Chem.*, **23,** 636 (1951).

FOR FURTHER READING

Bennett, C. A. and N. L. Franklin, *Statistical Analysis in Chemistry and the Chemical Industry*, John Wiley and Sons, New York, 1954.

Young, H. D., *Statistical Treatment of Experimental Data*, McGraw-Hill Book Co., New York, 1962.

Beveridge, W. I. B., *The Art of Scientific Investigation*, 3rd ed., Random House, New York, 1957.

Problems

1. These values were obtained in five determinations of the normality of an HCl solution: N = 0.0535, 0.0527, 0.0531, 0.0536, 0.0521. Calculate the mean, standard deviation, and standard deviation of the mean.

2. The saponification equivalent of an ester was determined to be, in five trials, 163.2, 162.3, 162.8, 161.5, 164.6. Give 95% confidence limits for the mean saponification equivalent of this ester.

3. The precision of the weighing, transfer, and titration steps of an analytical procedure were evaluated; it was found that the standard deviation of weighing was 0.2 mg; of transfer 0.1 mg; and of titration 0.5 mg. What was the standard deviation of the overall analytical method?

4. Four determinations of a molar absorptivity gave the results 3835, 3760, 3810, and 3845. Would the analyst be justified in rejecting the most discordant result?

A VOLUMETRIC TECHNIQUES AND CALCULATIONS

A.1 Experimental Techniques and Equipment

Safety in the Laboratory. Pharmaceutical analytical work is not particularly dangerous, and the precautions familiar from the general chemistry and organic chemistry laboratories will protect against possible accidents in this type of experimentation. Some of the important points will nevertheless be repeated here in the form of guidelines.

(*a*) Always wear eye protection in a laboratory! An ordinary pair of eyeglasses is sufficient protection for most operations in the laboratory, but safety goggles are available in the stockroom and should be worn if glasses are not available or for dangerous operations. It is especially important for wearers of contact lenses to have their eyes protected at all times, because it is very difficult to cleanse the eye with a contact lens in place. For any chemical splash in the eyes the best immediate treatment is copious washing with water. This should be followed by prompt emergency treatment by a physician.

(*b*) Learn where the laboratory safety equipment is located; this includes the first aid cabinet, fire extinguishers, showers and eye wash stations, protective masks, fire blankets, and emergency exits.

(*c*) Never taste chemicals. When it is necessary to smell a chemical do so with great caution.

(*d*) Use fume hoods when working with noxious vapors or solvents (such as pyridine, mercaptans, and large quantities of benzene, chloroform, acetic acid, etc.).

(*e*) Never pipet toxic or corrosive liquids by mouth; use a pipet bulb.

(*f*) When inserting glass tubing or a thermometer into a rubber stopper use water or glycerol as a lubricant and protect the hands, in case of breakage, with a towel.

(*g*) Do not use an open flame in the presence of flammable liquids.

(*h*) Flush aqueous solutions down the sink with plenty of water. Do not put organic solvents in the sink, but dispose of them in containers provided for this purpose.

General neatness and cleanliness in the laboratory are not only conducive to better analytical results, but also tend to reduce the frequency of minor accidents such as spills.

Drying Chemicals. Adsorbed moisture can be removed from most solids by heating 1–2 hr in an oven at 100–110°C. If the substance contains water of crystallization this treatment should not be used, since some, but probably not all, of this water might be lost. If a substance is chemically unstable it also cannot be dried in this way.

Drying is best accomplished, for small amounts of solids, in weighing bottles. After removal from the oven, the weighing bottle and its cover are placed in a desiccator. The cover is placed on the bottle only after the contents are cool. The function of the desiccator is to keep the environment dry by means of a desiccant such as calcium sulfate, calcium chloride, or phosphorus pentoxide. Some analysts use concentrated sulfuric acid as a desiccant, but it is too dangerous to be recommended.

If a substance is too unstable to be dried by heating, it can be placed in a desiccator over P_2O_5 at room temperature or, even better, can be subjected to reduced pressure by connecting a vacuum desiccator to a vacuum pump.

Remember that drying is essentially a process of distillation; in order for a chemical to be dried, a "trap" or "sink" must be provided for the water; this is the function of the desiccant. It is fruitless to attempt to dry a substance by connecting a desiccator to a water aspirator.

Weighing Samples. Most analytical balances now in use are single-pan balances with dials indicating the weight in the range 0.1–100 g; an optical scale indicates the weight to the milligram level, and tenths of a milligram are estimated on this scale with a vernier. Specific instructions in the use of the balance will be provided by the instructor. The following suggestions are of general applicability.

The sample weight (actually mass) as determined on an analytical balance is obtained as the difference between two separate measurements. One satisfactory way to weigh a sample is to place the weighing bottle containing the substance on the balance pan and to obtain its weight. Then an appropriate amount of the substance is removed from the bottle and transferred to a suitable flask. The weighing bottle with its contents is now reweighed, and the sample weight is obtained as the difference between these two measurements. This method is quite efficient if several samples of the same substance are being weighed, since the "after" weighing for the first sample is also the "before" weighing for the second sample, and so on.

Another technique is to weigh an empty container (beaker, flask, watch glass, weighing boat, etc.) on the balance pan, then to deliver an appropriate amount of the sample substance into this container and to reweigh it. The sample weight is again obtained by difference. Never place any chemical directly on the balance pan.

The temperature of any object placed on the pan must be the same as the balance temperature. It is good practice to handle with tongs all containers being weighed, but in fact glass vessels can be handled by hand if the skin is clean and dry and if such handling is minimal. (This applies only to weighings on an ordinary analytical balance, that is, with sensitivity of the order 0.1 mg.) The gloved hand is a good way to handle objects while weighing.

Volatile liquids can be difficult to weigh. Relatively nonvolatile liquids like water can be weighed successfully in stoppered flasks, but organic liquids may evaporate during the weighing process. A good method for weighing small quantities (2–10 mmole) of volatile liquids is with a syringe. Plastic 1 cm^3 disposable tuberculin syringes, supplied with needle and a needle cap, are effective for those liquids that do not interact with the plastic. The syringe is filled with the liquid, the needle cap is put in place, and the entire assembly is weighed. Then an appropriate amount of liquid is discharged from the syringe into a sample flask, the needle cap is replaced immediately, and a second weighing is made. Of course evaporation from the sample flask must be prevented, for example, by delivering the sample into excess reagent, etc.

When making replicate determinations the analyst can choose between weighing out separate samples for each analysis, or weighing out a single large sample, which is made into a solution from which known fractions (*aliquots*) are drawn for analysis. The first method is exemplified by the directions for standardizing sodium hydroxide in Experiment 1.1; the second method is suggested for the standardization of EDTA in Experiment 4.1. In general the first procedure, weighing of separate samples, is to be preferred because it provides better opportunity for detecting systematic errors or a serious weighing error. The second method is preferable if each individual sample size needed is too small for accurate weighing.

Pipets. Known volumes of solutions usually are transferred from one vessel to another by means of a transfer pipet, the most commonly available sizes being for 1, 2, 5, 10, 20, 25, and 50 ml volumes. Pipets are calibrated by the manufacturer in accordance with National Bureau of Standards specifications; the allowed error limits depend upon the pipet size. These limits can be found in the USP and the NF. Pipets are calibrated *to deliver* (TD) the specified volume of water at a given temperature, usually 20°C, within the permitted limits. The analyst can check this calibration by weighing water delivered from the pipet, but for ordinary analytical work such recalibration is seldom carried out. The accuracy of delivery depends on reproducing the conditions of calibration, however, so for temperatures appreciably different from 20°C or for nonaqueous solutions the error introduced may be significant, and recalibration may be necessary.

Use the pipet as follows. Extend the clean dry pipet tip into the solution and draw liquid above the calibration mark. It is best to use a pipet bulb for this purpose; a bulb must certainly be used for any toxic or corrosive liquid (e.g., acids, bases, oxidizing agents, drugs). Hold the column of liquid in place by pressing a finger to the top of the pipet, and remove the pipet from the solution. With a clean tissue paper, wipe excess liquid from the outside of the pipet tip. Touch the tip to the inside of a clean waste vessel and, with the pipet in a vertical position, carefully allow liquid to run from the pipet, by letting air into the top, until the bottom of the meniscus just touches the calibration mark.

Place the filled pipet over the vessel into which the solution will be discharged. Remove the finger at the top of the pipet, allowing the liquid to flow freely, with the pipet in a vertical position. Touch the pipet tip to the side of the vessel and hold the pipet in this position about 20 sec. This completes the transfer. Do not blow out the liquid remaining in the tip.

It is best not to remove solution directly from a stock bottle by pipet, because of the possibility of contaminating the bulk of the solution. Instead pour some solution into a flask or beaker, and pipet portions from this. Discard any excess solution.

Volumetric Flasks. Volumetric flasks are calibrated *to contain* (TC) a specified volume at a given temperature; the common sizes of flasks are 10, 25, 50, 100, 250, 500, and 1000 ml. They are used for the preparation of solutions.

Most of these flasks are too large or too heavy to serve as weighing containers, so samples often are weighed into smaller containers and then transferred quantitatively to the flask with the aid of the solvent. The solution should be mixed well before its final dilution to the calibration mark. If necessary, it must be brought to room temperature, and finally solvent is added carefully until the bottom of the meniscus just touches the mark. The stopper is inserted and the solution is well mixed by repeatedly inverting the flask. It is a common mistake to mix the solution inadequately.

Burets and Titrations. A buret is a glass cylinder calibrated in milliliters and fractions of milliliters, and fitted with a stopcock at its lower end to control the flow of liquid. The most common sizes are 10, 25, and 50 ml burets. Their primary function is to deliver accurately measured volumes of solutions in titrations; they are also very effective replacements for pipets. With proper care and use, burets perform these roles very well.

It is first necessary to clean the buret and to grease the stopcock. First remove the stopcock and clean it and the bore of all residual grease by wiping them with a tissue soaked in petroleum ether. Then thoroughly wash the buret and stopcock in water and detergent. Rinse well, and observe the manner in which water flows on the interior of the buret; it is necessary that the surface drain evenly, without uneven patches of wetting. If further cleaning is necessary, set up the buret in a buret clamp, insert the stopcock (without grease), and fill the buret with warm chromic acid cleaning solution* (heated on a hot plate). After this treatment rinse the buret well with distilled water.

Next grease the stopcock. Thoroughly dry the stopcock and bore, and apply stopcock grease, using a boiling stick or other applicator, in several strips lengthwise on the stopcock. Press the stopcock firmly in the bore, then rotate it a few times. Remove the stopcock and, with a pipe cleaner, clean out any grease that has entered the hole. Replace the stopcock and affix the retainer spring or washer. A clean buret can be stored full of distilled water, with a cork on the upper end. When emptying a buret, always run the liquid out through the stopcock; otherwise some stopcock grease may be deposited on the buret walls. If a bit of stopcock grease should become detached and plug the buret tip, it often can be dislodged with a fine wire; the first (E) string of a guitar or the first (D) or fifth (G) strings of a banjo have the necessary strength and fineness.

For use in a titration, fill the buret with titrant by pouring from a small beaker or through a small funnel. Run titrant through the stopcock and flush out any air bubbles in the buret tip below the stopcock. Fill the buret to somewhere between the 0.00 and 1.00 ml marks; for most titrations there is no point in bringing the liquid exactly to the 0.00 ml mark. Instead, measure the volume reading before titration and at the end point, and subtract to find the titration end point volume. For experiments such as potentiometric titrations, in which many readings of volume are made during a titration, it is most convenient to begin the titration exactly at 0.00.

After the end point has been reached, allow several seconds for titrant to drain down the buret wall before making the volume reading. For clear titrants measure the volume at the bottom of the meniscus; a white card held behind the buret will reveal the meniscus. The volume should be estimated to within 0.01 ml.

Throughout the titration the sample solution must be stirred. This is best done with a magnetic stirrer, but it can also be done manually. In this case the flask is held in the right hand (for a right-handed person) and the stopcock is manipulated with the left hand; the technique is best demonstrated by the laboratory instructor. Erlenmeyer flasks are the best vessels into which to titrate; the 125 ml and 250 ml size will usually be satisfactory. For potentiometric titrations 250 ml beakers are suitable. Occasionally during titrations

* Prepared by slowly adding 1500 ml of concentrated sulfuric acid to a solution of 200 g of sodium dichromate in 100 ml of water.

with aqueous solutions the sides of the flask should be washed down with water, which is conveniently done by means of a plastic squeeze bottle of water.

The size of sample to take for titration is determined in part by the capacity of the buret. It is desirable not to have to refill the buret during the titration; but it is also desirable to utilize the full capacity of the buret so as to reduce the relative error of the volume measurement. The sample size is therefore selected so that roughly 80% of the buret capacity is utilized. For example, if 0.1 *N* titrant is being added from a 25 ml buret, the sample size should be about 2 meq, since this will consume about 20 ml of titrant.

During all experimental operations it is good practice to cover open vessels with stoppers, corks, or watch glasses. The buret can be covered with a small inverted beaker. This practice retards evaporation, limits access by the atmosphere, and prevents contamination by airborne particles.

Recording Data. All data obtained in the laboratory should be directly written into a bound (not looseleaf or spiral) notework. Do not write on loose sheets of paper, meaning to transfer the data later; one reason is that such loose pieces of paper may be lost, and another is that this is a time-wasting procedure. It is less important that the data book be neat (though neatness certainly is desirable) than that it be complete. If an entry is later determined to be in error, simply draw a line through it and give an explanation nearby; do not erase or obliterate the entry. Do not remove pages. Date all entries.

These are among the kinds of information that should be entered in the data book:

(*a*) References to procedures used, such as to textbooks or other literature, and a brief description of the procedure.
(*b*) All balance and buret readings (concise tables can be constructed).
(*c*) Identity, source, and related information for all chemicals used.
(*d*) Identity of instruments used.
(*e*) All raw experimental data, such as pH, absorbance, temperature, etc., depending upon the nature of the experiment.
(*f*) Typical calculations.
(*g*) Summary and conclusions.

The details of procedure should be sufficiently precise to allow recalculations to be performed at a later date. In general, the criterion to be used as a guide is that one should never rely on memory to recover a significant point for later use or interpretation. The data book should include an index or table of contents to help in locating specific experiments, standardization of solutions, frequently used procedures, etc.

All solutions prepared for use in analytical procedures should be labeled by glass-marking wax pencil, felt-tip marker, or paper labels; the pressure-sensitive type of label is convenient. Include on the label the identity of the solution, its concentration, your initials, the date, and the page of your notebook describing its preparation. An instructor would be justified in discarding any unlabeled solutions.

A.2 Calculations

Expression of Concentration. Solution concentrations can be expressed on a physical basis (weight or volume), the common forms being these:

(*a*) Percent by weight: the number of grams of solute contained in 100 g of solution. The concentrations of strong acids, as available commercially, are expressed in this way.

(*b*) Percent by volume: the number of milliliters of solute contained in 100 ml of solution; this is a common way of specifying solution composition of mixtures of miscible liquids.

(*c*) Percent weight/volume (w/v): the number of grams of solute contained in 100 ml of solution. This is usually encountered in describing the composition of solutions of solids in liquids.

Some related concentration units are milligram percent (mg%), which is the number of mg of solute contained in 100 ml of solution, and the concentration in parts per million (ppm), the number of grams of solute contained in 10^6 g of solution.

One form of concentration scale can be converted into another if the solution density is known.

The chemical methods of expressing concentration are based upon chemical formula or combining power:

(*a*) Molarity (M): the number of moles of solute contained in 1000 ml of solution.

(*b*) Normality (N): the number of equivalents of solute contained in 1000 ml of solution. For the definition of equivalent see Chapters 1 and 5. The normality of a solution is always equal to an integer times its molarity.

(*c*) Formality (F): used by some authors to denote the number of formula weights of solute contained in 1000 ml of solution. The purpose is to make a distinction between actual equilibrium concentration of a chemical species and the total analytical concentration of the solute giving rise to that species.

(*d*) Molality (m): the number of moles of solute per 1000 g of solvent.

The molarity and normality are temperature dependent, since they are based on volume; the molality is independent of temperature.

The physical and chemical concentration scales can be interconverted by interconverting weights and moles. A given weight (actually mass) of a pure substance can be expressed in terms of gram-molecular weights (moles) or gram-equivalent weights (equivalents) of a compound or gram-atomic weights of an element. The conversion formula can be obtained by establishing a proportion. Suppose it is desired to calculate the number of moles represented by w g of a substance with molecular weight MW g. Then these parallel statements can be made:

If MW g equals 1 mole

Then w g equals x mole

or

$$\frac{\mathrm{MW}}{w} = \frac{1}{x}$$

$$x = \frac{w}{\mathrm{MW}}$$

The same approach can be used for converting weight to equivalents. The following important formulas will be frequently needed:

$$\text{No. of moles} = \frac{\text{weight in g}}{\mathrm{MW}} \tag{A.1}$$

$$\text{No. of millimoles} = \frac{\text{weight in mg}}{\mathrm{MW}} \tag{A.2}$$

$$\text{No. of equivalents} = \frac{\text{weight in g}}{\mathrm{EW}} \tag{A.3}$$

$$\text{No. of milliequivalents} = \frac{\text{weight in mg}}{\mathrm{EW}} \tag{A.4}$$

The symbol EW represents equivalent weight.

EXAMPLE A.1. Calculate the approximate molarity of concentrated hydrochloric acid.

Concentrated hydrochloric acid has a concentration of about 38.0% by weight, and its density is about 1.19. 100 g of solution therefore contains 38.0 g of HCl, and the volume of this amount of solution is 100/1.19 = 84.0 ml (since density = weight per unit volume). Using the method of proportions shown earlier, we find that (38.0)(100)/84.0 = 45.2 g of HCl are contained in 100 ml, or 452 g in 1000 ml of the solution. The MW of HCl is 36.46, so

452 g of HCl is 452/36.46 moles = 12.4 moles. Concentrated hydrochloric acid is therefore about 12.4 *M*.

Preparation of Solutions. Solutions are prepared by dissolving a known weight of solute in enough solvent to make the desired volume of solvent, or by dilution of a more concentrated solution. To prepare a solution of a given molarity by the first method, convert the number of moles needed to the corresponding weight, and dissolve this weight in solvent to make the suitable volume. Thus to prepare 500 ml of 0.3 *M* NaCl, one-half of 0.3 mole of NaCl, or (0.3)(58.45)/2 = 8.768 g, is dissolved in enough water to make 500 ml; a 500 ml volumetric flask is used for this operation. This calculation illustrates a use of Eq. A.1.

The preparation of solutions by dilution is very simple. It is based upon the calculation of the number of equivalents (or moles) of solute in a given volume of solution of known normality (or molarity). From the definitions of normality and molarity, the important formulas A.5 and A.6 are obtained, where volumes V are in milliliters, and meq represents milliequivalents of solute.

$$\text{No. of meq} = VN \tag{A.5}$$

$$\text{No. of mmoles} = VM \tag{A.6}$$

It is convenient to work with meq and mmoles in volumetric analysis.

In the dilution of a solution, the total number of milliequivalents in the volume of concentrated solution must be equal to the total number of milliequivalents in the final diluted solution, since only solvent is added. Therefore

$$\text{meq of solute in conc soln} = N_c V_c$$

$$\text{meq of solute in dil soln} = N_d V_d$$

$$N_c V_c = N_d V_d \tag{A.7}$$

EXAMPLE A.2. Give directions for the preparation of 2 liters of approximately 0.1 *N* hydrochloric acid from concentrated hydrochloric acid.

Equation A.7 is applied, with $N_d = 0.1$, $V_d = 2000$, $N_c = 12.4$ (see Example A.1), giving $V_c = 16.1$. Therefore proceed by diluting about 16 ml of concentrated hydrochloric acid to 2000 ml with water.

Titration Calculations. At the equivalence point of a titration the number of milliequivalents contained in the titrant solution added is equal to the number of milliequivalents contained in the sample solution taken, by definition. This equality provides the basis of titrimetric analysis. The end point is the experimental estimate of the equivalence point. At the end point, then (assuming negligible error in locating the end point),

$$\text{Meq of titrant} = \text{meq of sample}$$

But from Eq. A.5, meq of titrant $= V_t N_t$, where V_t is the number of milliliters of titrant required to reach the end point and N_t is the titrant normality. Therefore,

$$\text{Meq of sample} = V_t N_t \tag{A.8}$$

The next step in the calculation depends upon the manner in which the sample was taken and the information desired. If the sample was an accurately measured volume V_s of a solution whose concentration N_s is to be determined by titration, we can write meq of sample $= V_s N_s$, from which Eq. A.8 leads to

$$V_s N_s = V_t N_t \tag{A.9}$$

EXAMPLE A.3. A 25.00 ml portion of sulfuric acid solution was titrated with 0.1050 *N* sodium hydroxide, 23.45 ml of titrant being required. What is the normality of the acid solution?

Using Eq. A.9 with $V_t = 23.45$ ml, $N_t = 0.1050$, $V_s = 25.00$ ml gives $N_s = 0.0985$ as the normality of the sulfuric acid.

Note that Eq. A.9 can be rearranged to $V_t/V_s = N_s/N_t$, from which the relative concentrations of two solutions can be determined even without knowing the absolute concentration of either of them. Note also that it is irrelevant whether or not additional solvent was added to the titration flask before or during titration, since such addition in no way alters the number of milliequivalents of sample in the flask.

If the sample that was titrated was originally weighed out and then dissolved (in some unknown volume of solvent) in order to titrate it, the titration result is treated in this way. Equation A.8 still applies, but the number of milliequivalents of sample is given by Eq. A.4. Therefore, at the end point,

$$\frac{\text{Weight of sample in mg}}{\text{EW}} = V_t N_t \tag{A.10}$$

If the sample was a weighed portion of a primary standard substance, Eq. A.10 can be used to find N_t, that is, to standardize the titrant. Alternatively, if N_t is known, the equation can be used to determine the purity of sample substance taken, or, if the sample is known to be pure, its EW can be determined.

EXAMPLE A.4. A 0.8168 g sample of primary standard potassium biphthalate (EW 204.2) was titrated to the phenolphthalein end point with 41.03 ml of sodium hydroxide solution. Calculate the normality of the titrant solution.

From Eq. A.4, 4.00 meq of potassium biphthalate were taken. Applying Eq. A.8 with $V_t = 41.03$ gives $N_t = 0.0975$.

EXAMPLE A.5. 0.2212 g of potassium bicarbonate was titrated with 20.30 ml of 0.1091 *N* HCl. Calculate the purity of the sample.

From Eq. A.5, (20.23)(0.1091) = 2.207 meq of HCl were consumed in the titration, and Eq. A.10 can be applied with EW = 100.1, giving 0.2209 g of $KHCO_3$ found. The percent purity is given by

$$\% \text{ purity} = \frac{\text{wt found}}{\text{wt taken}} \times 100 \tag{A.11}$$

or 99.86% in this case.

EXAMPLE A.6. A 0.2261 g sample of a pure weak base of unknown identity was titrated with 18.03 ml of 0.1026 *N* acetous perchloric acid. What is the equivalent weight of the base?

Equation A.10 is applied, with sample weight 226.1 mg, $V_t = 18.03$ ml, and $N_t = 0.1026$, giving EW = 122.2.

All these titration calculations have been developed for direct titrations, for which only a single titrant is involved, and Eq. A.8 is fairly obvious. For more complicated analyses the method of calculation can be more readily comprehended with the aid of titration diagrams, which are line charts showing the relationship of sample and titrant graphically. In these diagrams the number of milliequivalents of any substance is represented by the length of a line. For example, Fig. A.1*a* shows a titration diagram for a direct titration of a sample of potassium biphthalate (KHP) with sodium hydroxide. The lengths of the lines are proportional to number of milliequivalents, so it is immediately clear that meq of potassium biphthalate = meq of sodium hydroxide. Figure A.1*b* shows a direct titration incorporating a blank titration, which corrects for the consumption of titrant by solvent impurities, indicator, etc. If I represents the milliequivalents of titrant consumed in the blank titration and II the milliequivalent consumed in the sample titration, evidently meq of sample = II − I, or meq of sample = $(V_{\text{sample}} - V_{\text{blank}})N_t$.

Figure A.1*c* is the diagram of a back-titration of a sample of ephedrine. First a known volume of standard HCl, in excess of that required to react with the ephedrine, is added; then the excess HCl is back-titrated with standard NaOH. From the diagram it is seen that meq of ephedrine = II − I, or meq of ephedrine = $V_{\text{HCl}}N_{\text{HCl}} - V_{\text{NaOH}}N_{\text{NaOH}}$.

Now let us incorporate a blank titration into the back-titration analysis, using the same system as in Fig. A.1*c*. The procedure is to add the same

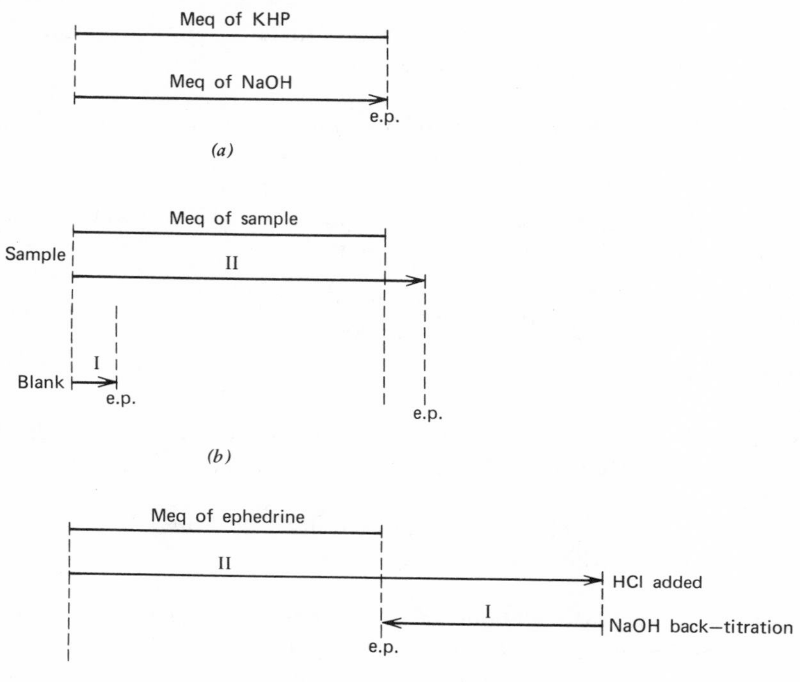

Fig. A.1. Examples of titration diagrams. The lengths of lines are proportional to milliequivalents of reactants, and the locations of titration end points (e.p.) are shown. (*a*) Direct titration; (*b*) direct titration including a blank titration; (*c*) back-titration.

volume of the same HCl solution in the blank as was used in the sample, and to back-titrate with the same solution of NaOH in both cases. If an impurity is present in the solvent, the number of milliequivalents of NaOH used in the blank back-titration will not exactly equal the milliequivalents of HCl added. There are two possibilities: the impurity can consume acid or it can consume base.

Figure A.2 is a titration diagram for this analysis in which the impurity consumes acid. Let milliequivalents of impurity be denoted V. Then from the blank titration diagram, V = III − IV. The fundamental assumption in carrying out a blank titration is that the magnitude of the blank consumption is identical in both the blank and the sample titrations. Thus from the sample titration diagram in Fig. A.2,

$$\begin{aligned}\text{Meq of ephedrine} &= \text{I} - (\text{II} + \text{V}) \\ &= (\text{I} - \text{II}) - (\text{III} - \text{IV})\end{aligned}$$

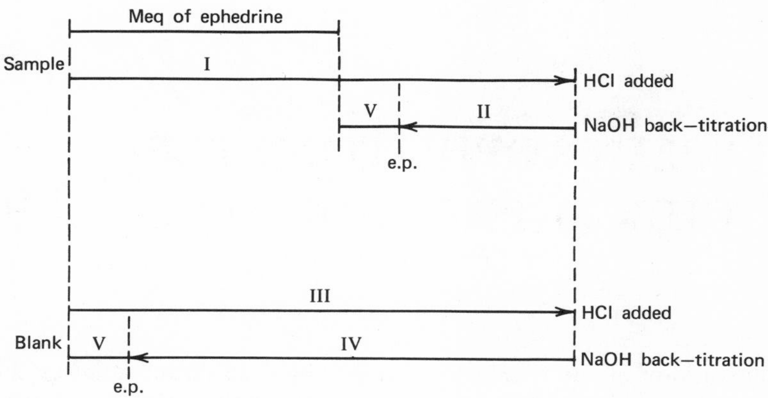

Fig. A.2. Titration diagram of a back-titration including a blank determination.

But, from the way in which the analysis is carried out, I = III; therefore

$$\text{Meq of ephedrine} = \text{IV} - \text{II}$$

(It can be shown that the same expression is obtained if the impurity consumes base.) An interesting feature of this result is that the quantities II and IV can be calculated from a knowledge of the volumes and normality of the back-titrant (NaOH) alone; as long as the same volume of the same HCl solution is added in both the sample and the blank, its concentration and volume do not enter the calculation.

B SPECTROPHOTOMETER CHECK PROCEDURES

The validity of the numbers generated by a spectrophotometer should occasionally be verified by measurements of materials with known spectral properties. Some simple checks are described here; for further discussion see Lothian* or Edisbury.†

B.1 The Wavelength Scale

For wavelength calibration in the uv and visible regions several standards have been suggested: (1) the emission spectrum of mercury, available as a special lamp for some instruments; (2) emission lines of hydrogen (or deuterium), observed in the output of the standard uv light source; (3) the absorption spectrum of holmium oxide as a glass or a solution; (4) the vapor spectrum of benzene. For a quick check the last of these is convenient in a chemical laboratory. Place a small drop of pure benzene in the bottom of a 1 cm silica cell, stopper the cell, and scan the uv spectrum slowly. A recording spectrophotometer will give a trace like Fig. 8.10*a*; a manual spectrophotometer will produce "kicks" in the needle reading corresponding to the sharp absorption maxima. According to ASTM specifications,‡ the eight most prominent peaks in the spectrum appear at these wavelengths (in nm): 236.35, 241.59, 247.10, 248.08, 252.86, 253.90, 258.90, 259.98. Agreement should be within the wavelength accuracy range specified by the instrument manufacturer; this accuracy is about 0.5 nm for many spectrophotometers.

Infrared spectrophotometers are calibrated against absorption bands of polystyrene, indene, or 1,2,4-trichlorobenzene.

* Lothian, G. F., *Absorption Spectrophotometry*, 3rd ed., Adam Hilger Ltd., London, 1969, Chap. 10.

† Edisbury, J. R., *Practical Hints on Absorption Spectrometry*, Plenum Press, New York, 1967, Chaps. 15, 16.

‡ *Manual on Recommended Practices in Spectrophotometry*, 3rd ed., American Society for Testing and Materials, Philadelphia, 1969, p. 70.

B.2 The Absorbance Scale

Several absorbance standards have been proposed, but there is no full agreement on their "true" absorbance values. For practical purposes, however, adequate checks can be made with some simple solutions. Prepare accurately a 1% (w/v) solution of the best reagent grade potassium nitrate (KNO_3) in distilled water, measure the absorbance at 302 nm, and calculate $A_{1\,cm}^{1\%}$; this value should be 0.70–0.71.

Wavelength (nm)	Absorbance	Wavelength	Absorbance	Wavelength	Absorbance
220	0.446	300	0.149	375	0.991
225	0.221	302.2	0.113	380	0.932
230	0.171	305	0.079	385	0.824
235	0.210	310	0.048	390	0.695
240	0.295	313.2	0.043	395	0.532
245	0.396	315	0.046	400	0.396
250	0.496	320	0.064	404.7	0.288
253.6	0.554	325	0.095	410	0.199
255	0.572	330	0.149	420	0.124
260	0.633	334.2	0.208	430	0.084
265	0.695	335	0.222	435.8	0.066
270	0.745	340	0.316	440	0.054
275	0.757	345	0.428	450	0.033
280	0.712	350	0.559	460	0.018
285	0.590	355	0.701	470	0.009
290	0.428	360	0.830	480	0.004
295	0.273	365	0.936	490	0.001
296.7	0.223	370	0.987	500	0.000

A check over a wide range of wavelengths can be made with an alkaline solution of potassium chromate.* Two alternative preparations, which yield identical solutions, are available.

Procedure I. Dissolve 0.0400 g of reagent grade K_2CrO_4 in enough 0.05 *N* KOH to make exactly 1 liter. The 0.05 *N* KOH is prepared by dissolving 3.3 g of reagent potassium hydroxide (85% KOH) in enough distilled water to make 1 liter.

Procedure II. Dissolve 0.0303 g of reagent grade $K_2Cr_2O_7$ in enough 0.05 *N* KOH to make 1 liter. This reacts according to the equation $K_2Cr_2O_7 + 2KOH = 2K_2CrO_4 + H_2O$, giving the equivalent of 0.0400 g of K_2CrO_4.

* Haupt, G. W., *J. Res. Natl. Bur. Stand.*, **48,** 414 (1952).

The solution should be stored in an ordinary glass bottle with glass stopper, and should not be unnecessarily exposed to light. The solution should not be poured from the bottle, but should be withdrawn by pipet without disturbing any sediment that forms. For calibration below 260 nm this solution may be regarded as stable for a 6 month period. For measurements above 260 nm the solution is stable for at least 5 years.

The absorbance of this standard solution should be measured in a 1.00 cm cell against distilled water as a solvent blank; the solution temperature should be close to 25°C. The "correct" values are given in the table. Marked discrepancies usually indicate either maladjustment of the wavelength scale or excessive stray light.

Linearity of the detector response can be established by measuring the absorbance of one of these solutions at two or more path lengths.

ANSWERS TO PROBLEMS

Chapter 1

1. (*a*) pH = 4.35; (*b*) pH = 0.00; (*c*) pH = 9.44; (*d*) pH = 7.06; (*e*) pH = 2.84
2. (*a*) 1.12×10^{-4} *N*; (*b*) 1.41×10^{-7} *N*; (*c*) 3.02×10^{-13} *N*; (*d*) 1.00×10^{-8} *N*; (*e*) 5.01×10^{-9} *N*
3. (*a*) $K_b = 1.62 \times 10^{-6}$
4. (*a*) pH = 2.70; (*b*) pH = 2.70; (*c*) pH = 10.97; (*d*) pH = 5.28; (*e*) pH = 12.70
5. pH = 4.28
6. ΔpH = −0.60
7. 55.5 *M*
8. pH = 6.98
9. 0.1514 *N*
10. EW = 154.9
11. pH = 8.56
12. (*a*) 0.9887 g; (*b*) 73.02%
13. (*a*) $K = 1.74 \times 10^9$; (*b*) $K = 6.93 \times 10^5$
14. (*a*) pH = 12.26; (*b*) $pK_b = 9.48$
15. pH = 6.92
16. 0.494 g
17. (*a*) Both are $\frac{1}{15}$ *M*; (*b*) pH = 7.17
18. 0.1594 *N*
19. pH = 6.62
21. 0.0382 *M*
22. (*a*) $[H^+] + [BH^+] = [OH^-] + [X^-]$
    (*b*) $[H^+] = [OH^-] + [HA^-] + 2[A^{2-}]$
    (*c*) $[H^+] + [K^+] = [OH^-] + [CH_3COO^-]$
23. $[H^+]^3 + (K_a + b)\,[H^+]^2 - (K_a c - K_a b + K_w)\,[H^+] - K_a K_w = 0$
24. (*a*) $\sigma = pK_a{}^0 - pK_a$
    (*b*) $\sigma(H) = 0.00$
    $\rho(p\text{-}NO_2) = +0.78$
    $\rho(m\text{-}NH_2) = -0.59$
    (*c*) Plus

Chapter 2

1. 42.3 ml
2. 0.4922 *N*

3. 0.1497 N
4. (*a*) $[H^+] = (K_{HClO_4}C_{HClO_4})^{1/2}$
   (*b*) 0.5 unit
   (*c*) 1.0 unit
6. 25.23 mg
7. 29.8 mg per tablet
8. 93.45%
9. 80.92%

Chapter 3

1. 27.8 mg
2. 2.5×10^{-10} M
4. (*a*) 0.01; (*b*) 1.10×10^{-6} M; (*c*) 99.2%
5. (*a*) 520.8 mg; (*b*) 518.7 mg
6. $s^{3/2} = \frac{1}{2}K_{sp}^{1/2}(1 + [H^+]/K_a)$
7. 10^{-3} M
8. (*a*) 1.47×10^{-4} M; (*b*) 1.78×10^{-5} M; (*c*) 1.26×10^{-7} M
9. 1.23×10^{-2} M
10. $s = (K_{sp}/256)^{1/5}$
11. pH 8
13. $AgBr(8.95 \times 10^{-7}\ M)$, $Zn(OH)_2(1.71 \times 10^{-5}\ M)$,
    $BaCO_3(8.95 \times 10^{-5}\ M)$, $Al(OH)_3(1.1 \times 10^{-4}\ M)$,
    $CaF_2(2.15 \times 10^{-4}\ M)$

Chapter 4

1. (*a*) $K = K_1K_2$; (*b*) $K = 8 \times 10^7$
2. pZn = 9.03
3. (*a*) 1.70; (*b*) 2.44; (*c*) 8.44; (*d*) 14.70
4. 0.06625 M
8. (*a*) 25; (*b*) 2.549 mg
9. (*a*) 1.70; (*b*) 2.08; (*c*) 5.04; (*d*) 7.10

Chapter 5

1. (*a*) $Cr_2O_7^{2-} + 6Fe^{2+} + 14H^+ = 2Cr^{3+} + 6Fe^{3+} + 7H_2O$
   (*b*) $ClO_3^- + 3Sn^{2+} + 6H^+ = Cl^- + 3Sn^{4+} + 3H_2O$
   (*c*) $2MnO_4^- + 5H_2C_2O_4 + 6H^+ = 2Mn^{2+} + 10CO_2 + 8H_2O$
   (*d*) $PbO_2 + 2I^- + 4H^+ = Pb^{2+} + I_2 + 2H_2O$
   (*e*) $Cr_2O_7^{2-} + 6V^{3+} + 2H^+ = 2Cr^{3+} + 6VO^{2+} + H_2O$
   (*f*) $3OBr^- + 2NH_3 = 3Br^- + N_2 + 3H_2O$
   (*g*) $KIO_3 + N_2H_4 + 2HCl = ICl + N_2 + KCl + 3H_2O$
   (*h*) $H_2O_2 + 2I^- + 2H^+ = I_2 + 2H_2O$
2. 4.945 g
3. 41.97 ml
5. (*a*) 1.701 mg; (*b*) 7.496 mg; (*c*) 15.191 mg; (*d*) 4.945 mg; (*e*) 6.405

Chapter 6

1. (*a*) 0.1097 N
2. (*a*) 0.2 M; (*b*) 0.3 M; (*c*) 0.05 M
3. $pK'_a = 4.710$; $pK_a = 4.756$
4. $\Delta E = 4.13$ mV
5. (*a*) 50.0 ml; (*b*) $[Sn^{4+}] = 0.025\ M$, $[Fe^{2+}] = 0.05\ M$, $[Sn^{2+}] = 2.5 \times 10^{-9}$ M, $[Fe^{3+}] = 5 \times 10^{-9}\ M$
6. $\Delta G^0 = -30.0$ kcal/mole; $K = 10^{22}$
7. -0.10 V
8. (*b*) $E = +1.71$ V
9. (*a*) $Ni^{2+}(0.015\ M) \rightleftharpoons Ni^{2+}(0.15\ M)$
   (*b*) E = -0.03 V
   (*c*) No
10. $pK_{sp} = 10.85$
11. pH = 2.66; $pK'_a = 3.92$
12. (*a*) $E^0 = +0.74$ V, log K = 62.7; (*b*) $[Fe^{2+}] = 3.55 \times 10^{-13}\ M$
13. $E = +0.39$ V

Chapter 7

1. (*a*) $I = 3.56$; (*b*) $D = 0.86 \times 10^{-5}$ cm^2/sec
5. -0.54 V

Chapter 8

1. $\lambda = 2500$ Å or 2.50×10^{-5} cm;
   wave number = 40,000 cm^{-1}; $\nu = 1.20 \times 10^{15}$ Hz;
   $E = 7.96 \times 10^{-12}$ erg/photon; $E = 114.3$ kcal/einstein
2. (*a*) $\epsilon = 1.32 \times 10^4$; (*c*) 84.2%
3. (*b*) $A^{1\%}_{1\,cm} = 10.5$; (*c*) $\epsilon = 474$; (*d*) 90.2%
4. $pK'_a = 3.66$
5. $\epsilon_{239} = 1.37 \times 10^4$; $\epsilon_{315} = 7.89 \times 10^3$
6. (*a*) $A = 3.00$; (*b*) $A = 0.602$; (*c*) $A = 0.125$; (*d*) $A = 0.004$
7. (*a*) $T = 0.966$; (*b*) $T = 0.316$; (*c*) $T = 0.100$; (*d*) $T = 0.050$; (*e*) $T = 0.00316$
9. (*a*) $\epsilon = A^{1\%}_{1\,cm} \dfrac{MW}{10}$; (*b*) $A^{1\%}_{1\,cm} = 1254$; (*c*) $\epsilon = 5.18 \times 10^3$
10. Wave number = $10^4/\lambda$
11. (*a*) Compound X; (*b*) $3.87 \times 10^{-5}\ M$
12. (*a*) $\epsilon_{245} = 8.72 \times 10^3$; (*b*) $A_{245} = 0.264$
13. (*a*) $A = 0.800$; (*b*) $c = 2.54 \times 10^{-4}\ M$; (*c*) $A = 0.824$
14. 500 mg
15. $E_1/E_2 = \lambda_2/\lambda_1$
17. (*a*) 1.00 ml; (*b*) $A = 0.0, 0.6, 1.4, 2.0, 2.0$
18. 59.3
19. 9.85×10^3
20. $A = 0.488$

Chapter 9

2. 89.4%

Chapter 10

1. $n = 1.4233$; $v = 2.108 \times 10^{10}$ cm/sec
2. 21.52 ml

Chapter 11

1. $[\alpha]_D^{20} = -25.2^0$
2. $\alpha = -1.02^0$
4. $K = 1.75$
6. (*a*) $[\Phi] = M[\alpha]/100$; (*b*) $[\Phi] = +605.4^0$
8. Compound C

Chapter 12

1. 1:4:6:4:1
3. $\sigma_{TMS} > \sigma_{sample}$, so $\nu_{sample} - \nu_{TMS} > 0$
4. For $I = \frac{1}{2}$, $m = +\frac{1}{2}, -\frac{1}{2}$; for $I = 1$, $m = +1, 0, -1$; for $I = \frac{3}{2}$, $m = +\frac{3}{2}, +\frac{1}{2}, -\frac{1}{2}, -\frac{3}{2}$
5. The actual spectra show:
   (*a*) Triplet at $\delta 1.32$, quartet at $\delta 4.20$
   (*b*) Doublet at $\delta 1.27$, triplets at $\delta 2.72$ and 3.74, septet at $\delta 5.08$; the relative integrated intensities of these multiplets are 6:2:2:1, respectively
   (*c*) Singlets at $\delta 2.20$, 2.33, and 6.80 with relative intensities 3:6:2, respectively
8. Doublet at $\delta 0.89$ (CH_3); singlet at $\delta 1.93$ (CH_3CO); doublet at $\delta 3.80$ (CH_2)
9. $\Delta\nu/J = (243 - 73)/7.0 = 28.3$

Chapter 13

1. $R \approx 240$
2. $CH_2{=}NH_2^+$ (*m/e* 30) and $CH_2{=}OH^+$ (*m/e* 31)
3. *n*-Butanol
4. *m/e* 43, 58, 85, 100
7. $ClCH_2COOH$, monochloroacetic acid

Chapter 14

2. (*a*) 0.9798; (*b*) 0.9769; (*c*) Witch hazel water

Chapter 15

2. (*a*) 85.0%; (*b*) 11.8 mg/ml; (*c*) 4.7 mg/ml
3. 83.6% pure; solubility = 4.35 mg/ml

Chapter 16

1. 90.7 mg
2. $K = 4.05$
4. 102.5 mg
7. 17 extractions
8. $A = 1.744$
9. 120 mg
10. (*a*) r_{max} (acetanilide) = 9.0, r_{max} (aspirin) = 4.0; (*b*) 2.39 mg

11. 318 mg
12. $K = 0.267$
14. (*a*) $K_{AB} = C_A/C_B$; $K_{BC} = C_B/C_C$; $K_{AC} = C_A/C_C$
    (*b*) $K_{AB} = K_{AC}/K_{BC}$
    (*c*) $p_A = \dfrac{K_{AB}V_A}{K_{AB}V_A + V_B + V_C/K_{BC}}$
15. $K = 8.62$
16. (*a*) 1.591 g; (*b*) 1.480 g
18. Tubes 23.4 and 42.4
19. $K = 0.25, 1.0, 4.0$
20. 0.0379
21. $K = 0.224$; 1.24
24. (*b*) 48.8 mg; (*c*) Tubes 184–216

Chapter 17

1. For A, $K = 8.5$, $R = 0.29$; for B, $K = 14.0$, $R = 0.20$; for C, $K = 25.5$, $R = 0.12$
2. Less than pK_a
5. Compound Y, $V_R = 13.5$ ml; compound Z, $V_R = 18.5$ ml
6. (*a*) $V_M = 12$ ml; (*b*) 22 ml, 37 ml
7. $V_S = 15$ ml, $V_M = 25$ ml
8. $r = 4\left(\dfrac{R_A + R_B}{R_A - R_B}\right)^2$
9. $R = 1/(1 + k')$
14. (*a*) $R_f(\text{A}) = 0.80$, $R_f(\text{B}) = 0.68$; (*b*) $R_s = 1.58$
15. (*a*) 30 ml, 40 ml; (*b*) 10 ml; (*c*) 196 plates; (*d*) $H = 5.1$ mm
16. (*a*) $v = (B/C)^{1/2}$; (*b*) $H_{\min} = A + 2(BC)^{1/2}$
17. (*a*) $t_R = 21$ min, 30 min; $V_R = 31.5$ ml, 45.0 ml
    (*b*) $H = 2.34$ mm; 171 plates
    (*c*) $R_s = 1.40$

Chapter 18

1. $R_s = 1.1$
2. $\alpha = (t_B - t_M)/(t_A - t_M)$;
   $(\alpha - 1)/\alpha = (t_B - t_A)/(t_B - t_M)$
3. t_R(heroin) = 11.34 min, t_R(methadone) = 3.30 min, etc.
4. About 970 plates
5. 13.5 min

Chapter 19

1. 24.06%
2. 11.36%
4. 40.01%

Chapter 20

2. 10.03 mg
3. 89.10%

Chapter 21

1. Ethanol: percent hydroxyl, 37; hydroxyl value, 1220; EW, 46
   1,3-Dihydroxypropane: percent hydroxyl, 44.7; hydroxyl value, 1476; EW, 38
2. 94.25%
5. *p*-acetaminophen (*p*-hydroxyacetanilide)
6. 298 mg/tablet
7. 6.21 mg of H_2O/ml
8. 5.59%
9. 47.2%
10. 1.92%

Chapter 22

1. 68.28%
2. (*a*) 238.21 − 58.08 = 180.13
   (*b*) 238.21/58.08 = 4.10 g
   (*c*) 0.145 g/ml
5. 36.7%

Chapter 23

1. 208.7
2. 67.6%
3. Monoethyl fumarate and monethyl maleate are two possibilities
7. 83.44%
8. *A*, nicotinamide; *B*, nicotinic acid; *C*, nikethamide
9. pH 10.8

Chapter 24

1. 27.83 mg
3. Compound II
6. *p*-Aminosalicylic acid
7. 411.8 mg/tablet
8. *A*, procaine; *B*, *p*-aminobenzoic acid

Chapter 25

2. EW = MW/6

Chapter 26

3. A1, benzoic acid
   A2, thiopental, phenol
   A3, testosterone
   B, dextroamphetamine, atropine
4. *p*-Acetaminophen

Chapter 27

1. $m = 0.0530$, $s = 6.2 \times 10^{-4}$, $s_m = 2.8 \times 10^{-4}$
2. 162.9 ± 1.4
3. 0.55 mg

Index

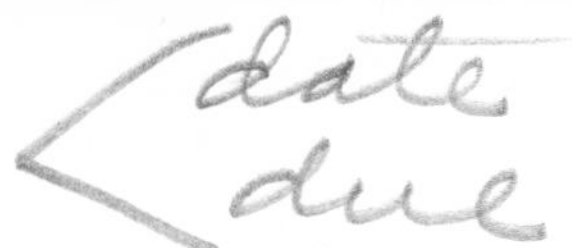

COMMON LOGARITHMS

N	0	1	2	3	4	5	6	7	8	9
10	0000	0043	0086	0128	0170	0212	0253	0294	0334	0374
11	0414	0453	0492	0531	0569	0607	0645	0682	0719	0755
12	0792	0828	0864	0899	0934	0969	1004	1038	1072	1106
13	1139	1173	1206	1239	1271	1303	1335	1367	1399	1430
14	1461	1492	1523	1553	1584	1614	1644	1673	1703	1732
15	1761	1790	1818	1847	1875	1903	1931	1959	1987	2014
16	2041	2068	2095	2122	2148	2175	2201	2227	2253	2279
17	2304	2330	2355	2380	2405	2430	2455	2480	2504	2529
18	2553	2577	2601	2625	2648	2672	2695	2718	2742	2765
19	2788	2810	2833	2856	2878	2900	2923	2945	2967	2989
20	3010	3032	3054	3075	3096	3118	3139	3160	3181	3201
21	3222	3243	3263	3284	3304	3324	3345	3365	3385	3404
22	3424	3444	3464	3483	3502	3522	3541	3560	3579	3598
23	3617	3636	3655	3674	3692	3711	3729	3747	3766	3784
24	3802	3820	3838	3856	3874	3892	3909	3927	3945	3962
25	3979	3997	4014	4031	4048	4065	4082	4099	4116	4133
26	4150	4166	4183	4200	4216	4232	4249	4265	4281	4298
27	4314	4330	4346	4362	4378	4393	4409	4425	4440	4456
28	4472	4487	4502	4518	4533	4548	4564	4579	4594	4609
29	4624	4639	4654	4669	4683	4698	4713	4728	4742	4757
30	4771	4786	4800	4814	4829	4843	4857	4871	4886	4900
31	4914	4928	4942	4955	4969	4983	4997	5011	5024	5038
32	5051	5065	5079	5092	5105	5119	5132	5145	5159	5172
33	5185	5198	5211	5224	5237	5250	5263	5276	5289	5302
34	5315	5328	5340	5353	5366	5378	5391	5403	5416	5428
35	5441	5453	5465	5478	5490	5502	5514	5527	5539	5551
36	5563	5575	5587	5599	5611	5623	5635	5647	5658	5670
37	5682	5694	5705	5717	5729	5740	5752	5763	5775	5786
38	5798	5809	5821	5832	5843	5855	5866	5877	5888	5899
39	5911	5922	5933	5944	5955	5966	5977	5988	5999	6010
40	6021	6031	6042	6053	6064	6075	6085	6096	6107	6117
41	6128	6138	6149	6160	6170	6180	6191	6201	6212	6222
42	6232	6243	6253	6263	6274	6284	6294	6304	6314	6325
43	6335	6345	6355	6365	6375	6385	6395	6405	6415	6425
44	6435	6444	6454	6464	6474	6484	6493	6503	6513	6522
45	6532	6542	6551	6561	6571	6580	6590	6599	6609	6618
46	6628	6637	6646	6656	6665	6675	6684	6693	6702	6712
47	6721	6730	6739	6749	6758	6767	6776	6785	6794	6803
48	6812	6821	6830	6839	6848	6857	6866	6875	6884	6893
49	6902	6911	6920	6928	6937	6946	6955	6964	6972	6981
50	6990	6998	7007	7016	7024	7033	7042	7050	7059	7067
51	7076	7084	7093	7101	7110	7118	7126	7135	7143	7152
52	7160	7168	7177	7185	7193	7202	7210	7218	7226	7235
53	7243	7251	7259	7267	7275	7284	7292	7300	7308	7316
54	7324	7332	7340	7348	7356	7364	7372	7380	7388	7396